Hearing: An Introduction to Psychological and Physiological Acoustics

5th Edition

Stanley A. Gelfand

Department of Linguistics and Communication Disorders
Queens College of the City University of New York
Flushing, New York
Ph.D. Program in Speech-Language-Hearing Sciences, and Au.D. Program
Graduate School of the City University of New York
New York, New York, USA

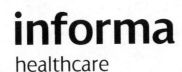

First published in 2010 by Informa Healthcare, Telephone House, 69-77 Paul Street, London EC2A 4LQ, UK.

Simultaneously published in the USA by Informa Healthcare, 52 Vanderbilt Avenue, 7th Floor, New York, NY 10017, USA.

Informa Healthcare is a trading division of Informa UK Ltd. Registered Office: 37–41 Mortimer Street, London W1T 3JH, UK. Registered in England and Wales number 1072954.

A CIP record for this book is available from the British Library.

Library of Congress Cataloging-in-Publication Data available on application

ISBN-13: 9781420088656

Orders may be sent to: Informa Healthcare, Sheepen Place, Colchester, Essex CO3 3LP, UK
Telephone: +44 (0)20 7017 5540
Email: CSDhealthcarebooks@informa.com
Website: http://informahealthcarebooks.com/

For corporate sales please contact: CorporateBooksIHC@informa.com
For foreign rights please contact: RightsIHC@informa.com
For reprint permissions please contact: PermissionsIHC@informa.com

To Janice
In Loving Memory

Contents

Preface .... *vii*

1. **Physical Concepts**   *1*

2. **Anatomy**   *20*

3. **Conductive Mechanism**   *51*

4. **Cochlear Mechanisms and Processes**   *72*

5. **Auditory Nerve**   *103*

6. **Auditory Pathways**   *122*

7. **Psychoacoustic Methods**   *146*

8. **Theory of Signal Detection**   *160*

9. **Auditory Sensitivity**   *166*

10. **Masking**   *187*

11. **Loudness**   *207*

12. **Pitch**   *218*

13. **Binaural and Spatial Hearing**   *231*

14. **Speech and Its Perception**   *257*

Author Index *282*
Subject Index *301*

Preface

This is the fifth edition of a textbook intended to provide beginning graduate students with an introduction to the sciences of hearing, as well as to provide an overview of the field for more experienced readers. The need for a current text has been expanded by the advent and wide acceptance of the professional doctorate in audiology, the Au.D. However, an interest in hearing is by no means limited to audiologists and includes readers with widely diverse academic backgrounds. Among them one finds psychologists, speech-language pathologists, physicians, deaf educators, industrial hygienists, and engineers, among others. The result is a frustrating dilemma in which a text will likely be too basic for some of its intended readers and too advanced for others. Thus, the idea is to provide a volume sufficiently detailed to serve as a core text for graduate students with a primary interest in hearing, at the same time avoiding a reliance on scientific or mathematical backgrounds not shared by those with different kinds of academic experiences.

Hearing science is an exciting area of study because of its broad, interdisciplinary scope, and even more because it is vital and dynamic. Research continuously provides new information to expand on the old and also causes us to rethink what was once well established. The reader (particularly the beginning student) is reminded that new findings occasionally disprove the "laws" of the past. Thus, this textbook should be treated as a first step; it is by no means the final word.

This edition of *Hearing* was strongly influenced by extensive comments and suggestions from colleagues and graduate students. As a result of their input, material has been updated and added, and a number of new and revised figures have been included; however, the fundamental characteristics of the prior editions have been maintained wherever possible. These include the basic approach, structure, format, and the general (and often irregular) depth of coverage, the provision of references at the end of each chapter, and liberal references to other sources for further study. As one might expect, the hardest decisions involved choosing material that could be streamlined, replaced, or omitted, keeping the original orientation and flavor of the book, and avoiding a "state-of-the-art" treatise.

It is doubtful that all of the material covered in this text would be addressed in a single, one semester course. It is more likely that this book might be used as a core text for a two-course sequence dealing with psychological and physiological acoustics, along with appropriately selected readings from the research literature and state-of-the-art books. Suggested readings are provided in context throughout the text to provide a firm foundation for further study.

My sincerest thanks are expressed to the numerous colleagues and students who provided me with valuable suggestions that have been incorporated into this and prior editions. I am especially indebted to my current and former colleagues and students in the Department of Linguistics and Communication Disorders at Queens College, the Ph.D. Program in Speech-Language-Hearing Sciences and the Au.D. Program at the City University of New York Graduate Center, and at the East Orange Veterans Affairs Medical Center. Thank you all for being continuous examples of excellence and for your valued friendships. I am also grateful to the talented and dedicated staff of *Informa Healthcare*, who contributed so much to this book and graciously arranged for the preparation of the indices and the proofreading of the final page proofs.

At the risk of inadvertently omitting several, I would like to thank the following people for their advice, inspiration, influence, and support, which have taken forms too numerous to mention: Sandra Beberman, Moe Bergman, Arthur Boothroyd, Helen Cairns, Joseph Danto, Daniel Falatko, Lillian and Sol Gelfand, Irving Hochberg, Gertrude and Oscar Katzen, Arlene Kraat, Aimee Laussen, John Lutolf, Harriet Marshall-Arnold, Maurice Miller, Neil Piper, Teresa Schwander, Stanley Schwartz, Shlomo Silman, Carol Silverman, Harris, Helen and Gabe Topel, Robert Vago, Barbara Weinstein, and Mark Weiss. Very special gratitude is expressed to Harry Levitt, who will always be my professor.

Finally, my deepest gratitude goes to Janice, the love of my life, whose memory will always be a blessing and inspiration; and to my wonderful children, Michael, Jessica, Joshua, and Erin, for their love, support, confidence, and unparalleled patience.

Stan Gelfand

1   Physical Concepts

This book is concerned with hearing, and what we hear is sound. Thus, both intuition and reason make it clear that a basic understanding of the nature of sound is prerequisite to an understanding of audition. The study of sound is acoustics. An understanding of **acoustics**, in turn, rests upon knowing several fundamental physical principles. This is so because acoustics is, after all, the physics of sound. We will therefore begin by reviewing a number of physical principles so that the following chapters can proceed without the constant need for the distracting insertions of basic definitions and concepts. The material in this chapter is intended to be a review of principles that were previously learned. Therefore, the review will be rapid and somewhat cursory, and the reader may wish to consult the American National Standard addressing acoustical terminology and a physics or acoustics textbook for a broader coverage of these topics (e.g., Pearce and David, 1958; van Bergeijk et al., 1960; Peterson and Gross, 1972; Beranek, 1986; Everest, 2000; Kinsler et al., 1999; Speaks, 1960; Rossing et al., 2002; Hewitt, 2005; Young and Freedman, 2007),[1] as well as the American National Standard addressing acoustical terminology (ANSI, 2004).

PHYSICAL QUANTITIES

Physical quantities may be thought of as being basic or derived, and as either scalars or vectors. The **basic quantities** of concern here are **time**, **length (distance)**, and **mass**. The **derived quantities** are the results of various combinations of the basic quantities (and other derived quantities), and include such phenomena as velocity, force, and work. If a quantity can be described completely in terms of *just* its *magnitude* (size), then it is a **scalar**. Length is a good example of a scalar. On the other hand, a quantity is a **vector** if it needs to be described by *both* its *magnitude* and its *direction*. For example, if a body moves 1 m from point x_1 to point x_2, then we say that it has been displaced. Here, the scalar quantity of length becomes the vector quantity of **displacement** when both magnitude and direction are involved. A derived quantity is a vector if any of its components is a vector. For example, force is a vector because it involves the components of mass (a scalar) and acceleration (a vector). The distinction between scalars and vectors is not just some esoteric concept. One must be able to distinguish between scalars and vectors because they are manipulated differently in calculations.

The basic quantities may be more or less appreciated in terms of one's personal experience and are expressed in terms of conventionally agreed upon units. These units are values that are measurable and repeatable. The unit of **time (t)** is the **second (s)**, the unit of **length (L)** is the **meter (m)**, and the unit of **mass (M)** is the **kilogram (kg)**. There is a common misconception that mass and weight are synonymous. This is actually untrue. Mass is related to the density of a body, which is the same for that body no matter where it is located. On the other hand, an object's weight is related to the force of gravity upon it so that weight changes as a function of gravitational attraction. It is a common knowledge that an object weighs more on the earth than it would on the moon, and that it weighs more at sea level than it would in a high-flying airplane. In each of these cases, the mass of the body is the same despite the fact that its weight is different.

A brief word is appropriate at this stage regarding the availability of several different systems of units. When we express length in meters and mass in kilograms, we are using the units of the *Système International d'Unités*, referred to as the **SI** or the **MKS system**. Here, MKS stands for *meters*, *kilograms*, and *seconds*. An alternative scheme using smaller metric units coexists with MKS, which is the **cgs system** (for *centimeters*, *grams*, and *seconds*), as does the English system of weights and measures. Table 1.1 presents a number of the major basic and derived physical quantities we will deal with, their units, and their conversion factors.[2]

Velocity (v) is the speed at which an object is moving and is derived from the basic quantities of displacement (which we have seen is a vector form of length) and time. On average, velocity is the distance traveled divided by the amount of time it takes to get from the starting point to the destination. Thus, if an object leaves point x_1 at time t_1 and arrives at x_2 at time t_2, then we can compute the average velocity as

$$v = \frac{(x_2 - x_1)}{(t_2 - t_1)}. \qquad (1.1)$$

If we call $(x_2 - x_1)$ displacement (x) and $(t_2 - t_1)$ time (t), then, in general we have

$$v = \frac{x}{t}. \qquad (1.2)$$

Because displacement (x) is measured in meters and time (t) in seconds, velocity is expressed in meters per second (m/s).

---

[1] Although no longer in print, the interested student may be able to find the classical books by Pearce and David (1958), van Bergeijk et al. (1960), and Peterson and Gross (1972) in some libraries.

[2] The student with a penchant for trivia will be delighted to know the following details: (1) The reference value for 1 kg of mass is that of a cylinder of platinum–iridium alloy kept in the International Bureau of Weights and Measures in France. (2) One second is the time needed to complete 9,192,631,700 cycles of the microwave radiation that causes a change between the two lowest energy states in a cesium atom. (3) One meter is 1,650,763.73 times the wavelength of orange-red light emitted by krypton-86 under certain conditions.

Table 1.1 Principal Physical Quantities

Quantity	Formula	SI (MKS) units	cgs units	Equivalent values
Time (t)	t	Second (s)	s	
Mass (M)	M	Kilogram (kg)	Gram (g)	1 kg = 1000 g
Displacement (x)	x	Meter (m)	Centimeter (cm)	1 m = 100 cm
Area (A)	A	m^2	cm^2	1 m^2 = 10^4 cm^2
Velocity (v)	v = x/t	m/s	cm/s	1 m/s = 100 cm/s
Acceleration (a)	$a = v/t = x/t^2$	m/s^2	cm/s^2	1 m/s^2 = 100 cm/s^2
Force (F)	F = Ma = Mv/t	Newton (N), kg·m/s^2	Dyne (d), g·cm/s^2	1 N = 10^5 d
Work (w)	w = Fx	Joule (J), N·m	erg, d·cm	1 J = 10^7 erg
Power (P)	P = w/t = Fx/t = Fv	Watt (W)	Watt (W)	1 W = 1 J/s = 10^7 erg/s
Intensity (I)	I = P/A	W/m^2	W/cm^2	Reference values: 10^{-12} W/m^2 or 10^{-16} W/cm^2
Pressure (p)	p = F/A	Pascal (Pa), N/m^2	Microbar (μbar) d/cm^2	Reference values: 2×10^{-5} N/m^2 (μPa) or 2×10^{-4} d/cm^2 (μbar)[a]

[a]The reference value for sound pressure in cgs units is often written as 0.0002 dynes/cm^2.

In contrast to **average velocity**, as just defined, **instantaneous velocity** is used when we are concerned with the speed of a moving body at a *specific moment* in time. Instantaneous velocity reflects the speed at some point in time when the displacement and time between that point and the next one approaches zero. Thus, students with a background in mathematics will recognize that instantaneous velocity is equal to the derivative of displacement with respect to time, or

$$v = \frac{dx}{dt}. \qquad (1.3)$$

As common experience verifies, a fixed speed is rarely maintained over time. Rather, an object may speed up or slow down over time. Such a change of velocity over time is **acceleration (a)**. Suppose we are concerned with the average acceleration of a body moving between two points. The velocity of the body at the first point is v_1 and the time as it passes that point is t_1. Similarly, its velocity at the second point and the time when it passes this point are, respectively, v_2 and t_2. The **average acceleration** is the difference between these two velocities divided by the time interval involved:

$$a = \frac{(v_2 - v_1)}{(t_2 - t_1)} \qquad (1.4)$$

or, in general:

$$a = \frac{v}{t}. \qquad (1.5)$$

If we recall that velocity corresponds to displacement divided by time (Eq. 1.2), we can substitute x/t for v so that

$$a = \frac{\frac{x}{t}}{t} = \frac{x}{t^2}. \qquad (1.6)$$

Therefore, acceleration is expressed in units of meters per second squared (m/s^2) or centimeters per second squared (cm/s^2).

The acceleration of a body at a given moment is called its **instantaneous acceleration**, which is the derivative of velocity with respect to time, or

$$a = \frac{dv}{dt}. \qquad (1.7)$$

Recalling that velocity is the first derivative of displacement (Eq. 1.3), and substituting, we find that acceleration is the second derivative of displacement:

$$a = \frac{d^2x}{dt^2}. \qquad (1.8)$$

Common experience and Newton's first law of motion tell us that if an object is not moving (is at rest), then it will tend to remain at rest, and that if an object is moving in some direction at a given speed, then it will tend to continue doing so. This phenomenon is **inertia**, which is the property of mass to continue doing what it is already doing. An outside influence is needed to make a stationary object move, or to change the speed or the direction of a moving object. That is, a **force (F)** is needed to overcome the body's inertia. Because a change in speed is acceleration, we may say that force is that which causes a mass to be accelerated, that is, to change its speed or direction. The amount of force is equal to the product of mass and acceleration (Newton's second law of motion):

$$F = Ma. \qquad (1.9)$$

Recall that acceleration corresponds to velocity over time (Eq. 1.5). Substituting v/t for a (acceleration) reveals that force can also be defined in the form:

$$F = \frac{Mv}{t}, \qquad (1.10)$$

where **Mv** is the property of **momentum**. Stated in this manner, force is equal to momentum over time.

Because force is the product of mass and acceleration, the amount of force is measured in kg·m/s^2. The unit of force is the **newton (N)**, which is the force needed to cause a 1-kg mass to be accelerated by 1 kg·m/s^2 (i.e., 1 N = 1 kg·m/s^2). It would thus take a 2-N force to cause a 2-kg mass to be accelerated by 1 m/s^2, or a 1-kg mass to be accelerated by 2 kg·m/s^2. Similarly, the force required to accelerate a 6-kg mass by 3 m/s^2 would be 18 N. The unit of force in cgs units is the **dyne**, where 1 dyne = 1 g·cm/s^2 and 10^5 dynes = 1 N.

Actually, many forces tend to act upon a given body at the same time. Therefore, the force referred to in Eqs. 1.9 and 1.10 is actually the resultant or the net force, which is the net effect of all forces acting upon the object. The concept of net force is clarified by a few simple examples: If two forces are both pushing on a body in the same direction, then the net force would be the sum of these two forces. (For example, consider a force of 2 N that is pushing an object toward the north, and a second force of 5 N that is also pushing that object in the same direction. The net force would be 2 N + 5 N, or 7 N and the direction of acceleration would be to the north.) Alternatively, if two forces are pushing on the same body but in opposite directions, then the net force is the difference between the two, and the object will be accelerated in the direction of the greater force. (Suppose, for example, that a 2-N force is pushing an object toward the east and a 5-N force is simultaneously pushing it toward the west. Then the net force would be 5 N − 2 N, or 3 N, which would cause the body to accelerate toward the west.)

If two equal forces push in opposite directions, then the net force would be zero, in which case there would be no change in the motion of the object. This situation is called **equilibrium**. Thus, under conditions of equilibrium, if a body is already moving, it will continue in motion, and if it is already at rest, it will remain still. That is, of course, what Newton's first law of motion tells us.

Experience, however, tells us that a moving object in the real world tends to slow down and will eventually come to a halt. This occurs, for example, when a driver shifts to "neutral" and allows his car to coast on a level roadway. Is this a violation of the laws of physics? Clearly, the answer is no. The reason is that in the real world a moving body is constantly in contact with other objects or mediums. The sliding of one body against the other constitutes a force opposing the motion, called **friction** or **resistance**. For example, the coasting automobile is in contact with the surrounding air and the roadway; moreover, its internal parts are also moving one upon the other.

The opposing force of friction depends on two factors. Differing amounts of friction occur depending upon what is sliding on what. The magnitude of friction between two given materials is called the **coefficient of friction**. Although the details of this quantity are beyond current interest, it is easily understood that the coefficient of friction is greater for "rough" materials than for "smooth" or "slick" ones.

The second factor affecting the force of friction is easily demonstrated by an experiment the reader can do by rubbing the palms of his hands back and forth on one another. First rub slowly and then rapidly. Not surprisingly, the rubbing will produce heat. The temperature rise is due to the conversion of

the mechanical energy into heat as a result of the friction, and will be addressed again in another context. For the moment, we will accept the amount of heat as an indicator of the amount of friction. Note that the hands become hotter when they are rubbed together more rapidly. Thus, the amount of friction is due not only to the coefficient of friction (R) between the materials involved (here, the palms of the hands), but also to the velocity (v) of the motion. Stated as a formula, the force of friction (F) is thus

$$F = Rv. \tag{1.11}$$

A compressed spring will bounce back to its original shape once released. This property of a deformed object to return to its original form is called **elasticity**. The more elastic or stiff an object, the more readily it returns to its original form after being deformed. Suppose one is trying to compress a coil spring. It becomes increasingly more difficult to continue squeezing the spring as it becomes more and more compressed. Stated differently, the more the spring is being deformed, the more it opposes the applied force. The force that opposes the deformation of a spring-like material is called the **restoring force**.

As the example just cited suggests, the restoring force depends on two factors: the elastic modulus of the object's material and the degree to which the object is displaced. An **elastic modulus** is the ratio of stress to strain. **Stress** (s) is the ratio of the applied force (F) to the area (A) of an elastic object over which it is exerted, or

$$s = \frac{F}{A} \tag{1.12}$$

The resulting relative displacement or change in dimensions of the material subjected to the stress is called **strain**. Of particular interest is **Young's modulus**, which is the ratio of compressive stress to compressive strain. **Hooke's law** states that stress and strain are proportional within the elastic limits of the material, which is equivalent to stating that a material's elastic modulus is a constant within these limits. Thus, the restoring force (F) of an elastic material that opposes an applied force is

$$F = Sx \tag{1.13}$$

where S is the stiffness constant of the material and x is the amount of displacement.

The concept of "work" in physics is decidedly more specific than its general meaning in daily life. In the physical sense, **work** (w) is done when the application of a force to a body results in its displacement. The amount of work is therefore the product of the force applied and the resultant displacement, or

$$w = Fx \tag{1.14}$$

Thus, work can be accomplished only when there is displacement: If the displacement is zero, then the product of force and displacement will also be zero no matter how great the force. Work is quantified in newton-meters (N·m), and the unit of work is the **joule (J)**. Specifically, one joule (1 J) is equal to

1 N·m. In the cgs system, work is expressed in **ergs**, where 1 erg corresponds to 1 dyne-centimeter (1 d·cm).

The capability to do work is called **energy**. The energy of an object in motion is called **kinetic energy**, and the energy of a body at rest is its **potential energy**. **Total energy** is the body's kinetic energy plus its potential energy. Work corresponds to the change in the body's kinetic energy. The energy is not consumed, but rather is converted from one form to the other. Consider, for example, a pendulum that is swinging back and forth. Its kinetic energy is greatest when it is moving the fastest, which is when it passes through the midpoint of its swing. On the other hand, its potential energy is greatest at the instant that it reaches the extreme of its swing, when its speed is zero.

We are concerned not only with the amount of work, but also with how fast it is being accomplished. The rate at which work is done is **power (P)** and is equal to work divided by time,

$$P = \frac{w}{t} \qquad (1.15)$$

in joules per second (J/s). The **watt (W)** is the unit of power, and 1 W is equal to 1 J/s. In the cgs system, the watt is equal to 10^7 ergs/s.

Recalling that w = Fx, Eq. 1.15 may be rewritten as

$$P = \frac{Fx}{t} \qquad (1.16)$$

If we now substitute v for x/t (based on Eq. 1.2), we find that

$$P = Fv \qquad (1.17)$$

Thus, power is equal to the product of force and velocity.

The amount of power per unit of area is called **intensity (I)**. In formal terms,

$$I = \frac{P}{A} \qquad (1.18)$$

where I is intensity, P is power, and A is area. Therefore, intensity is measured in watts per square meter (W/m²) in SI units, or in watts per square centimeter (W/cm²) in cgs units. Because of the difference in the scale of the area units in the MKS and cgs systems, we find that 10^{-12} **W/m²** corresponds to 10^{-16} **W/cm²**. This apparently peculiar choice of equivalent values is being provided because they represent the amount of intensity required to just barely hear a sound.

An understanding of intensity will be better appreciated if one considers the following. Using for the moment the common-knowledge idea of what sound is, imagine that a sound source is a tiny pulsating sphere. This *point source* of sound will produce a sound wave that will radiate outward in every direction so that the propagating wave may be conceived of as a sphere of ever-increasing size. Thus, as distance from the point source increases, the power of the sound will have to be divided over the ever-expanding surface. Suppose now that we measure how much power registers on a one-unit area of this surface at various distances from the source. As the overall size of the sphere is getting larger with distance from the source, so this one-unit sam-ple must represent an ever-decreasing proportion of the total surface area. Therefore, less power "falls" onto the same area as the distance from the source increases. It follows that the magnitude of the sound appreciated by a listener would become less and less with increasing distance from a sound source.

The intensity of a sound decreases with distance from the source according to an orderly rule as long as there are no reflections, in which case a **free field** is said to exist. Under these conditions, increasing the distance (D) from a sound source causes the intensity to decrease to an amount equal to 1 over the square of the change in distance $(1/D^2)$. This principle is known as the inverse-square law. In effect, the **inverse square law** says that doubling the distance from the sound source (e.g., from 1 to 2 m) causes the intensity to drop to $1/2^2$ or 1/4 of the original intensity. Similarly, tripling the distance causes the intensity to fall to $1/3^2$, or 1/9, of the prior value; four times the distance results in $1/4^2$, or 1/16, of the intensity; and a 10-fold increase in distance causes the intensity to fall $1/10^2$, or 1/100, of the starting value.

Just as power divided by area yields intensity, so force (F) divided by area yields a value called **pressure (p)**:

$$p = \frac{F}{A} \qquad (1.19)$$

so that pressure is measured in N/m² or in dynes/cm². The unit of pressure is called the **pascal (Pa)**, where 1 Pa = 1 N/m². As for intensity, the softest audible sound can also be expressed in terms of its pressure, for which 2×10^{-5} **N/m²** and 2×10^{-4} **dynes/cm²** are equivalent values.

DECIBEL NOTATION

The range of magnitudes we concern ourselves with in hearing is enormous. As we shall discuss in Chapter 9, the sound pressure of the loudest sound that we can tolerate is on the order of 10 million times greater than that of the softest audible sound. One can immediately imagine the cumbersome task that would be involved if we were to deal with such an immense range of numbers on a linear scale. The problems involved with and related to such a wide range of values make it desirable to transform the absolute physical magnitudes into another form, called **decibels (dB)**, which make the values both palatable and rationally meaningful.

One may conceive of the decibel as basically involving two characteristics, namely, ratios and logarithms. First, the value of a quantity is expressed in relation to some meaningful baseline value in the form of a ratio. Because it makes sense to use the softest sound one can hear as our baseline, we use the intensity or pressure of the softest audible sound as our reference value.

As introduced earlier, the **reference sound intensity** is 10^{-12} W/m², and the equivalent **reference sound pressure** is 2×10^{-5} N/m². Also, recall that the equivalent corresponding values in cgs units are 10^{-16} W/cm² for sound intensity and 2×10^{-4}

dynes/cm^2 for sound pressure. The appropriate reference value becomes the denominator of our ratio, and the absolute intensity or pressure of the sound in question becomes the numerator. Thus, instead of talking about a sound having an absolute intensity of 10^{-10} W/m^2, we express its intensity relatively in terms of how it relates to our reference, as the ratio:

$$\frac{\left(10^{-10}\,\text{W/m}^2\right)}{\left(10^{-12}\,\text{W/m}^2\right)},$$

which reduces to simply 10^2. This intensity ratio is then replaced with its common logarithm. The reason is that the linear distance between numbers having the same ratio relationship between them (say, 2:1) becomes wider when the absolute magnitudes of the numbers become larger. For example, the distance between the numbers in each of the following pairs increases appreciably as the size of the numbers becomes larger, even though they all involve the same 2:1 ratio: 1:2, 10:20, 100:200, and 1000:2000. The logarithmic conversion is used because equal ratios are represented as equal distances on a logarithmic scale.

The decibel is a relative entity. This means that the decibel in and of itself is a dimensionless quantity, and is meaningless without knowledge of the reference value, which constitutes the denominator of the ratio. Because of this, it is necessary to make the reference value explicit when the magnitude of a sound is expressed in decibel form. This is accomplished by stating that the magnitude of the sound is whatever number of decibels with respect to the reference quantity. Moreover, it is a common practice to add the word "level" to the original quantity when dealing with decibel values. Intensity expressed in decibels is called **intensity level (IL)**, and sound pressure in decibels is called **sound pressure level (SPL)**. The reference values indicated above are generally assumed when decibels are expressed as **dB IL** or **dB SPL**. For example, one might say that the intensity level of a sound is "50 dB *re*: 10^{-12} W/m^2" or "50 dB IL."

The general formula for the decibel is expressed in terms of power as

$$PL_{dB} = 10 \cdot \log\left(\frac{P}{P_0}\right) \tag{1.20}$$

where P is the power of the sound being measured, P_0 is the reference power to which the former is being compared, and PL is the **power level**. Acoustical measurements are, however, typically made in terms of intensity or sound pressure. The applicable formula for decibels of intensity level is thus:

$$IL_{dB} = 10 \cdot \log\left(\frac{I}{I_0}\right) \tag{1.21}$$

where I is the intensity (in W/m^2) of the sound in question, and I_0 is the reference intensity, or 10^{-12} W/m^2. Continuing with the example introduced above, where the value of I is 10^{-10} W/m^2,

we thus find that

$$\begin{aligned} IL_{dB} &= 10 \cdot \log\left(\frac{10^{-10}\,\text{W/m}^2}{10^{-12}\,\text{W/m}^2}\right) \\ &= 10 \cdot \log 10^2 \\ &= 10 \times 2 \\ &= 20\,\text{dB} \quad re: 10^{-12}\,\text{W/m}^2 \end{aligned}$$

In other words, an *intensity* of 10^{-10} W/m^2 corresponds to an **intensity level** of 20 dB *re*: 10^{-12} W/m^2, or 20 dB IL.

Sound intensity measurements are important and useful, and are preferred in certain situations. [See Rassmussen (1989) for a review of this topic.] However, most acoustical measurements involved in hearing are made in terms of sound pressure, and are thus expressed in decibels of **sound pressure level**. Here, we must be aware that intensity is proportional to pressure squared:

$$I \propto p^2 \tag{1.22}$$

and

$$p \propto \sqrt{I} \tag{1.23}$$

As a result, converting the dB IL formula into the equivalent equation for dB SPL involves replacing the intensity values with the squares of the corresponding pressure values. Therefore

$$SPL_{dB} = 10 \cdot \log\left(\frac{p^2}{p_0^2}\right) \tag{1.24}$$

where p is the measured sound pressure and p_0 is the reference sound pressure (2×10^{-5} N/m^2). This formula may be simplified to

$$SPL_{dB} = 10 \cdot \log\left(\frac{p}{p_0}\right)^2 \tag{1.25}$$

Because the logarithm of a number squared corresponds to two times the logarithm of that number ($\log x = 2 \cdot \log x$), the square may be removed to result in

$$SPL_{dB} = 10 \cdot 2 \cdot \log\left(\frac{p}{p_0}\right) \tag{1.26}$$

Therefore, the simplified formula for decibels of SPL becomes

$$SPL_{dB} = 20 \cdot \log\left(\frac{p}{p_0}\right) \tag{1.27}$$

where the value of 20 (instead of 10) is due to having removed the square from the earlier described version of the formula. (One *cannot* take the intensity ratio from the IL formula and simply insert it into the SPL formula, or vice versa. The square root of the intensity ratio yields the *corresponding* pressure ratio, which must be then placed into the SPL equation. Failure to use the proper terms will result in an erroneous doubling of the value in dB SPL.

By way of an example, a sound pressure of 2×10^{-4} N/m^2 corresponds to a SPL of 20 dB (*re*: 2×10^{-5} N/m^2), which may

5

be calculated as follows:

$$SPL_{dB} = 20 \cdot \log \left(\frac{2 \times 10^{-4}\,N/m^2}{2 \times 10^{-5}\,N/m^2} \right)$$
$$= 20 \cdot \log 10^1$$
$$= 20 \times 1$$
$$= 20\,dB \quad re: 10^{-5}\,N/m^2$$

What would happen if the intensity (or pressure) in question were the same as the reference intensity (or pressure)? In other words, what is the dB value of the reference itself? In terms of intensity, the answer to this question may be found by simply using 10^{-12} W/m^2 as both the numerator (I) and denominator (I_0) in the dB formula; thus

$$IL_{dB} = 10 \cdot \log \left(\frac{10^{-12}\,W/m^2}{10^{-12}\,W/m^2} \right) \qquad (1.28)$$

Because anything divided by itself equals 1, and the logarithm of 1 is 0, this equation reduces to:

$$IL_{dB} = 10 \cdot \log 1$$
$$= 10 \times 0$$
$$= 0\,dB \quad re: 10^{-12}\,W/m^2$$

Hence, 0 dB IL is the intensity level of the reference intensity. Just as 0 dB IL indicates the intensity level of the reference intensity, so 0 dB SPL similarly implies that the measured sound pressure corresponds to that of the reference

$$SPL_{dB} = 20 \cdot \log \left(\frac{2 \times 10^{-5}\,N/m^2}{2 \times 10^{-5}\,N/m^2} \right) \qquad (1.29)$$

Just as we saw in the previous example, this equation is solved simply as follows:

$$SPL_{dB} = 20 \cdot \log 1$$
$$= 20 \times 0$$
$$= 0\,dB \quad re: 10^{-5}\,N/m^2$$

In other words, 0 dB SPL indicates that the pressure of the sound in question corresponds to the reference sound pressure of 2×10^{-5} N/m^2. Notice that 0 dB does *not* mean "no sound." Rather, 0 dB implies that the quantity being measured is equal to the reference quantity. Negative decibel values indicate that the measured magnitude is smaller than the reference quantity.

Recall that sound intensity drops with distance from the sound source according to the inverse-square law. However, we want to know the effect of the inverse-square law in terms of *decibels of sound pressure level* because sound is usually expressed in these terms. To address this, we must first remember that pressure is proportional to the square root of intensity. Hence, pressure decreases according to the inverse of the distance change (1/D) instead of the inverse of the square of the distance change (1/D^2). In effect, the *inverse-square law* for *intensity* becomes an *inverse-distance law* when we are dealing with *pressure*. Let us assume a doubling as the distance change, because this is the most useful relationship. We can now calculate the size of the decrease in decibels between a point at some distance from the sound source (D$_1$, e.g., 1 m) and a point at twice the distance (D$_2$, e.g., 2 m) as follows:

$$\text{Level drop in SPL} = 20 \cdot \log(D_2/D_1)$$
$$= 20 \cdot \log(2/1)$$
$$= 20 \cdot \log 2$$
$$= 20 \times 0.3$$
$$= 6\,dB$$

In other words, the inverse-square law causes the sound pressure level to decrease by 6 dB whenever the distance from the sound source is doubled. For example, if the sound pressure level is 60 dB at 1 m from the source, then it will be $60-6 = 54$ dB when the distance is doubled to 2 m, and $54-6 = 48$ dB when the distance is doubled again from 2 to 4 m.

HARMONIC MOTION AND SOUND

What is sound? It is convenient to answer this question with a formally stated sweeping generality. For example, one might say that sound is a form of vibration that propagates through a medium (such as air) in the form of a wave. Although this statement is correct and straightforward, it can also be uncomfortably vague and perplexing. This is so because it assumes a knowledge of definitions and concepts that are used in a very precise way, but which are familiar to most people only as "gut-level" generalities. As a result, we must address the underlying concepts and develop a functional vocabulary of physical terms that will not only make the general definition of sound meaningful, but will also allow the reader to appreciate its nature.

Vibration is the to-and-fro motion of a body, which could be anything from a guitar string to the floorboards under the family refrigerator, or a molecule of air. Moreover, the motion may have a very simple pattern as produced by a tuning fork, or an extremely complex one such as what one might hear at lunchtime in an elementary school cafeteria. Even though few sounds are as simple as that produced by a vibrating tuning fork, such an example provides what is needed to understand the nature of sound.

Figure 1.1 shows an artist's conceptualization of a vibrating tuning fork at different moments of its vibration pattern. The heavy arrow facing the prong to the reader's right in Fig. 1.1a represents the effect of applying an initial force to the fork, such as by striking it against a hard surface. The progression of the pictures in the figures from (a) through (e) represents the movements of the prongs as time proceeds from the moment that the outside force is applied.

Even though both prongs vibrate as mirror images of one another, it is convenient to consider just one of them for the time being. Figure 1.2 highlights the right prong's motion after being struck. Point C (center) is simply the position of the prong at rest. Upon being hit (as in Fig. 1.1a) the prong is pushed, as

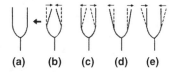

Figure 1.1 Striking a tuning fork (indicated by the heavy arrow) results in a pattern of movement that repeats itself over time. One complete cycle of these movements is represented from frames (a) through (e). Note that the two prongs move as mirror images of one another.

shown by arrow 1, to point L (left). The prong then bounces back (arrow 2), picking up speed along the way. Instead of stopping at the center (C), the rapidly moving prong overshoots this point. It now continues rightward (arrow 3), slowing down along the way until it comes to a halt at point R (right). It now reverses direction and begins moving leftward (arrow 4) at an ever-increasing speed so that it again overshoots the center. Now, again following arrow 1, the prong slows down until it reaches a halt at L, where it reverses direction and repeats the process.

The course of events just described is the result of applying a force to an object having the properties of elasticity and inertia (mass). The initial force to the tuning fork displaces the prong. Because the tuning fork possesses the property of elasticity, the deformation caused by the applied force is opposed by a restoring force in the opposite direction. In the case of the single prong in Fig. 1.2, the initial force toward the left is opposed by a restoring force toward the right. As the prong is pushed farther to the left, the magnitude of the restoring force increases relative to the initially applied force. As a result, the prong's movement is slowed down, brought to a halt at point L, and reversed in direction. Now, under the influence of its elasticity, the prong starts moving rightward. Here, we must consider the mass of the prong.

As the restoring force brings the prong back toward its resting position (C), the inertial force of its mass causes it to increase in speed, or accelerate. When the prong passes through the resting position, it is actually moving fastest. Here, inertia does not permit the moving mass (prong) to simply stop, so instead it

overshoots the center and continues its rightward movement under the force of its inertia. However, the prong's movement is now resulting in deformation of the metal again once it passes through the resting position. Elasticity therefore comes into play with the buildup of an opposing (now leftward) restoring force. As before, the restoring force eventually equals the applied (now inertial) force, thus halting the fork's displacement at point R and reversing the direction of its movement. Here, the course of events described above again comes into play (except that the direction is leftward), with the prong building up speed again and overshooting the center (C) position as a result of inertia. The process will continue over and over again until it dies out over time, seemingly "of its own accord."

Clearly, the dying out of the tuning fork's vibrations does not occur by some mystical influence. On the contrary, it is due to **resistance**. The vibrating prong is always in contact with the air around it. As a result, there will be **friction** between the vibrating metal and the surrounding air particles. The friction causes some of the mechanical energy involved in the movement of the tuning fork to be converted into heat. The energy that has been converted into heat by friction is no longer available to support the to-and-fro movements of the tuning fork. Hence, the oscillations die out, as continuing friction causes more and more of the energy to be converted into heat. This reduction in the size of the oscillations due to resistance is called **damping**.

The events and forces just described are summarized in Fig. 1.3, where the tuning fork's motion is represented by the curve. This curve represents the displacement to the right and left of the center (resting) position as the distance above and below the horizontal line, respectively. Horizontal distance from left to right represents the progression of time. The initial dotted line represents its initial displacement due to the applied force. The elastic restoring forces and inertial forces of the prong's mass are represented by arrows. Finally, damping is shown by the reduction in the displacement of the curve from center as time goes on.

The type of vibration just described is called **simple harmonic motion (SHM)** because the to-and-fro movements repeat themselves at the same rate over and over again. We will discuss the nature of SHM in greater detail below with respect to the motion of air particles in the sound wave.

The tuning fork serves as a sound source by transferring its vibration to the motion of the surrounding air particles (Fig. 1.4). (We will again concentrate on the activity to the right of the fork, remembering that a mirror image of this pattern occurs to the left.) The rightward motion of the tuning fork prong displaces air molecules to its right in the same direction as the prong's motion. These molecules are thus displaced to the right of their resting positions, thereby being forced closer and closer to the particles to their own right. In other words, the air pressure has been increased above its resting (ambient or atmospheric) pressure because the molecules are being compressed. This state is clearly identified by the term "**compression**." The amount of compression (increased air pressure) becomes greater as the

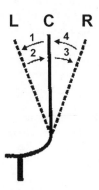

Figure 1.2 Movements toward the right (R) and left (L) of the center (C) resting position of a single tuning fork prong. The numbers and arrows are described in the text.

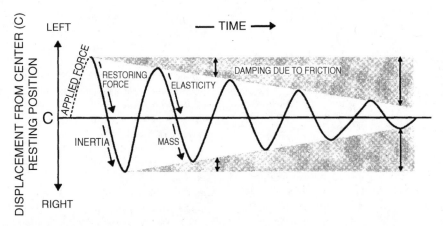

Figure 1.3 Conceptualized diagram graphing the to-and-fro movements of the tuning fork prong in Fig. 2. Vertical distance represents the displacement of the prong from its center (C) or resting position. The dotted line represents the initial displacement of the prong as a result of some applied force. Arrows indicate the effects of restoring forces due to the fork's elasticity, and the effects of inertia due to its mass. The damping effect due to resistance (or friction) is shown by the decreasing displacement of the curve as time progresses and is highlighted by the shaded triangles (and double-headed arrows) above and below the curve.

tuning fork continues displacing the air molecules rightward; it reaches a maximum positive pressure when the prong and air molecules attain their greatest rightward amplitude.

The prong will now reverse direction, overshoot its resting position, and then proceed to its extreme leftward position. The compressed air molecules will also reverse direction along with the prong. The reversal occurs because air is an elastic medium, so the rightwardly compressed particles undergo a leftward restoring force. The rebounding air molecules accelerate due to mass effects, overshoot their resting position, and continue to an extreme leftward position. The amount of com-

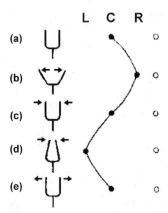

Figure 1.4 Transmittal of the vibratory pattern from a tuning fork to the surrounding air particles. Frames represent various phases of the tuning fork's vibratory cycle. In each frame, the filled circle represents an air parti-cle next to the prong as well as its position, and the unfilled circle shows an air molecule adjacent to the first one. The latter particle is shown only in its resting position for illustrative purposes. Letters above the filled circle high-light the relative positions of the oscillating air particle [C, center (resting); L, leftward; R, rightward]. The line connecting the particle's positions going from frames (a) through (e) reveals a cycle of simple harmonic motion.

pression decreases as the molecules travel leftward, and falls to zero at the moment when the molecules pass through their resting positions.

As the air molecules move left of their ambient positions, they are now at an increasingly greater distance from the molecules to their right than when they were in their resting positions. Consequently, the air pressure is reduced below atmospheric pressure. This state is the opposite of compression and is called **rarefaction**. The air particles are maximally rarefied so that the pressure is maximally negative when the molecules reach the leftmost position. Now, the restoring force yields a right-ward movement of the air molecules, enhanced by the push of the tuning fork prong that has also reversed direction. The air molecules now accelerate rightward, overshoot their resting positions (when rarefaction and negative pressure are zero), and continue rightward. Hence, the SHM of the tuning fork has been transmitted to the surrounding air so that the air molecules are now also under SHM.

Consider now one of the air molecules set into SHM by the influence of the tuning fork. This air molecule will vibrate back and forth in the same direction as that of the vibrating prong. When this molecule moves rightward, it will cause a similar displacement of the particle to its own right. Thus, the SHM of the first air molecule is transmitted to the one next to it. The second one similarly initiates vibration of the one to its right, and so forth down the line.

In other words, each molecule moves to and fro around its own resting point, and causes successive molecules to vibrate back and forth around their own resting points, as shown schematically by the arrows marked "individual particles" in Fig. 1.5 Notice in the figure that each molecule stays in its own general location and moves to and fro about this aver-age position, and that it is the vibratory pattern, which is transmitted.

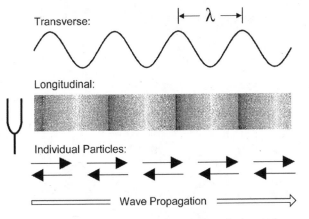

Figure 1.5   Transverse and longitudinal representations of a sinusoidal wave (illustrating points made in the text).

This propagation of vibratory motion from particle to particle constitutes the sound wave. This wave appears as alternating compressions and rarefactions radiating from the sound source as the particles transmit their motions outward and is represented in Fig. 1.5

The distance covered by one cycle of a propagating wave is called its **wavelength** (λ). If we begin where a given molecule is at the point of maximum positive displacement (compression), then the wavelength would be the distance to the next molecule, which is also at its point of maximum compression. This is the distance between any two successive positive peaks in the figure. (Needless to say, such a measurement would be equally correct if made between identical points on any two successive replications of the wave.) The wavelength of a sound is inversely proportional to its frequency, as follows:

$$\lambda = \frac{c}{f} \qquad (1.30)$$

where f is frequency and c is a constant representing the speed of sound. (The speed of sound in air approximates 344 m/s at a temperature of 20°C.) Similarly, frequency can be derived if one knows the wavelength, as:

$$f = \frac{c}{\lambda} \qquad (1.31)$$

Figure 1.5 reveals that the to-and-fro motions of each air molecule is in the same direction as that in which the overall wave is propagating. This kind of wave, which characterizes sound, is a **longitudinal wave**. In contrast to longitudinal waves, most people are more familiar with **transverse waves**, such as those that develop on the water's surface when a pebble is dropped into a still pool. The latter are called transverse waves because the water particles vibrate up and down around their resting positions at right angles (transverse) to the horizontal propagation of the surface waves out from the spot where the pebble hit the water.

Even though sound waves are longitudinal, it is more convenient to show them diagrammatically as though they were transverse, as in upper part of Fig. 1.5 Here, the dashed horizontal baseline represents the particle's resting position (ambient pressure), distance above the baseline denotes compression (positive pressure), and distance below the baseline shows rarefaction (negative pressure). The passage of time is represented by the distance from left to right. Beginning at the resting position, the air molecule is represented as having gone through one cycle (or complete repetition) of SHM at point 1, two cycles at point 2, three complete cycles at point 3, and four cycles at point 4.

The curves in Fig. 1.5 reveal that the **waveform** of SHM is a sinusoidal function and is thus called a **sinusoidal wave**, also known as a **sine wave** or a **sinusoid**. Figure 1.6 elucidates this concept and also indicates a number of the characteristics of sine waves. The center of the figure shows one complete cycle of SHM, going from points a through i. The circles around the sine wave correspond to the various points on the wave, as indicated by corresponding letters. Circle (a) corresponds to point a on the curve, which falls on the baseline. This point corresponds to the particle's resting position.

Circle (a) shows a horizontal radius (r) drawn from the center to the circumference on the right. Imagine as well a second radius (r′) that will rotate around the circle in a counterclockwise direction. The two radii are superimposed in circle (a) so that the angle between them is 0°. There is clearly no distance between these two superimposed lines. This situation corresponds to point a on the sine wave at the center of the figure. Hence, point a may be said to have an angle of 0°, and no displacement from the origin. This concept may appear quite vague at first, but it will become clear as the second radius (r′) rotates around the circle.

Let us assume that radius r′ is rotating counterclockwise at a *fixed speed*. When r′ has rotated 45°, it arrives in the position shown in circle (b). Here, r′ is at an angle of 45° to r. We will call this angle as the **phase angle** (θ), which simply reflects the degree of rotation around the circle, or the number of degrees into the sine wave at the corresponding point b. We now drop a vertical line from the point where r′ intersects the circle down to r. We label this line d, representing the vertical distance between r and the point where r′ intersects the circle. The length of this line corresponds to the displacement of point b from the baseline of the sine wave (dotted line at b). We now see that point b on the sine wave is 45° into the cycle of SHM, at which the displacement of the air particle from its resting position is represented by the height of the point above the baseline. It should now be clear that the sine wave is related to the degrees of rotation around a circle. The shape of the sine wave corresponds to the sine of θ as r′ rotates around the circle, which is simply equal to d/r′.

The positive peak of the sine wave at point c corresponds to circle (c), in which r′ has rotated to the straight up position. It is now at a 90° angle to r, and the distance (d) down to the

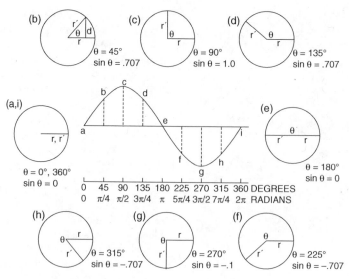

Figure 1.6   The nature of sinusoidal motion (see text).

horizontal radius (r) is the greatest. Here, we have completed a quarter of the wave and an arc equal to quarter the circumference of the circle. Notice now that further counterclockwise rotation of r' results in decreasing the distance (d) down to the horizontal, as shown in circle (d), as well as by the displacement of point d from the baseline of the sine wave. Note also that θ is now 135°. Here, the air particle has reversed direction and is now moving back toward the resting position. When the particle reaches the resting position (point e), it is again at no displacement. The zero displacement condition is shown in circle (e) by the fact that r and r' constitute a single horizontal line (diameter). Alternatively stated, r and r' intersect the circle's circumference at points that are 180° apart. Here, we have completed half of the cycle of SHM, and the phase angle is 180° and the displacement from the baseline is again zero.

Continuing rotation of r' places its intersection with the circumference in the lower left quadrant of the circle, as in circle (f). Now, θ is 225°, and the particle has overshot and is moving away from its resting position in the negative (rarefaction) direction. The vertical displacement from the baseline is now downward or negative, indicating rarefaction. The negative peak of the wave occurs at 270°, where displacement is maximum in the negative direction [point and circle (g)].

Circle (h) and point h show that the negative displacement has become smaller as the rotating radius passes 315° around the circle. The air particle has reversed direction again and is now moving toward its original position. At point i, the air particle has once again returned to its resting position, where displacement is again zero. This situation corresponds to having completed a 360° rotation so that r and r' are once again superimposed. Thus, 360° corresponds to 0°, and circle (i) is one and the same with circle (a). We have now completed one full cycle.

Recall that r' has been rotating at a fixed speed. It therefore follows that the number of degrees traversed in a given amount of time is determined by how fast r' is moving. If one complete rotation takes 1 s, then 360° is covered each second. It clearly follows that if 360° takes 1 s, then 180° takes 0.5 s, 90° takes 0.25 s, 270° takes 0.75 s, etc. It should now be apparent that the phase angle reflects the elapsed time from the onset of rotation. Recall from Fig. 1.3 that the **waveform** shows how particle displacement varies as a function of time. We may also speak of the horizontal axis in terms of phase, or the equivalent of the number of degrees of rotation around a circle. Hence, the **phase** of the wave at each of the labeled points in Fig. 1.6 would be 0° at a, 45° at b, 90° at c, 135° at d, 180° at e, 225° at f, 270° at g, 315° at h, and 360° at i. With an appreciation of phase, it should be apparent that each set of otherwise identical waves in Fig. 1.7 differs with respect to phase: (a) wave 2 is offset from wave 1 by

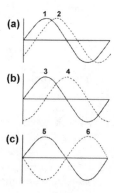

Figure 1.7   Pairs of sinusoidal waves of identical frequency differing in phase by (a) 45°, (b) 90°, and (c) 180°. The numbers serve only to identify the individual waves.

45°, (b) waves 3 and 4 are apart in phase by 90°, and (c) waves 5 and 6 are 180° out of phase.

We may now proceed to define a number of other fundamental aspects of sound waves. A cycle has already been defined as one complete repetition of the wave. Thus, four cycles of a sinusoidal wave were shown in Fig. 1.5 because it depicts four complete repetitions of the waveform. Because the waveform is repeated over time, this sound is said to be **periodic**. In contrast, a waveform that does not repeat itself over time would be called **aperiodic**.

The amount of time that it takes to complete one cycle is called its **period**, denoted by the symbol **t** (for time). For example, a periodic wave that repeats itself every millisecond is said to have a period of 1 ms, or t = 1 ms or 0.001 s. The periods of the waveforms considered in hearing science are overwhelmingly less than 1 s, typically in the milliseconds and even microseconds. However, there are instances when longer periods are encountered.

The number of times a waveform repeats itself per unit of time is its **frequency (f)**. The standard unit of time is the second; thus, frequency is the number of times a wave repeats itself in a second, or the number of **cycles per second (cps)**. By convention, the unit of cycles per second is the **hertz (Hz)**. Thus, a wave that is repeated 1000 times per second has a frequency of 1000 Hz, and the frequency of a wave that repeats at 2500 cycles per second is 2500 Hz.

If period is the time it takes to complete one cycle, and frequency is the number of cycles that occur each second, then it follows that period and frequency are intimately related. Consider a sine wave that is repeated 1000 times per second. By definition it has a frequency of 1000 Hz. Now, if exactly 1000 cycles take exactly 1 s, then each cycle must clearly have a duration of 1 ms, or 1/1000 s. Similarly, each cycle of a 250-Hz tone must last 1/250 s, or a period of 4 ms. Formally, then, frequency is the reciprocal of period, and period is the reciprocal of frequency:

$$f = \frac{1}{t} \tag{1.32}$$

and

$$t = \frac{1}{f} \tag{1.33}$$

It has already been noted that the oscillating air particle is moving back and forth around its resting or average position. In other words, the air particle's displacement changes over the course of each cycle. The magnitude of the air particle's displacement is called **amplitude**. Figure 1.8 illustrates a difference in the amplitude of a sinusoid, and contrasts this with a change in its frequency. In both frames of the figure, the tone represented by the finer curve has greater amplitude than the one portrayed by the heavier line. This is shown by the greater vertical distance from the baseline (amplitude) at any point along the horizontal axis (time). (Obviously, exceptions occur at those times when both curves have zero amplitudes.)

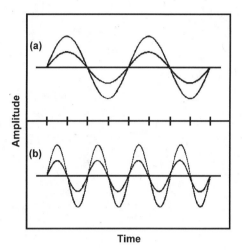

Figure 1.8 Within each frame (a and b), both sinusoidal waves have the same frequency, but the one depicted by the lighter curves has a greater amplitude than the one represented by the heavier curves. The curves in frame (b) have twice the frequency as those shown in frame (a).

At any given moment, the particle may be at its extreme positive or negative displacement from the resting position in one direction or the other, or it may be somewhere between these two extremes (including being at the resting position, where displacement is zero). Because each of these displacements is a momentary glimpse that holds true only for that instant, the magnitude of a signal at a given instant is aptly called its **instantaneous amplitude**.

Because the instantaneous amplitude changes from moment to moment, we also need to be able to describe the magnitude of a wave in more general terms. The overall displacement from the negative to positive peak yields the signal's **peak-to-peak amplitude**, while the magnitude from baseline to a peak is called the wave's **peak amplitude**. Of course, the actual magnitude is no more often at the peak than it is at any other phase of the sine wave. Thus, although peak amplitudes do have uses, we most often are interested in a kind of "average" amplitude that more reasonably reflects the magnitude of a wave throughout its cycles. The simple average of the sinusoid's positive and negative instantaneous amplitudes cannot be used because this number will always be equal to zero. The practical alternative is to use the **root-mean-square (rms) amplitude**. This value is generally and simply provided by measuring equipment, but it conceptually involves the following calculations: First, the values of all positive and negative displacements are squared so that all resulting values are positive numbers (and zero for those values that fall right on the resting position). Then the mean of all these values is obtained, and the rms value is finally obtained by taking the square root of this mean. The rms amplitude of a sinusoidal signal is numerically equal to 0.707 times the peak amplitude, or 0.354 times the peak-to-peak amplitude. Figure 1.9 illustrates the relationships among peak, peak-to-peak, and rms amplitudes.

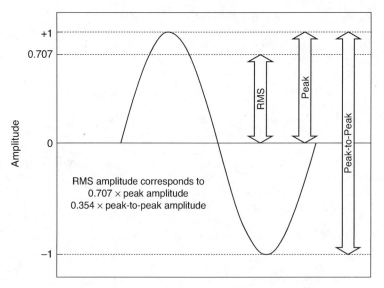

Figure 1.9 The relationships among the root-mean-square (rms), peak, and peak-to-peak amplitudes.

COMBINING WAVES

The sound associated with a sinusoidal wave is called a **pure tone**. Figure 1.10 shows what occurs when two sinusoids having the *same frequencies* and *amplitudes* are combined. In this case, the resulting wave will also be a pure tone, but the concepts illustrated in Fig. 1.10 reveal the principles that apply whenever waves are being combined. In Fig. 1.10a, the first and second sinusoids (labeled f_1 and f_2) are *in-phase* with each other. Here, the two waves are equal to one another in terms of (instantaneous) amplitude at every moment in time. The resulting wave (labeled $f_1 + f_2$) has twice the amplitude of the two components, but it is otherwise identical to them. This finding illustrates the central concept involved in combining waves: The amplitudes of the two waves being combined are *algebraically added to each other at every point along the horizontal (time) axis*. In the case of two identical, in-phase sinusoids, the resultant wave becomes twice as big at each point along the time axis and remains zero wherever the two waves have zero amplitudes. The latter occurs because the amplitudes of the two waves at the moments when they cross the baseline are zero; zero plus zero equals zero. For readily apparent reasons, the case shown in Fig. 1.10a is called **reinforcement**.

Figure 1.10b shows what happens when we combine two otherwise identical sinusoids that are *180° out of phase* with each other. This is, of course, the opposite of the relationship depicted in Fig. 1.10a. Here, wave f_1 is equal and opposite to wave f_2 at every moment in time. Algebraic addition under these circumstances causes the resulting amplitude to equal zero at all points along the horizontal (time) axis. Notice that the result $(f_1 + f_2)$ is complete **cancellation**.

If the two otherwise identical sinusoids are out of phase by a value other than 180°, then the shape of the resulting wave will depend upon how their amplitudes compare at each moment in time. The two sinusoids in Fig. 1.10c are 90° out of phase. The result of algebraically adding their magnitudes on a point-by-point basis is shown by wave $f_1 + f_2$ below the two original waves. In general, combining two identical sinusoids having the same frequency that are out of phase (except 180° out of phase) results in a sinusoid with the same frequency, but that is different in its phase and amplitude.

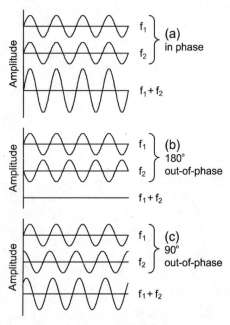

Figure 1.10 Combining sinusoids with equal frequencies and amplitudes that are (a) in phase, (b) 180° out of phase, and (c) 90° out of phase.

COMPLEX WAVES

Thus far, we have dealt only with the combination of sinusoids having the same frequency. What happens when we combined sinusoids that differ in frequency? When two or more pure tones are combined, the result is called a **complex** wave or a complex sound. The mechanism for combining waves of dissimilar frequencies is the same as what applies for those having the same frequency: *Any* two or more waves are combined by algebraically summing their instantaneous displacements on a point-by-point basis along the horizontal (time) axis, regardless of their individual frequencies and amplitudes or their phase relationships. However, the combination of waves having unequal frequencies will not yield a sinusoidal result. Instead, the result will depend upon the specifics of the sounds being combined.

Consider the three sinusoids at the top in Fig. 1.11, labeled f_1, f_2, and f_3. Note that the two cycles of f_1 are completed in the same time as four cycles of f_2 or six cycles of f_3. Thus, frequency of f_2 is *exactly* two times that of f_1, and the frequency of f_3 is *exactly* three times f_1. The actual frequencies of f_1, f_2, and f_3 could be any values meeting the described conditions; for example, 100, 200, and 300 Hz; 1000, 2000, and 3000 Hz, or 20, 40, and 60 Hz, etc. Because f_2 and f_3 are integral multiples of f_1, we say that they are **harmonics** of f_1. Hence, f_1, f_2, and f_3 constitute a harmonic series. The lowest frequency of this series is the **fundamental frequency**. Otherwise stated, harmonics are whole-number multiples of the fundamental frequency; the fundamental is the largest whole-number common denominator of its harmonics. Notice that the fundamental frequency (often written as $\mathbf{f_0}$) is also the first harmonic because its frequency is the value of the first harmonic, or $1 \times f_0$. Clearly, the harmonics are separated from one another by amounts equal to the fundamental frequency.

The lower three waves in Fig. 1.11 show what happens when f_1, f_2, and f_3 are combined in various ways. Notice that the combining of two or more sinusoidal waves differing in frequency generates a resultant wave that is no longer sinusoidal in character. Note, however, that the combined waveforms shown in this figure are still periodic. In other words, even though these combined waveforms are no longer sinusoidal, they still retain the characteristic of repeating themselves at regular intervals over time. Moreover, notice that all three waves ($f_1 + f_2$, $f_1 + f_3$, and $f_1 + f_2 + f_3$) repeat themselves with the same period as f_1, which is the lowest component in each case. These are examples of **complex periodic waves**, so called because (1) they are composed of more than one component and (2) they repeat themselves at regular time intervals. The lowest-frequency component of a complex periodic wave is its fundamental frequency. Hence, f_1 is the fundamental frequency of each of the complex periodic waves in Fig. 1.11 The period of the fundamental frequency constitutes the rate at which the complex periodic wave repeats itself. In other words, the time needed for one cycle of a complex periodic wave is the same as the period of its fundamental frequency.

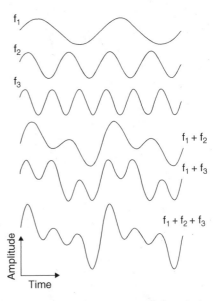

Figure 1.11 The in-phase addition of sinusoidal waves f_1, f_2, and f_3 into complex periodic waves, $f_1 + f_2$, $f_1 + f_3$, and $f_1 + f_2 + f_3$. The frequency of f_2 is twice that of f_1, and f_3 is three times the frequency of f_1. The frequency of f_1 is the fundamental frequency of each of the three complex periodic waves.

The example shown in Fig. 1.12 involves combining only odd harmonics of 1000 Hz (1000, 3000, 5000, and 7000 Hz) whose amplitudes become smaller with increasing frequency. The resulting complex periodic waveform becomes progressively squared off as the number of odd harmonics is increased, eventually resulting in the aptly named **square wave**. The complex periodic waveform at the bottom of the figure depicts the extent to which a square wave is approximated by the combination of the four odd harmonics shown above it.

The combination of components that are not harmonically related results in a complex waveform that does not repeat itself over time. Such sounds are thus called **aperiodic**. In the extreme case, consider a wave that is completely random. An artist's conceptualization of two separate glimpses of a random waveform is shown in Figs. 1.13 1.13a and 1.13b. The point of the two pictures is that the waveform is quite different from moment to moment. Over the long run, such a wave would contain all possible frequencies, and all of them would have the same average amplitudes. The sound described by such waveforms is often called **random noise** or **Gaussian noise**. Because all possible frequencies are equally represented, they are more commonly called **white noise** on analogy to white light. Abrupt sounds that are extremely short in duration must also be aperiodic because they are not repeated over time. Such sounds are called **transients**. The waveform of a transient is shown in Fig. 1.13c.

Because the **waveform** shows amplitude as a function of time, the frequency of a pure tone and the fundamental frequency of a complex periodic tone can be determined only indirectly by

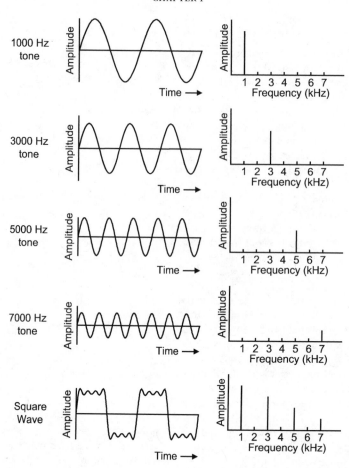

Figure 1.12 The addition of odd harmonics of 1000 Hz to produce a square wave. Waveforms (amplitude as a function of time) are shown in the left panels and corresponding spectra (amplitude as a function of frequency) are shown in the right panels.

examining such a representation, and then only if the time scale is explicit. Moreover, one cannot determine the frequency content of a complex sound by looking at its waveform. In fact, dramatically different waveforms result from the combination of the same component frequencies if their phase relationships are changed. Another means of presenting the material is therefore needed when one is primarily interested in information about frequency. This information is portrayed by the **spectrum,** which shows amplitude as a function of frequency. In effect, we are involved here with the issue of going between the time domain (shown by the waveform) and the frequency domain (shown by the spectrum). The underlying mathematical relationships are provided by **Fourier's theorem**, which basically says that a complex sound can be analyzed into its constituent sinusoidal components. The process by which one may break down the complex sound into its component parts is called **Fourier analysis**. Fourier analysis enables one to plot the spectrum of a complex sound.

The spectra of several periodic waves are shown in the right side of Fig. 1.12, and the spectrum of white noise is shown in

Fig. 1.13d. The upper four spectra in Fig. 1.12 corresponds, respectively, to the waveforms of the sinusoids to their left. The top wave is that of a 1000-Hz tone. This information is shown on the associated spectrum as a single (discrete) vertical line drawn at the point along the abscissa corresponding to 1000 Hz. The height of the line indicates the amplitude of the wave. The second waveform in Fig. 1.12 is for a 3000-Hz tone that has a lower amplitude than does the 1000-Hz tone shown above it. The corresponding spectrum shows this as a single vertical line drawn at the 3000-Hz location along the abscissa. Similarly, the spectra of the 5000- and 7000-Hz tones are discrete vertical lines corresponding to their respective frequencies. Notice that the heights of the lines become successively smaller going from the spectrum of the 1000-Hz tone to that of the 7000-Hz tone, revealing that their amplitudes are progressively lower.

The lowest spectrum in Fig. 1.12 depicts the complex periodic wave produced by the combination of the four pure tones shown above it. It has four discrete vertical lines, one each at the 1000-, 3000-, 5000-, and 7000-Hz locations. This spectrum approximates that of a square wave. The spectrum of a square

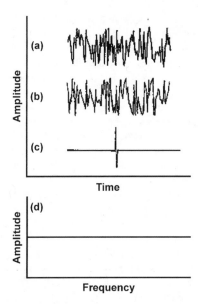

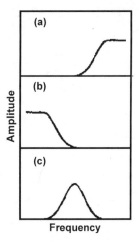

Figure 1.14 Continuous spectra of aperiodic sounds with (a) greater amplitude in the high frequencies, (b) greater amplitude in the lower frequencies, and (c) a concentration of energy within a given band of frequencies.

Figure 1.13 Artist's conceptualizations of the waveform of white noise as it might appear at two different times (a and b), and of a transient (c), along with the spectrum of white noise or a transient (d).

wave is composed of many discrete vertical lines, one each at the frequencies corresponding to odd multiples of its lowest (fundamental) component, with their heights decreasing as frequency increases.

To summarize, the spectrum of a periodic wave shows a vertical line at the frequency of each sinusoidal component of that wave, and the amplitude of each component is shown by the height of its corresponding line. Consequently, the spectrum of a periodic sound is referred to as a **discrete spectrum**. As should be apparent, the phase relationships among the various components are lost when a sound is represented by its spectrum.

Figure 1.13d shows the spectrum of white noise. Because white noise contains all conceivable frequencies, it would be a fruitless exercise to even try to draw individual (discrete) vertical lines at each of its component frequencies. The same point applies to the three spectra depicted in Fig. 1.14 shows the continuous spectra of aperiodic sounds that contain (1) greater amplitude in the higher frequencies, (2) greater amplitude in the lower frequencies, and (3) a concentration of energy within a particular range band (range) of frequencies.

FILTERS

The three spectra depicted in Fig. 1.14 may also be used to describe the manner in which a system transfers energy as a function of frequency. **Filters** are described according to the range of frequencies that they allow to *pass* as opposed to those that they *stop* or *reject*. Thus, Fig. 1.15a depicts a **high-pass filter** because the frequencies higher than a certain **cutoff frequency** are passed, whereas those below that cutoff frequency are stopped or rejected. On the other hand, Fig. 1.15b shows a **low-pass filter** because the frequencies lower than its cutoff frequency are passed whereas higher ones are rejected. A cutoff frequency is usually defined as the frequency where the power falls to half of its peak value. This location is called the **half-power point**. In decibels, the half-power point is 3 dB below that level of the peak, and is therefore also known as the **3-dB down point**.

Figure 1.15c illustrates a **band-pass filter** because the frequencies within the designated range are passed, whereas those below and above its lower and upper cutoff frequencies are rejected. A band-pass filter is usually described in terms of its **center frequency**, which is self-explanatory, and its **bandwidth**, which is how wide the filter is between its upper and lower cutoff frequencies. A filter that passes the frequencies above and below a certain band, but rejects the frequencies within that band is called a **band-reject filter** (Fig. 1.15d).

The sharpness with which a filter de-emphasizes the reject band is given by its **slope**, also know as its **rolloff**, **attenuation**, or **rejection rate**. The slope is usually expressed in *decibels per octave*. For example, a slope of 24 dB/octave means that the magnitude of the sound outside of the pass band is reduced at a rate of 24 dB for each doubling of frequency. Beginning at 1000 Hz, a 24-dB/octave rolloff rate would cause the signal to be reduced by 24 dB by 2000 Hz (an octave above 1000 Hz) and by an additional 24 dB by 4000 Hz (an octave above 2000 Hz). Besides using its slope, it is often convenient to describe the sharpness of tuning for a band-pass filter in terms of a value called **Q**, especially when comparing the characteristics of different filters. The Q of a filter is simply the ratio of its center frequency to its bandwidth.

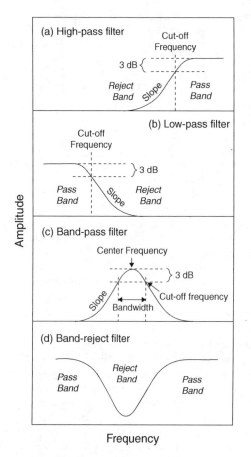

Figure 1.15 Examples of filters and some of their parameters: (a) high-pass filter, (b) low-pass filter, (c) band-pass filter, and (d) band-reject filter.

STANDING WAVES

Let us consider two situations. In the first situation, imagine the sound waves propagating rightward and leftward from a vibrating tuning fork placed in the center of a small room. These sound waves will hit and be reflected from the walls so that now there will also be reflected waves propagating in the opposite directions in addition to the original waves. (Considering for the moment only the right wall for simplicity, we can envision a rightward-going original wave and a leftward-going reflected wave.) The other situation involves plucking the center of a guitar string that is tied tautly at both ends. Here, the waves initiated by the pluck move outward toward each fixed end of the string, from which a reflected wave propagates in the opposite direction.

To reiterate, in both cases, just described, there are continuous original and continuous reflected waves moving toward one another. The reflected waves are equal in frequency to the original ones, and both the reflected and original waves are of course propagating at the same speed. Now, recall from prior discussion that two waves will interact with one another such that

their instantaneous displacements add algebraically. Thus, the net displacement (of the air particles in the room or of the string) at any moment that occurs at any point (in the room or along the string) will be due to how the superimposed waves interact. It turns out that the resultant wave produced by this interaction constitutes a pattern that f_1, f_2, and f_3 actually stands still even though it is derived from component waves which themselves are propagating. Hence, the points of maximum displacement (peaks of the waves) and no displacement (baseline crossings of the waves) will always occur at fixed locations in the room or along the string. This phenomenon is quite descriptively called a **standing wave**.

Because the vibration pattern of the string is easily visualized, we will refer only to the string as example for the remainder of the discussion, although these points apply similarly to the room example as well. The locations of no (zero) displacement in the standing wave pattern are called **nodes**, and the places of maximum displacement are thus called **antinodes**. Even brief consideration will reveal that the displacement must be zero at the two ends of the string, where they are tied and thus cannot move. (This corresponds to the hard walls of the room, which prevent the air molecules from being displaced.) Hence, nodes must occur at the two ends of the string. It follows that if there is a node at each end of the string, then there must be an antinode at the center of the string, halfway between the two nodes. This notion should not be surprising, because we already know that the zero displacements (at 0° and 180° phase) and maximum displacements (at 90° and 270° phase) alternate for any cycle of a sinusoid.

This standing wave pattern is depicted in Fig. 1.16a. Some thought will confirm that the arrangement just described (a node at each end an antinode at the center) constitutes the

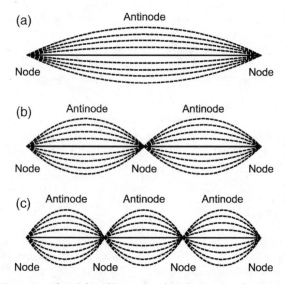

Figure 1.16 The (a) first, (b) second, and (c) third modes of a vibrating string.

longest possible standing wave pattern that can occur for any given string. We will call it the first **mode of vibration**. The figure also highlights the fact that this standing wave pattern comprises exactly one-half of a cycle (from 0° to 180°). Consequently, its length (L) corresponds to exactly one-half of a wavelength (λ), or L = λ/2. Its length therefore is equal to one-half of a wavelength (λ/2) of some frequency. This frequency, in turn, may be determined by applying the formula, f = c/λ (Eq. 1.31). By substitution, the frequency of the string's first mode of vibration would be c/2L (where L is the length of the string and c is the appropriate speed of the wave for that string[3]). It should now be apparent that the first mode of vibration corresponds to the fundamental frequency.

The standing wave just described is not the only one that can occur for the string, but rather is the longest one. Other standing waves may develop as well as long as they meet the requirement that nodes occur at the two tied ends of the string. Several other examples are shown in Fig. 1.16, which reveals that each of these standing wave patterns must divide the string into parts that are exactly equal in length to one another. Thus, there will be standing wave patterns that divide the string into exact halves, thirds, fourths, fifths, etc. These are the second, third, fourth, fifth, etc., modes of vibration. In turn, they produce frequencies, which are exact multiples (harmonics) of the fundamental frequency.

Suppose we were to set the air inside of a tube into vibration by, for example, blowing across the open end of the tube. If we were to do this experiment for several tubes, we would find that the shorter tubes make higher-pitch sounds than do the longer ones. We would also find that the same tube would produce a higher pitch when it is open at both ends than when it is open at only one end. The frequency(ies) at which a body or medium vibrates is referred to as its **natural** or **resonant** frequency(ies).

In the case of a column of air vibrating in a tube open at both ends, the greatest pressure and the least particle displacement can occur in the center of the tube, while the greatest displacement and thus lowest pressure can occur at the two open ends (Fig. 1.17a). This is analogous to the vibration of the string. One may understand this in the sense that going from one end of the tube to the other involves going from a pressure node to an antinode to a node (or from displacement antinode to node to antinode), or 180° of a cycle. This pattern is related to the out-of-phase reflection of the wave at the two ends of the tube so that the pattern is duplicated when the length of the tube is covered twice. Hence, the lowest (fundamental) frequency capable of covering the tube exactly twice in one cycle must have a wavelength twice the length of the tube. Thus, the lowest

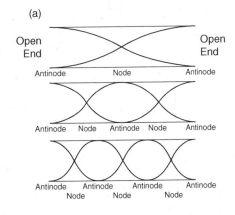

(a)

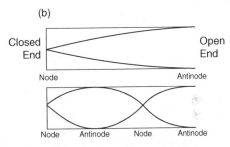

(b)

Figure 1.17   Standing waves in (a) a tube which is open at both ends (a half-wavelength resonator) and (b) a tube which is closed at one end and open at the other end (a quarter-wavelength resonator). *Source*: From Gelfand SA (2001). *Essentials of Audiology, Second Edition*. New York: Thieme Medical Publishers, with permission.

resonant frequency (f_1) of a tube open at both ends is the frequency whose wavelength is twice the length of the tube, or $f_1 = $ c/2L. Harmonics will occur at each multiple of this fundamental frequency.

Air vibration in a tube closed at one end is most restricted at the closed end, where pressure must thus be greatest and displacement the least (Fig. 1.17b). (Reflections at the closed end occur without phase reversal.) Thus, in terms of displacement, there must be a node at the closed end and an antinode at the open end. This means that the length of the tube corresponds to a quarter of a wavelength so that the lowest resonant frequency (f_1) of a tube closed at one end and open at the other is the one whose wavelength is four times the length of the tube, or $f_1 = $ c/4L. Since a node can occur at only one end, such a tube produces only the fundamental frequency and its odd harmonics (e.g., f_1, f_3, f_5, f_7, etc.).

IMPEDANCE

Impedance is the opposition to the flow of energy through a system. Some knowledge of impedance thus helps one to understand how a system transmits energy, and why it is more responsive to some frequencies than it is to others. We may generally define **impedance (Z)**, in **ohms**, as the ratio of force

---

[3] The speed of a wave along a vibrating string is not the same as for air. Instead, we would be dealing with the speed of a transverse wave along a string, which is the square root of the ratio of the string's tension (T) to its mass per unit area (M). Hence, the formula for the string's lowest resonant frequency actually would be f = $(1/2L)\sqrt{T/M}$.

to velocity:

$$Z = \frac{F}{v} \qquad (1.34)$$

Therefore, the greater the amount of force needed to result in a given amount of velocity, the greater the impedance of the system.

We may also consider impedance in terms of its components. These are shown in the form of a mechanical representation of impedance in Fig. 1.18 Here, we see that impedance (Z) is the interaction between **resistance (R)** and two kinds of **reactance (X)**, known as **positive** or **mass reactance (X_m)** and **negative** or **stiffness reactance (X_s)**. These components are, respectively, related to friction, mass, and stiffness. In the figure, mass is represented by the block, and stiffness is provided by the spring. Friction is represented in the figure by the irregular surface across which the mass (represented by a solid block) is moved.

Let us imagine that a sinusoidal force (represented by the arrow) is being applied to the system depicted in the illustration. Friction causes a portion of the energy applied to the system to be converted into heat. This dissipation of energy into heat is termed resistance. Resistance is not related to frequency and occurs in phase with the applied force. In contrast, reactance is the storage (as opposed to the dissipation) of energy by the system. Mass reactance is, of course, associated with the mass of the system (the block in Fig. 1.18). Since mass is associated with the property of inertia, the application of a force causes the mass to accelerate according to the familiar formula F = Ma (where F is force, M is mass, and a is acceleration). If the force is applied sinusoidally, then the mass reactance is related to frequency as

$$X_m = M \cdot 2\pi f \qquad (1.35)$$

where f is frequency. Thus, the magnitude of the mass reactance is directly proportional to frequency; that is, the higher the frequency, the greater the mass reactance. Since acceleration precedes force by a quarter-cycle, X_m will lead the applied force in phase by 90°. This is why X_m is termed positive reactance,

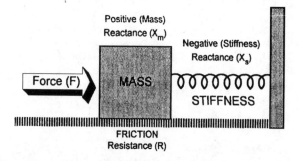

Figure 1.18 The components of impedance (Z) are friction or resistance (R), represented by the rough surface, mass (positive) reactance (X_m), represented by the block, and stiffness (negative) reactance (X_s), represented by the spring.

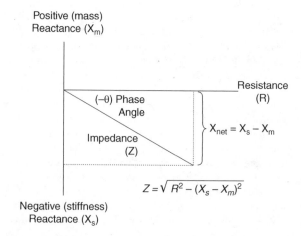

Figure 1.19 The relationships between impedance and its components.

and its value is shown in the positive direction on the y-axis in Fig. 1.19

Stiffness reactance is represented by the spring in Fig. 1.18 We will represent the stiffness as S. Applying a force compresses (displaces) the spring according to the formula F = Sx, where x is the amount of displacement. When the force is applied sinusoidally, then stiffness reactance is related to frequency as

$$X = \frac{S}{2\pi f} \qquad (1.36)$$

In other words, the amount of stiffness reactance is *inversely proportional* to frequency; that is, stiffness reactance goes down as frequency goes up. Since displacement follows force by a quarter-cycle, X_s lags behind the applied force in phase by 90°. It is thus called negative reactance and is plotted downward on the y-axis in Fig. 1.19 It should be apparent at this point that X_m and X_s are 180° out of phase with each other.

Because stiffness and mass reactance are 180° out of phase, a system's net reactance is equal to the difference between them ($X_m - X_s$). This relationship is illustrated in Fig. 1.19 for the condition where X_s exceeds X_m, which is the case for lower frequencies in the normal ear (see Chap. 3). Notice that the impedance (Z) is a vector, which results from the interaction between the resistance (R) and the **net reactance (X_{net})**. The negative phase angle ($-\theta$) in Fig. 1.19 shows that the net reactance is negative. The relationship among impedance, resistance, and reactance may now be summarized as follows:

$$Z = \sqrt{R^2 + (X_s - X_m)^2} \qquad (1.37)$$

Looking at the effect of frequency, we find that

$$Z = \sqrt{R^2 + \left(\frac{S}{2\pi f} - M \cdot 2\pi f \right)^2} \qquad (1.38)$$

The implication is that frequency counts. Because X_m is proportional to frequency, while X_s is inversely proportional to

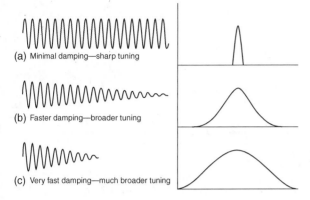

(a) Minimal damping—sharp tuning

(b) Faster damping—broader tuning

(c) Very fast damping—much broader tuning

Figure 1.20 Artist's conceptualizations of the relationship between the amount of damping (*left panels*) and the sharpness of tuning around the resonant frequency (*right panels*).

REFERENCES

American National Standards Institute, ANSI S1—1994 (R2004). 2004. *American National Standard Acoustical Terminology*. New York: ANSI.

Beranek LL. 1986. *Acoustics*. New York: American Institute of Physics.

Everest FA. 2000. *The Master Handbook of Acoustics, 4th ed*. New York: McGraw-Hill.

Gelfand SA. 2001. *Essentials of Audiology, 2nd ed*. New York: Thieme Medical Publishers.

Hewitt, PG 2005. *Conceptual Physics, 10th ed*. Boston, MA: Pearson Addison-Wesley.

Kinsler LE, Frey AR, Coopens AB, and Sanders JB. 1999. *Fundamentals of Acoustics, 4th ed*. New York, NY: Wiley.

Pearce JR, David EE Jr. 1958. *Man's World of Sound*. Garden City, New York, NY: Doubleday.

Peterson APG, Gross EE. 1972. *Handbook of Noise Measurement, 7th ed*. Concord, MA: General Radio.

Rassmussen G. Intensity—Its measurement and uses. *Sound Vibr* 1989; 23(3):12–21.

Rossing TD, Moore RF, Wheeler PA. 2002. *The Science of Sound, 3rd ed*. Boston, MA: Pearson Addison-Wesley.

Speaks CE. 1999. *Introduction to Sound: Acoustics for Hearing and Speech Sciences, 3rd ed*. San Diego, CA: Singular.

van Bergeijk WA, Pearce JR, David EE Jr. 1960. *Waves and the Ear*. Garden City, New York, NY: Doubleday.

Young HD, Freedman RA. 2007. *Sears and Zemansky's University Physics with Modern Physics, 12th ed*. Boston, MA: Pearson Addison-Wesley.

frequency, they should be equal at some frequency. This is the system's **resonant frequency**, at which the reactance components cancel each other out, leaving only the resistance component.

The amount of resistance is associated with how rapidly damping occurs, and it determines the sharpness of the tuning around the resonant frequency. This relationship is illustrated in Fig. 1.20 The less the resistance (i.e., the slower the damping), the more narrowly tuned the resonance is; the more resistance (i.e., the faster the damping), the broader the responsiveness of the system around the resonant frequency.

2 Anatomy

GROSS ANATOMY AND OVERVIEW

The auditory system comprises the ears and their connections to and within the central nervous system. From the standpoint of physical layout, the auditory system may be divided into the outer, middle, and inner ears; the auditory nerve; and the central auditory pathways. This section provides a very brief and simplified overview of the auditory system, in the hope that a brief glance at the forest will help the student avoid being blinded by the trees. Before proceeding, those not familiar with anatomical terminology should review the pictures in Fig. 2.1 and the definitions in Table 2.1, which summarize some of the terms used to describe the orientation of anatomical structures and the relationships among them.

The major divisions of the ear are shown in Fig. 2.2, and their relative positions within the head are given in Fig. 2.3. The **outer ear** is made up of the pinna (auricle) and ear canal (external auditory meatus). The eardrum (tympanic membrane) separates the outer and middle ears and is generally considered to be part of the latter. The **middle ear** also includes the tympanic (middle ear) cavity; the ossicular chain with its associated muscles, tendons, and ligaments; and the eustachian (auditory) tube. The **inner ear** begins at the oval window. It includes the sensory organs of hearing (the cochlea) and of balance (the semicircular canals, utricle, and saccule). While the balance system is certainly important, the concern here is hearing, and accordingly the balance apparatus is mentioned only insofar as it is directly associated with the auditory system.

The inner ear, beyond the oval window, is composed of the vestibule, the cochlea, and the vestibular apparatus. A membranous duct is continuous throughout these. In the cochlea, it separates the perilymph-filled scala vestibuli and scala tympani above and below from the endolymph-filled scala media between them. The scala media contains the organ of Corti, whose hair cells are the sensory receptors for hearing. When stimulated, the hair cells initiate activity in the auditory nerve fibers with which they are in contact. The **auditory nerve** leaves the inner ear through the internal auditory canal (internal auditory meatus), enters the brain at the angle of the pons and cerebellum, and terminates in the brainstem at the cochlear nuclei. We are now in the central auditory system.

TEMPORAL BONE

The ear is contained within the **temporal bone.** Knowledge of the major landmarks of this bone is thus important in understanding the anatomy and spatial orientation of the ear. The right and left temporal bones are two of the 22 bones that make up the skull. Eight of these bones (including the two temporal bones) contribute to the cranium, and the remaining 14 bones

form the facial skeleton. Figure 2.4 gives a lateral (side) view of the skull, emphasizing the temporal bone. The temporal bone forms the inferior portion of the side of the skull. It is bordered by the mandible, zygomatic parietal, sphenoid, and occipital bones. The temporal bone itself is divided into five anatomical divisions: the squamous, mastoid, petrous, and tympanic portions, and the anteroinferiorly protruding styloid process. These parts of the temporal bone, as well as its major landmarks, are shown in Fig. 2.5.

The **squamous portion** is the fan-shaped part of the temporal bone. It is quite thin, often to the point of being translucent. Its inferior surface forms the roof and part of the posterior wall of the ear canal. The **zygomatic process** protrudes forward from the squamous portion to meet the zygomatic bone. The fan-shaped squamous plate is also in contact with the sphenoid bone anteriorly and with the parietal bone superiorly and posteriorly. The mandible attaches to the temporal bone just anterior to the ear canal, near the base of the zygomatic process, forming the **temporomandibular joint.**

The **mastoid portion** lies behind and below the squamous and forms the posterior aspect of the temporal bone. The mastoid portion attaches to the parietal bone superiorly and to the occipital bone posteriorly. It projects downward to form the **mastoid process**, which appears as a somewhat cone-shaped extension below the base of the skull. The mastoid process contains interconnecting air cells of variable size, shape, and number. Continuous with these air cells is a cavity known as the **tympanic antrum**, which lies anterosuperior to the mastoid process. The antrum also connects with the **epitympanic recess (attic)** of the middle ear via the **aditus ad antrum.** The antrum is bordered inferiorly by the mastoid process, superiorly by the thin bony plate called the **tegmen tympani**, medially by the wall of the lateral **semicircular canal**, and laterally by the squamous part.

The **tympanic portion** of the temporal bone forms the floor as well as the anterior and inferoposterior walls of the ear canal. It is bordered superiorly by the squamous and petrous portions and by the mastoid process posteriorly. The lower part of the tympanic portion partially covers the **styloid process**, which is a thin, cylinder-like anteroinferior projection from the base of the temporal bone. The styloid process, which varies in length from as little as 5 mm to as much as 50 mm, is generally considered to be a separate portion of the temporal bone. Although it does not contribute to the hearing mechanism, per se, the styloid process is important as a connecting point for several muscles involved in speech production.

The **petrous portion** houses the sensory organs of hearing and balance and contains the **internal auditory canal**. It is medially directed and is fused at its base to the tympanic and squamous portions. The mastoid lies posterior to the petrous portion, and in fact develops from it postnatally. The details

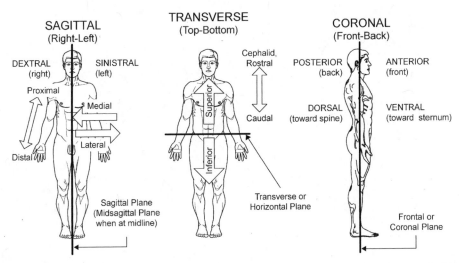

Figure 2.1 Commonly used anatomical orientations and directions. *Source*: From Gelfand (2001), *Essentials of Audiology, Second Edition*, by permission of Thieme Medical Publishers.

of the petrous portion are equivalent to those of the inner ear, discussed below.

OUTER AND MIDDLE EAR

Pinna

The **pinna (auricle)** is the external appendage of the ear. It is an irregularly shaped ovoid of highly variable size, which folds over the side of the head posteriorly, superiorly, and inferiorly. It is basically composed of skin-covered elastic cartilage, although it contains some grossly undifferentiated muscles that are of a completely vestigial nature in humans. The pinna has a number of extrinsic muscles as well, which are also essentially vestigial in humans.

The landmarks of the pinna are shown in Fig. 2.6. Most of its perimeter is demarcated by a ridge-like rim called the **helix**.

Table 2.1 Summary of Commonly Used Terms Describing Anatomical Planes, Orientations, and Directions

Term	Definition
Anterior	Front
Caudal	Toward the tail
Cephalad	Toward the head
Contralateral	Opposite side of the body
Coronal plane	Vertical plane separating the structure into front and back; frontal plane
Cranial	Toward the head
Dextral	Right
Distal	Away or further from a reference point (e.g., midline of the body)
Dorsal	Toward the spine (posterior in humans)
Homolateral	Same side of the body
Inferior	Below
Ipsilateral	Same side of the body
Lateral	Away from the midline (toward the side)
Medial	Toward the midline
Midsagittal plane	Sagittal plane at the midline
Posterior	Back
Proximal	Toward, closer to a reference point (e.g., midline of the body)
Rostral	Toward the head (toward the beak)
Sagittal plane	Vertical plane separating the structure into right and left
Sinistral	Left
Superior	Above
Transverse plane	Horizontal plane separating the structure into top and bottom; axial plane
Ventral	Toward the sternum (anterior in humans)

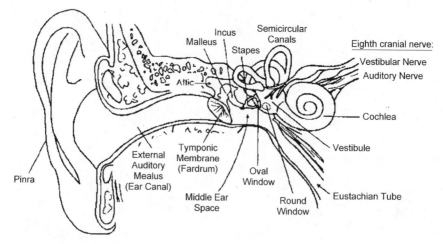

Figure 2.2 Cross-sectional view of the human ear.

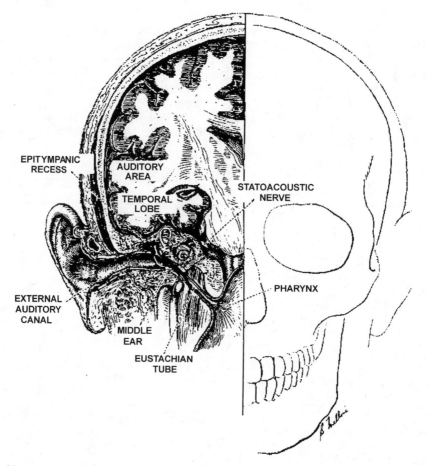

Figure 2.3 Structures of the ear in relation to the head. *Source*: Courtesy of Abbott Laboratories.

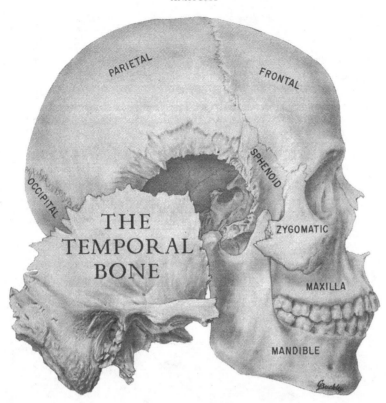

PARIETAL

FRONTAL

SPHENOID

OCCIPITAL

THE TEMPORAL BONE

ZYGOMATIC

MAXILLA

MANDIBLE

Figure 2.4 Lateral view of the skull emphasizing the position of the temporal bone. *Source*: From Anson and Donaldson (1967). *The Surgical Anatomy of the Temporal Bone and Ear*, Copyright © 1967 by W.B. Saunders, with permission.

If we first follow the helix posteriorly from the top of the ear, we see that it curves widely back and down to end in the **earlobe (lobule)** at the bottom of the pinna. Unlike the rest of the pinna, the lobe does not have any cartilage. Starting again from the apex of the helix, we see that it proceeds anteriorly and downward, and then turns posteriorly in a rather sharp angle to form the **crus of the helix**, which is an almost horizontal shelf at about the center of the pinna. The **scaphoid fossa** is a depression lying between the posterior portion of the helix posteriorly and a ridge called the **antihelix** anteriorly.

The **antihelix** is a ridge that runs essentially parallel to the posterior helix. Its upper end bifurcates to form two crura, a rather wide **superoposterior crus** and a narrower **anterior crus**, which ends under the angle where the helix curves backward. A triangular depression is thus formed by the two crura of the antihelix and the anterior part of the helix, and is called the **triangular fossa**. From the crura, the antihelix curves downward and then forward, and ends in a mound-like widening, the **antitragus**. Opposite and anterior to the antitragus is a backward-folding ridge called the **tragus**. The inferoanterior acute angle formed by the tragus and antitragus is called the **intertragal incisure**. The tragus, the antitragus, and the crus of the helix border a relatively large and cup-shaped depression called the **concha**. Sebaceous glands are present in the skin of

the concha as well as in the ear canal. At the bottom of the concha, protected by the tragus, is the entrance to the ear canal.

Ear Canal

The **ear canal (external auditory meatus)** leads from the concha to the eardrum and varies in both size and shape. The outer portion of the canal, about one-third of its length, is cartilaginous; the remaining two-thirds is **bony**. The canal is by no means straight; rather it is quite irregular in its course. It takes on a somewhat S-shaped form medially. It curves first anterosuperiorly, then posterosuperiorly, and finally anteroinferiorly. It is for this reason that the pinna must be pulled up and back in order for one to see the eardrum.

The ear canal has a diameter of about 0.7 cm at its entrance, with an average horizontal diameter of 0.65 cm and a mean vertical diameter of 0.9 cm (Wever and Lawrence, 1954). As would be expected from its irregular course, the length of the canal is not uniform. Instead, it is approximately 2.6 cm long posterosuperiorly and about 3.1 cm long inferoanteriorly (Donaldson and Miller, 1973). Also contributing to the greater length of the lower part of the ear canal is the oblique orientation of the eardrum as it sits in its **annulus** at the end of the canal.

The canal is lined with tight-fitting skin that is thicker in the cartilaginous segment than in the bony part. **Ceruminous (wax)**

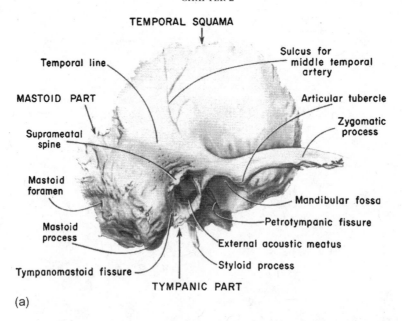

TEMPORAL SQUAMA

Temporal line

MASTOID PART

Suprameatal spine

Mastoid foramen

Mastoid process

Tympanomastoid fissure

Sulcus for middle temporal artery

Articular tubercle

Zygomatic process

Mandibular fossa

Petrotympanic fissure

External acoustic meatus

Styloid process

TYMPANIC PART

(a)

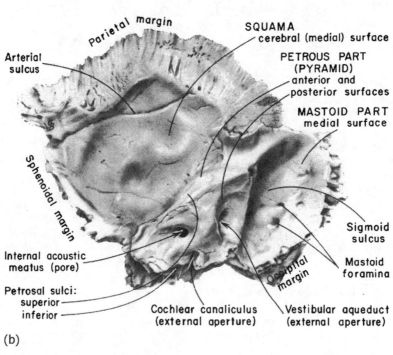

Parietal margin

Arterial sulcus

Sphenoidal margin

Internal acoustic meatus (pore)

Petrosal sulci:
superior
inferior

Cochlear canaliculus (external aperture)

SQUAMA
cerebral (medial) surface

PETROUS PART
(PYRAMID)
anterior and posterior surfaces

MASTOID PART
medial surface

Sigmoid sulcus

Mastoid foramina

Occipital margin

Vestibular aqueduct (external aperture)

(b)

Figure 2.5 Lateral (a) and medial (b) aspects of view of the temporal bone. *Source*: From Anson and Donaldson (1967). *The Surgical Anatomy of the Temporal Bone and Ear*, Copyright © 1967 by W.B. Saunders, with permission.

and **sebaceous (oil) glands** are plentiful in the cartilaginous segment and are also found on the posterior and superior walls of the bony canal. The wax and oil lubricate the canal and help to keep it free of debris and foreign objects. Tiny hairs similarly contribute to the protection of the ear from invasion.

Eardrum

The canal terminates at the **eardrum (tympanic membrane)**, which tilts laterally at the top, so as to sit in its annulus at an angle of about 55° to the ear canal (see Fig. 2.1). The membrane is quite thin and translucent, with an average thickness of approximately

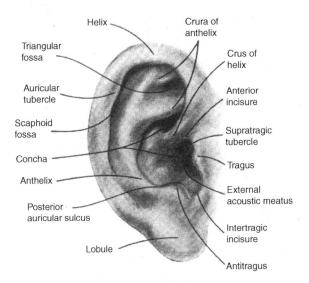

Figure 2.6 Landmarks of the pinna. *Source*: From Anson and Donaldson (1967). *The Surgical Anatomy of the Temporal Bone and Ear*, Copyright © 1967 by W.B. Saunders, with permission.

0.074 mm (Donaldson and Miller, 1973). It is elliptical in shape, with a vertical diameter of about 0.9 to 1.0 cm and a horizontal cross section of approximately 0.8 to 0.9 cm. The eardrum is concave outward, and the peak of this broad cone is known as the **umbo.** This inward displacement is associated with the drum's attachment to the **manubrium** of the **malleus**, the tip of which corresponds to the umbo (Fig. 2.7). In contact with the drum, the malleus continues upward in a direction corresponding to the 1-o'clock position in the right ear and the 11-o'clock position in the left. The **malleal prominence** of the malleus is formed by the lateral process of the malleus, from which run the **malleal folds**, which divide the drum into the **pars flaccida** above and the **pars tensa** below.

The eardrum is made up of four layers. The outermost layer is continuous with the skin of the ear canal, and the most medial layer is continuous with the mucous membrane of the middle ear. The pars flaccida is composed solely of these two layers. The pars tensa has two additional layers: a layer of radial fibers just medial to the skin layer, and a layer of nonradial fibers between the radial and mucous membrane layers.

Tympanic Cavity

The **middle ear cavity** or **tympanum** may be thought of schematically as a six-sided box or room. The lateral wall is the eardrum, and opposite to it the promontory of the basal cochlear turn forms the medial wall. Figure 2.8 shows such a schematic conceptualization of the right middle ear. The view is as though the lateral wall of the room (the eardrum, shown with the malleus attached to it) had been folded downward to reveal its contents. The front of the head would be toward the right in the drawing and the back of the head would be toward the left.

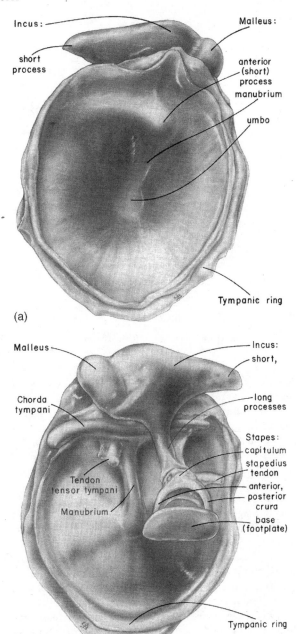

(a)

(b)

Figure 2.7 Lateral (a) and medial (b) aspects of the tympanic membrane and its connections to the ossicular chain. *Source*: From Anson and Donaldson (1967). *The Surgical Anatomy of the Temporal Bore and Ear*, Copyright © 1967 by W.B. Saunders, with permission.)

The roof of the middle ear is formed by the **tegmen tympani**, which separates the middle ear from the middle cranial fossa above. The floor of the tympanum separates it from the jugular bulb. In the anterior wall is the opening to the **eustachian tube**, and above it the canal for the tensor tympani muscle. The canal

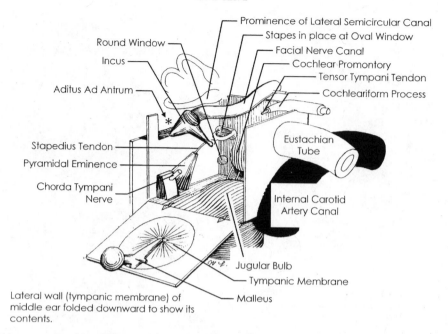

Figure 2.8 Schematic representation of the middle ear as though it were a room with its lateral wall (including the tympanic membrane with the malleus attached) folded downward. *Source*: Adapted from Proctor (1989), *Surgical Anatomy of the Temporal Bone*, by permission of Thieme Medical Publishers.

of the internal carotid artery lies behind the anterior wall, posteroinferior to the tubal opening. The posterior wall contains the **aditus ad antrum**, through which the upper portion of the middle ear called the **epitympanic recess or attic** communicates with the **mastoid antrum**. The posterior wall also contains the **fossa incudis**, a recess that receives the short process of the incus, and the **pyramidal eminence**, which houses the **stapedial muscle**. The **stapedial tendon** exits from the pyramidal prominence at its apex.

Returning to the medial wall, we see that the **oval window** is located posterosuperiorly to the **promontory**, while the **round window** is posteroinferior to the latter. Superior to the oval window lies the **facial canal prominence** with the **cochleariform process** on its anterior aspect. The **tendon** of the **tensor tympani muscle** bends around the cochleariform process to proceed laterally to the malleus.

The **eustachian tube**, also known as the **auditory tube**, serves to equalize the air pressure on both sides of the eardrum as well as allow for drainage of the middle ear by serving as a portal into the nasopharynx. Its principal features are highlighted in relation to the structures of the ear in Fig. 2.9. From its opening in the middle ear, the eustachian tube courses medially, downward at an angle of approximately 45°, and forward to exit into the nasopharynx via a prominence called the **torus tubarius**. The overall length of the tube is about 3.5 cm. The lateral first third of the eustachian tube beginning at the middle ear is surrounded by bone, whereas the remainder is enclosed within an incomplete ring of hook-shaped elastic cartilage, as illustrated in Fig. 2.9. The meeting of the **bony and cartilaginous portions** is called

the **isthmus**. At this point, the lumen of the tube may be as little as 1.0 to 1.5 mm compared to a diameter of about 3.0 to 6.0 mm at its opening into the middle ear. The cartilaginous part of the eustachian tube is normally closed (Fig. 2.10a), and it opens reflexively by action of the **tensor palatini muscle**, which

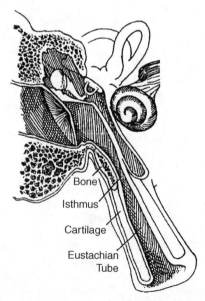

Figure 2.9 Orientation of the eustachian tube with respect to the ear. *Source*: Adapted from Hughes (1985), *Textbook of Otology*, by permission of Thieme Medical Publishers.

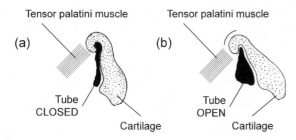

Figure 2.10 (a) Cross-section of the hook-shaped cartilage in the normally closed state of the tube. (b) Opening of the tube by action of the tensor palatini muscles, which uncurls the hook-shaped cartilage. *Source*: Adapted from Gelfand (2001), *Essentials of Audiology, Second Edition*, by permission of Thieme Medical Publishers.

uncurls the normally hook-shaped cartilages (Fig. 2.10b) in response to swallowing, yawning, sneezing, or shouting.

Ossicular Chain

Sound energy impinging upon the eardrum is conducted to the inner ear by way of the ossicles, which are the smallest bones in the body. There are three ossicles in each ear, the **malleus, incus, and stapes**; they are collectively referred to as the **ossicular chain**. Schematic illustrations of these bones are shown with the ossicular chain in place in Fig. 2.11. (Different and somewhat more life-like perspectives of the ossicles may also

be seen in Fig. 2.7.) Instead of being attached to the other bones of the skull, the ossicular chain is *suspended* in the middle ear by a series of ligaments, by the tendons of the two intratympanic muscles, and by the attachments of the malleus to the eardrum and of the stapes to the oval window.

The malleus is commonly called the hammer, although it more closely resembles a mace. It is the largest of the ossicles, being about 8 to 9 mm long and weighing approximately 25 mg. The head of the malleus is located in the epitympanic space, to which it is connected by its superior ligament. Laterally, the **manubrium** (handle) is embedded between the mucous membrane and fibrous layers of the eardrum. The anterior process of the malleus projects anteriorly from the top of the manubrium just below the neck. It attaches to the tympanic notch by its anterior ligament, which forms the axis of mallear movement. The malleus is connected to the tensor tympani muscle via a tendon, which inserts at the top of the manubrium.

The **incus** bears a closer resemblance to a tooth with two roots than to the more commonly associated anvil. It weighs approximately 30 mg and has a length of about 5 mm along its short process and about 7 mm along its long process. Its body is connected to the posteromedial aspect of the mallear head within the epitympanic recess. The connection is by a saddle joint, which was originally thought to move by a cog-like mechanism when the malleus was displaced (Helmholtz, 1868). However, subsequent research demonstrated that these

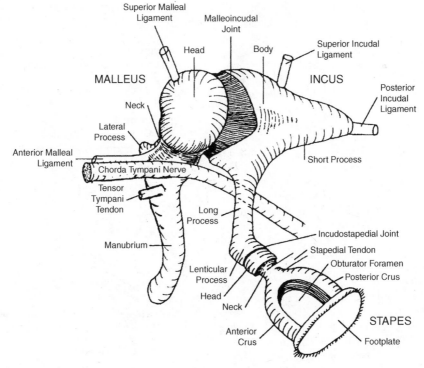

Figure 2.11 Schematic representation of the ossicular chain. *Source*: Adapted from Tos (1995), *Manual of Middle Ear Surgery, Vol 2*, by permission of Thieme Medical Publishers.

two bones move as a unit rather than relative to one another (Wever and Lawrence, 1954). The short process of the incus connects via its posterior ligaments to the fossa incudis on the posterior wall of the tympanic cavity. Its long process runs inferiorly, parallel to the manubrium. The end of the long process then bends medially to articulate with the head of the stapes in a true ball-and-socket joint.

The **stapes** (stirrup) is the smallest of the ossicles. It is about 3.5 mm high, and the footplate is about 3 mm long by 1.4 mm wide. It weighs on the order of 3 to 4 mg. The head of the stapes connects to the footplate via two crura. The anterior crus is straighter, thinner, and shorter than the posterior crus. The **footplate**, which encases the very fine stapedial membrane, is attached to the oval window by the annular ligament. The stapedius tendon inserts on the posterior surface of the neck of the stapes and connects the bone to the stapedius muscle.

Intratympanic Muscles

The middle ear contains two muscles, the tensor tympani and the stapedius (Figs. 2.7 and 2.8). The **stapedius muscle** is the smallest muscle in the body, with an average length of 6.3 mm and a mean cross-sectional area of 4.9 mm^2 (Wever and Lawrence, 1954). This muscle is completely encased within the pyramidal eminence on the posterior wall of the tympanic cavity and takes origin from the wall of its own canal. Its tendon exits through the apex of the pyramid and courses horizontally to insert on the posterior aspect of the neck of the stapes. Contraction of the stapedius muscle thus pulls the stapes posteriorly. The stapedius is innervated by the stapedial branch of the **seventh cranial (facial) nerve**.

The **tensor tympani muscle** has an average length of 25 mm and a mean cross-sectional area of approximately 5.85 mm^2 (Wever and Lawrence, 1954). The tensor tympani occupies an *osseous semicanal* on the anterior wall of the tympanum, just superior to the eustachian tube, from which it is separated by a thin bony shelf. The muscle takes origin from the cartilage of the auditory tube, from the walls of its own canal, and from the part of the sphenoid bone adjacent to the canal. Emerging from the canal, the tendon of the tensor tympani hooks around the **cochleariform process**, and inserts on the top of the manubrium of the malleus. Contraction of the tensor tympani thus pulls the malleus anteromedially, at a right angle to the uninterrupted motion of the ossicles. The tensor tympani muscle is innervated by the tensor tympani branch of the otic ganglion of the **fifth cranial (trigeminal) nerve**.

Both intratympanic muscles are completely encased within bony canals and attach to the ossicular chain by way of their respective tendons. Bekesy (1936) pointed out that this situation reduces the effects that muscular contractions might have upon the transmission of sound through the middle ear system. Contraction of either muscle increases the stiffness of the ossicular chain as well as of the eardrum. The stapedius muscle pulls posteriorly whereas the tensor tympani pulls anteromedially so that they might initially be thought to be antagonists.

However, the effect of these muscles is to lessen the amount of energy conducted by the ossicular chain, and they thus function as synergists with respect to hearing.

Of particular interest in this context is the **acoustic reflex**, which is the response of the intratympanic muscles to intense sound stimulation. It is generally accepted that the acoustic reflex *in humans is* due mainly, if not exclusively, to contraction of the *stapedius* muscle. In contrast, auditory activation of the tensor tympani muscle in humans occurs only for extremely intense sounds, as part of a *startle* response. The acoustic reflex arc is described in the context of the auditory pathways later in this chapter.

INNER EAR

Osseous and Membranous Labyrinths

The inner ear structures are contained within a system of spaces and canals, the **osseous** or **bony labyrinth**, in the petrous portion of the temporal bone. As shown in Fig. 2.12, these spaces and canals are grossly divided into three sections: the vestibule, the cochlea, and the semicircular canals. The oval window accepts the footplate of stapes and opens medially into the **vestibule**, which is about 4 mm in diameter and is somewhat ovoid in shape. The snail-shaped **cochlea** lies anterior and slightly inferior to the vestibule and is approximately 5 mm high and 9 mm in diameter at its base. Posterior to the vestibule are the three **semicircular canals**, lying at right angles to one another, each about 1 mm in diameter. The general shape of the bony labyrinth is followed by the enclosed **membranous labyrinth**, which contains the *end organs* of hearing and balance. The membranous labyrinth and its principal structures are illustrated in Fig. 2.13.

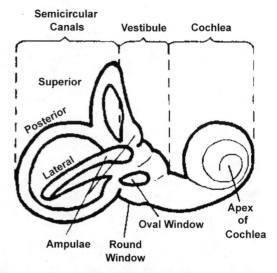

Figure 2.12 The osseous (bony) labyrinth.

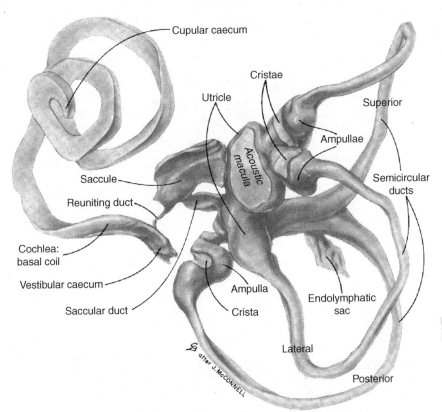

Figure 2.13   The membranous labyrinth. *Source*: From Donaldson and Miller (1973), Anatomy of the ear, in *Otolaryngology, Vol. 1*, Paparella and Schurnrick (eds.), Copyright © 1973 by W.B. Saunders (with permission).

Inner Ear Fluids

The spaces between the bony walls of the osseous labyrinth and the membranous labyrinth are filled with a fluid called **peri-lymph** or **perilymphatic fluid**, and the membranous labyrinth itself is mostly filled with **endolymph** or **endolymphatic fluid**.[1] Because they are located outside of any cells, perilymph and endolymph are referred to as **extracellular fluids**. In contrast, fluids contained within cells are called **intracellular fluids**. Smith Lowry, and Wu (1954) found that perilymph is chem-ically similar to other extracellular fluids (e.g., cerebrospinal fluid and blood serum) in the sense that it has a very high con-centration of sodium and a very low concentration of potas-sium. Oddly, they found that endolymph has just the opposite concentrations—it is high in potassium but low in sodium. In fact, endolymph has the distinction of being the only extra-cellular fluid in the body with this characteristic. Subsequent research has not only confirmed the different compositions of perilymph and endolymph, but has also richly expanded our knowledge about their composition and properties, relation-ships to other fluids and structures, as well as their roles in the cochlea.

The spaces within the organ of Corti itself are filled with perilymph-like fluid that diffuses across the basilar membrane from the scala tympani.[2] As a result, the cochlear hair cells and other structures within the organ of Corti are bathed in a sodium-rich fluid (Slepecky, 1996; Wangemann and Schacht, 1996). Tight junctions among the cells forming the reticular lamina (discussed below) isolate the endolymph above from the organ of Corti below.

The origins of perilymph and endolymph have been the sub-ject of controversy. Perilymph appears to be a derivative of the cerebrospinal fluid and/or the cochlear blood supply, and several lines of evidence have suggested that endolymph components may be derived from perilymph rather than from the blood. Overall, modern experiments disproved early ideas that these fluids are secreted at one site and flow longitudinally to another location, replacing them with the concept that the composi-tions of the inner ear fluids are maintained locally within the

---

[1] A third inner ear fluid called **intrastrial fluid** is found in the stria vascularis (see, e.g., Wangemann and Schacht, 1996).

[2] It was previously thought that the organ of Corti contained a distinct sodium-rich fluid called "cortilymph."

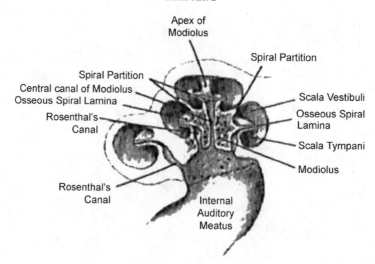

Figure 2.14 The modiolus. *Source*: Adapted from Proctor (1989), *Surgical Anatomy of the Ear and Temporal Bone*, by permission of Thieme Medical Publishers.

cochlea (e.g., Ohyama et al., 1998; Salt, 2001; Salt et al., 1986). Informative reviews are provided by Wangemann and Schacht (1996), Salt (2001), and Rask-Andersen, Schrott-Fisher, Pfaller, and Glueckert (2006).

The **cochlear aqueduct** leads from the vicinity of the round window in the scala tympani to the subarachnoid space medial to the dura of the cranium. Although the aqueduct leads from the perilymph-filled scala to the cerebrospinal fluid-filled subarachnoid space, it is not patent in many humans. Thus, it is doubtful that there is any real interchange between these two fluid systems. The **endolymphatic duct** leads from the membranous labyrinth within the vestibule to the **endolymphatic sac**. The sac is located partially between the layers of the dura in the posterior cranial fossa and partly in a niche in the posterior aspect of the petrous portion of the temporal bone.

Vestibular Organs

Returning to the structures of the inner ear, the vestibule contains two **vestibular** or **balance organs**, which are concerned with linear acceleration and gravity effects. These organs are the **utricle and saccule**. The **semicircular canals**, located behind the vestibule, widen anteriorly into five sac-like structures, which open into the somewhat elongated utricle. These widenings are the **ampullae**, and they contain the sensory receptors for rotational acceleration. (The interested reader is referred to any of the fine books listed in the References section for a detailed discussion of the balance system.) The most important connection between the areas of hearing and balance is the **ductus reuniens**, which joins the membranous labyrinth between the cochlea and the utricle.

Cochlea

The **cochlea** is the part of the inner ear concerned with hearing. An extensive albeit rather advanced review of cochlear anatomy

and physiology may be found in Dallos, Popper, and Fay (1996). The human cochlea is about 35 mm long and forms a somewhat cone-shaped spiral with about 2 3/4 turns. It is widest at the base, where the diameter is approximately 9 mm, and tapers toward the apex. It is about 5 mm high. The **modiolus** is the core, which forms the axis of the cochlear spiral, as illustrated in Fig. 2.14. Through the modiolus course the auditory nerve and the blood vessels that supply the cochlea. The osseous spiral lamina is a bony ramp-like shelf that goes up the cochlea around the modiolus much like the spiral staircase of a lighthouse, as illustrated in Fig. 2.15. Notice how the basilar membrane is attached to the osseous spiral lamina medially, as it proceeds up the cochlea. Figure 2.16 illustrates how the osseous spiral lamina

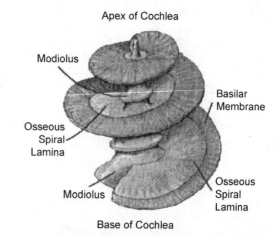

Figure 2.15 The osseous spiral lamina coils around the modiolus like the spiral staircase of a lighthouse. Notice how the basilar membrane is attached to osseous spiral lamina. *Source*: Adapted from Proctor (1989), *Surgical Anatomy of the Ear and Temporal Bone*, by permission of Thieme Medical Publishers.

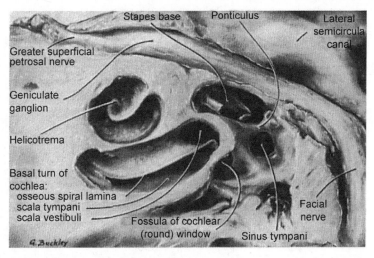

Figure 2.16   The osseous spiral lamina, scala vestibuli, scala tympani, and helicotrema. *Source*: From Anson and Donaldson (1967), *The Surgical Anatomy of the Temporal Bone and Ear*, Copyright © 1967, by W.B. Saunders with permission.

separates the scala vestibuli above from the scala tympani below. It also shows the orientation of the helicotrema at the apical turn, and the relationship between the round window and the scala tympani at the base of the cochlea.

It is easier to visualize the cochlea by imagining that the spiral has been uncoiled, as in Fig. 2.17. In this figure, the base of the cochlea is shown at the left and the apex at the right. We see three chambers: the **scala media**, **scala vestibuli**, and **scala tympani**. The scala media is self-contained and separates the other two. The scalae vestibuli and tympani, on the other hand, communicate with one another at the apex of the cochlea, through an opening called the **helicotrema**. The scala media is enclosed within the membranous labyrinth and contains endolymph, while the other two contain perilymph. The scala vestibuli is in contact with the stapes at the oval window, while the scala tympani has a membrane-covered contact with the middle ear at the round window. The scala media is separated from the scala vestibuli above by **Reissner's membrane**,

and from the scala tympani below by the **basilar membrane**. Reissner's membrane is only two cells thick and separates perilymph above from endolymph below without influencing the mechanical properties of the cochlea. In contrast, the basilar membrane plays a major role in cochlear functioning. Bekesy (1960/1989) reported that the basilar membrane is approximately 32 mm long, and that it tapers from about 0.5 mm wide at the apex to about 0.1 mm wide near the stapes at its base. Figures 2.15 and 2.17 illustrate how the basilar membrane gets progressively wider going from the base to the apex. Furthermore, it is thicker at the base than at the apex. Central to its role in cochlear functioning, the basilar membrane is stiffest at its base and becomes progressively less stiff toward the apex (Bekesy, 1960/1989).

The structures and orientation of the **scala media** are shown schematically in Fig. 2.18. The scala media is attached medially to the osseous spiral lamina, just described, and laterally to the outer wall of the cochlea by a fibrous connective tissue

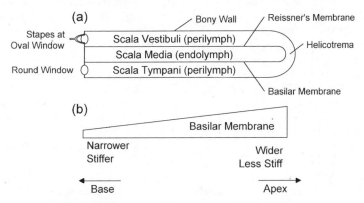

Figure 2.17   Schematic representations of the uncoiled cochlea. (a) Side view showing the three chambers. (b) Top view looking down on the basilar membrane (cochlear partition).

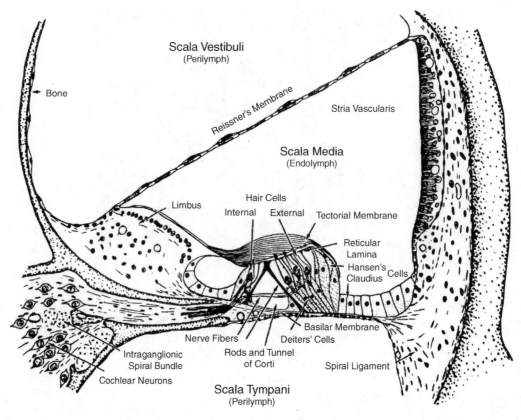

Figure 2.18 Cross-section of the organ of Corti. *Source*: From Davis (1962), with permission.

called the **spiral ligament**. Looking first at the osseous spiral lamina (toward the left in the figure), we see that this bony shelf is actually composed of two plates, separated by a space through which fibers of the auditory nerve pass. These fibers enter via openings called the **habenula perforata**. Resting on the osseous spiral lamina is a thickened band of periosteum, the **limbus**. Reissner's membrane extends from the top of the inner aspect of the limbus to the outer wall of the canal. The side of the limbus facing the organ of Corti is concave outward. The **tectorial membrane** is attached to the limbus at the upper lip of this concave part, forming a space called the **internal spiral sulcus**. The basilar membrane extends from the lower lip of the limbus to the spiral ligament at the outer wall of the duct. The spiral ligament itself has been described in considerable detail (Henson et al., 1984; Morera et al., 1980; Takahashi and Kimura, 1970); it is involved in the metabolic activities of the inner ear in addition to its role as a crucial supporting structure.

The basilar membrane has two sections. The inner section extends from the osseous spiral lamina to the outer pillars and is relatively thin. The remainder is thicker and extends to the spiral ligament. These two sections are called the **zona arcuata** and the **zona pectinata**, respectively. Sitting on the basilar membrane is the end organ of hearing—the organ of Corti. The width,

thickness, and orientation of the basilar membrane and the organ of Corti on it vary along the course of the cochlear duct (Lim, 1980).

The **organ of Corti** runs longitudinally along the basilar membrane. Grossly, it is made up of a single row of **inner hair cells (IHCs)**, three rows of **outer hair cells (OHCs)** (though as many as four or five rows have been reported in the apical turn), the **pillar cells** forming the **tunnel of Corti**, and various **supporting cells** (see Slepecky, 1996, for a detailed review). The tunnel pillars contribute considerably to the rigidity of the zona arcuata of the basilar membrane (Miller, 1985).

This tunnel separates the IHCs from the OHCs. Each of the approximately 3500 IHCs is supported by a **phalangeal cell** that holds the rounded base of the IHC as in a cup. There are about 12,000 OHCs, shaped like test tubes, which are supported by **Deiters' cells**. The closeup drawing of the organ of Corti in Fig. 2.19 shows that the IHCs are surrounded by supporting cells. In contrast, the OHCs are attached to the Deiters' cells below and the reticular lamina above, but their sides are not in contact with other cells.

Between the inner and outer hair cells are the tilted and rather conspicuous pillars (rods) of Corti, which come together at their tops to enclose the triangular tunnel of Corti. Fibers of

TECTORIAL MEMBRANE

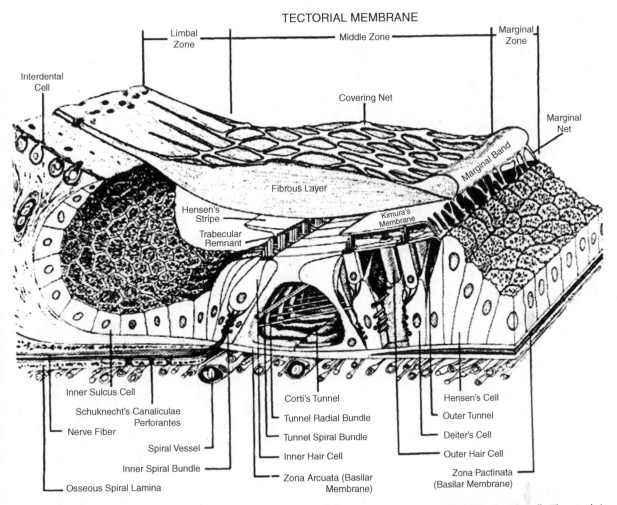

Figure 2.19 Schematic drawing of the organ of Corti and the tectorial membrane. The inner hair cells are surrounded by supporting cells. The outer hair cells attach to the Deiters' cells below and the reticular lamina above, but their lateral aspects do not make contact with other cells. *Source*: From Lim (1980) with permission of *J Acoust Soc Am*.

the eighth cranial (auditory) nerve traverse the tunnel to contact the OHCs. Just lateral to Deiters' cells are several rows of tall, supporting cells called **Hensen's cells**. Lateral to these are the columnar **Claudius cells**, which continue laterally to the spiral ligament and the stria vascularis.

The **reticular lamina** is made up of the tops of the hair cells (cuticular plates; see below) along with the upward-extending processes of the phalangeal and Deiters' cells. *Tight junctions* between the apical parts of these cells provide a barrier that isolates the endolymph-filled portions of the scala media from the structures and spaces of the organ of Corti. The distinctive surface pattern of the reticular lamina is shown in Fig. 2.20. The pillar cells maintain a strong structural attachment between the reticular lamina above and the basilar membrane below, and thus the reticular lamina provides a source of support for the hair cells at their upper surfaces. This relationship is exemplified in Fig. 2.21, showing the OHCs and Deiters' cells in the reticular lamina, as well as the stereocilia of the hair cells protruding through the lamina.

The **tectorial membrane** (Fig. 2.19) extends from its medial connection to the upper lip of the limbus, courses over the hair cells, and then connects laterally to the Hensen's (and perhaps to the most lateral Deiters') cells by a border or marginal net. Its connection to the limbus is a strong and robust one; however, the attachment of the tectorial membrane to the Hensens cells is quite fragile. The undersurface of the main body of the tectorial membrane (fibrous layer) is marked by Hensen's stripe located above the inner hair cells. Informative reviews of the tectorial membrane are provided by Steel (1983, 1985) and Lim (1986a).

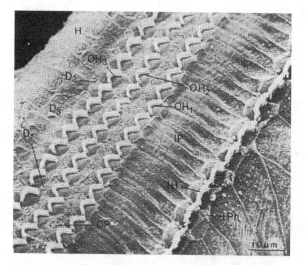

Figure 2.20 The upper surface of the organ of Corti (chinchilla) showing the stereocilia of the inner and outer hair cells protruding through the reticular lamina. The outside aspect (toward the spiral ligament) is at the left, and the medial side (toward the modiolus) is at the right. Landmarks indicated are the Hensen's cells (H), three rows of Deiters' cells (D_1, D_2, D_3), and outer hair cells (OH_1, OH_2, OH_3), outer (OP) and inner (UP) pillar cells, inner hair cells (UH), and inner phalangeal cells (UPh). *Source*: From *Hearing Research* 22, Lim (Functional structure of the organ of Corti: a review, 117–146, © 1986) with kind permission from Elsevier Science Publishers-NL, Sara Burgerhartstraat 25, 1055 KV Amsterdam, The Netherlands.

The tectorial membrane is frequently described as being ribbon-like in appearance, although Fig. 2.19 shows that this is really not the case. Instead, the tectorial membrane has a gelatinous consistency containing various proteins, mainly collagen II, which is arranged in fibers going across the tectorial

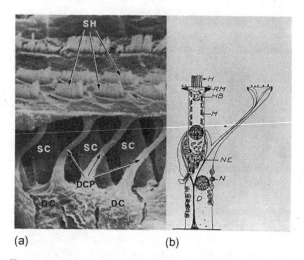

(a)   (b)

Figure 2.21 Scanning electron micrograph (a) and schematic diagram (b) of Deiters' cells, outer hair cells, and the reticular lamina. *Abbreviations*: DC, Deiters' cell; DCP, phalange of Deiters' cell; SC, sensory (outer hair) cell; SH, sensory hairs (stereocilia). *Source*: From Engstrom and Wersall (1958) by permission of Academic Press.

membrane (Thalmann et al., 1987, 1993). Notice also that it is topped by a covering net. The collagen II provides the tecorial membrane with tensile strength (Zwislocki et al., 1988). The collagen fibers in the part of the tectorial membrane overlying the OHCs become increasingly tightly packed going from the apex toward the base of the cochlea, and its stiffness changes going up the length of the cochlea from stiffest at the base to least stiff at the apex (Gueta et al., 2006, 2007).

The **stria vascularis** contains a rich network of capillaries and is attached to the spiral ligament on the lateral wall of the scala media. Structurally, the stria vascularis is composed of three layers having characteristic cell types (e.g., Slepecky, 1996). The hexagonal **marginal cells** face into the scala media. Next are irregular **intermediate cells**, which have projections into the marginal layer. Finally, there are rather flat **basal cells**, which are in contact with the spiral ligament. The stria vascularis maintains the electrochemical characteristics of the endolymph, and in particular is viewed as the source of its high concentration of potassium as well as the endocochlear potential discussed in Chapter 4 (see Wangemann and Schacht, 1996, for an in-depth discussion).

The **blood supply** to the cochlea is well described (see, e.g., Axelsson and Ryan, 2001; Slepecky, 1996). It follows a course of successive arterial branches, going from the **basilar artery** to the **anterior inferior cerebellar artery**, to the **labyrinthine (internal auditory) artery,** to the **common cochlear artery**, and finally to the **spiral modiolar artery**. As its name implies, the spiral modiolar artery follows a corkscrew-like course up the modiolus from the base to the apex of the cochlea, as shown in Fig. 2.22a. The distribution of the blood supply to the structures in the cochlear duct is illustrated in Fig. 2.22b. Notice that the system involves one branch supplying the spiral ligament above the point of attachment of Reissner's membrane, the capillary network within the stria vascularis, and the spiral prominence, as well as a second branch feeding the limbus and a plexus under the basilar membrane. Venous drainage of the cochlea is into the internal auditory vein.

Hair Cells

There are roughly 12,000 **outer hair cells** (OHC) and 3500 **inner hair cells** (IHC) in each ear, averaging (with considerable variability among people) about 86 IHCs and 343 OHCs per millimeter of cochlear length (Ulehlova et al., 1987; Wright, 1981; Wright et al., 1987).

The inner and outer hair cells were shown in relation to the cross-section of the organ of Corti in Fig. 2.17. A closer look at these cells is provided in Fig. 2.23. The hair cells are so-named because of the presence of cilia on their upper surfaces. Notice in Fig. 2.23 that the upper surface of each hair cell contains a thickening called the **cuticular plate**, which is topped by three rows of **stereocilia**, as well as a noncuticular area that contains the **basal body** of a rudimentary **kinocilium**.

The structures and interrelationships of the cuticular plate and stereocilia have been described by many researchers

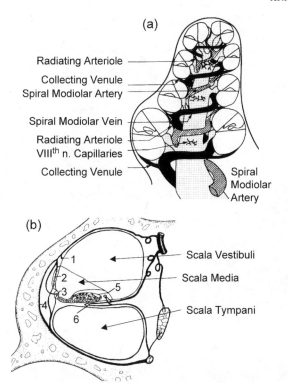

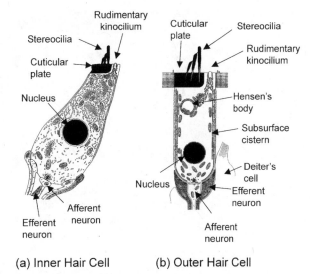

(a) Inner Hair Cell   (b) Outer Hair Cell

Figure 2.23 Schematic representation of (a) an inner hair cell and (b) an outer hair cell (see text). *Source*: Used with permission from Lim D J (1986b), Effects of noise and ototoxic drugs at the cellular level in the cochlea: A review. *Am J Otolaryngol* 7, 73–99.

Figure 2.22 Cochlear blood supply: (a) Modiolar view emphasizing the spiral modiolar artery (crosshatched) and the spiral modiolar vein (black). *Source*: Adapted from Axelsson A and Ryan AF (2001), with permission. (b) Cross-sectional view of the cochlear duct emphasizing distribution of blood supply to the spiral ligament above Reissner's membrane (1), stria vascularis (2), spiral prominence (3), limbus (5), and (6) basilar membrane. Also shown are terminal branches to collecting venules (4). *Source*: Adapted from Lawrence (1973), Inner ear physiology, in *Otolaryngology, Vol. 1*, Paparella and Schumrick (eds.), Copyright © 1973 by W.B. Saunders with permission.

(e.g., Crawford and Fettiplace, 1985; Flock and Cheung, 1977; Flock et al., 1981; Hirokawa and Tilney, 1982; Tilney et al., 1980; Tilney and Tilney, 1986). The stereocilia are composed of bundles of actin filaments and are encased in plasma membranes. The actin filaments are extensively cross-linked, and the cuticular plate into which the stereocilia rootlets are planted is similarly made up of a mosaic of cross-linked actin filaments. The filaments of the stereocilia rootlets extend into the cuticular plate, where fine cross bridges also interconnect the rootlet and cuticular plate filaments.

The stereocilia are arranged in a W-shaped pattern on the OHCs and a very wide "U" or "W" shape on the IHCs, as shown in Fig. 2.20. The base of the "W" faces away from the modiolus (or toward the outer wall of the duct). The stereocilia themselves taper toward the base. When the stereocilia are displaced, they remain stiff, bending at the tapered base in response to physical stimulation (Flock et al., 1977; Flock and Strelioff, 1984; Strelioff and Flock, 1984).

Figure 2.24 shows closeup views of the stereocilia bundles from all three rows of OHCs and also for IHCs. The figure highlights the tapering of stereocilia heights from row to row on each hair cell, with the tallest row toward the outer wall of the duct (or away from the modiolus). At least the tallest stereocilia of the OHCs are firmly attached to the undersurface of the tectorial membrane; however, the IHC stereocilia are not attached to Hensen's stripe, or their attachment is tenuous if it does exist (see, e.g., Slepecky, 1996; Steel, 1983, 1985).

The height (length) of the stereocilia increases going from the base (high-frequency end) to the apex (low-frequency end) of the cochlea in many species (Fettiplace and Fuchs, 1999; Lim, 1986b; Saunders et al., 1985; Tilney and Saunders, 1983; Weiss et al., 1976; Wright, 1984). In humans, Wright (1984) found that the longest IHC stereocilia increased linearly from about 4 to 5 μm near the base to about 7 to 8 μm near the apex. The length of the OHC stereocilia also increased with distance up the cochlear duct, although there was more variability and the relationship was not linear.

A particularly interesting aspect of the hair cell stereocilia may be seen in Fig. 2.23. Looking back to this figure, one may notice that the stereocilia are joined by tiny lines. These lines represent filaments that serve as cross-links among the stereocilia. These cross-links occur in both inner and outer hair cells (Flock et al., 1977; Flock and Strelioff, 1984; Furness and Hackney, 1986; Osborne et al., 1988; Pickles et al., 1984; Rhys Evans et al., 1985; Strelioff and Flock, 1984; Vollrath, Kwan, and Corey, 2007). Different types of cross-links occur between the stereocilia of both inner and outer hair cells and are variously named according to their locations and configurations (Figs. 2.25–2.28). Thus, **shaft connectors** go between the main

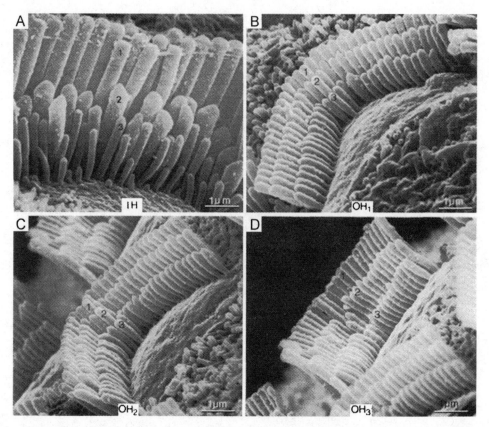

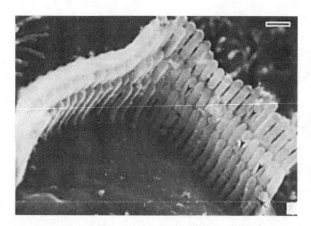

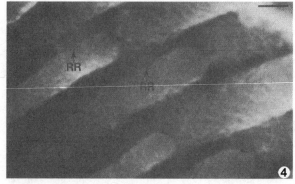

Figure 2.24 Close-up views of the stereocilia bundles of inner (a) and outer (b–d) hair cells demonstrating the decreasing cilia heights from row to row (numbered 1 to 3). *Source*: From *Hearing Research* 22, Lim (Functional structure of the organ of Corti: A review, 117–146, © 1986) with kind permission from Elsevier Science Publishers-NL, Sara Burgerhartstraat 25, 1055 KV Amsterdam, The Netherlands.

Figure 2.25 Side-to-side (arrows) and tip-links (tip-to-side) cross-links on OHCs. *Source*: From *Hearing Research* 21, Furness and Hackney (High-resolution scanning-electron microscopy of stereocilia using the osmium-thiocarbohydrazide coating technique, © 1986) with kind permission from Elsevier Science Publishers-NL, Sara Burgerhartstraat 25, 1055 KV Amsterdam, The Netherlands.

Figure 2.26 Row-to-row cross-links (RR) on OHCs. *Source*: From *Hearing Research* 21, Furness and Hackney (High-resolution scanning-electron microscopy of stereocilia using the osmium-thiocarbohydrazide coating technique, © 1986) with kind permission from Elsevier Science Publishers-NL, Sara Burcrerhartstraat 25, 1055 KV Amsterdam, The Netherlands.

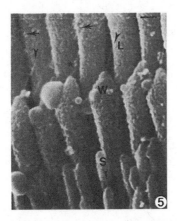

Figure 2.27 Inner hair cell stereocilia showing examples of side-to-side cross links (arrows) and tip-links (arrowheads), which may be relatively long (L) or short (S). *Source*: From *Hearing Research* 21, Furness and Hackney (High-resolution scanning-electron microscopy of stereocilia using the osmium-thiocarbohydrazide coating technique, 1986) with kind permission from Elsevier Science Publishers-NL, Sara Burgerhartstraat 25, 1055 KV Amsterdam, The Netherlands.

shafts of the stereocilia; **ankle connectors** are links between the tapered bottoms of the stereocilia; **side-to-side cross-links** join stereocilia that are juxtaposed within the same row; **row-to-row cross-links** go from stereocilia in one row to adjacent ones in the next row.[3] Finally, **tip links** (also known as **tip-to-side** or **upward-pointing cross-links**) go from the tips of stereocilia in a shorter row upward to the sides of the stereocilia in the adjacent taller row and plays a central role in the functioning of the hair cells. As we shall see in Chapter 4, bending of the stereocilia toward the outer wall of the duct stretches these tip links, which in turn open mechanoelectrical transduction pores at the tops of the shorter stereocilia, triggering the hair cell's response (Fettiplace and Hackney, 2006; Vollrath et al., 2007; Beurg et al., 2009).

The structures of the hair cells and their orientation in the organ of Corti reflect their function as sensory receptors, which transduce the mechanical signal carried to them into electrochemical activity. Yet, the contrasting structures and associations of the inner and outer hair cells reflect functional differences between them. Even a casual look at Fig. 2.23 reveals that the test tube–shaped OHCs are very different from the flask-shaped IHCs. Many of these characteristics are associated with the unique property of OHC **electromotility**, their ability to contract and expand, which is central to the active cochlear processes discussed in Chapter 4. For example, OHCs contain **contractile proteins** (e.g., actin, fibrin, myosin, tropomyosin, tubulin) in their cell bodies and cell membranes, stereocilia,

---

[3] Horizontal top connectors going between the apical ends of the cilia have been described in the mouse cochlea (Goodyear, Marcotti, Kros, and Richardson, 2005).

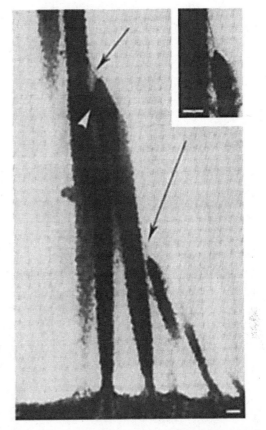

Figure 2.28 Tip-links (arrows) on an outer hair cell. The white arrowhead shows a row-to-row link. *Inset*: close-up of a tip-link. *Source*: From *Hearing Research* 15, Pickles, Comis, and Osborne (Cross links between stereocilia in the guinea pig organ of Corti, and their possible relation to sensory transduction, 103–112, © 1984) with kind permission from Elsevier Science Publishers-NL Sara Burgerhartstraat 25, 1055 KV Amsterdam, The Netherlands.

and cuticular plates (e.g., Flock, 1980; Flock et al., 1982, 1986; Slepecky, 1996; Slepecky et al., 1988). A more apparent difference pertains to the arrangement of their intracellular structures. Notice that the intracellular structures are distributed throughout the IHC, which is the typical arrangement. In contrast, the nucleus and many organelles in the OHC tend to be concentrated toward the bottom and top of the cell, leaving the cytoplasm between these areas relatively free of cellular structures (Brownell, 1990).

The lateral walls of the OHCs are particularly interesting. They are composed of three layers, as illustrated in Fig. 2.29 (e.g., Brownell and Popel, 1998; Dallos, 1992; Holley, 1996; Slepecky, 1996). The outside layer is the cell's **plasma membrane**, and the inside layer comprises the **subsurface cisternae**. Between them is the **cortical lattice**, which is a matrix composed of parallel rows of actin filaments going circumferentially around the tube-shaped cell, with spectrin cross-links between them. The actin filaments appear to be attached to the outer surface

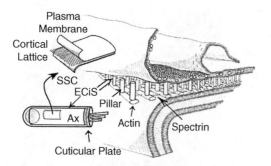

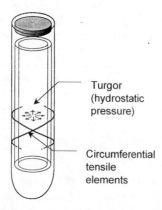

Figure 2.29 The lateral wall of the outer hair cell is composed of the subsurface cisternae on the inside, the plasma membrane on the outside, and a filamentous matrix between them (see text). *Abbreviations*: Ax, axial core of the hair cell; ECiS, extra-cisternal space; SSC, subsurface cisternae. *Source*: Adapted from Brownell and Popel (1998), Electrical and mechanical anatomy of the outer hair cell, in *Psychophysical and Physiological Advances in Hearing*, Palmer et al. (eds.), copyright © 1998 by Whurr, with permission.

of the subsurface cisternae, and they are attached to the plasma membrane by **pillars**. The actin filaments are slanted at about 15° (instead of horizontal) so that they go around the cell in the form of a helix (Fig. 2.30). The OHC's cytoplasm provides positive hydrostatic pressure (turgor) within the cell, and its test tube–like shape is maintained by the tension of the matrix of structures in its lateral walls (Fig. 2.30).

INNERVATION

The sensory hair cells of the cochlea interact with the nervous system by way of the **auditory (cochlear) branch** of the **eighth cranial (vestibulocochlear or statoacoustic) nerve**. The auditory nerve was probably first described in the 1500s by Falloppia. However, its structure and connections have become well defined only during the 20th century. A com-

Figure 2.30 Schematic illustration of the hydrostatic pressure (or turgor) of the cytoplasm of an OHC and the matrix of circumferential tensile elements of its lateral walls. *Source*: Adapted from Brownell (1990), with permission.

prehensive discussion of the auditory nerve, its relationship to the cochlea, and its central projections are provided by Ryugo (1992).

There are approximately 30,000 neurons in the human auditory nerve, and approximately 50,000 or more cochlear neurons in the cat (Engstrom and Wersall, 1958; Furness and Hackney, 1986). These neurons are primarily afferents, which carry sensory information up from the hair cells, but they also include efferents, which descend from the brainstem to the cochlea. The efferent fibers of the auditory nerve represent the terminal portion of the **olivocochlear bundle**, described later in this chapter. The cell bodies of the afferent auditory neurons constitute the spiral ganglia, residing in Rosenthal's canal in the modiolus. These neurons may be myelinated or unmyelinated before exiting through the habenula perforata, but all auditory nerve fibers are unmyelinated once they enter the organ of Corti. Figure 2.31 shows how the auditory nerve and spiral ganglia relate to a cross section of the cochlear duct.

Most sensory neurons are bipolar, so called because the cell body is located part way along the axon, as illustrated in Fig. 2.32. Auditory neurons are of this general type. More specifically, the cells of the spiral ganglia are composed of at least two distinctive types. Spoendlin (1969, 1971, 1978) demonstrated that approximately 95% of these cells are *relatively large, myelinated, bipolar* neurons. Spoendlin classified these cells as type I auditory neurons. In contrast, he found that roughly 5% of the spiral ganglion cells were relatively *small, unmyelinated*, and tended to be *pseudo-monopolar* in structure. These spiral ganglion cells were classified as type II auditory neurons. These two types of auditory neurons are illustrated in the lower left hand portion in Fig. 2.33.

Upon exiting the habenula perforata into the organ of Corti, the now unmyelinated neural fibers follow different routes to distribute themselves asymmetrically between the inner and outer hair cells, as shown schematically in Figs. 2.33 and 2.34. About 95% of these fibers are inner radial fibers, which course directly out to innervate the *inner* hair cells. The remaining 5%, consist of 2500 to 3000 outer spiral fibers that cross the tunnel of Corti as *basal fibers*, and then turn to follow a route of about 0.6 mm toward the base as the *outer spiral bundle*. These outer spiral fibers then make their way up between the Deiters' cells to synapse with the *outer* hair cells.

Innervation patterns are very different for inner and outer hair cells. Each inner hair cell receives a fairly large number of radial fibers. Each IHC in the cat cochlea receives an exclusive supply of 10 to 30 afferent fibers, with fewer toward the apex and more toward the base (Liberman, Dodds, and Pierce, 1990; Spoendlin, 1978). In contrast, outer spiral bundle gives off collaterals so that each neural fiber innervates several outer hair cells (up to 10 toward the base, and about 10–20 toward the apex), and each OHC receives collaterals from roughly 10 neurons. In humans, IHCs receive about 10 afferents throughout the cochlea, and some fibers branch at their ends to synapse with two or three IHCs instead of to just one (Nadol, 1983a).

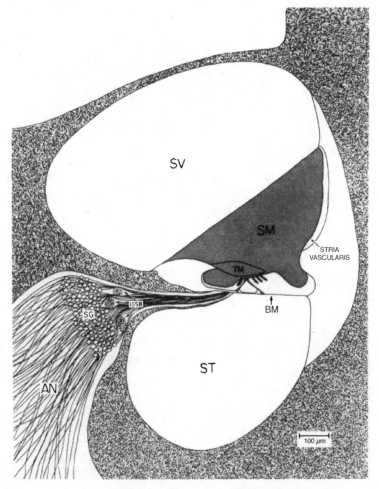

Figure 2.31 Relationship of the auditory nerve to a cross-section of the cochlear duct (cat). *Abbreviations*: AN, auditory nerve; SG, spiral ganglion; IGSB, intraganglionic spiral bundle primarily composed of efferents; TM, tectorial membrane; BM, basilar membrane; SV, SM, ST, scalae vestibuli, media, and tympani, respectively. *Source*: From *Hearing Research* 22, Kiang, Liberman, Sewell, and Guinan (Single unit clues to cochlear mechanisms, 171–182, © 1984) with kind permission from Elsevier Science Publishers-NL, Sara Burgerhartstraat 25, 1055 KV Amsterdam, The Netherlands.

Human OHCs typically receive 4 to 6 afferent fibers (Nadol, 1983b).

Liberman (1982) traced the courses of single auditory neurons by marking them with horseradish peroxidase (HRP). All of the type I auditory neurons he labeled with intracellular injections of HRP could be traced to radial fibers going to IHCs. Kiang et al. (1982) injected HRP into the auditory nerve within the internal auditory canal. They were then able to trace the courses of 50 radial and 11 outer spiral fibers. Their HRP labeling studies confirmed earlier conjectures by Spoendlin (1971, 1978) that the large caliber (over 2 μm), bipolar type I cells continue as radial fibers in the organ of Corti; and that the small caliber (under 1 μm), pseudomonopolar type II cells correspond to the outer spiral fibers (see Figs. 2.32 and 2.33).

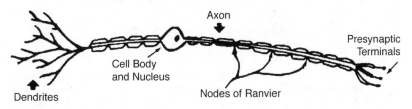

Figure 2.32 Schematic drawing of a typical bipolar sensory neuron.

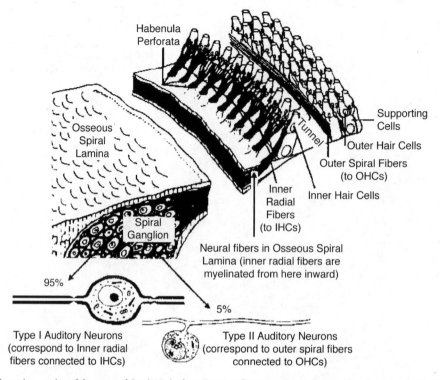

Figure 2.33 The afferent innervation of the organ of Corti. Notice how Type I auditory neurons in the spiral ganglion continue in the organ of Corti as inner radial fibers to inner hair cells, and Type II auditory neurons continue as outer spiral fibers to outer hair cells. Examples of Type I and Type II neurons are illustrated in the lower left-hand section of the drawing. *Source*: Adapted from drawings by Spoendlin H. The afferent innervation of the cochlea, in *Electrical Activity of the Auditory Nervous System*, R.F. Naunton and C. Fernandez (eds.), Copyright © 1978 by Academic Press, with permission.

As illustrated in Fig. 2.35, Liberman and Simmons (1985) demonstrated that a given inner hair cell makes contact with three types of radial fibers, differing in terms of their average diameters, cellular characteristics, and spontaneous firing rates (see Chap. 5). Moreover, these three types of radial fibers attach to the IHC at characteristic locations. The thickest fibers (having the highest spontaneous rates) always attach on the surface of the IHC, which is toward the OHCs. The thinnest and medium thickness fibers (having low and medium spontaneous rates, respectively) attach to the IHC on the surface facing toward the modiolus.

Efferent Innervation of the Hair Cells
Other kinds of neurons are also found in the organ of Corti. Figures 2.34 and 2.36 show that two different types of fibers can be identified with respect to their nerve endings (Engstrom, 1958; Smith and Sjostrand, 1961). One group of cells has smaller nonvesiculated endings. These are afferent (ascending sensory) neurons.

The second group of cells has larger vesiculated endings and is derived from the **efferent** (descending) neurons of the **olivocochlear bundle** (see below). The vesiculated endings contain *acetylcholine*. Various studies found degeneration of these vesiculated units when parts of the descending olivocochlear bundle

were cut (Smith and Rasmussen, 1963; Spoendlin and Gacek, 1963). However, no degeneration was found to occur for the nonvesiculated afferent neurons. The endings of the efferent fibers are in direct contact with the OHCs, whereas they terminate on the afferent neural fibers of the IHCs rather than on these sensor cells themselves (Fig. 2.36). This suggests that the efferents act directly upon the OHCs (presynaptically), but that they act upon the associated afferent fibers of the IHCs (postsynaptically). The density of efferent fibers is substantially greater for the OHCs than for the IHCs. Furthermore, there is greater efferent innervation for the OHCs at the base of the cochlea than at the apex, and this innervation of the OHCs also tapers from the first row through the third.

CENTRAL AUDITORY PATHWAYS

The auditory (or cochlear) nerve appears as a twisted trunk—its core is made up of fibers derived from the apex of the cochlea, and its outer layers come from more basal regions. The nerve leaves the inner ear via the internal auditory meatus and enters the brainstem at the lateral aspect of the lower pons. We are now in the **central auditory nervous system**, or the **central auditory pathways**, the major aspects of which are outlined in

(a)

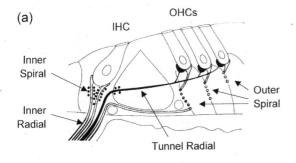

(b)

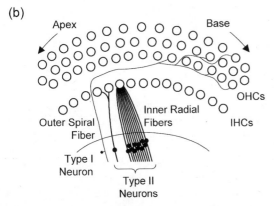

Figure 2.34 (a) Afferent and efferent innervation of the organ of Corti. *Source*: Adapted from Spoendlin (1975) with permission. Efferent fibers are shown in black. (b) Arrangement of Type I and Type II afferent auditory nerve fibers to inner and outer hair cells [based on findings of Spoendlin (1975) and Nadol (1983a)].

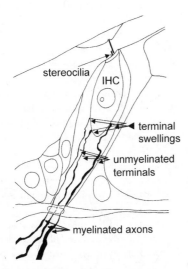

Figure 2.35 The thickest radial fibers attach to the IHC surface facing the OHCs, whereas the thinnest and medium thickness fibers attach on the surface toward the modiolus. *Source*: From Liberman and Simmons (1985), with permission of *J Acoust Soc Am*.

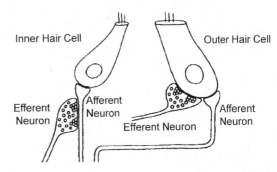

Figure 2.36 Relationship between afferent and efferent neural fibers and the inner and outer hair cells. *Source*: Adapted from Spoendlin (1975), with permission.

this section. Although not addressed here, interested students will find a summary of the neurotransmitters associated with the auditory system in Table 2.2. In addition, many sources are available to those wishing to pursue a more detailed coverage of the anatomy and physiology of the auditory pathways (e.g., Ehret and Romand, 1997; Møller, 2000; Musiek and Baran, 2007; Popper and Fay, 1992; Webster, Popper and Fay, 1992; Altschuler, Bobbin, Clopton, and Hoffman, 1991; Winer, 1992).

Afferent Pathways

The major aspects of the ascending central auditory pathways are shown schematically in Fig. 2.37. The fibers of the auditory nerve constitute the first-order neurons of the ascending central auditory pathways. The number of nerve fibers associated with the auditory system increases dramatically going from the auditory nerve to the cortex. For example, the rhesus monkey has roughly 30,000 cells in its auditory nerve, compared to approximately 10 million at the auditory cortex (Chow, 1951).

Upon entering the brainstem, the auditory nerve fibers synapse with cells in the **cochlear nuclei**, constituting the first level of way stations in the central auditory nervous system. Comprehensive discussions of the cochlear nuclei and their synaptic connections may be found in Cant (1992) and Ryugo (1992). The cochlear nuclei are composed of three main sections: the **anterior ventral cochlear nucleus (AVCN)**, the **posterior ventral cochlear nucleus (PVCN)**, and the **dorsal cochlear nucleus (DCN)**. The incoming type I auditory neurons (originating from the inner hair cells) bifurcate into ascending branches to the AVCN and descending branches to the PVCN and DCN. [Type II auditory neurons also project to the cochlear nuclei, following paths parallel to the type I fibers, but they terminate in different cellular regions (Leak-Jones and Snyder, 1982; Ruggero et al., 1982; Ryugo, 1992).] Auditory neurons arising from the more basal (higher frequency) areas of the cochlea terminate in the dorsomedial parts of the cochlear nuclei, and fibers from the more apical (lower frequency) parts of the cochlea go to the ventrolateral parts of these nuclei. Frequency–place relationships extend throughout the central

Table 2.2 Likely/Possible Neurotransmitters in the Auditory Nervous System

Location	Neurotransmitter(s)	Reference examples
Auditory nerve	Aspartate, glutamate	Wenthold (1978), Romand and Avan (1997)
Cochlear nucleus	Ach, aspartate, GABA, glutamate, glycine	Godfrey et al. (1990), Wenthold et al. (1993), Romand and Avan (1997)
Superior olivary complex	Aspartate (in MSO), GABA, glutamate (in MSO), glutamate decarboxylase, glycine (in LSO)	Wenthold (1991), Helfert and Aschoff (1997)
Lateral lemniscus	GABA, glycine	Helfert and Aschoff (1997)
Inferior colliculus	GABA, glutamate decarboxylase, glycine	Faingold et al. (1989), Wynne et al. (1995)
Medial geniculate	GABA, glutamate	Li et al. (1995), Schwartz et al. (2000)
Auditory cortex	Ach, GABA, glutamate, noradrenoline, serotonin	Metherate and Ashe (1995), Metherate and Hsieh (2003)
Medial olivocochlear bundle	Ach, CGRP, GABA	Sahley et al. (1997)
Lateral olivocochlear bundle	Ach, CGRP, dopamine, dynorphin, enkephalin, GABA, urocortin	Fex and Altschuler (1981), Sahley et al. (1997), Gil-Loyzaga et al. (2000)

Abbreviations: Ach, acetylcholine; CGRP, calcitonin gene-related peptide; GABA, γ-aminobutyric acid; LSO, lateral superior olive; MSO, medial superior olive.

auditory nervous system and are covered in the discussion of *tonotopic organization* in Chapter 6.

Second-order neurons arise from the cochlear nuclei to proceed up the auditory pathways. Some fibers ascend ipsilaterally, but most cross the midline and ascend along the contralateral pathway. The **ventral acoustic stria** arises from the AVCN, forming the **trapezoid body**. The fibers of the trapezoid body *decussate* [cross to the opposite side to synapse with the nuclei of the contralateral superior olivary complex (SOC) or to ascend

in the lateral lemniscus]. Other fibers of the trapezoid body terminate at the SOC on the ipsilateral side and at the trapezoid nuclei. The PVCN gives rise to the **intermediate acoustic stria** (of Held), which contralateralizes to ascend in the lateral lemniscus of the opposite side. The **dorsal acoustic stria** (of Monakow) is made up of fibers projecting from the DCN, which cross to the opposite side and ascend in the contralateral lateral lemniscus.

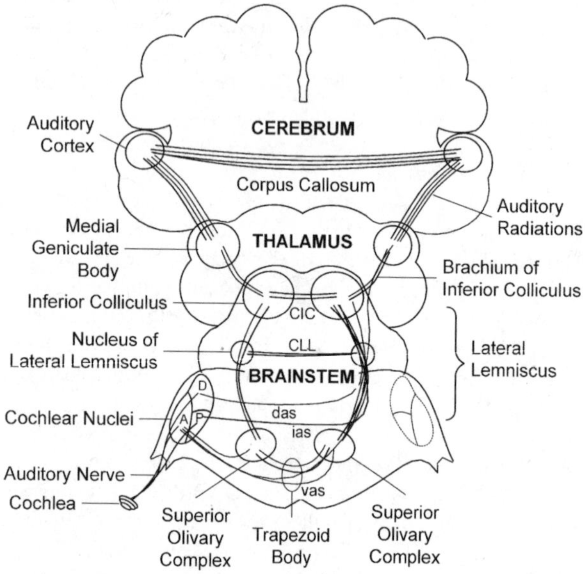

The **superior olivary complex** constitutes the next way station in the auditory pathway and is distinguished as the first (lowest) level that receives information originating from both sides of the head (*bilateral representation*). The SOC is made up of the **medial superior olive (MSO)**, the **lateral superior olive (LSO)**, and the **medial nucleus of the trapezoid body (MNTB)**, as well as rather diffuse accumulations of cell bodies known as the **periolivary nuclei** (Helfert and Aschoff, 1997; Moore, 1987, 2000; Schwartz, 1992). Each MSO receives bilateral inputs from the right and left AVCNs, and then projects to the ipsilateral inferior colliculus via the lateral lemniscus on its own side. The LSO also receives inputs directly from the AVCN on the same side as well as from the opposite AVCN via the ipsilateral MNTB. In turn, the LSO projects bilaterally to the inferior colliculi via the lateral lemnisci on both sides. As just implied, the MNTB receives its input from the opposite AVCN and then projects to the LSO on its own side. Although similar to the SOCs of lower mammals, the human SOC has a relatively smaller LSO, more prominent periolovary cell groups, and the TB does not appear to be organized into a identifiable nucleus (Moore, 2000).

The **lateral lemniscus (LL)** is the pathway from the lower nuclei of the auditory pathway just described to the level of the inferior colliculus and has been described in some detail (e.g., Brunso-Bechtold, Thompson, and Masterton, 1981; Ferraro and Minckler, 1977a; Glendenning, Brunso-Bechtold, Thompson, and Masterton, 1981; Helfert and Aschoff, 1997; Moore, 1987; Schwartz, 1992). Each lateral lemniscus includes neural

Figure 2.37 Schematic representation of the major aspects of the ascending central auditory pathways. *Abbreviations*: A, anterior ventral cochlear nucleus; P, posterior ventral cochlear nucleus; D, dorsal cochlear nucleus; CIC, commissure of the inferior colliculus; CLL, commissure of the lateral lemniscus; das, dorsal acoustic stria; ias, intermediate acoustic stria; vas, ventral acoustic stria.

fibers originating from the cochlear nuclei and superior olivary complexes on both sides, as well as fibers arising from the nuclei of the LL itself. The LL principally includes a **ventral nucleus (VNLL)** and a **dorsal nucleus (DNLL)**, which have typically been described, although an intermediate nucleus has also been described. However, Ferraro and Minckler (1977a) reported that the nuclei of the human LL are somewhat dispersed into scattered cell clusters among the lemniscal fibers, and that a clear-cut demarcation between them could not be found. Communication between the lateral lemnisci of the two sides occurs via the **commissural fibers of Probst**.

The majority of the ascending fibers from the LL project to the **inferior colliculi (IC)**, which are large nuclei on the right and left sides of the midbrain (see, e.g., Ehret and Romand, 1997; Oliver and Huerta, 1992; Oliver and Morest, 1984). The divisions of the IC have been variously described based on different anatomical and physiological methods (e.g., Morest and Olivers, 1984; Rockel and Jones, 1973a, 1973b). The **central nucleus** of the IC is the principal way station for auditory signals arising from the LL, while its **dorsal cortex** and **pericentral** and **external (lateral) nuclei** interact with the central nucleus as well as being involved in many interconnections with other neural systems. Hence, the IC plays a role in multisensory integration. Communication between the inferior colliculi of the two sides occurs via the **commissure of the inferior colliculus**. The auditory pathway continues from the IC to the medial geniculate body (MGB) of the thalamus by way of the **brachium of the inferior colliculus**, which also includes ascending fibers that bypass the IC (Ferraro and Minckler, 1977b). See Oliver and Huerta (1992) for a comprehensive review of the anatomy of the inferior colliculus.

The **medial geniculate body** is the highest subcortical way station of the auditory pathway, which has been described in great detail by Winer (1984, 1985, 1991, 1992). Unlike other way stations along the ascending auditory pathway, all fibers reaching the MGB will synapse here. Moreover, the right and left MGBs are not connected by commissural pathways. Each MGB is composed of **ventral**, **dorsal**, and **medial divisions**, which are relatively similar in humans and other mammals. The ventral division receives auditory signals from the central nucleus of the IC (and nonauditory inputs from the reticular nucleus of the thalamus and the ventrolateral medullary nucleus). It projects mainly to the primary auditory cortex, as well as to some other cortical auditory areas. The dorsal division receives auditory signals from the IC and nonauditory information from a variety of brainstem and thalamic inputs and projects mainly to the auditory association cortex as well as to a wide variety of other cortical sites. The medial division receives a wide range of both auditory inputs (from the IC, perolivary nuclei of the SOC, and the ventral nucleus of the LL) and multisensory nonauditory inputs (from the spinal cord, superior colliculus, vestibular nuclei, and spinal cord), and projects to diverse areas of the cortex, including the somatosensory and prefrontal cortices. The **auditory (geniculocortical** or **thalamocortical)**

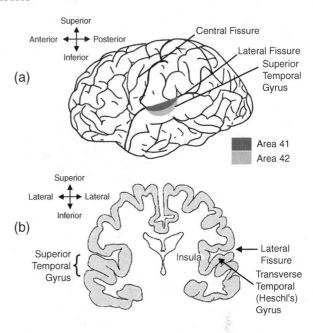

Figure 2.38 Lateral (a) and coronal (b) representations of the human brain illustrating the locations of the primary and secondary auditory areas.

radiations project ipsilaterally from the MGB to the **auditory cortex**, which is located in the temporal lobe.

The **auditory cortex** occupies a band of tissue along the superior border of the temporal lobe just below the **lateral (Sylvian) fissure**, largely involving the **transverse temporal (Heschl's) gyrus** and the posterior two-thirds of the **superior temporal gyrus** (Fig. 2.38) The traditional view of the auditory cortex distinguishes between the primary auditory and auditory association cortices. The **primary auditory cortex (koniocortex)**, or **area AI**, mainly involves Heschl's gyrus located within the lateral fissure, and roughly corresponds to **area 41** in the classic Brodmann classification system. Area AI is largely surrounded by the **auditory association cortex (parakoniocortex)**, or **area AII**, which is mainly situated on parts of the posterior transverse and superior temporal gyri, more-or-less corresponding to Brodmann **area 42**. A more precise description of the auditory cortex is still evolving, with current descriptions of the anatomy expressed in terms of **core** regions and secondary **belt** regions (e.g., Galaburda and Sanides, 1980; Hackett, Preuss, and Kaas, 2001; Rivier and Clark, 1997; Wallace, Johnson, and Palmer, 2002). For example, Wallace et al. (2002) integrated their findings with those of Rivier and Clark (1997) to delineate the anatomical regions in the human auditory cortex illustrated in Fig. 2.39. The figure identifies two core regions surrounded by six belt regions. The **core regions** are (filled with dots in the figure) include (a) the primary auditory area (**AI**) involving the posteriomedial two-thirds of Heschl's gyrus, and (b) a narrow lateroposterior area (**LP**) adjacent to it and abutting Heschl's sulcus. The surrounding **belt regions** (filled with lines

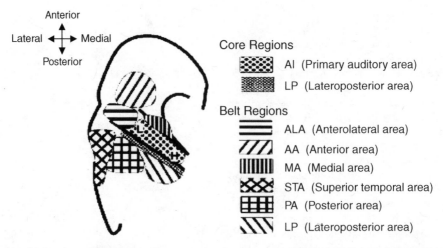

Core Regions

▦ AI (Primary auditory area)

▦ LP (Lateroposterior area)

Belt Regions

≡ ALA (Anterolateral area)

▧ AA (Anterior area)

▥ MA (Medial area)

⋈ STA (Superior temporal area)

⊞ PA (Posterior area)

▨ LP (Lateroposterior area)

Figure 2.39 The core and belt regions of the human auditory cortex based on the combined findings of Rivier and Clarke (1997) and Wallace et al. (2002). Dots represent core regions; lines and cross-hatching represent belt regions. *Abbreviations*: AI, primary auditory area; LP, lateroposterior area; ALA, anterolateral area; AA, anterior area; MA, medial area; LA, lateral area (lateral to LP); PA, posterior area; STA, superior temporal area; L, responsive to low frequencies; H, responsive to high frequencies. *Source*: From Wallace et al. (2002), Histochemical identification of cortical areas, *Experimental Brain Research*, Vol 143, p. 506, Fig. 6A, ©2002, used with kind permission of Springer Science+Business Media.

and cross-hatching in the figure) include the (a) anterolateral area (**ALA**) on the posterior third of Heschl's gyrus, (b) anterior area (**AA**) anterior to area AI, (c) medial area (**MA**) anteromedial to AI, (d) lateral area (**LA**) lateral to LP, (e) posterior area (**PA**) posterior to LP, and (f) a superior temporal area (**STA**).

The fiber connections between the medial geniculate body and auditory cortex have been described based on findings in various animals and humans (e.g., Diamond et al., 1958; Mesulam and Pandya, 1973; Niimi and Matsuoka, 1979; Ravizza and Belmore, 1978; Rose and Woolsey, 1949, 1958; Winer et al., 1977). The principal connections are from the ventral division of the MGB to area AI; however, there are also connections from other parts of the MGB to many of the areas that respond to auditory stimulation, such as areas AII and Ep, among others.

As suggested in the previous paragraph, areas AI and AII are by no means the only cortical locations that respond to sound. Additional cortical auditory areas have been known for some time (e.g., Reale and Imig, 1980; Rose, 1949; Rose and Woolsey, 1958), and are discussed further in Chapter 6. Communication between right and left auditory cortices occurs via the **corpus callosum** (e.g., Karol and Pandya, 1971; Musiek and Baran, 2007; Pandya et al., 1969).

In contrast to the principal afferent auditory pathway from the cochlea to the primary auditory cortex (AI), as in Fig. 2.37, those involving more diverse connections and leading to other areas have been identified as the **nonclassical (adjunct) auditory pathways** (see, Aitkin, 1986; Ehret and Romand, 1997; Møller, 2000). This include the **diffuse system** from IC to the dorsal division of the MGB, and then to auditory association cortex (AII); and the **polysensory system**, which goes from the IC (including visual and somatosensory inputs) to the medial division of the MGB, and then projecting to sites such as

the anterior auditory field of the cortex, the thalamic reticular nucleus, and the limbic system.

Acoustic Reflex Arc

The **acoustic reflex** was mentioned earlier in this chapter and is addressed in some detail in Chapter 3. The **acoustic reflex arc** has been described in detail (Borg, 1973; Lyons, 1978) and is shown schematically in Fig. 2.40. The afferent (sensory) leg of the reflex arc is the **auditory nerve**, and the efferent (motor) legs are the **seventh cranial (facial) nerve** to the stapedius muscle and the **fifth cranial (trigeminal) nerve** to the tensor tympani. We will trace the pathways for just the **stapedius reflex**, which constitutes the acoustic reflex in humans (see Chap. 3).

The afferent leg of the reflex goes from the stimulated cochlea via the auditory nerve to the ipsilateral VCN. From

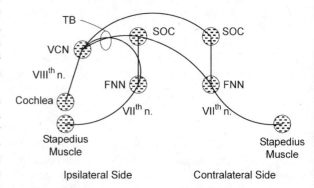

Figure 2.40 Schematic diagram of the crossed and uncrossed acoustic (stapedius) reflex pathways. *Abbreviations*: FNN, facial nerve nucleus; SOC, superior olivary complex; TB, trapezoid body; VCN, ventral cochlear nucleus.

there, second-order neurons pass through the trapezoid body leading to two uncrossed and two crossed pathways. One of the **uncrossed pathways** goes from the VCN to the facial nerve nucleus, from which motor neurons go to the stapedius muscle on the same side. The other uncrossed pathway goes from the VCN to the ipsilateral SOC, from which third-order neurons go to the facial nerve nucleus. From there, motor neurons proceed to the ipsilateral stapedius muscle.

One of the **crossed pathways** goes from the ipsilateral VCN to the ipsilateral SOC, from which third-order neurons cross the midline to the facial nerve nucleus on the opposite side. From there, the facial nerve goes to the stapedius muscle on the side opposite the stimulated ear. The other crossed pathway goes from the ipsilateral VCN to the contralateral SOC, and then to the facial nerve nucleus on that side (opposite to the stimulated cochlea). The facial nerve then proceeds to the stapedius muscle contralateral to the stimulated cochlea.

Efferent Pathways

As described above, descending efferent fibers enter the inner ear and make contact with the OHCs directly and with the IHCs indirectly via synapses with their associated afferent fibers. These fibers are the cochlear terminations of the **olivocochlear bundle (OCB)**. The OCB is sometimes referred to as *Rasmussen's bundle* because it was originally characterized in 1946 by Rasmussen. Since then, the OCB has been described in considerable detail (e.g., DeVenecia, Liberman, Guinan, and Brown, 2005; Guinan, 1996, 2006; Guinan et al., 1983, 1984; Liberman and Brown, 1986; Luk et al., 1974; Robertson, 1985; Strutz and Spatz, 1980; Warr, 1978, 1992).

The general organization of the olivocochlear pathway system is depicted in Fig. 2.41. It is made up of neurons derived from the regions of the **medial superior olive (MSO)** and the **lateral superior olive (LSO)** on both sides. The neurons of the OCB enter the inner ear along with the vestibular branch of the auditory nerve, and then enter the cochlea to distribute themselves to the inner and outer hair cells.

Figure 2.40 shows that we are really dealing with two efferent systems rather than one. The **lateral olivocochlear (LOC) system**, or **uncrossed olivocochlear bundle (UOCB)**, is made up of efferent fibers derived from the vicinity of the lateral superior olive. These unmyelinated, small diameter fibers project to the ipsilateral cochlea, where they synapse with the afferents of the inner hair cells. A comparably small number of myelinated fibers from the ipsilateral medial superior olive go to outer hair cells on the same side.

The **medial olivocochlear (MOC) system** or **crossed olivocochlear bundle (COCB)** involves large-diameter, myelinated neurons originating from the vicinity of the medial superior olive. These cross the midline of the brainstem at the level of the fourth ventricle and eventually terminate directly upon the outer hair cells on the opposite side. (A few unmyelinated fibers from the lateral superior olivary area also cross the midline, going to the contralateral inner hair cells.)

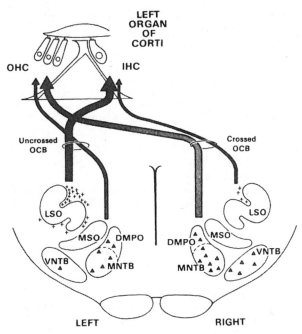

Figure 2.41 Schematic representation of the crossed and uncrossed olivocochlear bundles. As suggested by the wider lines, the crossed OCB goes mainly from the MSO to the contralateral OHCs, and the uncrossed OCB goes mainly from the LSO to the ipsilateral IHCs. *Abbreviations*: OCB, olivocochlear bundle; LSO, lateral superior olive; MSO, medial superior olive; DMPO, dorsal periolivary nucleus; MNTB, medial nucleus of trapezoid body; VNTB, ventral nucleus of trapezoid body; triangles, large OCB neurons; crosses, small OCB neurons. *Source*: Adapted from Warr (1978), The olivocochlear bundle: Its origins and terminations in the cat, in *Evoked Electrical Activity in the Auditory Nervous System*, R.E Naunton and C. Fernandez (eds.), Copyright © 1978 by Academic Press.

In addition to the olivocochlear systems, other efferent connections have been demonstrated coming from the inferior colliculus, the nuclei of the lateral lemniscus, and possibly the cerebellum (e.g., Harrison and Howe, 1974; Huffman and Henson, 1990; Rasmussen, 1967), as well as descending fibers that may also provide cortical feedback and/or control over lower centers including, for example, corticofugal pathways to the inferior colliculus and to the medial geniculate (e.g., Anderson et al., 1980; Diamond et al., 1969; Oliver and Huerta, 1992; Rockel and Jones, 1973a, 1973b; Winer, 1992; Winer et al., 1977).

REFERENCES

Aitkin, J. 1986. *The Auditory Midbrain*. Clifton, NJ: Humana Press.

Anderson, RA, Snyder, RL, Merzenich, MM. 1980. The tonotopic organization of corticocollicular projections from physiologically identified loci in AI, AII, and anterior cortical fields of the cat. *J Comp Neurol* 191, 479–494.

Anson, BJ, Donaldson, JA. 1967. *The Surgical Anatomy of the Temporal Bone and the Ear*. Philadelphia, PA: Saunders.

Axelsson, A, Ryan, AF. 2001. Circulation of the inner ear: I. Comparative study of the vascular anatomy in the mallalian cochlea. In: AF Jahn, J Santos-Sacchi (eds.), *Physiology of the Ear*, 2nd ed. San Diego: Singular, 301–320.

Bekesy, G. 1936. Zur Physik des Mittelohres und uber das Horen bei fehlerhaftem Trommelfell. *Akust Zeitschr* i, 13–23.

Bekesy, G. 1960/1989. *Experiments in Hearing*. New York: McGraw-Hill. [Republished by the Acoustical Society of America].

Beurg, M, Fettiplace, R, Nam, J-H, Ricci, AJ. 2009. Localization of inner hair cell mechanotransducer channels using high-speed calcium imaging. *Nature Neurosci* 12, 553–558.

Borg, E. 1973. On the neuronal organization of the acoustic middle ear reflex: A physiological and anatomical study. *Brain Res* 49, 101–123.

Brodmann, K. 1909. Vergleichende Lokalisantionlehre der Grosshirnrinde in ihren Preinzipien dargestellt auf Grund des Zellenbaues. Leipzig: Barth.

Brownell, WE. 1990. Outer hair cell electromotility and otoacoustic emissions. *Ear Hear* 11, 82–92.

Brownell, WE, Popel, AS. 1998. Electrical and mechanical anatomy of the outer hair cell. In: AR Palmer, A Rees, AQ Summerfield, R Meddis (eds.), *Psychophysical and Physiological Advances in Hearing*. London: Whurr, 89–96.

Brunso-Bechtold, JK, Thompson, GC, Masterton, RB. 1981. HRP study of the organization of the auditory afferents ascending to central nucleus of inferior colliculus in cat. *J Comp Neurol* 197, 705–722.

Cant, NB. 1992. The cochlear nucleus: Neuronal types and their synaptic organization. In: WB Webster, AN Popper, RF Fay (eds.), *The Mammalian Auditory Pathway: Neuroanatomy*. New York: Springer-Verlag, 66–116.

Chow, K. 1951. Numerical estimates of the auditory central nervous system of the monkey. *J Comp Neurol* 95,159–175.

Crawford, AC, Fettiplace, R. 1985. The mechanical properties of ciliary bundles of turtle cochlear hair cells. *J Physiol* 364, 359–379.

Dallos, P. 1992. The active cochlea. *J Neurosci* 12, 4575–4585.

Dallos, P, Popper, AN, Fay, RR (eds.) (1996). *The Cochlea*. New York, NY: Springer-Verlag.

Davis, H. 1962. Advances in the neurophysiology and neuroanatomy of the cochlea. *J Acoust Soc Am* 34, 1377–1385.

DeVenecia, RK, Liberman, MC, Guinan, JJ Jr, Brown, MC. 2005. Medial olivocochlear reflex interneurons are located in the posteroventral cochlear nucleus: A kainic acid lesion study in guinea pigs. *J Comp Neurol* 487, 345–360.

Diamond, IT, Chow, KL, Neff, WD. 1958. Degeneration of caudal medial geniculate body following cortical lesion ventral to auditory area II in the cat. *J Comp Neurol* 109, 349–362.

Diamond, IT, Jones, EG, Powell, TPS. 1969. The projection of the auditory cortex upon the diencephalon and brain stem in the cat. *Brain Res* 15, 305–340.

Donaldson, JA, Miller, JM. 1973. Anatomy of the ear. In: MM Paparella, DA Shumrick (eds.), *Otolaryngology Vol. 1: Basic Sciences and Related Disciplines*. Philadelphia, PA: Saunders, 75–110.

Ehret, G, Romand, R, eds. 1997. *The Central Auditory Pathway*. New York, NY: Oxford University Press.

Engstrom, H. 1958. On the double innervation of the inner ear sensory epithelia. *Acta Otol* 49, 109–118.

Engstrom, H, Wersäll, J. 1953. Structure and innervation of the inner ear sensory epithelia. *Int Rev Cytol* 7, 535–585.

Engstrom, H, Wersall, J. 1958. Structure and innervation of the inner ear sensory epithelia. *Int Rev Cytol* 7, 535–585.

Faingold, CL, Gehlbach, G, Caspary, DM. 1989. On the role of GABA as an inhibitory *neurotransmitter* in *inferior colliculus* neurons: iontophoretic studies. Brain Res 500, 302–312.

Ferraro, JA, Minckler, J. 1977a. The human auditory pathways: A quantitative study: The human lateral lemniscus and its nuclei. *Brain Lang* 4, 277–294.

Ferraro, JA, Minckler, J. 1977b. The human auditory pathways: A quantitative study: The brachium of the inferior colliculus. *Brain Lang* 4, 156–164.

Fettiplace, R, Fuchs, PA. 1999. Mechanisms of hair cell tuning. *Ann Rev Physiol* 61, 809–834.

Fettiplace, R, Hackney, CM. 2006. The sensory and motor roles of auditory hair cells. *Nat Rev Neurosci* 7(1), 19–29.

Fex, J, Altschuler, RA. 1981. Enkephalin-like immuno reactivity of olivocochlear nerve fibers in cochlea of guinea pig and cat. *Proc Natl Acad Sci U S A* 78, 1255–1259.

Flock, A. 1980. Contractile proteins in hair cells. *Hear Res* 2, 411–412.

Flock, A, Bretscher, A, Weber, K. 1982. Immunohistochemical localization of several cytoskeletal proteins in inner ear sensory and supporting cells. *Hear Res* 7, 75–89.

Flock, A, Cheung, HC. 1977. Actin filaments in sensory hairs of inner ear receptor cells. *J Cell Biol* 75, 339–343.

Flock, A, Cheung, HC, Utter, G. 1981. Three sets of actin filaments in sensory hairs of the inner ear: Identification and functional organization determined by gel electrophoresis, immunofluorescence, and electron microscopy. *J Neurocytol* 10, 133–147.

Flock, A, Flock, B, Murray, E. 1977. Studies on the sensory hairs of receptor cells in the inner ear. *Acta Otol* 83, 85–91.

Flock, A, Flock, B, Ulfendahl, M. 1986. Mechanisms of movement in outer hair cells and a possible structural basis. *Arch Otoryhinolaryngol* 243, 83–90.

Flock, A, Strelioff, D. 1984. Studies on hair cells in isolated coils from the guinea pig cochlea. *Hear Res* 15, 11–18.

Frommer, GH. 1982. Observations of the organ of Corti under in vivo-like conditions. *Acta Otol* 94, 451–460.

Furness, DN, Hackney, CM. 1985. Cross links between stereocilia in the guinea pig cochlea. *Hear Res* 18, 177–188.

Furness, DN, Hackney, CM. 1986. High-resolution scanning-electron microscopy of stereocilia using the osmium-thiocarbohydrazide coating technique. *Hear Res* 21, 243–249.

Galaburda, A, Sanides, F. 1980. Cytoarchitectonic organization of the *human auditory* cortex. *J Comp Neurol* 190, 597–610.

Gelfand, SA. 2001. *Essentials of Audiology*, 2nd ed. New York, NY: Thieme Medical Publishers.

Gil-Loyzaga, P, Bartolome, V, Vicente-Torres, A, Carricondo, F. 2000. Serotonergic innervation of the organ of Corti. *Acta Otolaryngol* 120, 128–132.

Glendenning, KK, Brunso-Bechtold, JK, Thompson, GC, Masterton, RB. 1981. Ascending afferents to the nuclei of the lateral lemniscus. *J Comp Neurol* 197, 673–703.

Godfrey, D, Beranek, K, Carlson, L, Parli, J, Dunn, J, and Ross, C. 1990. Contribution of centrifugal innervation to choline acetyltransferase activity in the cat cochlear nucleus. *Hear Res* 49, 259–280.

Goodyear, RJ, Marcotti, W, Kros, CJ, Richardson, GP. 2005. Development and properties of stereociliary link types in hair cells of the mouse cochlea. *J Comp Neurol* 485, 75–85.

Gueta, R, Barlam, D, Shneck, RZ, Rousso, I. 2006. Measurement of the mechanical properties of isolated tectorial membrane using atomic force microscopy. *Proc Natl Acad Sci USA* 103, 14790–14795.

Gueta, R, Tal, E, Silberberg, Y, Rousso, I. 2007. The 3D structure of the tectorial membrane determined by second-harmonic imaging microscopy. *J Struct Biol* 159, 103–110

Guinan, JJ Jr. 1996. Physiology of olivocochlear efferents. In: P Dallos, AN Popper, RR Fay (eds.), *The Cochlea*. New York, NY: Springer-Verlag, 435–502.

Guinan, JJ Jr. 2006. Olivocochlear efferents: Anatomy, physiology, function, and the measurement of efferent effects in humans. *Ear Hear* 27, 589–607.

Guinan, JJ, Warr, WB, Norris, BE. 1983. Differential olivocochlear projections from lateral vs medial zones of the superior olivary complex. *J Comp Neurol* 221, 358–370.

Guinan, JJ, Warr, WB, Norris, BE. 1984. Topographic organization of the olivocochlear projections from the lateral and medial zones of the superior olivary complex. *J Comp Neurol* 226, 21–27.

Hackett, TA, Preuss, TM, Kaas, JH. 2001. Architectonic identification of the core region in auditory cortex of macaques, chimpanzees, and humans. *J Comp Neurol* 441, 197–222.

Harrison, JM, Howe, ME. 1974. Anatomy of the descending auditory system (mammalian). In: WD Keidel, WD Neff (eds.), *Handbook of Sensory Physiology*, V5/1. Berlin, Germany: Springer, 363–388.

Helfert, RH, Aschoff, A. 1997. Superior olivary complex and nuclei of the lateral lemniscus. In: G Ehret, R Romand (eds.), *The Central Auditory System*. New York, NY: Oxford University Press, 193–258.

Helmholtz, H. 1868. Die Mechanik der Gehorknochelchen und des Trommelfells. *Pflugers Arch Physiol* 1, 1–60.

Henson, MM, Henson, OW Jr, Jenkins, DB. 1984. The attachment of the spiral ligament to the cochlear wall: Anchoring cells and the creation of tension. *Hear Res* 16, 231–242.

Hirokawa, N, Tilney, LG. 1982. Interactions between actin filaments and between actin filaments and membranes in quick-frozen and deeply etched hair cells of the chick ear. *J Cell Biol* 95, 249–261.

Holley, MC. 1996. Cochlear mechanics and micromechanics. In: P Dallos, AN Popper, RR Fay (eds.), *The Cochlea*. New York, NY: Springer-Verlag, 386–434.

Holton, T, Hudspeth, AJ. 1983. A micromechanical contribution to cochlear tuning and tonotopic organization. *Science* 222, 508–510.

Huffman, RF, Henson, OW Jr. 1990. The descending auditory pathway and acousticomotor systems: Connections with the inferior colliculus. *Brain Res Rev* 15, 295–323.

Hughes, GB. 1985. *Textbook of Otology*. New York, NY: Thieme Medical Publishers.

Jepsen, O. 1963. Middle-ear muscle reflexes in man. In: J Jerger (ed). *Modern Developments in Audiology*. New York, NY: Academic Press, 194–239.

Karol, EA, Pandya, DN. 1971. The distribution of the corpus callosum in the rhesus monkey. Brain 94, 471–486.

Kiang, NYS, Rho, JM, Northrop, CC, Liberman, MC, Ryugo, DK. 1982. Hair-cell innervation by spiral ganglion cells in adult cats. *Science* 217, 175–177.

Lawrence, M. 1966. Effects of interference with terminal blood supply on the organ of Corti. *Laryngoscope* 76, 1318–1337.

Lawrence, M. 1973. Inner ear physiology. In: MM Paparella, DA Shumrick (eds.), *Otolaryngology Vol. 1: Basic Sciences and Related Disciplines*. Philadelphia, PA: Saunders, 275–298.

Leak-Jones, PA, Synder, RL. 1982. Uptake transport of horseradish peroxidase by cochlear spiral ganglion neurons. *Hearing Res* 8, 199–223.

Li, XF, Phillips, R, LeDouz, JE. 1995. NMDA and non-MNDA receptors contribue to synaptic transmission between the medial geniculate body and the lateral nucleus of the amygdala. *Exp Brain Res* 105, 87–100.

Liberman, MC. 1982. Single-neuron labeling in the cat auditory nerve. *Science* 216, 1239–1241.

Liberman, MC, Brown, MC. 1986. Physiology and anatomy of single olivocochlear neurons in the cat. *Hear Res* 24, 17–36.

Liberman, MC, Dodds, LW, Pierce, S. 1990. Afferent and efferent innervation of the cat cochlea: Quantitative analysis with light and electron microscopy. *J Comp Neurol* 301, 443–460.

Liberman, MC, Simmons, DD. 1985. Applications of neural labeling to the study of the peripheral auditory system. *J Acoust Soc Am* 78, 312–319.

Lim, DJ. 1980. Cochlear anatomy related to cochlear microphonics. A review. *J Acoust Soc Am* 67, 1686–1695.

Lim, DJ. 1986a. Functional structure of the organ of corti: A review. *Hear Res* 22, 117–146.

Lim, DJ. 1986b. Effects of noise and ototoxic drugs at the cellular level in cochlea: A review. *Am J Otol* 7, 73–99.

Lim, DJ, Melnick, W. 1971. Acoustic damage of the cochlea: A scanning and transmission electron microscope observation. *Arch Otol* 94, 294–305.

Luk, GD, Morest, DK, McKenna, NM. 1974. Origins of the crossed olivocochlear bundle shown by an acid phophatase method in the cat. *Ann Otol* 83, 382–392.

Lyons, MJ. 1978. The central location of the motor neurons to the stapedius muscle in the cat. *Brain Res* 143, 437–444.

Mesulam, MM, Pandya, DN. 1973. The projections of the medial geniculate complex within the Sylvian fissure of the rhesus monkey. *Brain Res* 60, 315–333.

Metherate, R, Ashe, JH. 1995. Synaptic interactions involving *acetylcholine*, glutamate, and GABA in rat *auditory cortex*. *Exp Brain Res* 107, 59–72.

Metherate, R, Hsieh, CY. (2003). Regulation of glutamate synapses by nicotinic *acetylcholine* receptors in *auditory cortex*. *Neurobiol Learn Mem* 80, 285–290.

Miller, CE. 1985. Structural implications of basilar membrane compliance measurements. *J Acoust Soc Am* 77, 1465–1474.

Møller, AR. 2000. *Hearing: Its Physiology and Pathophysiology*. San Diego, CA: Academic Press.

Moore, JK. 1987. The human auditory brain stem: A comparative review. *Hear Res* 29, 33–43.

Moore, JK. 2000. Organization of the human superior olivary complex. *Microsc Res Tech* 51, 403–412.

Morera, C, DalSasso, A, Iurato, S. 1980. Submicroscopic structure of the spiral ligament in man. *Rev Laryngol* 101, 73–85.

Morest, DK, Oliver, DL. 1984. The neuronal architecture of the inferior colliculus in the cat: Defining the functional anatomy of the auditory midbrain. *J Comp Neurol* 222, 209–236.

Musiek, FE, Baran, JA. 2007. *The Auditory System: Anatomy, Physiology, and Clinical Correlates*. Boston: Allyn & Bacon.

Nadol, JB Jr. 1983a. Serial section reconstruction of the neural poles of hair cells in the human organ of Corti. I. Inner hair cells. *Laryngoscope* 93, 599–614.

Nadol, JB Jr. 1983b. Serial section reconstruction of the neural poles of hair cells in the human organ of Corti. II. Outer hair cells. *Laryngoscope* 93, 780–791.

Niimi, K, Matsuoka, H. 1979. Thalamocortical organization of the auditory system in the cat studied by retrograde axonal transport of horseradish peroxidase. *Adv Anat Embryol Cell Biol* 57, 1–56.

Ohyama, K, Salt, AN, Thalmann, R. 1998. Volume flow rate of perilymph in the guinea-pig cochlea. *Hear Res* 35, 119–129.

Oliver, DL, Huerta, MF. 1992. Inferior and superior colliculi. In: WB Webster, AN Popper, RF Fay (eds.), *The Mammalian Auditory Pathway: Neuroanatomy*. New York, NY: Springer-Verlag, 168–221.

Oliver, DL, Morest, DK. 1984. The central nucleus of the inferior colliculus in the cat. *J Comp Neurol* 222, 237–264.

Osborne, M, Comis, SD, Pickles, JO. 1988. Further observations on the fine structure of tip links between stereocilia of the guinea pig cochlea. *Hear Res* 35, 99–108.

Pandya, DN, Hallett, M, Mukherjee, S. 1969. Intra- and interhemispheric connections of neocortical auditory system in the rhesus monkey. *Brain Res* 14, 49–65.

Pickles, JO, Comis, SD, Osborne, MR. 1984. Cross links between stereocilia in the guinea-pig organ of Corti, and their possible relation to sensory transduction. *Hear Res* 15, 103–112.

Popper, AN, Fay RF, (eds). 1992. *The Mammalian Auditory Pathway: Neurophysiology*. New York, NY: Springer-Verlag.

Proctor, B. 1989. *Surgical Anatomy of the Ear and Temporal Bone*. New York, NY: Thieme Medical Publishers.

Rask-Andersen, H, Schrott-Fisher, A, Pfaller, K, Glueckert, R. 2006. Perilymph/modiolar communication routes in the human cochlea. *Ear Hear* 27, 457–465.

Rasmussen, GL. 1946. The olivary peduncle and other fiber projections of the superior olivary complex. *J Comp Neurol* 84, 141–219.

Rasmussen, GL. 1967. Efferent connections of the cochlear nucleus. In: AB Graham (ed.), *Sensorineural Hearing Processes and Disorders*. Boston, MA: Little, Brown.

Ravizza, RJ, Belmore, SM. 1978. Auditory forebrain: Evidence from anatomical and behavioral experiments involving human and animal subjects. In: RB Masterson (ed.), *Handbook of Behavioral Neurobiology*. New York, NY: Plenum Press, 459–501.

Reale, RA, Imig, TJ. 1980. Tonotopic organization in the auditory cortex of the cat. *J Comp Neurol* 192, 265–291.

Rhys Evans, RH, Comis, SD, Osborne, MR, Pickles, JO, Jefferies, DJR. 1985. Cross links between stereocilia in the human organ of Corti. *J Laryngol Otol* 99, 11–20.

Rivier, F, Clarke, S. 1997. Cytochrome oxidase, acetylcholinesterase, and NADPH-diaphorase staining in *human supratemporal* and insular cortex: Evidence for multiple auditory areas. *Neuroimage* 6, 288–304.

Robertson, D. 1985. Brainstem localization of efferent neurons projecting to the guinea pig cochlea. *Hear Res* 20, 79–84.

Rockel, AJ, Jones, EG. 1973a. The neuronal organization of the inferior colliculus of the adult cat. I. The central nucleus. *J Comp Neurol* 147, 22–60.

Rockel, AJ, Jones, EG. 1973b. The neuronal organization of the inferior colliculus of the adult cat: II. The pericentral nucleus. *J Comp Neurol* 147, 301–334.

Romand, R, Avan, P. 1997. Anatomical and functional aspects of the cochlear nucleus. In: G Ehret, R Romand (eds.), *The Central Auditory System*. New York, NY: Oxford University Press, 97–192.

Rose, JE. 1949. The cellular structure of the auditory region of the cat. *J Comp Neurol* 91, 409–439.

Rose, JE, Woolsey, CN. 1949. The relations of thalamic connections, cellular structure and evokable electrical activity in the auditory region of the cat. *J Comp Neurol* 91, 441–466.

Rose, JE, Woolsey, CN. 1958. Cortical connections and functional organization of the thalamic auditory system of the cat. In: HF Harlow, CN Woolsey (eds.), *Biological and Biochemical Bases of Behavior*. Madison, WI: University of Wisconsin Press, 127–150.

Ruggero, MA, Santi, PA, Rich NC. 1982. Type II cochlear ganglion cells in the chinchilla. *Hearing Res* 8, 339–356.

Ryugo, DK. 1992. The auditory nerve: Peripheral innervation, cell body morphology, and central projections. In: WB Webster, AN Popper, RF Fay (eds.), *The Mammalian Auditory Pathway: Neuroanatomy*. New York, NY: Springer-Verlag, 23–65.

Sahley, SL, Nodar, RH, Musiek, FE. 1997. *Efferent Auditory System*. San Diego, CA: Singular.

Salt, AN. 2001. Dynamics of the inner ear fluids. In: AF. Jahn, J Santos-Sacchi (eds.), *Physiology of the Ear*, 2nd ed. San Diego, CA: Singular, 333–355.

Salt, AN, Thalmann, R, Marcus, DC, Bohne, BA. 1986. Direct measurement of longitudinal endolymph flow rate in the guinea pig cochlea. *Hear Res* 23, 141–151.

Saunders, JC, Schneider, ME, Dear, SR. 1985. The structure and function of actin in hair cells. *J Acoust Soc Am* 78, 299–311.

Schwartz, DW, Tennigkeit, F, Puil, E. 2000. Metabotropic transmitter actions in auditory thalamus. *Acta Otolaryngol* 120, 251–254.

Schwartz, IR. 1992. The superior olivary complex and lateral lemniscal nuclei. In: WB Webster, AN Popper, RF Fay (eds.), *The Mammalian Auditory Pathway: Neuroanatomy*. New York, NY: Springer-Verlag, 117–167.

Slepecky, NB. 1996. Structure of the mammalian cochlea. In: P Dallos, AN Popper, RR Fay (eds.), *The Cochlea*. New York, NY: Springer-Verlag, 44–129.

Slepecky, NB, Ulfendahl, M, Flock, A. 1988. Effects of caffeine and tetracaine on outer hair cell shortening suggest intracellular calcium involvement. *Hear Res* 32, 11–32.

Smith, CA, Lowry, OH, Wu, M-L. 1954. The electrolytes of the labyrinthine fluids. *Laryngoscope* 64, 141–153.

Smith, CA, Rasmussen, GL. 1963. Recent observations on the olivocochlear bundle. *Ann Otol* 72, 489–506.

Smith, CA, Sjostrand, F. 1961. Structure of the nerve endings of the guinea pig cochlea by serial sections. *J Ultrasound Res* 5, 523–556.

Spoendlin, H. 1969. Innervation of the organ of Corti of the cat. *Acta Otol* 67, 239–254.

Spoendlin, H. 1971. Degeneration behavior in the cochlear nerve. *Arch Klin Exp Ohren Nasen KehlkopfFeilkd* 200, 275–291.

Spoendlin, H. 1975. Neuroanatomical basis of cochlear coding mechanisms. *Audiology* 14, 383–407.

Spoendlin, H. 1978. The afferent innervation of the cochlea. In: RF Naunton, C Fernandez (eds.), *Evoked Electrical Activity in the Auditory Nervous System*. London, UK: Academic Press, 21–41.

Spoendlin, H. 1979. Neural connection of the outer hair-cell system. *Acta Otol* 87, 381–387.

Spoendlin, H. 1981. Differentiation of cochlear afferent neurons. *Acta Otol* 91, 451–456.

Spoendlin, H. 1982. Innervation of the outer hair cell system. *Am J Otol* 3, 274–278.

Spoendlin, H, Gacek, RR. 1963. Electromicroscopic study of the efferent and afferent innervation of the organ of Corti. *Ann Otol* 72, 660–686.

Steel, KR. 1983. The tectorial membrane of mammals. *Hear Res* 9, 327–359.

Steel, KR. 1985. Composition and properties of mammalian tectorial membrane. In: DG Drescher (ed.), *Auditory Biochemistry*. Springfield, IL: Charles C. Thomas, 351–365.

Strelioff, D, Flock, A. 1984. Stiffness of sensory-cell hair bundles in the isolated guinea pig cochlea. *Hear Res* 15, 19–28.

Strutz, J, Spatz, W. 1980. Superior olivary and extraolivary origin of centrifugal innervation of the cochlea in guinea pig: A horseradish peroxadase studys. *Neurosci Lett* 17, 227.

Takahashi, T, Kimura, RS. 1970. The ultrastructure of the spiral ligament in the Rhesus monkey. *Acta Otol* 69, 46–60.

Thalmann, I, Machiki, K, Calabro, A, Hascall, VC, Thalmann, R. 1993. Uronic acid-containing glycosaminoglycans and keratan sulfate are present in the tectorial membrane of the inner ear: Functional implications. *Arch Biochem Biophys* 307, 391–393.

Thalmann, I, Thallinger, G, Comegys, TH, Crouch, EC, Barret, N, Thalmann, R. 1987. Composition and supramolecular organization of the tectorial membrane. *Laryngoscope* 97, 357–367.

Tilney, LG, DeRosier, DJ, Mulroy, MJ. 1980. The organization of actin filaments in the skeleton of cochlear hair cells. *J Cell Biol* 86. 244–259.

Tilney, LG, Saunders, JC. 1983. Actin filaments, stereocilia, and hair cells of bird cochlea. I. Length, number, width, and distribution of stereocilia of each hair cell are related to the position of the hair cell on the cochlea. *J Cell Biol* 96, 807–821.

Tilney, LG, Tilney, MS. 1986. Functional Organization of the Cytoskeleton. *Hear Res* 22, 55–77.

Tos, M. 1995. *Manual of Middle Ear Surgery: Vol. 2, Mastoid Surgery and Reconstructive Procedures*. New York, NY: Thieme Medical Publishers.

Ulehlova, J, Voldrich, L, Janisch, R. 1987. Correlative study of sensory cell density and cochlear length in humans. *Hear Res* 28, 149–151.

Vollrath, MA, Kwan, KY, Corey, DP. 2007. The micromachinery of mechanotransduction in hair cells. *Ann Rev Neurosci* 30, 339–365.

Wallace, MN, Johnson, PW, Palmer, AR. 2002. Histochemical identification of cortical areas in the *auditory region* of the human brain. *Exp Brain Res* 143, 499–508.

Wangemann, P, Schacht, J. 1996. Cochlear homeostasis. In: P Dallos, AN Popper, RR Fay (eds.), *The Cochlea: Handbook of Auditory Research*. Vol. 8. New York: Springer Verlag, 130–185.

Warr, WB. 1978. The olivocochlear bundle: Its origins and terminations in the cat. In: RF Naunton, C Fernandez (eds.), *Evoked Electrical Activity in the Auditory Nervous System*. New York, NY: Academic Press, 43–65.

Warr, WB. 1992. Organization of the olivocochlear efferent systems in mammals. In: WB Webster, AN Popper, RF Fay (eds.), *The Mammalian Auditory Pathway: Neuroanatomy*. New York, NY: Springer-Verlag, 410–448.

Wbarnes, WT, Magoun, HW, Ranson, SW. 1943. The ascending auditory projection in the brainstem of the monkey. *J Comp Neurol* 79, 129–152.

Webster, WB, Popper, AN, Fay, RF, (eds.). 1992. *The Mammalian Auditory Pathway: Neuroanatomy*. New York, NY: Springer-Verlag.

Weiss, TE, Mulroy, MJ, Turner, RG, Pike, CL. 1976. Tuning of single fibers in the cochlear nerve of the alligator lizards: Relation to receptor morphology. *Brain Res* 115, 71–90.

Wenthold, RJ. 1978. Glutamic acid and apartic acid in subdivisions of the cochlear nucleus after auditory nerve lesion. *Brain Res* 143, 544–548.

Wenthold, RJ. 1991. Neurotransmitters of the brainstem auditory nuclei. In: RA Altschuler, RP Bobbin, BM Clopton, DW Hoffman (eds.), *Neurobiology of Hearing: The Central Auditory System*. New York, NY: Raven, 121–140.

Wenthold, R, Hunter, C, Petralia, R. 1993. Excitatory amino acid in the rat cochlear nucleus. In: M Murchan, J Juis, D Godfrey, F Mugnaina (eds.), *The Mammalian Cochlear Nuclei: Organization and Function*. New York, NY: Plenum, 179–194.

Wever, EG, Lawrence, M. 1954. *Physiological Acoustics*. Princeton, NJ: Princeton University Press.

Winer, JA. 1984. The human medial geniculate body. *Hear Res* 15, 225–247.

Winer, JA. 1985. The medial geniculate body of the cat. *Adv Anat Embryol Cell Biol* 86, 1–98.

Winer, JA. 1991. Anatomy of the medial geniculate body. In: RA Altschuler, RP Bobbin, BM Clopton, DW Hoffman (eds.), *Neurobiology of Hearing, Vol. 2. The Central Auditory System*. New York, NY: Springer-Verlag.

Winer, JA. 1992. The functional architecture of the medial geniculate body and the primary auditory cortex. In: WB Webster, AN Popper, RF Fay (eds.), *The Mammalian Auditory Pathway: Neuroanatomy*. New York, NY: Springer-Verlag, 222–409.

Winer, JA, Diamond, IT, Raczkowski, D. 1977. Subdivisions of the auditory cortex of the cat: The retrograde transport of horseradish peroxidase to the medial geniculate body and posterior thalamic nuclei. *J Comp Neurol* 176, 387–417.

Wright, A. 1981. Scanning electron microscopy of the human cochlea—The organ of Corti. *Arch Otorhinolaryngol* 230, 11–19.

Wright, A. 1984. Dimensions of the cochlear stereocilia in man and the guinea pig. *Hear Res* 13, 89–98.

Wright, A, Davis, A, Bredberg, G, Ulehlova, L, Spencer, H. 1987. Hair cell distributions in the normal human cochlea. *Acta Otol Suppl* 444, 1–48.

Wynne, B, Harvey, AR, Robertson, D, and Sirinathsinghji, DJ. 1995. *Neurotransmitter* and neuromodulator systems of the rat *inferior colliculus* and auditory brainstem studied by in situ hybridization. *J Chem Neuroanat* 9, 289–300.

Zwislocki, JJ, Chamberlain, SC, Slepecky, NB. 1988. Tectorial membrane 1: Static mechanical properties in vivo. *Hear Res* 33, 207–222.

3 Conductive Mechanism

This chapter deals with the routes over which sound is conducted to the inner ear. The first section is concerned with the usual air conduction path through the outer and middle ear. The second section briefly discusses the bone conduction route. In the last section, we shall address the acoustic reflex.

OUTER EAR

We cannot discuss the contributions of the outer ear *per se* without being aware that the sounds we hear are affected by the entire acoustical path from the sound source to our ears. This path includes the effects of the listener him- or herself. For example, the head casts an acoustical shadow (analogous to an eclipse) when it is between the sound source and the ear being tested. This **head shadow** is significant for frequencies over about 1500 Hz because their wavelengths are small compared to the size of the head. Moreover, the sound entering the ear canal is affected by reflections and diffractions associated with the head, pinna, and torso. Hence, the issue of spatial orientation comes into play, and with it the need for a way to describe the direction of a sound source. Many of these matters are discussed in Chapter 13. For now, it should suffice to know that the *horizontal direction* of a source is given as an angle called **azimuth**, where 0° is straight ahead, 180° is straight back, and 90° is off to one side; and that the *vertical direction* (along the medial plane from front to back) is given by an angle called **elevation**, where 0° is straight ahead, 180° is straight back, and 90° is directly above.

Pinna

The **pinna** has traditionally been credited with funneling sounds into the ear canal and enhancing localization. It has been demonstrated, however, that hearing sensitivity is not affected when the pinna is excluded from sound conduction by bypassing it with tubes into the canal and by filling its depressions (Bekesy and Rosenblith, 1958). Thus, the sound collecting/funneling function is not significant for the human pinna. The pinna's greatest contribution to hearing is actually in the realm of sound source *localization* (see Chap. 13).

The pinna influences localization because its depressions and ridges filter the high-frequency aspects of the signal (over about 4000 Hz) in a way that depends on the direction of the sound (e.g., Shaw, 1997). The spectral variations introduced by the pinna are important directional cues for determining the *elevation* of a sound source and *front/back* distinctions, and contribute to *extracranialization*, or the perception that a sound source is outside of the head (Plenge, 1974 ; Blauert, 1997). Pinna effects are particularly important when one must localize sounds while listening with only one ear (monaurally), because monaural hearing precludes the use of the interaural differences

available during binaural hearing, and when the sound source is in the *medial plane* of the head, where interaural differences are minimized because the sound source is equidistant from both ears. These effects are readily shown by increases in the number of localization errors that are made when the various depressions of the pinna are filled (e.g., Gardner and Gardner, 1973 ; Oldfield and Parker, 1984).

Ear Canal

The tympanic membrane is located at the end of the ear canal rather than flush with the surface of the skull. Sounds reaching the eardrum are thus affected by the acoustic characteristics of the ear canal. The ear canal may be conceived of as a tube open at one end and closed at the other. Such a tube resonates at the frequency with a wavelength four times the length of the tube. Because the human ear canal is about 2.3 cm long, its resonance should occur at the frequency corresponding to a wavelength of 9.2 cm, that is, at about 3800 Hz. One could test this hypothesis by directing a known sound into a sound field, and then monitoring the sound pressure at the eardrum of a subject sitting in that sound field. This test has been done in various ways in many studies. Figure 3.1 shows the results of three classic studies in the form of head-related transfer functions (Wiener and Ross, 1946 ; Shaw, 1974 ; Mehrgardt and Mellert, 1977). A **transfer function** shows the relationship between the input to a system and its output. The **head-related transfer function (HRTF)** shows how sounds presented from a particular direction are affected by the entire path from the loudspeaker to the eardrum. The HRTFs in the figure show how sounds presented from a speaker directly in front of the subject (0° azimuth) are affected by the ear canal. The common finding of these functions is a wide resonance peak in from roughly 2000 to 5000 Hz, which is due to the resonance of the ear canal. It does not resemble the sharp resonance of a rigid tube. However, the ear canal is an irregular rather than a simple tube, and the drum and canal walls are absorptive rather than rigid. These factors introduce damping. Group (averaged) data are also shown in the figure. Because resonant frequency depends on canal length, variations in ear canal length among subjects will widen and smooth the averaged function. The important point, however, is that the resonance characteristics of the canal serve to boost the level of sounds in the mid-to-high frequencies by as much as about 15 dB at the eardrum compared to the sound field.

Stinton and Lawton (1989) reported very accurate geometric specifications of the human ear canal based upon impressions taken from cadavers. They found considerable diversity from canal to canal, resulting in differences greater than 20 dB for the higher frequencies, particularly over 10,000 Hz. Considerable variability in the dimensions of the skull, dimensions of pinna structures, etc., which influence HRTFs, has also been reported by Middlebrooks (1999) .

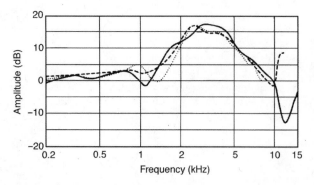

Figure 3.1 Head-related transfer functions for sounds presented from directly in front of the listener (0° azimuth) from three studies [Wiener and Ross (1946), *dotted line*; Shaw (1974), *dashed line*; Mehrgardt and Mellert (1977), *solid line*]. *Source*: From Mehrgardt and Mellert (1977), with permission of *J Acoust. Soc. Am.*

Head-related transfer functions depend on the direction of the sound source. The fundamental nature of this azimuth effect is illustrated for two representative directions in Fig. 3.2. Here, we are concerned with the sound reaching the right eardrum when it is presented from a loudspeaker at an azimuth of 45° to the right compared to being presented from a speaker at 45° to the left. The right ear is the **near ear** when the sound comes from the right (same side of the head), and it is the **far ear** when the sound comes from the left (the opposite side of the head). Note that the sound level increases going from the far ear, and that there are differences in the details of the shapes

of the two curves. Physical factors of this type provide the basis for sound localization in space (see Chap. 13).

Middle Ear

Sound reaches the ear by way of the air, a gas. On the other hand, the organ of Corti is contained within the cochlear fluids, which are physically comparable to seawater. The difference between these media is of considerable import to hearing, as the following example will show. Suppose you and a friend are standing in water at the beach. He is speaking, and in the middle of his sentence you dunk your head under the water. However loud and clear your friend's voice was a moment ago, it will be barely, if at all, audible while your head is submerged. Why?

The answer to this question is really quite straightforward. Air offers less opposition, or **impedance**, to the flow of sound energy than does seawater. Because the water's impedance is greater than that of the air, there is an impedance mismatch at the boundary between them. Airborne sound thus meets a substantial increase in the opposition to its flow at the water's surface, and much of the energy is reflected back rather than being transmitted through the water. The impedance mismatch between the air and cochlear fluids has the same effect. The middle ear system serves as an **impedance-matching transformer** that makes it possible for the sound energy to be efficiently transmitted from the air to the cochlea.

As with any other system, the impedance of the conductive system is due to its stiffness, mass, and resistance. Figure 3.3 is a block diagram of the conductive mechanism with respect to its impedance components, based on conceptualizations by

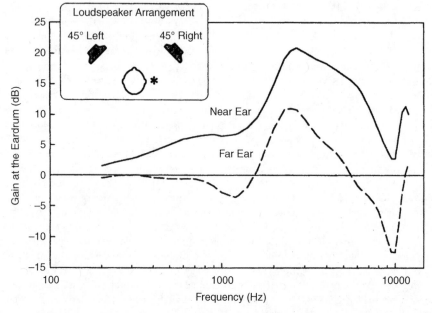

Figure 3.2 Head-related transfer functions resulting from the presentation of sound from loudspeakers located on the same ("near ear") and opposite ("far ear") sides of the head. Insert: loudspeaker arrangement associated with the transfer functions. *Source*: Based on data derived from Shaw (1974) and Shaw and Vaillancourt (1985).

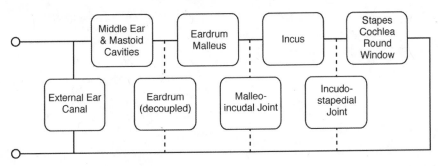

Figure 3.3 Block diagram of the components contributing to the impedance of the ear, based on various diagrams by Zwislocki (1962, 1976) and Bennett (1984).

Zwislocki (1962, 1976) and Bennett (1984) . The leftmost box, labeled "external ear canal," represents the stiffness reactance contributed by the external auditory meatus. One may think of the upper row of boxes as the line of energy flow from the eardrum to the cochlea, and of the boxes coming down from them via dotted lines as the ways in which energy is shunted from the system. The first box represents the middle ear cavities, which contribute significantly to the stiffness of the system. Actually, the impedance of the middle ear space (including the mastoid air cells) is controlled by compliance up to about 500 Hz, but becomes complicated at higher frequencies (Stepp and Voss, 2005). The next two boxes, "eardrum/malleus" and "eardrum (decoupled)," should be thought of together. The former represents the proportion of sound energy transmitted from the drum to the malleus. It includes the inertia of the malleus; the elasticity of the drum, tensor tympani muscle, and mallear ligaments; and the friction caused by the strain on these structures. "Eardrum (decoupled)" is the proportion of energy diverted from the system when the drum vibrates independently (decoupled from) the malleus, which occurs particularly at high frequencies. The box labeled "incus" is the effective mass of the incus and the stiffness of its supporting ligaments. The energy lost at the two ossicular joints is represented by the boxes labeled "malleoincudal joint" and "incudostapedial joint," which shunt energy off the main line of the diagram. The last box shows the effects of the stapes, cochlea, and round window in series. The attachments of the stapes as well as the round window membrane contribute to the stiffness component. Most of the ear's resistance is attributable to the cochlea. Zwislocki (1975) pointed out that a major effect of this resistance is to smooth out the response of the middle ear by damping the free oscillations of the ossicular chain.

Middle Ear Transformer Mechanism

The ratio between the impedances of the cochlear fluids and the air is approximately 4000:1. To find out how much energy would be transmitted from the air to the cochlea without the middle ear, we apply the simple formula $T = 4r/(r + 1)^2$, where T is transmission and r is the ratio of the impedances. The result is approximately 0.001. In other words, only about 0.1%

of the airborne energy would be transmitted to the cochlea, while about 99.9% would be reflected back. This corresponds to a 40-dB drop going from the air to the cochlea.

The middle ear "steps up" the level of airborne sound to overcome the impedance mismatch between the air and cochlear fluids. As we shall see in the next chapter, early place theory held that the middle ear transformer mechanism was the source of various nonlinearities in hearing, such as the perception of combination tones (Helmholtz, 1868). These *distortion products* of the middle ear's hypothetical nonlinear response were ostensibly transmitted to the cochlea, where the nonlinearities were analyzed according to the place principle as though they were present in the original signal. However, Wever and Lawrence (1954) demonstrated that the middle ear mechanism actually performs its function with elegant linearity, and we must accordingly regard it as a linear transformer, and look elsewhere (to the cochlea) for the sources of nonlinear distortions.

Several factors, discussed below, contribute to the transformer function of the middle ear. They include the area ratio of the eardrum to the oval window, the curved-membrane mechanism of the eardrum, and the lever action of the ossicular chain.

Area Ratio

We know that pressure (p) is equal to force (F) per unit area (A), or p = F/A. If we therefore exert the same pressure over two areas, one of which is five times larger than the other, then the pressure on the smaller surface will be five times greater. Examples of the fundamental principle are shown in Fig. 3.4a.

Wever and Lawrence (1954) reported that the area of the human eardrum is roughly 64.3 mm², whereas Bekesy (1941) estimated its area to be about 85 mm². Regardless of which estimate is used, it is clear that the area of the eardrum is substantially larger than that of the oval window, which is commonly accepted to be only 3.2 mm². Using the values by Wever and Lawrence for purposes of illustration, the ratio of the area of the eardrum to that of the oval window area would be 64.3/3.2 = 20.1 to 1, as shown in Fig. 3.4b. If we assume that the ossicles act as a simple rigid connection between the two membranes,

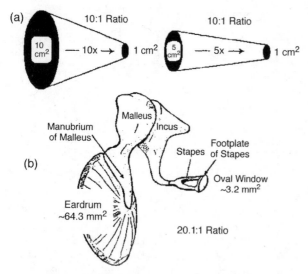

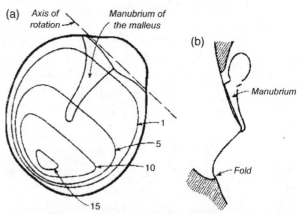

Figure 3.6 (a) Equal relative eardrum displacement contours for a 2000-Hz stimulus. Numbers indicate the relative amplitudes. (b) Cross-section of the tympanic membrane showing a loose-fitting inferior edge. *Source*: From Bekesy (1941).

Figure 3.4 (a) Conceptual representation of the area ratio. (b) Determination of the overall area ratio using values by Wever and Lawrence (1954); using Bekesy's (1941) values and applying the effective area result in different estimates of the area ratio (see text).

then this area ratio would cause the pressure to be amplified by a factor of 20.1 going from the tympanic membrane to the oval window.

Curved-Membrane Mechanism

Helmholtz (1868) suggested that the eardrum contributes to the effectiveness of the middle ear transformer by a form of lever action, according to the curved-membrane principle (Fig. 3.5). The eardrum's rim is firmly attached to the annulus and curves down to the attachment of the malleus, which is mobile, as in the figure. A given force increment thus displaces the membrane with greater amplitude than it displaces the manubrium. Because the products of force and distance (amplitude of displacement) on both legs of the lever are equal ($F_1 D_1 = F_2 D_2$), the smaller distance traveled by the manubrium is accompanied by a much greater force. In this way, Helmholtz proposed that lever action of the eardrum would result in an amplification of force to the ossicles.

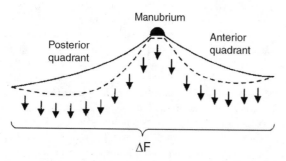

Figure 3.5 The curved-membrane principle (see text). *Source*: Adapted from Tonndorf and Khanna (1970), with permission of *Ann. Otol.*

Subsequent experiments led to the abandonment of this principle, since studies of drum movement were inconsistent with it, and since Helmholtz's results were not replicated (Wever and Lawrence, 1954). Bekesy (1941) used a capacitance probe to measure human eardrum displacement at various frequencies. The capacitance probe used a very fine wire as one plate of a capacitor and the drum surface as the other plate. Sound causes the drum to vibrate, which in turn varies its distance from the wire. If a current is passed through this capacitor, the movement of the drum will affect current flow. Monitoring the current flow at different spots on the drum enabled Bekesy to determine its displacement with considerable accuracy.

Figure 3.6a shows Bekesy's results for a 2000-Hz tone in the form of equal displacement contours. For frequencies up to approximately 2000 Hz, the eardrum moved as a stiff plate or piston, hinged superiorly at the axis of the ossicles. The greatest displacement occurred inferiorly. Bekesy attributed the drum's ability to move in this manner, without significant deformation, to a highly elastic or loose-fitting fold at its inferior edge (Fig. 3.6b). Above about 2000 Hz the tympanic membrane's stiffness broke down, and movement of the manubrium lagged behind that of the membrane rather than being synchronized with it. The stiffly moving portion of the drum had an area of 55 mm^2 out of a total area of 85 mm^2. This area constitutes an **effective area** for the eardrum of about 55 mm^2/85 mm^2 = 65% of its total area. Using Bekesy's values, the ratio of the area of the entire eardrum to the area of the oval window would be 85 mm^2/3.2 mm^2 = 26.6 to 1. However, applying the eardrum's 65% effective area to the overall ratio results in an *effective* area ratio of 26.6 × 0.65 = 17.3 to 1.

The role of the eardrum was reevaluated by Tonndorf and Khanna (1970), who used time-averaged holography to study eardrum movement in the cat. Time-averaged holography is an optical method that reveals equal-amplitude (or isoamplitude) contours as alternating bright and dark lines on a vibrating

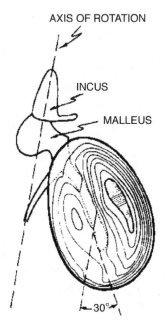

AXIS OF ROTATION

INCUS

MALLEUS

30°

Figure 3.7 Vibration patterns of the cat's eardrum in response to a 600-Hz tone. *Source*: From Tonndorf and Khanna (1970), with permission of *Ann. Otol.*

membrane. Figure 3.7 shows the isoamplitude contours for a 600-Hz tone. These contours show that the eardrum actually does not move as a stiff plate. Instead, there are two areas of peak displacement revealing a buckling effect in the eardrum vibration pattern that is consistent with Helmholtz's curved-membrane concept. This mode of vibration is seen up to about 1500 Hz. The pattern becomes more restricted at higher frequencies, and increasingly complex subpatterns occur in the vibrations as frequency rises above 3000 Hz. The curved-membrane principle contributes to the middle ear transformer ratio by a factor of 2.0 based upon the cat data. If we accept an area ratio of 34.6 to 1 for the cat, then the middle ear transfer ratio as of this point becomes 34.6 × 2.0 = 69.2 to 1. This value must be multiplied by the lever ratio of the ossicles to arrive at the final transformer ratio of the middle ear.

Ossicular Lever

Helmholtz (1868) proposed that nonlinear distortions are introduced by the ossicular chain, and are largely due to what he conceived of as a cogwheel articulation between the malleus and incus. This situation would allow for relative movement in one direction at the malleoincudal joint. The resulting distortions would stimulate the cochlea at places corresponding to the receptors for those frequencies, as though they were present in the original signal. Barany (1938) demonstrated, however, that except during intense stimulation these two bones are rigidly fixed at the malleoincudal joint and move as a unit in response to sound stimulation.

Bekesy (1936) reported that the stapes moves differently in response to moderate and intense stimulation in human cadavers, as illustrated in Fig. 3.8. At moderate intensities, the stapedial footplate rocks with a piston-like motion in the oval window, with greater amplitude anteriorly (Fig. 3.8a). Intense stimulation results in rotation of the footplate around its longitudinal axis (Fig. 3.8b). Rocking of the stapes around the longitudinal axis substantially reduces the energy transmitted to the cochlea. However, Guinan and Peake (1967) have shown that the cat stapes maintains essentially piston-like movements even at very high intensities, at least for low frequencies.

It has been known for a long time that the ossicular chain rotates around its axis, illustrated in Fig. 3.9 (top), which corresponds to a line through the long process of the malleus and the short process of the incus (Barany, 1938). Measurements using advanced optical techniques have revealed that the motion of the malleus is frequency-dependent, so that its vibratory pattern is essentially in one dimension below 2500 Hz, but involves an elliptical path in all three dimensions, as opposed to having a single axis above 2500 Hz (Decraemer, Khanna, and Funnell, 1991, 1994).

The ossicular chain is delicately balanced around its center of gravity so that the inertia of the system is minimal (Barany, 1938). As a result, the ossicular chain acts as a lever about its axis (Fig. 3.9). The malleus constitutes the longer leg of this ossicular lever and the incus constitutes the shorter leg. The lever ratio is on the order of 1.3 to 1 in humans and 2.2 to 1 in cats. However, the actual lever ratio is smaller, because of the interaction of the curvature of the eardrum and the length of the ossicular chain lever (Tonndorf and Khanna, 1970).

Recall that the drum curves more toward the umbo, and may be regarded as a curved string. The transformer ratio of a curved string decreases as the curvature becomes stronger (1/curvature). On the other hand, the transformer ratio of the ossicular lever increases with length. Note in Fig. 3.10 that the ossicular lever is long (with respect to the point of attachment of the malleus on the drum) where the curvature is strong, and that it is short where the curvature is small. This interaction results in an essentially constant lever ratio, with a value of about 1.4 for the cat ossicular chain.

We may now apply the ossicular lever ratio to the intermediate solution of 69.2 obtained so far for the cat's middle ear transfer ratio. The final ratio becomes 69.2 × 1.4 = 96.9 to 1. The ratio is converted into decibels as follows: 20 × log 96.9 = 39.7 dB. This value closely approximates the 40-dB loss that results when the cat's middle ear is completely obliterated (Tonndorf, Khanna, and Fingerhood, 1966). Using an effective area ratio of 26.6, an eardrum buckling factor of 2.0 and an ossicular lever ratio of 1.3, the human middle ear transformer ratio may be estimated at approximately 26.6 × 2 × 1.3 = 69.2 to 1, which corresponds to 20 × log 69.2 = 36.8 dB. As illustrated in Fig. 3.11, actual middle ear transformer ratios fall short of these values, and they depend considerably upon frequency. That the actual boost provided by the conductive

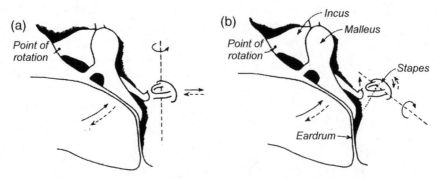

Figure 3.8 The nature of stapes movement in cadavers in response to stimuli presented at (a) moderate levels and (b) very intense levels. *Source*: From Bekesy (1936).

system does not achieve the values based on the calculations is probably due to transmission losses. Rosowski (1991) estimated that the efficiency of the human middle ear system peaks at about 0.4 in the vicinity of 900 Hz, and then decreases for higher frequencies, and averages approximately 0.2 in the cat.

Middle Ear Response

Figure 3.11, based on Nedzelnitsky's (1980) data from cats, provides an example of a middle ear transfer function. The middle ear transfer function makes a substantial contribution to the shapes of minimal audibility curves (see Chap. 9). These curves show the amount of sound energy needed to reach the threshold of hearing as a function of frequency.

Bekesy (1941) reported that the resonant frequency of the middle ear is in the 800 to 1500 Hz region. Recall that resonance occurs when mass and stiffness reactance are equal, canceling out. Impedance is then entirely composed of resistance, and accordingly the opposition to energy flow is minimal at the resonant frequencies. Møller (1960) found the major resonance

peak of the middle ear to be about 1200 Hz, with a smaller resonance peak around 800 Hz. Normal ear reactance and resistance values based on 20 studies are summarized in Fig. 3.12 (Margolis, VanCamp, Wilson, and Creten, 1985). Note that the ear's impedance results primarily from negative reactance up to about 800 Hz. This effect is due to the middle ear mechanism itself, which is stiffness controlled below the resonant frequency. There is virtually no reactance between about 800 Hz and roughly 5000–6000 Hz, indicating that energy transmission from the eardrum to the cochlea is maximal in this range. Positive reactance takes over at higher frequencies as a result of the effective mass of the drum and ossicles. We thus expect sound transmission through the middle ear to be frequency-dependent with emphasis on the midfrequencies; and the minimal audibility curves of the ear should reflect this relation.

The cat's middle ear transfer function and behavioral thresholds are compared in Fig. 3.13. The open circles in Fig. 3.13 show the middle ear transfer function based on data from anesthetized cats (Dallos, 1973). The filled circles are the behavioral

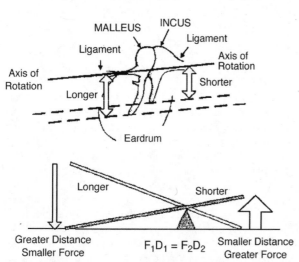

Figure 3.9 The axis of rotation of the ossicular chain and the ossicular lever mechanism. Based in part on drawings by Barany (1938) and Bekesy (1941).

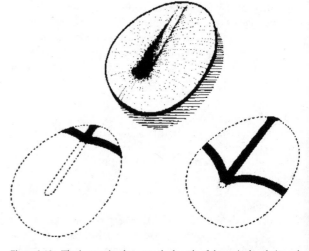

Figure 3.10 The interaction between the length of the ossicular chain and the inverse of the eardrum curvature. *Source*: From Tonndorf and Khanna (1970), with permission of *Ann. Otol.*

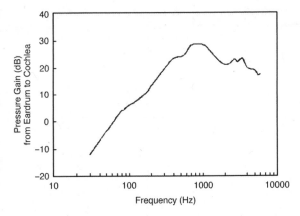

Figure 3.11 The middle ear transfer function from the tympanic membrane to the cochlear fluids as a function of frequency. *Source*: Adapted from Nedzelnitsky (1980), with permission of *J. Acoust. Soc. Am.*

flattened by the averaging among subjects; the transfer function is from a single representative animal. In addition, there is a peak at around 4000 Hz in the middle ear response of anesthetized animals, which is much smaller when they are awake due to damping of the system by the tonus of the stapedius muscle. A second factor has to do with the effects of head diffraction, the pinna, and the ear canal, as discussed in the section on the outer ear in this chapter. These effects are accounted for by viewing the behavioral thresholds in terms of the sound pressure level (SPL) near the eardrum at threshold, as is shown by the filled triangles in Fig. 3.13. The relationship of the threshold curve to the transfer function is closer when considered in these terms. The disparity between the transfer function and thresholds below about 1000 Hz is reconciled by correcting the transfer function for the input impedance of the cochlea (open triangles).

These factors show a considerable degree of correspondence between the middle ear transfer function and the threshold curve, at least for the cat. Reasonable agreement between the transfer function based upon a model of the middle ear and the threshold curve has also been shown for humans (Zwislocki, 1975). Thus we find that the impedance-matching job of the middle ear is accomplished quite well for the midfrequencies, although the frequency-dependent nature of the middle ear reduces its efficiency at higher and lower frequencies.

thresholds of waking cats in a sound field (Miller et al., 1963). The binaural threshold and transfer function are generally similar, but the threshold curve is steeper at low frequencies and flatter at high. This may reflect several factors (Simmons, 1964; Wiener et al., 1966; Dallos, 1970, 1973): First, since the thresholds show mean group data, the curve is probably somewhat

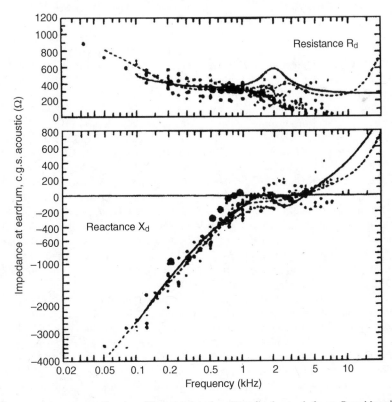

Figure 3.12 Acoustic resistance and reactance as a function of frequency based on 20 studies (see text). *Source*: From Margolis, Van Camp, Wilson, and Creten (1985), with permission.

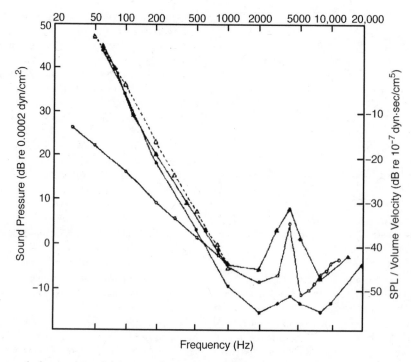

Figure 3.13 Middle ear transfer function (*open circles*) compared to behavioral thresholds (*closed circles*) and sound pressure level (SPL) at the eardrum (*closed triangles*) in cats. *Source*: From Dallos (1973), *The Auditory Periphery*, copyright © 1973 by Academic Press.

BONE CONDUCTION

Until now we have dealt with the usual route from the air to the cochlea. The discussion would be incomplete, however, without at least a brief consideration of bone conduction—the transmission of sound to the cochlea by the bones of the skull. For this to occur, a sound must be strong enough to cause the bones to vibrate, or else the stimulus must be delivered by way of a vibrator applied to the skull. The impedance mismatch between air and bone is even greater than between air and cochlear fluid: An airborne sound must exceed the air conduction threshold by at least 50 to 60 dB before the bone conduction threshold is reached (Bekesy, 1948). Direct stimulation with a vibrator is routinely employed in audiological evaluations to separate hearing losses attributable to the outer and/or middle ear from those due to impairments of the sensorineural mechanisms.

Two classic experiments proved that both air conduction and bone conduction initiate the same traveling waves in the cochlea (see Chap. 4). Bekesy (1932) showed that air- and bone-conduction signals cancel one another when their phases and amplitudes are appropriately adjusted. Lowy (1942) demonstrated that this cancellation occurs in the cochlea, since repetition of the Bekesy experiment on guinea pigs resulted in cancellation of the cochlear microphonic. (The cochlear microphonic is an electrical potential that reflects the activity of the hair cells; see Chap 4.) The implications of these experiments are monumental, since they demonstrate that the final activity

in the cochlea is the same regardless of the mode of entry of the sound. Furthermore, this result gives support to the use of bone conduction as an audiological tool, and the results of which can validly be compared with those of air conduction in determining the locus of a lesion (assuming appropriate calibration of both signals).

Bekesy (1932) found that below 200 Hz the human skull vibrates as a unit (Fig. 3.14a). At about 800 Hz, the mode of vibration changes (Fig. 3.14b), and the front and back of the head vibrate in opposite phase to one another, with a nodal line of compression between them. At about 1600 Hz, the head begins to vibrate in four segments (Fig. 3.14c).

Tonndorf and colleagues (1966, 1968) demonstrated that the mechanism of bone conduction includes contributions from the outer, middle, and inner ear. For clarity, let us look at these components, beginning with the inner ear.

Compressional bone conduction is illustrated in Fig. 3.15. Vibration of the temporal bone results in alternate compression and expansion of the cochlear capsule. Because the cochlear fluids are incompressible, there should be bulging at compliant points. Bulging would occur at the oval and round windows without displacement of the cochlear partition if both windows were equally compliant (Fig. 3.15a). However, since the round window is much more compliant than the oval window, compression of the cochlear capsule pushes the fluid in the scala vestibuli downward, displacing the basilar membrane as shown in Fig. 3.15b. This effect is reinforced, since the sum of the

Bone Vibrator at Forehead

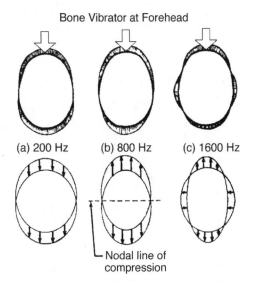

(a) 200 Hz (b) 800 Hz (c) 1600 Hz

Nodal line of compression

Figure 3.14 Patterns of skull vibration at (a) 200 Hz, (b) 800 Hz, and (c) 1600 Hz, in response to a bone conduction stimulus being applied to the forehead. *Source*: Adapted from Bekesy (1932).

surface area of the vestibule and the surface area of the scala vestibuli is greater than that of the scala tympani (Fig. 3.15c). The possibility of a "third window" for the release of this pressure is provided by the cochlear aqueduct.

Tonndorf (1962), however, found that the primary mechanism of bone conduction in the inner ear involves distortional vibrations of the cochlear capsule, which are synchronous with the signal (Fig. 3.16). **Distortional bone conduction** occurs because the volume of the scala vestibuli is greater than that of the scala tympani, so that distortions of the cochlear capsule result in compensatory displacements of the cochlear

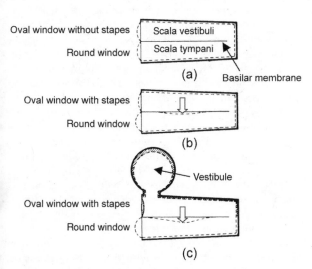

Figure 3.15 Compressional bone conduction (see text). *Source*: Adapted from Bekesy (1932).

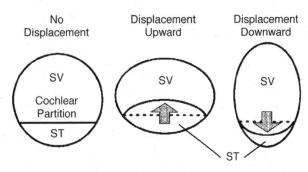

Figure 3.16 Effects of distortional vibrations on displacement of the cochlear partition. *Source*: Adapted from Tonndorf (1962), with permission of *J. Acoust. Soc. Am.*

partition even in the absence of compliant windows. The above-mentioned "windows effects" modify the distortional component.

The contribution of the middle ear to bone conduction is often known as **inertial** or **ossicular-lag bone conduction**, and was demonstrated by Barany (1938). Recall that the ossicles move from side to side rather than front to back. Barany found that for low frequencies bone conduction was maximal when a vibrator was applied to the side of the head and was minimal when it was applied to the forehead. This occurs because the lateral placement vibrates the skull in the direction of ossicular movement (Fig. 3.17a), whereas frontal placement vibrates the skull perpendicular to their movement (Fig. 3.17b). In other words, the signal was transmitted best when it was applied in the direction of rotation of the ossicular chain about its axis. The mechanism is as follows: Because the ossicles are suspended analogously to pendulums, as shown in Fig. 3.17, their inertia causes them to move relative to the skull when the latter is vibrated. Inertial bone conduction, then, stimulates the cochlea by the relative movement of the skull and ossicles, and the effect of which is a rocking motion of the stapes at the oval window.

The middle ear component of bone conduction is of particular interest in otosclerosis, a disorder in which hearing loss

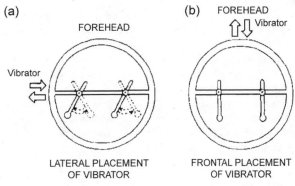

Figure 3.17 Inertial (ossicular lag) bone conduction: (a) lateral placement of the bone vibrator; (b) forehead placement. *Source*: Abstracted from Barany (1938).

results from fixation of the stapes in the oval window. A hearing loss results because the fixated stapedial footplate cannot effectively transmit energy to the cochlea. Although one might expect bone conduction to be impaired at low frequencies, the elevated bone-conduction threshold occurs at about 2000 Hz. This phenomenon is called *Carhart's notch* (Carhart, 1950). Bone conduction is impaired at 2000 Hz, because this is the resonant frequency of the ossicular chain in humans (Tonndorf, 1966).[1]

The contribution of the outer ear to bone conduction is often called osseotympanic bone conduction. It occurs because the vibration of the skull leads to the radiation of sound energy into the ear canal from its walls, and is principally due to vibrations of the cartilaginous portion of the canal (Naunton, 1963; Stenfelt et al., 2003). These radiations then stimulate the eardrum and finally the cochlea along the familiar air-conduction route. The outer ear component is emphasized at low frequencies during occlusion of the cartilaginous part of the ear canal, called the **occlusion effect**. According to Tonndorf (1966), this enhancement of the low frequencies is not appreciated when the ear is unoccluded because the open ear canal acts as a high-pass (lowcut) filter. However, closing off the canal removes the high-pass filter so that the lows are not lost. Another explanation attributes the occlusion effect to differences in the resonances of the ear canal when it is open and closed (Huizing, 1960).

In summary, the bone-conduction mechanism appears to be primarily due to distortion of the inner ear capsule, to the relative movements of the skull and ossicles due to the inertial lag of the latter, and to the sound radiated into the ear canal from its walls. Tonndorf (1966) found in cats that the outer and middle ear components are dominant below about 1000 Hz, but that all three mechanisms are about equally important in the range of 1000 to 6000 Hz, as illustrated in Fig. 3.18. However, findings in human cadavers have suggested that the outer ear component is not significant when the ears are open, although it becomes dominant when the ears are occluded (Stenfelt et al., 2003).

THE ACOUSTIC REFLEX

The contraction of the middle ear muscles in response to relatively intense sound stimulation is known as the **acoustic reflex**. Early experiments on dogs revealed bilateral tensor tympani contractions when either ear was stimulated by intense sound (Hensen, 1878; Pollack, 1886). It was later demonstrated that the stapedius muscles also respond bilaterally to sound stimulation in cats and rabbits (Kato, 1913). However, whether the acoustic reflex in humans is due to contractions of one or both of the intratympanic muscles has been the subject of some controversy.

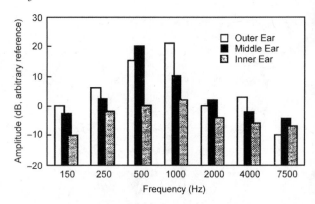

Figure 3.18 The relative contributions of the inner, middle, and outer ear components of bone conduction. *Source*: Adapted from Tonndorf et al. (1966).

Direct observation through perforated eardrums revealed stapedius muscle contractions in humans as a consequence of intense sound stimulation (Lüscher, 1929; Lindsay et al., 1936; Potter, 1936). Terkildsen (1957, 1960) indirectly examined middle ear muscle activity by monitoring changes in air pressure in the ear canal in response to sound stimulation. Stapedius contraction would result in an outward movement of the drum, while tensor concentration would pull the drum inward (see Chap. 2). The drum movement, in turn, results in changes in ear canal pressure. Terkildsen could thus infer the nature of muscle activity by monitoring the air pressure in the ear canal during sound stimulation. Most of his subjects manifested an outward deflection of the drum, suggesting that the stapedius muscle was active. There were, however, some cases showing tensor activity as well (inward drum displacement). Similar findings were reported by Mendelson (1957, 1961).

Perhaps the greatest contribution to what is known about the acoustic reflex comes from measurements of acoustic impedance at the plane of the eardrum using impedance bridges and subsequent instruments. The mechanical acoustic impedance bridge was first applied to the study of the acoustic reflex by Metz (1946) and was improved upon and made clinically efficient by Zwislocki (1963). An electroacoustic impedance bridge was introduced by Terkildsen and Nielsen (1960). Almost all acoustic reflex research since the introduction of the electroacoustic device has used this method or variations of it. The main principle is straightforward: Because contractions of the intratympanic muscles stiffen the middle ear system (including the drum), the impedance is increased. (The reflex primarily affects the compliance component of impedance rather than resistance, because the system is stiffened.) It is this change in acoustic impedance that is measured by the device.

Let us now consider how the ear's impedance can be used to infer information about the activities of one intratympanic muscle versus the other. In the normal ear, we really cannot tell whether the acoustic reflex is due to contractions of the stapedius and/or of the tensor. However, if the reflex is present

---

[1] The resonant frequency was about 1500 Hz in temporal bones from cadavers of individuals averaging 74 years old (Stenfelt et al., 2002).

when the stapedius muscle is intact but not when the muscle (or its reflex arc or attachment) is impaired, then we may conclude that the stapedius muscle contributes to the acoustic reflex in humans. The same argument applies to the tensor tympani.

Several studies have demonstrated that the acoustic reflex is absent when there is pathology affecting the stapedius muscle (Jepsen, 1955; Klockhoff, 1961; Feldman, 1967). However, the acoustic reflex was still obtained in two cases of tensor tympani pathology (Jepsen, 1955). It might be added at this point that a measurable tensor tympani reflex is known to occur as part of a startle reaction to very intense sound (Djupesland, 1964), or in response to a jet of air directed into the eye (Klockhoff, 1961). Based on these observations, one is drawn to conclude that in humans the acoustic reflex is a *stapedius* reflex.

Reflex Parameters

Several parameters of the acoustic reflex should be discussed before describing its effect upon energy transmission through the ear, or its suggested roles within the auditory system. The possible relationship between the acoustic reflex and loudness will also be considered.

We have been referring to the acoustic reflex as occurring in response to "intense" sound stimulation. Let us now examine just how intense a sound is needed. With a reasonable amount of variation among studies, the acoustic reflex thresholds in response to pure-tone signals from 250 to 4000 Hz range from 85- to 100-dB SPL (Metz, 1952; Møller, 1962; Jepsen, 1963; Jerger, 1970; Margolis and Popelka, 1975; Wilson and McBride, 1978; Silman, Popelka, and Gelfand, 1978; Gelfand, 1984). The reflex threshold is approximately 20 dB lower (better) when the eliciting stimulus is broadband noise (Peterson and Liden, 1972; Margolis and Popelka, 1975; Silman et al., 1978; Gelfand, 1984). In general, the reflex response is obtained at a lower intensity when it is monitored in the ear being stimulated (the ipsilateral or uncrossed acoustic reflex) instead of in the opposite ear (the contralateral or crossed acoustic reflex) (Møller, 1961; Green and Margolis, 1984). For an extensive discussion of the acoustic reflex threshold and its parameters, see the review by Gelfand (1984).

The lower reflex threshold for broadband noise than for tones suggests that the acoustic reflex is related to the bandwidth of the stimulus. Flottrop et al. (1971) studied this relationship by measuring acoustic reflex thresholds elicited by successively wider bands of noise and complex tones. They found that the increasing bandwidth did not cause the threshold to differ from its value for a pure-tone activator until a certain bandwidth was exceeded. At this point there was a clear-cut break, after which increasing the bandwidth resulted in successively lower reflex thresholds. Similar results were found by Popelka, Karlovich, and Wiley (1974). In addition, Djupesland and Zwislocki (1973) found that increasing the separation in frequency between the two tones in a two-tone complex caused a lowering of the reflex threshold once a particular bandwidth was exceeded. These findings suggest that there is a **critical band** for the acoustic

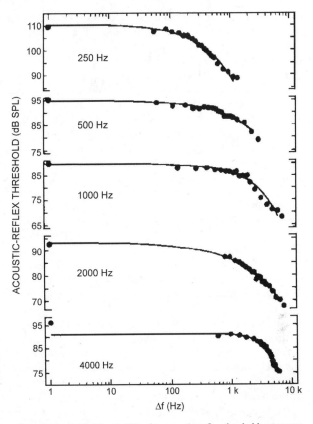

Figure 3.19 Critical bandwidths for acoustic reflex thresholds at center frequencies of 250 to 4000 Hz. Dots to the left of the functions show the corresponding pure-tone reflex thresholds. *Source*: From Popelka et al. (1976), with permission of *J. Acoust. Soc. Am.*

reflex, beyond which widening of the bandwidth results in lower thresholds.

Although the existence of a critical bandwidth was a consistent finding in the noise and two-tone studies, the thresholds were lower for noise. Popelka, Margolis, and Wiley (1976) replicated this work using tone complexes made up of many components that were equally spaced (on a logarithmic scale) in frequency. Their findings, which are shown in Fig. 3.19, confirm the critical band phenomenon. The width of the critical band (shown by the break from the horizontal on each function in Fig. 3.19) increases with center frequency. It is important to note that the critical bandwidth for the acoustic reflex is substantially wider than the psychoacoustic critical bands discussed in chapters that follow. However, Hellmann and Scharf (1984) pointed out that the differences between acoustic reflex and psychoacoustic critical bands may not be as substantial as has been supposed.

The acoustic reflex does not occur instantaneously upon the presentation of the activating signal. Instead, a measurable impedance change is observed after a **latency**, the length of which depends on both the intensity and frequency of the stimulus. Metz (1951) found that this latency decreased from about 150 ms at 80 dB above the threshold of hearing [dB sensation level (SL)] to 40 m at 100-dB SL in response to a 1000-Hz activating signal. Møller (1958) reported latencies of 25 to 130 ms for 500-Hz and 1500-Hz pure-tones. As a rule, latencies were shorter for 1500 Hz than for 500-Hz tones. Dallos (1964) found a similar inverse relationship between activator intensity and reflex latency for white noise. Hung and Dallos (1972) found that acoustic reflex latencies were shorter for noise signals than for pure-tones, with the longest latencies for tones below 300 Hz. The shortest latencies, on the order of 20 ms, were in response to noise activators.

These measurements were based upon changes in acoustic impedance. However, the latency of the impedance change reflects the *mechanical* response of the middle ear rather than of the *neural transport time* for the reflex arc alone (Borg, 1976). Zakrisson, Borg, and Blom (1974) found that the electromyographic (EMG) response of the stapedius muscle in humans is as short as 12 ms. They also reported that the EMG threshold is about 6 dB lower than that for the impedance change measured as the lowest stimulus level needed to yield 10% of the maximum response. Because we are concerned with the effect of the acoustic reflex on the transmission of energy through the middle ear (at least in this context), we are most interested in the mechanical-response latency. However, one should be aware that changes in muscle potentials occur in the stapedius prior to the measured impedance change.

We have already seen that acoustic reflex latency shortens with increasing stimulus intensity. Similarly, increasing stimulus level also causes an increase in reflex magnitude, which is the amount of impedance change associated with the reflex (Metz, 1951; Møller, 1958; Silman et al., 1978; Gelfand et al., 1981; Silman and Gelfand, 1981; Silman, 1984) and a faster rise time of the reflex response (Dallos, 1964; Hung and Dallos, 1972). The relationship between stimulus level and the resulting reflex magnitude is called the **acoustic reflex growth function**.

The acoustic reflex growth function has been studied in response to pure-tones and wide- and narrowband noise activating signals (Møller, 1962; Dallos, 1964; Hung and Dallos, 1972; Wilson and McBride, 1978; Silman et al., 1978; Gelfand et al., 1981; Silman and Gelfand, 1981; Silman, 1984). The reflex growth functions of four subjects studied by Hung and Dallos (1972) are presented in Fig. 3.20. It illustrates that the growth of acoustic reflex magnitude is essentially linear for pure-tones as high as about 120-dB SPL. The functions for wideband noise are essentially linear up to approximately 110-dB SPL. These data are substantially supported by the other studies cited. Thus, acoustic reflex magnitude tends to increase linearly with a stimulus intensity of 85- to 120-dB SPL for tones and roughly 70- to 110-dB SPL for wideband noise. Saturation occurs at higher levels.

Møller (1961, 1962) reported steeper reflex growth functions with increasing frequency in the 300- to 1500-Hz range. Flottrop et al. (1971) found greater impedance changes at 250 Hz than

at 4000 Hz. They also reported that although signals at 1000 and 2000 Hz elicited the same maximum reflex magnitude as at 250 Hz, about 10 dB more (re: reflex threshold) was needed for the two higher frequencies. Furthermore, while some have suggested that a 2000-Hz tone elicits the greatest impedance change (e.g., Kaplan, Gilman, and Dirks, 1977), others suggest that 1000-Hz and wideband stimuli produce maximal responses (Cunningham, 1976; Wilson and McBride, 1978). On the other hand, Borg and Møller (1968) found no significant differences in the slopes of acoustic reflex growth functions in the range from 500 to 3000 Hz in laboratory animals. It thus appears that a clear-cut relationship between activator frequency and reflex magnitude is not fully established.

Temporal summation deals with the relationship between stimulus duration and intensity when the time frame is less than about 1 s (see Chap. 9). It is most easily understood by example. Suppose a subject's threshold for a tone that lasts 200 ms happens to be 18 dB. Will the threshold remain at 18 dB when the same tone is presented for only 20 ms? It is found that when the 20-ms tone is used the threshold changes to 28 dB. (A similar trade-off is needed to maintain the stimulus at a constant loudness. This illustrates the general psychoacoustic observation that when a signal is shortened by a factor of 10 (e.g., from 200 to 20 ms), the signal level must be increased by as much as 10 dB to offset the decade decrease in duration. This relationship is understandably called a **time-intensity trade**.

Temporal summation also occurs for the acoustic reflex (Djupesland and Zwislocki, 1971; Djupesland et al., 1973; Woodford et al., 1975; Jerger et al., 1977; Gelfand et al., 1981). However, it appears that the amount of intensity change needed to counteract a given decrease in stimulus duration is greater for the acoustic reflex than for psychoacoustic phenomena. Figure 3.21 summarizes the general nature of temporal summation for the acoustic reflex (Woodford et al., 1975). Unfortunately, there are rather large differences between the results of various studies reporting the intensity needed to offset a given duration change. For example, decreasing the duration of a 2000-Hz tone from 100 to 10 ms was offset by an increase in stimulus level by about 25 dB in one study (Djupesland and Zwislocki, 1971) as opposed to roughly 15 dB in another (Woodford et al., 1975). In the 500- to 4000-Hz range, Djupesland et al. (1973) studied the time-intensity trade-off relation for the acoustic reflex with one-octave wide noise bands. They used as their comparison point the stimulus level/duration needed to maintain the reflex magnitude at half the maximum impedance change. Djupesland et al. found that a 10-fold decrease in duration was offset by a 20- to 25-dB increase in signal level. In contrast, Gnewikow [1974, cited by Jerger et al. (1977)] found that a 12- to 23-dB intensity increase was needed to offset decade reductions in duration for 500- and 4000-Hz pure-tones. Jerger et al. (1977) found less temporal summation than the other studies, as shown in Fig. 3.22 for 500-, 1000-, 2000-, and 4000-Hz stimuli. Note that the amount of temporal integration increases with frequency, which

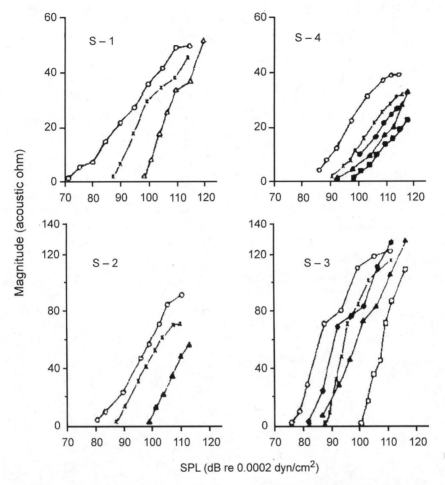

Figure 3.20 Reflex growth functions for wideband noise (*open circles*) and pure-tones (250 Hz, *open squares*; 300 Hz, *filled squares*; 500 Hz, *filled triangles*; 600 Hz, *open tri angles*; 1000 Hz, *crosses*; 1500 Hz, *filled circles*). *Source*: From Hung and Dallos (1972), with permission of *J. Acoust. Soc. Am.*

is a common finding among studies. Jerger et al. (1977) suggested that at least some of the differences are due to problems associated with the "visual detection threshold" (the smallest noticeable impedance change on a meter or oscilloscope), and with "constant percentage of maximum impedance change" methods (Djupesland et al., 1973) of obtaining the data.

Early studies on laboratory animals showed that the degree of muscle contraction due to the acoustic reflex decreases as stimulation is prolonged (Kato, 1913; Lorente de Nó, 1935). This decrease in acoustic reflex magnitude over time is referred to as **reflex decay** or **adaptation**, and it has been found in humans (Dallos, 1964; Borg, 1968; Tietze, 1969a,1969b; Wiley and Karlovich, 1975; Kaplan, Gilman, and Dirks, 1977; Wilson, McCollough, and Lilly, 1984a; Wilson, Shanks, and Lilly 1984b). An extensive review of this topic is provided by Wilson et al. (1984b). In spite of differences among studies, the common finding is that reflex adaptation increases as the frequency of a pure-tone stimulus is raised.

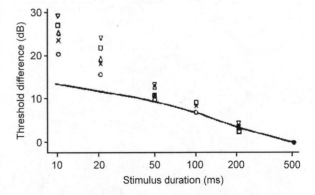

Figure 3.21 Temporal summation for the acoustic reflex threshold. This figure shows the trade-off between activator signal duration and level at 500 Hz (*crosses*), 1000 Hz (*circles*), 2000 Hz (*triangles*), 3000 Hz (*squares*), and 4000 Hz (*inverted triangles*). A typical psychoacoustic temporal summation function is represented by the solid line for comparison. *Source*: From Woodford, Henderson, Hamernick, and Feldman (1975), with permission.

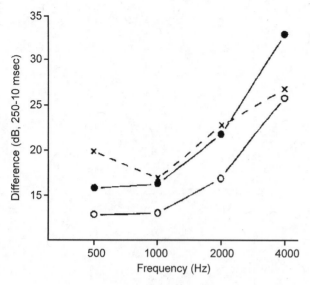

Particular attention should be given to the findings of Kaplan et al. (1977), who studied acoustic reflex adaptation to pure-tones of 500 to 4000 Hz, which were presented at levels of 6, 12, and 18 dB above the reflex threshold. Figure 3.23 summarizes their median data at three sensation levels re: reflex threshold, with stimulus frequency as the parameter. [**Sensation level (SL)** more properly refers to the number of dB above one's threshold of *hearing*. However, in the context of the acoustic reflex, SL is also used to refer to the number of dB above the *reflex* threshold.] There is greater reflex adaptation as frequency increases. Also, adaptation tends to begin sooner after stimulus onset for higher frequencies. These data are normalized in Fig. 3.24, in which the point of greatest impedance change is given a value of 100% and the other points are shown as percentages of the maximum impedance change. In this plot, the data are shown separately at each frequency, with the suprathreshold level as the parameter. In addition to clearly showing the frequency effect, Fig. 3.24 demonstrates that the course of the adaptation function is similar at various levels above reflex threshold, at least up to +18 dB.

Tietze (1969a,1969b) proposed that the course of acoustic reflex adaptation could be described by the time constants of reflex rise time and adaptation. These time constants refer

Figure 3.22 Temporal summation for the acoustic reflex at four frequencies obtained by Jerger et al. (1977) (*open circles*), Gnewikow (1974) (*filled circles*), and Woodford et al. (1975) (*crosses*). *Source*: From Jerger, Mauldin, and Lewis (1977). Temporal summation of the acoustic reflex, *Audiology* 16, 177–200, with permission.

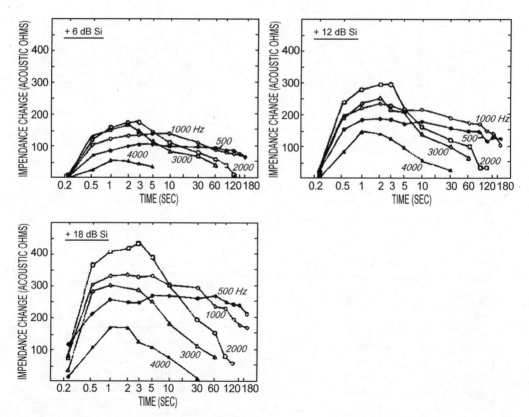

Figure 3.23 Median absolute impedance change (in acoustic ohms) as a function of time for three levels above the acoustic reflex threshold. *Source*: From Kaplan et al. (1977), with permission of *Ann. Otol.*

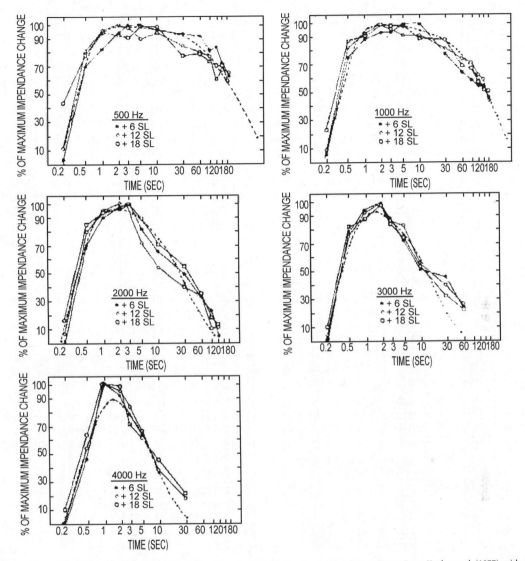

Figure 3.24 Median normalized impedance change (in percent) as a function of time for each frequency. *Source*: From Kaplan et al. (1977), with permission of *Ann. Otol.*

respectively to how long it takes for reflex magnitude to attain 63% of the maximum value (rise) and then to decrease to 63% of it (adaptation); both are measured from the moment of acoustic reflex onset. The time constants are functions of frequency. Tietz's model describes reflex adaptation by the formula

$$Zn = \frac{1}{1 - \tau_{an}/\tau_{ab}} \left[\exp\left(-t/\tau_{ab}\right) - \exp\left(-t/\tau_{an}\right) \right] \quad (3.1)$$

where Zn is the normalized maximum impedance change; τ_{an} and τ_{ab} are the time constants of reflex rise and adaptation, respectively; and t is the time (in seconds) of reflex rise from onset. Kaplan et al. (1977) applied this formula to their data, using the ratio τ_{an}/τ_{ab} to generate the dotted lines in Fig. 3.24.

(Note that, except at high frequencies where rapid adaptation reduces the maximum impedance change, τ_{an} is generally quite small relative to τ_{ab}.) As Fig. 3.24 shows, the data of Kaplan et al. support the exponential adaptation predicted by Tietze's model.

Loudness is the perceptual correlate of the intensity of the acoustic stimulus (see Chap. 11); other things being equal, loudness increases as stimulus level is increased. An aberration of the intensity–loudness relationship is found in patients with cochlear disorders. Once the signal is increased above the impaired threshold of such an ear, the loudness grows at a faster rate than normal in response to increasing stimulus level. This is called **loudness recruitment**. What has the acoustic reflex to do with loudness and recruitment? Because both loudness and the acoustic reflex are related to stimulus intensity, at least some association between them is understandable. The question is whether the acoustic reflex is a function of loudness.

Metz (1952) obtained acoustic reflex thresholds at lower SLs from patients with presumably cochlear sensorineural hearing loss than from normal subjects. In other words, the spread between the threshold of hearing and the acoustic reflex threshold was smaller for those with the hearing losses. Because the impaired subjects also had loudness recruitment, Metz proposed that the lower SL of the reflex reflected recruitment. In other words, it was argued that the acoustic reflex was elicited by the loudness of the signal. Jepsen (1963) also attributed acoustic reflex findings in patients with sensorineural hearing losses to be the result of recruitment.

The relationship between loudness and the acoustic reflex, however, is not nearly as clear-cut as these early findings suggest. Ross (1968) compared the equal-loudness and equal-reflex contours of four subjects. The contours were similar for two, while the others had systematic differences between the loudness and acoustic reflex contours (the loudness curves were flatter). Ross suggested that the latter two equal-loudness contours might have been aberrant, but in fact they were quite similar to those reported by Fletcher and Munson (1933), among others.

Margolis and Popelka (1975) compared the loudness of a variety of stimuli set to the acoustic reflex threshold level. There was a range of about 17 dB in the loudness levels, suggesting that the acoustic reflex is not a manifestation of a critical loudness level. Block and Wightman (1977) suggested that the loudness–reflex relationship is supported by their finding of similarly shaped equal-loudness and equal-reflex contours. However, they often found that the same reflex magnitude was elicited by stimulus levels as much as 10 dB apart. Such a spread corresponds to a doubling of loudness (Stevens, 1956); in this light, their findings appear to support rather than refute those of Margolis and Popelka. The substantially wider critical bands for the acoustic reflex than for loudness discussed previously provide a further basis for questioning the concept that the acoustic reflex is loudness-based.

Returning to patient data, Beedle and Harford (1973) found steeper acoustic reflex growth functions for normal ears than for ears with cochlear dysfunction. This result is, of course, inconsistent with a loudness basis for the reflex. The impact of their data, however, was impaired by the fact that their normal subjects averaged 24 years old, compared to 47 years old for the pathological group. The reflex growth functions of age-matched normal and hearing-impaired subjects were studied by Silman, Popelka, and Gelfand (1978). Examples of their findings are shown in Fig. 3.25. If the reflex were loudness-determined, then the function for the impaired groups, although displaced along the intensity axis, would be expected to approach the normal curves at higher stimulus levels. This expectation is based on the notion that loudness recruitment should result in equal loudness for both groups at equal suprathreshold levels. Equal loudness would in turn elicit equal reflex magnitudes at those levels. As Fig. 3.25 shows, this was not the case.

Hellman and Scharf (1984) argued that the case against a loudness–reflex relationship is not as convincing as it might seem. Just two examples will be briefly mentioned. Consider first the material in Fig. 3.25, just discussed. These data could be explained by the fact that both loudness and reflex magnitude increase as power functions of the stimulus level at the SPLs where these functions are obtained. Second, they demonstrated that for given subjects, equally loud sounds elicited equal reflex magnitudes when the criteria were defined precisely.

Given that both loudness and the acoustic reflex reflect the neural coding of the stimulus level at the periphery, it is thus understandable that the two phenomena should be related. The controversial and unresolved issue is whether one is dependent upon the other. It is apparent that the acoustic reflex is largely stimulus-dependent. Furthermore, it should not be surprising that the parameters of the reflex response reflect the sensory (and neural) processing of relatively intense stimulation. It is equally apparent that the acoustic reflex is a feedback or control mechanism, although its exact purpose(s) remains unclear. Given these points, what effect does the acoustic reflex have on energy transmission through the conductive mechanism?

Recall that the acoustic reflex stiffens the conductive mechanism so that sound is reflected at the eardrum (Dallos, 1964). Because the effect of stiffness is inversely related to frequency, we would expect the acoustic reflex to affect middle ear transmission most strongly at lower frequencies.

Smith (1943) and Reger (1960) compared the pure-tone thresholds of human subjects to the thresholds during voluntary contractions of the middle ear muscles. Thresholds were shifted by about 20 to 40 dB at 125 to 500 Hz, and by 15 dB at 1000 Hz, and there was little or no change at higher frequencies. While the expected frequency relation is maintained, voluntary contractions may not yield the same transmission loss as the acoustic reflex (Reger, 1960). Perhaps the most impressive data on how the acoustic reflex affects middle ear transmission come from animal studies.

The transmission loss produced by the acoustic reflex has been studied in animals by monitoring the resulting changes in the magnitude of the cochlear microphonic (e.g., Simmons, 1959; Møller, 1964, 1965; Nuttall, 1974). (The cochlear microphonic is an electrical potential of the cochlea, which is proportional to the intensity of the stimulus over a wide dynamic range; it is discussed in the next chapter.) Figure 3.26 shows the changes in the cochlear microphonic magnitude as a function of frequency due to stapedius muscle contraction in the cat, obtained by Møller (1965). He found that impedance change data and cochlear microphonic findings in response to the acoustic reflex were within 5 dB over a substantial portion of the frequency range. The figure shows that the acoustic reflex affects primarily the frequencies below about 2000 Hz. Low-frequency changes have also been reported in response to contractions of the tensor tympani muscle (e.g., Starr, 1969; Nuttall, 1974).

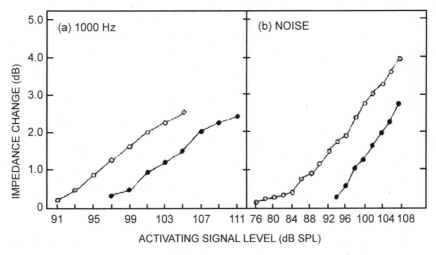

Figure 3.25 Reflex growth as a function of activator level in dB SPL for (a) a 1000-Hz tone and (b) a broadband noise. Open symbols, normal ears; closed symbols, impaired ears. *Source*: Adapted from Silman, Popelka, and Gelfand (1978).

Several studies have addressed the effects of middle ear muscle contractions on absolute thresholds and loudness in humans (Smith, 1946; Loeb and Riopelle, 1960; Morgan and Dirks, 1975; Morgan, Dirks, and Kamm, 1978; Rabinowitz, 1976), albeit with mixed results. For example, Rabinowitz (1976) reported a 10-dB change in the low-frequency transmission characteristics of the middle ear due to the acoustic reflex, but Morgan et al. (1978) found that absolute thresholds were not affected by the acoustic reflex. Morgan and Dirks (1975) found that the acoustic reflex caused a change in the loudness of a test tone presented to the opposite ear when the reflex-eliciting stimulus was greater than 100-dB SPL, but not for lower activator levels.

Middle Ear Muscle Theories

There are many theories and speculations about the purpose of the middle ear muscles and the acoustic reflex. Space and scope preclude more than a cursory review here; and the reader

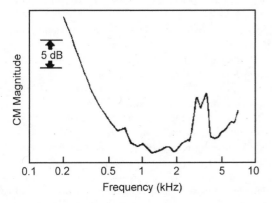

Figure 3.26 Effect of the acoustic reflex on transmission in the cat's middle ear. *Source*: Adapted from Møller (1965), with permission.

should see the discussions by Simmons (1964); Jepsen (1963); and Borg, Counter, and Rosler (1984).

Because the reflex is elicited by relatively high stimulus levels and its magnitude grows with increasing stimulus level, one would expect that a primary purpose of the acoustic reflex would be protection of the cochlea from damaging stimulation. This *protection theory* is limited by the latency and adaptation of the reflex, causing it to respond too slowly to sudden sounds, and making it inefficient against prolonged sounds. Nevertheless, protection against injury to hearing is still a beneficial effect of the acoustic reflex, even if it is not the main purpose.

The *accommodation theory* states that the action of the two middle ear muscles modifies the conductive mechanism so as to optimize the absorption of sound energy. According to the *ossicular fixation theory*, the intratympanic muscles help keep the ossicles in proper position and appropriately rigid, particularly at high frequencies, where acceleration is great. Other theories have asserted that these muscles contribute to changes in labyrinthine pressure and to the formation of aural overtones.

Simmons (1964) found a sharp antiresonance peak around 4000 Hz in the middle ear transmission function of cats whose intratympanic muscles were removed, as well as in normal cats under anesthesia. Normal, waking cats whose intratympanic muscles have normal tonus showed greatly reduced dips in this region. In his *perceptual theory*, Simmons reasoned that tonus of the middle ear muscles smoothes the frequency response of the conductive system. He suggested that modulation of muscle tonus would have the effect of enhancing attention by changing the intensity and frequency characteristics of environmental sounds. This modulation would be analogous to the constant motion of the extraocular muscles in vision. Also, several skeletal movements as well as unexpected and novel environmental sounds elicit the acoustic reflex. Because the reflex mainly attenuates low frequencies, and most of an organism's own physiological noises are low in frequency, such a reflex response would have the effect of reducing the animal's internal noise. A better signal-to-noise ratio would result, which is of obvious importance to the survival of any species, whether predator or prey. This idea agrees with Borg's (1976) position that the qualitative purpose of the acoustic reflex is to attenuate low-frequency sounds, thereby improving the auditory system's dynamic range.

The *desensitization–interference–injury protection theory* proposed by Borg et al. (1984) explained that the middle ear muscles and the acoustic reflex have multiple purposes: (1) Contractions of the intratympanic muscles are elicited by eating, talking, yelling, and other vocalizations. The muscle contractions alleviate *desensitization* because they reduce the noises produced by these activities, which would have otherwise compromised the alertness and the sensitivity to salient aspects of the acoustical environment. (2) *Interference* is reduced because contractions of the middle ear muscles cause the low frequencies to be attenuated, thereby reducing the extent to which they mask the higher frequencies (e.g., reducing the masking produced by one's own speech). (3) Finally, middle ear muscle contractions provide *injury protection* by attenuating intense sounds reaching the inner ear.

REFERENCES

Barany, E. 1938. A contribution to the physiology of bone conduction. *Acta Otol* Suppl 26, 1–223.

Beedle, RK, Harford, ER. 1973. A comparison of acoustic reflex growth in normal and pathological ears. *J Speech Hear Res* 16, 271–280.

Bekesy, G. 1932. Zur Theorie des Hören bei der Schallaufnahme durch Knochenleitung. *Ann Physik* 13, 111–136.

Bekesy, G. 1936. Zur Physik des Mittelohres und über das Hören bei fehlerhaftem Trommelfell. *Akust Zeitschr* 1, 13–23.

Bekesy, G. 1941. Über die Messung der Schwingungsamplitude der Gehörknöchelchen mittels einer kapazitiven Sonde. *Akust Zeitschr* 6, 1–16.

Bekesy, G. 1948. Vibrations of the head in a sound field and its role in hearing by bone conduction. *J Acoust Soc Am* 20, 749–760.

Bekesy, G. 1960/1989. *Experiments in Hearing*. New York, NY: McGraw-Hill. [Republished by the Acoustical Society of America].

Bekesy, G, Rosenblith, WA. 1958. The mechanical properties of the ear. In: SS Stevens (ed.), *Handbook of Experimental Psychology*. New York, NY: Wiley, 1075–1115.

Bennett, M. 1984. Impedance concepts relating to the acoustic reflex. In: S Silman (ed.), *The Acoustic Reflex*. New York, NY: Academic Press, 35–61.

Blauert, J. 1997. *Special Hearing: The Psychophysics of Human Sound Localization*. Revised Edition. Cambridge, MA: MIT Press.

Block, MG, Wightman, FL. 1977. A statistically based measure of the acoustic reflex and its relation to stimulus loudness. *J Acoust Soc Am* 61, 120–125.

Borg, E. 1968. A quantitative study of the effects of the acoustic stapedius reflex on sound transmission through the middle ear. *Acta Otol* 66, 461–472.

Borg, E. 1976. Dynamic characteristics of the intra-aural muscle reflex. In: AS Feldman, LA Wilber (eds.), *Acoustic Impedance and Admittance*. Baltimore: Williams Wilkins, 236–299.

Borg, E, Counter, SA, Rosler, G. 1984. Theories of middle-ear muscle function. In: S Silman (ed.), *The Acoustic Reflex*. New York, NY: Academic Press, 63–99.

Borg, E, Møller, A. 1968. The acoustic middle ear reflex in man and in anesthetized rabbits. *Acta Otol* 65, 575–585.

Bosatra, A, Russolo, M, Silverman, CA. 1984. Acoustic—reflex latency: State of the art. In: S Silman (ed.), *The Acoustic Reflex*. New York, NY: Academic Press, 301–328.

Carhart, R. 1950. Clinical application of bone conduction audiometry. *Arch Otol* 51, 798–808.

Cunningham, D. 1976. Admittance values associated with acoustic reflex decay. *J Acoust Soc Am* 1, 197–205.

Dallos, P. 1964. Dynamics of the acoustic reflex: Phenomenological aspects. *J Acoust Soc Am* 36, 2175–2183.

Dallos, P. 1970. Low-frequency auditory characteristics: Species dependencies. *J Acoust Soc Am* 48, 489–499.

Dallos, P. 1973. *The Auditory Periphery*. New York, NY: Academic Press.

Decraemer, WF, Khanna, SM, Funnell, WRL. 1991. Malleus vibration mode changes with frequency. *Hear Res* 54, 305–318.

Decraemer, WF, Khanna, SM, Funnell, WRL. 1994. A method for determining three-dimensional vibration in the ear. *Hear Res* 77, 19–37.

Djupesland, G. 1964. Middle ear muscle reflexes elicited by acoustic and nonacoustic stimulation. *Acta Otol* Suppl 188, 287–292.

Djupesland, G, Sundby, A, Flottrop, G. 1973. Temporal summation in the acoustic stapedius reflex mechanism. *Acta Otol* 76, 305–312.

Djupesland, G, Zwislocki, J. 1971. Effect on temporal summation on the human stapedius reflex. *Acta Otol* 71, 262–265.

Djupesland, G, Zwislocki, J. 1973. On the critical band in the acoustic stapedius reflex. *J Acoust Soc Am* 54, 1157–1159.

Dutsch, L. 1972. The threshold of the stapedius reflex for pure-tone and noise stimuli. *Acta Otol* 74, 248–251.

Feldman, A. 1967. A report of further impedance studies of the acoustic reflex. *J Speech Hear Res* 10, 616–622.

Fletcher, H, Munson, WA. 1933. Loudness: Its definition, measurement and calculation. *J Acoust Soc Am* 5, 82–108.

Flottrop, G, Djupesland, G, Winther, F. 1971. The acoustic stapedius reflex in relation to critical bandwidth. *J Acoust Soc Am* 49, 457–461.

Gardner, MB, Gardner, RS. 1973. Problems of localization in the medial plane: Effect of pinnae cavity occlusion. *J Acoust Soc Am* 53, 400–408.

Gelfand, SA. 1984. The contralateral acoustic—reflex threshold. In: S Silman (ed.), *The Acoustic Reflex*. New York, NY: Academic Press, 137–186.

Gelfand, SA, Silman, S, Silverman, CA. 1981. Temporal summation in acoustic reflex growth functions. *Acta Otol* 91, 177–182.

Green, KW, Margolis, RH. 1984. The ipsilateral acoustic reflex. In: S Silman (ed.), *The Acoustic Reflex*. New York, NY: Academic Press, 275–299.

Guinan, J, Peake, WT. 1967. Middle ear characteristics of anesthetized cats. *J Acoust Soc Am* 41, 1237–1261.

Hellman, R, Scharf, B. 1984. Acoustic reflex and loudness. In: S Silman (ed.), *The Acoustic Reflex*. New York, NY: Academic Press, 469–516.

Helmholtz, H. 1868. Die Mechanik der Gehorknochelchen und des Trommelfells. *Pflugers Arch Ges Physiol I*, 1–60.

Hensen, V. 1878. Beobachtungen uber die Thatigkeit des Trommellspanners bei Hund und Katze. *Arch Anat Physiol II*, 312–319.

Huizing, EH. 1960. Bone conduction—The influence of the middle ear. Acta Otol Suppl 155, 1–99.

Hung, I, Dallos, P. 1972. Study of the acoustic reflex in human beings: I. Dynamic characteristics. *J Acoust Soc Am* 52, 1168–1180.

Jepsen, O. 1955. *Studies on the acoustic stapedius reflex in man: Measurements of the acoustic impedance of the tympanic membrane in normal individuals and in patients with peripheral facial palsy* [Thesis], Universitetsforlaget, Aarhus, Denmark.

Jepsen, O. 1963. The middle ear muscle reflexes in man. In: J Jerger (ed.), *Modern Developments in Audiology*. New York, NY: Academic Press, 194–239.

Jerger, J. 1970. Clinical experience with impedance audiometry. *Arch Otol* 92, 311–321.

Jerger, J, Mauldin, L, Lewis, N. 1977. Temporal summation of the acoustic reflex. *Audiology* 16, 177–200.

Kaplan, H, Gilman, S, Dirks, D. 1977. Properties of acoustic reflex adaptation. *Ann Otol* 86, 348–356.

Kato, T. 1913. Zur Physiologie der Binnenmuskeln des Ohres. *Pflugers Arch Physiol* 150, 569–625.

Klockhoff, I. 1961. Middle-ear muscle reflexes in man. *Acta Otol Suppl.* 164.

Lindsay, JR, Kobrack, H, Perlman, HB. 1936. Relation of the stapedius reflex to hearing sensitivity in man. *Arch Otol* 23, 671–678.

Loeb, M, Riopelle, AJ. 1960. Influence of loud contralateral stimulation on the threshold and perceived loudness of low-frequency tones. *J Acoust Soc Am* 32, 602–610.

Lorente de Nó, R. 1935. The function of the central acoustic nuclei examined by means of the acoustic reflexes. *Laryngoscope* 45, 573–595.

Lowy, K. 1942. Cancellation of the electrical cochlear response with air- and bone-conduction. *J Acoust Soc Am* 14, 156–158.

Luscher, E. 1929. Die Function des Musculus stapedius beim Menschen. *Zeitschr Hals Nasen Ohrenheilk* 23, 105–132.

Margolis, R, Popelka, G. 1975. Loudness and the acoustic reflex. *J Acoust Soc Am* 58, 1330–1332.

Margolis, RH, Van Camp, J, Wilson, RH, Creten, WL. 1985. Multifrequency tympanometry in normal ears. *Audiology* 24, 44–53.

Mehrgardt, S, Mellert, V. 1977. Transformation characteristics of the external human ear. *J Acoust Soc Am* 61, 1567–1576.

Mendelson, ES. 1957. A sensitive method for registration of human intratympanic muscle reflexes. *J Appl Physiol* 11, 499–502.

Mendelson, ES. 1961. Improved method for studying tympanic reflexes in man. *J Acoust Soc Am* 33, 146–152.

Metz, O. 1946. The acoustic impedance measured on normal and pathological ears. *Acta Otol* 63(Suppl), 3–254.

Metz, O. 1951. Studies on the contraction of the tympanic muscles as indicated by changes in impedance of the ear. *Acta Otol* 39, 397–405.

Metz, O. 1952. Threshold of reflex contractions of muscles of the middle ear and recruitment of loudness. *Arch Otol* 55, 536–593.

Middlebrooks, JC. 1999. Individual differences in external ear transfer functions reduced by scaling in frequency. *J Acoust Soc Am* 106, 1480–1492.

Miller, JD, Watson, CS, Covell, WP. 1963. Deafening effects of noise on the cat. *Acta Otol* 176(Suppl), 1–91.

Møller, A. 1958. Intra-aural muscle contraction in man examined by measuring acoustic impedance of the ear. *Laryngoscope* 68, 48–62.

Møller, A. 1961. Bilateral contraction of the tympanic muscles in man examined by measuring acoustic impedance-change. *Ann Otol* 70, 735–753.

Møller, AR. 1960. Improved technique for detailed measurements of the middle ear impedance. *J Acoust Soc Am* 32, 250–257.

Møller, AR. 1962. The sensitivity of contraction of tympanic muscle in man. *Ann Otol* 71, 86–95.

Møller, AR. 1964. Effects of tympanic muscle activity on movement of the ear drum, acoustic impedance, and cochlear microphonics. *Acta Otol* 58, 525–534.

Møller, AR. 1965. An experimental study of the acoustic impedance and its transmission properties *Acta Otol* 60, 129–149.

Morgan, DE, Dirks, DD. 1975. Influence of middle ear muscle contraction on pure-tone suprathreshold loudness judgments. *J Acoust Soc Am* 57, 411–420.

Morgan, D.E, Dirks, DD, Kamm, C. 1978. The influence of middle-ear contraction on auditory threshold for selected pure-tones. *J Acoust Soc Am* 63, 1896–1903.

Nedzelnitsky, V. 1980. Sound pressures in the basal turn of the cat cochlea. *J Acoust Soc Am* 68, 1676–1689.

Naunton, R. 1963. The measurement of hearing by bone conduction. In: J Jerger (ed.), *Modern Developments in Audiology*. New York, NY: Academic Press, 1–29.

Nuttall, AL. 1974. Tympanic muscle effects on middle-ear transfer characteristic. *J Acoust Soc Am* 56, 1239–1247.

Oldfield, SR, Parker, PA. 1984. Acuity of sound localization: A topography of auditory space. II. Pinna cues absent. *Perception* 13, 601–617.

Peterson, JL, Liden, G. 1972. Some static characteristics of the stapedial muscle reflex. *Audiology* 11, 97–114.

Plenge, G. 1974. On the difference between localization and lateralization. *J Acoust Soc Am* 56, 944–951.

Pollack, J. 1886. Uber die Function des Musculus tensor tympani. *Med Jahrbuch* 82, 555–582.

Popelka, G, Karlovich, R, Wiley, T. 1974. Acoustic reflex and critical bandwidth. *J Acoust Soc Am* 55, 883–885.

Popelka, G, Margolis, R, Wiley, T. 1976. Effects of activating signal bandwidth on acoustic-reflex thresholds. *J Acoust Soc Am* 59, 153–159.

Potter, AB 1936. Function of the stapedius muscle. *Ann Otol* 45, 639–643.

Rabinowitz, WM. 1976. *Acoustic-Reflex Effects on the Input Admittance and Transfer Characteristics of the Human Middle-Ear* [unpublished Ph.D. Dissertation]. Cambridge, MA: MIT Press.

Reger, SN. 1960. Effect of middle ear muscle action on certain psycho-physical measurements. *Ann Otol* 69, 1179–1198.

Rosowski, JJ. 1991. The effects of external- and middle-ear filtering on auditory threshold and noise-induced hearing loss. *J Acoust Soc Am* 90, 124–135.

Ross, S. 1968. On the relation between the acoustic reflex and loudness. *J Acoust Soc Am* 43, 768–779.

Shaw, EAG. 1974. Transformation of sound pressure level from the free field to the eardrum in the horizontal plane. *J Acoust Soc Am* 56, 1848–1861.

Shaw, EAG. 1997. Acoustical features of the external ear. In: R Gilkey, T Anderson (eds.), *Binaural and Spacial Hearing in Real and Virtual Environments*. Hillsdale, NJ: Erlbaum, 25–47.

Shaw, EAG, Vaillancourt, MM. 1985. Transformation of sound-pressure level from the free field to the eardrum presented in numerical form. *J Acoust Soc Am* 78, 1120–1123.

Silman, S. 1984. Magnitude and growth of the acoustic reflex. In: S Silman (ed.), *The Acoustic Reflex*. New York, NY: Academic Press, 225–274.

Silman, S, Gelfand, SA. 1981. Effect of sensorineural hearing loss on the stapedius reflex growth function in the elderly. *J Acoust Soc Am* 69, 1099–1106.

Silman, S, Popelka, S, Gelfand, SA. 1978. Effect of sensorineural hearing loss on acoustic stapedius reflex growth functions. *J Acoust Soc Am* 64, 1406–1411.

Simmons, FB 1959. Middle ear muscle activity at moderate sound levels. *Ann Otol* 68, 1126–1143.

Simmons, FB. 1964. Perceptual theories of middle ear function. *Ann Otol* 73, 724–740.

Smith, HD. 1943. Audiometric effects of voluntary contraction of the tensor tympani muscle. *Arch Otol* 38, 369–373.

Smith, HD. 1946. Audiometric effects of voluntary contraction of the tensor tympani muscles. *Arch Otol* 38, 369–372.

Starr, A. 1969. Regulatory mechanisms of the auditory pathway. In: S Locke (ed.), *Modern Neurology*. Boston, MA: Little, Brown.

Stenfelt, S, Hato, N, Goode, RL. 2002. Factors contributing to bone conduction: The middle ear. *J Acoust Soc Am* 111, 947–959.

Stenfelt, S, Wild, T, Hato, N, Goode, RL. 2003. Factors contributing to bone conduction: The outer ear. *J Acoust Soc Am* 113, 902–913.

Stepp, CE, Voss, SE. (2005). Acoustics of the human middle-ear air space. *J Acoust Soc Am* 118, 861–871.

Stevens, SS. 1956. The direct estimation of sensory magnitude—Loudness. *Am J Psychol* 69, 1–25.

Stinton, MR, Lawton, DW. 1989. Specification of the geometry of the human ear canal for the prediction of sound-pressure level distribution. *J Acoust Soc Am* 85, 2492–2530.

Terkildsen, K. 1957. Movements of the eardrum following interaural muscle reflexes. *Arch Otol* 66, 484–488.

Terkildsen, K. 1960. Acoustic reflexes of the human musculus tensor tympani. *Acta Otol* Suppl. 158, 230–236.

Terkildsen, K, Nielsen, SS. 1960. An electroacoustic measuring bridge for clinical use. *Arch Otol* 72, 339–346.

Tietze, G. 1969a. Zum zeitverhalten des akustischen reflexes bei reizung mit dauertonen. *Arch Klin Exp Ohren Nasen Kehlkoopfheilkd* 193, 43–52.

Tietze, G. 1969b. Einge eigenschaften des akustischen reflexes bei reizung mit tonimpulsen. *Arch Klin Exp Ohren Nasen KehlkopfFeilkd* 193, 53–69.

Tonndorf, J. 1962. Compressional bone conduction in cochlear models. *J Acoust Soc Am* 34, 1127–1132.

Tonndorf, J. 1966. Bone conduction: Studies in experimental animals—A collection of papers. *Acta Otol* Suppl 213, 1–32.

Tonndorf, J. 1968. A new concepts of bone conduction. *Arch Otol* 87, 49–54.

Tonndorf, J, Khanna, SM. 1970. The role of the tympanic membrane in middle ear transmission. *Ann Otol* 79, 743–753.

Tonndorf, J, Khanna, SM, Fingerhood, BJ. 1966. The input impedance of the inner ear in cats. *Ann Otol* 75, 752–763.

Wever, EG, Lawrence, M. 1954. *Physiological Acoustics*. Princeton, NJ: Princeton University Press.

Wiener, FN, Pfeiffer, RR, Backus, ASN. 1966. On the pressure transformation by the head and auditory meatus of the cat. *Acta Otol* 61, 255–269.

Wiener, FM, Ross, DA. 1946. The pressure distribution in the auditory canal in a progressive sound field. *J Acoust Soc Am* 18, 401–408.

Wiley, TL, Karlovich, TS. 1975. Acoustic reflex response to sustained signals. *J Speech Hear Res* 18, 148–157.

Wilson, RH, McBride, LM. 1978. Threshold and growth of the acoustic reflex. *J Acoust Soc Am* 63, 147–154.

Wilson, RH, McCollough, JK, Lilly, DJ. 1984a. Acoustic reflex adaptation: Morphology and half-life data for subjects with normal hearing. *J Speech Hear Res* 27, 586–595.

Wilson, RH, Shanks, JE, Lilly, DJ. 1984b. Acoustic-reflex adaptation. In: S Silman (ed.), *The Acoustic Reflex*. New York, NY: Academic Press, 329–386.

Woodford, C, Henderson, D, Hamernick, R, Feldman, A. 1975. Threshold duration function of the acoustic reflex in man. *Audiology* 14, 53–62.

Zakrisson, JE, Borg, E, Blom, S. 1974. The acoustic impedance change as a measure of stapedius muscle activity in man: A methodological study with electromyography. *Acta Otol* 78, 357–364.

Zwislocki, J. 1962. Analysis of the middle-ear function. Part I: Input impedance. *J Acoust Soc Am* 34, 1514–1523.

Zwislocki, J. 1963. An acoustic method for clinical examination of the ear. *J Speech Hear Res* 6, 303–314.

Zwislocki, J. 1975. The role of the external and middle ear in sound transmission. In: DB Tower, EL. Eagles (eds.), *The Nervous System. Vol. 3: Human Communication and Its Disorders.* New York, NY: Raven Press, 45–55.

Zwislocki, J. 1976. The acoustic middle ear function. In: AS Feldman, LA, Wilber (eds.), *Acoustic Impedance and Admittance—The Measurement of Middle Ear Function.* Baltimore, MD: Williams & Wilkins. 66–77.

4   Cochlear Mechanisms and Processes

We have already discussed the manner in which the conductive mechanism influences the signal and transmits it to the inner ear. In this chapter we will concentrate upon the sensory mechanism. The cochlea may be conceived of as a transducer that converts the vibratory stimulus into a form usable by the nervous system. However, this is far from the whole picture. We shall see that the cochlea performs a considerable amount of analysis, that it is the major source of aural distortion, and that it is involved in processes that are active as well as passive.

Before proceeding to examine the processes of the cochlea, it is desirable to briefly review the traditional theories of hearing as well as some principles of sensory receptor action. These two topics provide a useful general framework as well as an important historical perspective within which the student can consider the material that follows.

CLASSICAL THEORIES OF HEARING

The study of the auditory system is practically and historically intertwined with the traditional theories of hearing. Broadly speaking, these theories fall into two general categories—place (resonance) theories and frequency (temporal, periodicity) theories—as well as the combined place-frequency theory. A detailed review of these theories goes beyond the current scope or intent; the student is referred to Wever's classical work *Theory of Hearing Hearing* (1949) for an excellent review of these theories.

Classical Resonance Theory

Although place or resonance theories existed since the beginning of the 1600s, modern versions began with the **resonance theory** proposed by Helmholtz (1870). Helmholtz relied to a large extent upon **Ohm's auditory law** and **Müller's doctrine of specific nerve energies**. Ohm's auditory law states that the ear performs a Fourier analysis upon complex periodic sounds; that is, that it breaks the complex wave down into its components regardless of their phase relationships. A major problem with Ohm's auditory law is that it precludes temporal analysis. We shall see, however, that the auditory system is sensitive to temporal as well as frequency parameters. Müller's doctrine refers to the specificity of the different senses. It states that the neural signal coming from the ear is interpreted as sound whether the actual stimulus was a tone or a blow to the head; the eye elicits a visual image whether the stimulus is light or pressure on the eyeball, etc. The doctrine appears to hold on the periphery, although there are dramatic commonalities among the various senses in terms of their fundamental principles of operation (see section "Action of Sensory Receptors," below) and central mechanisms.

The resonance place theory proposed by Helmholtz assumes that the basilar membrane is composed of a series of tuned segments, each of which resonates in response to a particular frequency. Thus, an incoming stimulus results in the vibration of those parts of the basilar membrane whose natural frequencies correspond to the components of the stimulus. Since these resonators are arranged by place along the cochlear partition, the precise place of the vibrating segment would signal the existence of a component at the natural frequency of that location. Nonlinear distortions introduced by the ear (such as combination tones due to the interaction of two stimulus tones, or harmonics of the stimulus tone) were viewed as being generated by a nonlinear response of the middle ear mechanism. These distortion products are then transmitted to the cochlea, where they cause vibrations at the places whose resonant frequencies correspond to the frequency of the combination tone (or harmonic). The distortion product is thus perceived as though it were present in the original signal.

Such a strict resonance theory is faced with several serious problems. To begin with, in order to account for the sharp frequency tuning of the inner ear, the theory demands that the basilar membrane contains segments that are under differing amounts of tension in a manner analogous to the tension on variously tuned piano strings. However, Bekesy (1948)[1] demonstrated that the basilar membrane is under no tension at all.

A second problem is that resonance theory cannot account for the perception of the "missing fundamental," the phenomenon in which the presence of only the harmonics of tone (e.g., 1100, 1200, and 1300 Hz) results in the perception of the fundamental frequency (100 Hz), even though the latter is not physically present. (The missing fundamental is discussed in Chap. 12.)

Resonance theory is also plagued by the relationship between the sharpness of a system's tuning and the persistence of its response. In order for the ear to achieve the required fine frequency discriminations, the various segments of the basilar membrane must be sharply tuned. In other words, they could each respond only to a very narrow range of frequencies. A segment could not respond to higher or lower frequencies, or else the necessary discriminations would be impossible. The problem is that such a narrowly tuned system must have very low damping—its response will take a relatively long time to die away after the stimulus stops. In other words, if there were sharp tuning of the resonators along the basilar membrane, then their responses would persist long after the stimulus had ceased. This situation would cause an interminable echo in our ears, precluding any functional hearing. On the other hand, if the resonators were less sharply tuned, they would not have the

---

[1] The student will find much of Bekesy's work is conveniently reproduced in his book, *Experiments in Hearing* (1960/1989).

persistence problem, but they would be unable to support the necessary fine frequency discriminations.

The resonance theory ascribed the perception aural distortions to nonlinear processes taking place in the middle ear. However, as we saw in the last chapter, it is now known that the middle ear operates in a manner that is astoundingly linear. Moreover, we shall see later in this chapter that the inner ear is the site of active processes, and that most nonlinear distortions are attributable to the cochlea.

Traveling Wave Theory

A variety of other place theories followed that of Helmholtz. Of particular interest is the **traveling wave theory** of Nobel laureate Georg von Bekesy. The traveling wave theory has been confirmed by many investigators using a multiplicity of approaches and is discussed later in this chapter.

Classical Temporal Theories

The classical **temporal (frequency) theories** proposed that the peripheral hearing mechanism does not perform a frequency analysis, but rather that it transmits the signal to the central auditory nervous system for processing. Such theories have been referred to as "telephone theories" by analogy with the manner in which a telephone signal is transmitted. Although there are several such theories, Rutherford's (1886) **telephone theory**, proposed not long after Helmholtz described the resonance theory, has been the best known. It proposed that the cochlea is not frequency-sensitive along its length, but rather that all parts respond to all frequencies. The job of the hair cells is simply to transmit all parameters of the stimulus waveform to the auditory nerve, and analysis is performed at higher levels.

Because a neuron can respond only in an all-or-none manner, the only way in which it can of itself transmit frequency information is to discharge the same number of times per second as there are cycles in the stimulus (e.g., it must fire 720 times per second to transmit 720-Hz tone). Classical temporal theory thus presumes that auditory nerve fibers can fire fast enough to represent this information. There is no problem at low frequencies; however, an upper limit on the number of discharges per second is imposed by the absolute refractory period of the neuron. The **absolute refractory period** is the time required after discharging for the cell to re-establish the polarization it needs to fire again; it lasts about 1 ms. The fiber cannot fire during the absolute refractory period, no matter how intensely stimulated. This period is followed by a relative refractory period during which the neuron will respond provided the stimulus is strong enough. The 1-ms absolute refractory period corresponds to a maximum firing rate of 1000 times per second. Thus, simple frequency theory is hard pressed to explain how sounds higher in frequency than about 1000 Hz can be transmitted by the auditory nerve and perceived by the listener.

A second problem of the telephone theories is that damage to the basal part of the cochlea results in high-frequency hearing loss. This is contradictory to frequency theory, which states that

Pure Tone Signal:

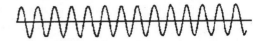

Neural Firing Patterns:

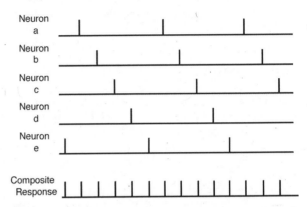

Figure 4.1 Diagrammatic representation of the volley principle (see text). *Source*: Based on various drawings by Wever and colleagues.

the different parts of the cochlea are not differentially sensitive to frequency. Furthermore, we shall see that there is actually a remarkable degree of frequency selectivity along the cochlear partition.

We shall see in Chapter 5 that the discharges of auditory nerve fibers do appear to follow the periodicity of the stimulus for frequencies as high as about 4000 to 5000 Hz. However, these responses are probabilistic rather than one-to-one.

Place-Volley Theory

Instead of suggesting that any one neuron must carry the entire information burden, Wever's (1949) **volley principle** states that groups of fibers cooperate to represent the stimulus frequency in the auditory nerve. This is shown in Fig. 4.1. The sinusoid (sound wave) at the top of the figure has a frequency too high to be represented by a series of spike discharges from a single auditory nerve fiber. Instead, fibers work in groups so that in the total response of the group there is a spike corresponding to each cycle of the stimulus. This cooperation is accomplished by having each individual neuron respond to cycles separated by some interval. In Fig. 4.1 this interval is every 5 cycles. Thus, fiber a discharges in response to cycles 1, 6, and 11; fiber b to cycles 2, 7, and 12; fiber c to 3, 8, and 13; etc. The result is that each cycle is represented by a spike in the combined response of the fiber group (bottom line in the figure).

Even at this early point it should be apparent that neither the place nor temporal theory alone can explain the selectivity of the ear. Instead, both mechanisms are operative. A periodicity mechanism is most important for low frequencies, while a place mechanism is paramount for high-frequency representation (Wever, 1949; Wever and Lawrence, 1954). The question is not one of where the "cutoff points" are, because these do not exist. As we shall see in the following chapters, place coding below approximately 300 to 400 Hz is too broad to reasonably account for frequency discrimination, and periodicity coding is not supported for frequencies above roughly 4000 to 5000 Hz. Frequency coding in the wide range between these two extremes appears to involve the interaction of both mechanisms.

ACTION OF SENSORY RECEPTORS

The auditory system is one of several specialized sensory systems. Although there is specificity of the senses at the periphery, there are nevertheless remarkable similarities among them. The following is a brief overview of sensory receptor action, with particular reference to the ear (Davis, 1961; Grundfest, 1971; Tonndorf, 1975).

Davis (1961) proposed a general plan of sensory action, which is outlined schematically in Fig. 4.2. This model describes how external stimulus energy is transmitted and coded into a form which is usable by the central nervous system. The **sensory neuron** is common to all sensory systems, although specialized receptor cells (sense organs) and accessory structures may or may not be present, and are different for the various senses. In the ear, the conductive mechanisms and the parts of the cochlea

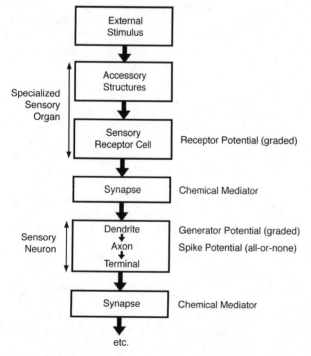

Figure 4.2 General plan of sensory receptor action (efferent feedback not shown) as described by Davis (1961).

other than the hair cells constitute the accessory structures. The hair cells are the specialized receptors for hearing.

The accessory structures assist in the action of the sense organ, but do not actually enter directly into the sensory transduction process per se. In other words, the conductive and cochlear structures help the hair cell to do its job, but are not themselves receptors. In the ear, the accessory structures carry out a large variety of vital functions. They receive, amplify, and analyze the stimulus, and convert it into a form usable by the hair cells. They may also perform feedback and inhibitory functions (under the control of efferent neurons), and protect the sensory receptors from external damage.

The sensory receptor cell transduces the stimulus and transmits it to the afferent neuron, which is an electrochemical event. Electrical potentials associated with this process can be detected within the hair cells and outside of them as receptor potentials. These **receptor potentials** are graded, meaning that their magnitudes depend upon the intensity of the stimulus. The receptor cell also emits a chemical mediator that is transmitted across the synapse between the hair cell and the afferent neuron. It is this chemical mediator that excites the neuron.

Exactly what substance constitutes the **neurotransmitter** from the hair cells to the *afferent* auditory neurons is still not firmly established. However, the amino acid **glutamate** is the most likely candidate. **Acetylcholine** is accepted as the principal *efferent* mediator in the cochlea, although others have also been identified [γ-aminobutyric acid (GABA), calcium gene-related peptide, dynorphin, and enkephalins]. Detailed discussion of neurotransmitters in the cochlea may be found in several informative reviews (Klink, 1986; Eybalin, 1993; Sewell, 1996; Wangemann and Schacht, 1996).

The neuron's dendrite receives an amount of chemical mediator from the hair cell, which elicits a graded **postsynaptic potential**. The postsynaptic potential is called a generator potential because it provides the electrical stimulus that triggers the all-or-none spike discharges from the axon. When the magnitude of the generator potential is great enough, it activates the axon, which in turn produces the **spike potential** (nerve impulse). The material in Chapter 5 on the activity of the auditory nerve is based upon these **action potentials**. This impulse travels down the axon to its terminus, where the presynaptic endings emit a chemical mediator. This chemical mediator crosses the synaptic junction to excite the dendrites of the next neuron, and the process is repeated.

THE TRAVELING WAVE

Classical resonance theory envisioned the basilar membrane to be under varying degrees of tension along its length to account for frequency tuning by place. However, Bekesy (1948) demonstrated that the basilar membrane is not under tension at all. Instead, its elasticity per unit area is essentially uniform, while there is a widening of the basilar membrane with distance along

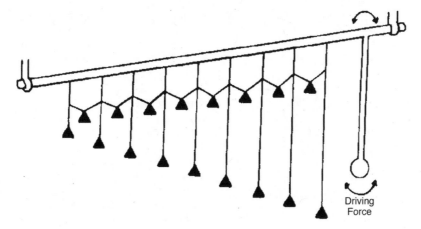

Figure 4.3   Pendulum analogy of traveling wave motion. *Source*: Based on various drawings by Bekesy.

the cochlea from base to apex (see Chap. 2). This widening of the basilar membrane results in a gradation of *stiffness* along the cochlear partition such that the membrane is about 100 times stiffer near the stapes than at the helicotrema (Naidu and Mountain, 1998). Because of this **stiffness gradient**, stimulation of the cochlea results in the formation of a pressure wave that travels from the base to the apex. In fact, this **traveling wave** proceeds toward the helicotrema regardless of where the stimulus is applied.

Before examining the details of the traveling wave, let us explore why it occurs. To begin with, the wavelengths of all audible sounds are much larger than the length of the outstretched cochlea. The result is that the pressure exerted on the cochlear partition is uniform over its length. The stiffness gradient of the basilar membrane causes it to act as a series of low-pass filters. Thus, no matter where applied, successively higher frequencies can only initiate vibrations of the cochlear partition closer and closer to the base, where they fall within the pass-band. Because the partition's impedance is composed of both stiffness and resistive components toward the base, and virtually only resistance toward the apex, the traveling wave is propagated up the partition from places of greater impedance to places of lesser impedance. The speed of the traveling wave decreases with distance from the stapes as it proceeds up the cochlear duct (Bekesy, 1960/1989).

The **pendulum analogy** suggested by Bekesy (1960/1989) should make the nature of the traveling wave clear. Suppose there is a rod to which a series of progressively longer pendulums are attached (Fig. 4.3). Each pendulum has its own natural frequency: the shorter the string, the higher the resonant frequency. We may think of each pendulum as representing a place along the basilar membrane, with the lengths of the pendulum strings corresponding to the stiffness gradient. A driving force is supplied by swinging the heavy pendulum rigidly attached to the rod. If the rod is rotated back and forth at a particular frequency, the resulting stimulus is applied over the entire rod just as the pressure from a sound stimulus is exerted over the

entire cochlear duct. The motion of the rod will cause each pendulum to swing at the stimulus frequency. Of course, the closer the natural frequency of a particular pendulum is to the frequency being applied to the rod, the larger will be its amplitude of swing. There will thus be a particular pendulum that swings with maximum amplitude for each frequency applied to the rod, and changing the frequency at which the rod rocks will move the location of maximum swing to the pendulum whose resonant frequency corresponds to the new stimulus frequency. Note at this point that each pendulum is connected to its neighbor so that the vibrations of the pendulums interact. The different string lengths cause phase differences between the pendulums, which produces waves. The result is that a sinusoidal motion applied to the rod causes a wave that travels from shorter (higher frequency) to longer (lower frequency) pendulums, with the maximum of the wave occurring at the pendulum that resonates at the frequency of the stimulus.

Let us now proceed to the vibration pattern of the basilar membrane in response to sinusoidal stimulation. The abscissa in Fig. 4.4 is distance (in mm) from the stapes along the basilar membrane, and the ordinate is amplitude of membrane displacement. Two types of information are shown in this figure.

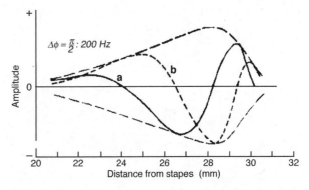

Figure 4.4   Traveling wave pattern for a 200-Hz tone. *Source*: From Bekesy (1947) with permission of *J. Acoust. Soc. Am.*

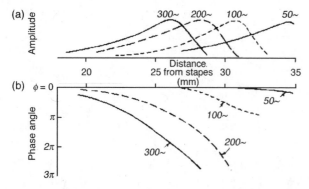

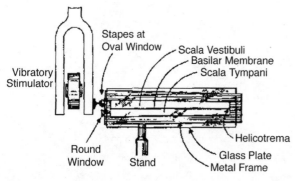

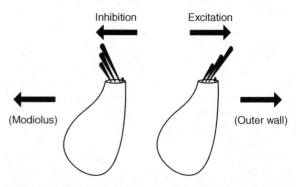

Figure 4.5 Traveling wave envelopes (a) and phase curves (b) for several low frequencies. *Source*: From Bekesy (1947) with permission of *J. Acoust. Soc. Am.*

The outer dashed lines represent the **envelope** of the **traveling wave** as a whole. This envelope outlines the displacement of the cochlear partition during an entire cycle of the wave. Note that the **displacement pattern** builds gradually with distance from the stapes, reaches a maximum in the vicinity of 28 to 29 mm, and then decays rapidly beyond the point of maximal displacement. The **peak** of the **traveling wave envelope** occurs at the place along the basilar membrane where vibration is greatest in response to the stimulus frequency (200 Hz in this case). The traveling wave envelopes for several low frequencies are shown in Fig. 4.5. Observe that these low frequencies result in displacement patterns covering most of the basilar membrane, although the places of maximum vibration move toward the base with increasing frequency. Standing waves do not arise because there are virtually no reflections from the apical end of the cochlear duct. For very low frequencies (50 Hz), the entire membrane vibrates in phase so that no traveling wave arises. For higher frequencies, however, notice that there is an increasing phase lag with distance from the stapes; this lag reflects the increasing propagation time and shortening wavelength as the wave proceeds toward the apex. Bekesy also used **cochlear models** like the one illustrated in Fig. 4.6 to observe the nature of the traveling wave. Models of this type were based on the known

properties of the cochlear duct and greatly facilitated experimental manipulations and measurements.

Figure 4.4 also shows the peak-to-peak amplitudes of membrane displacement at two discrete phases of the wave cycle. For simplicity, assume that the solid line a occurs at 0° (time zero) and that the dashed line b occurs at 90° (1/4-cycle later). The difference between the two instantaneous displacements depends on what phase of the cycle the wave is in. A full cycle would include a complex set of **instantaneous displacement** patterns back and forth within the traveling wave envelope, which would begin and end at the solid curve a we have designated as our reference for 0° phase. If one imagines this series of instantaneous displacement curves in rapid succession (as in a motion picture with a successive phase in each frame), then the resulting image would be a traveling wave with a maximum at the place shown by the peak of the envelope.

HAIR CELL ACTIVATION

A primary task is to determine exactly what it is that stimulates the hair cells of the organ of Corti. It is firmly established that hair cells transduce mechanical into electrochemical activity when their stereocilia are bent (e.g., Hudspeth and Corey, 1977; Hudspeth and Jacobs, 1979; Hudspeth, 1982, 1985; Roberts et al., 1988; Pickles and Corey, 1992). Flock (1971) demonstrated that sensory hair cells like those in the cochlea are activated (excited) when their stereocilia are bent in a particular direction, whereas inhibition occurs when they are bent in the opposite direction. *Excitation* is associated with an increase in the firing rate of the auditory neurons connected to the hair cell, and *inhibition* is associated with a decrease in their firing rates (these concepts will become clearer in Chap. 5). The effects of the direction of stereocilia bending are illustrated in Fig. 4.7. Here we see that bending of the stereocilia *toward* the tallest row results in *excitation*, while bending *away* from the tallest row is *inhibitory*. Recall that the tall row of stereocilia (as well as the base of their W- or U-shaped arrangement on the

Figure 4.6 An example of a cochlear model used by Bekesy (1928).

Figure 4.7 Bending of the stereocilia toward the tall row of stereocilia (toward the outer wall of the duct) causes excitation, and bending of the stereocilia away from the tall row (toward the modiolus) causes inhibition.

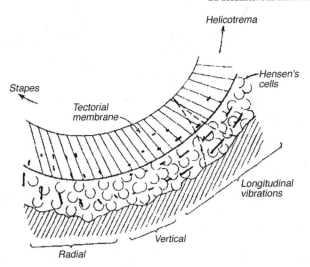

Figure 4.8 Schematic diagram showing radial and longitudinal shearing observed by Bekesy in the vicinity of the traveling wave peak. *Source*: From Bekesy (1953) with permission of *J. Acoust. Soc. Am.*

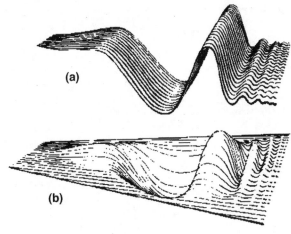

Figure 4.9 Vibration patterns of the basilar membrane that would be expected if it vibrated (a) like an unconstrained ribbon, and (b) when it is constrained by its lateral attachments. *Source*: From Tonndorf (1960) with permission of *J. Acoust. Soc. Am.*

hair cells) is *toward* the *outside* of the cochlear duct, *away* from the *modiolus*. Therefore, from the standpoint of orientation within the cochlea, the process of hair cell activation involves the bending of the stereocilia toward the outer wall or away from the modiolus.

Having established that the mechanical stimulus to the sensory cells is to bend their stereocilia away from the modiolus, we are left with two key questions. First, how does the mechanical activity along the cochlear partition get translated into such bending forces upon the sensory hairs? Second, what is it about the bending of these cilia, which causes the hair cells to become activated?

Bending of the hair cell stereocilia toward and away from the modiolus involves a motion that is *across* the cochlear duct, that is, in the *radial* direction. Yet, the traveling wave runs longitudinally in the direction of the cochlear duct. Bekesy (1953) demonstrated that such radial motion is actually achieved in the vicinity of the traveling wave peak. Specifically, he observed that the nature of the shearing force changes at different locations along the traveling wave envelope. As shown in Fig. 4.8, the shearing vibrations basal to the point of maximal displacement (toward the stapes) were found to be in the radial direction, as required to eventuate the properly oriented stimulation of the stereocilia. The shearing forces apical to the peak of the traveling wave (toward the helicotrema) were in the longitudinal direction, that is, in the direction followed by the cochlear duct.

Tonndorf (1960) explained how this change from longitudinal to radial shearing can come about. Figure 4.9a shows how the basilar membrane might move if it were like a freely vibrating ribbon. Note how the pattern is all in the longitudinal direction. However, this is not the case. Instead, the membrane is actually constrained on both sides by its attachments to the walls

of the cochlea. The result is a vibration pattern more like the one depicted in Fig. 4.10b, which is based upon observations of the instantaneous pattern in a cochlear model. Notice that the vibrations under these lateral constraints induce radially directed forces on the basal (high frequency) side of the travel-

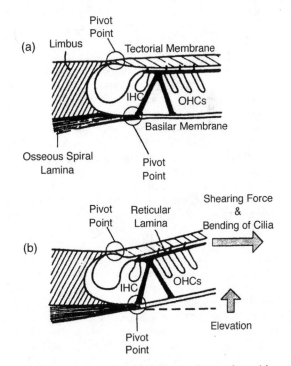

Figure 4.10 Relative positions of the basilar membrane and tectorial membrane (a) at rest, and (b) duration elevation toward the scala vestibuli. *Source*: Based on Davis, 1958. Davis' (1958) model calls for upward deflection to result in outward bending of the stereocilia, as shown in frame (b).

ing wave peak. In the cochlea, these forces would be across the direction of the duct.

Having established a mechanism to generate radial forces, we may focus on how these forces are caused to act upon the hair cells. It has long been established that the bending of the hair cell stereocilia in the proper direction (away from the modiolus) occurs when the cilia are sheared between the tectorial membrane above and the reticular lamina below. Recall here that the hair cells are seated in a complex system of supporting cells on the basilar membrane with the reticular lamina on top and with their cilia associated in various ways with the tectorial membrane (Chap. 2). The shearing effect takes place because the tectorial and basilar membranes are hinged at different points. Specifically, although the basilar membrane extends from the bottom of the osseous spiral lamina, the tectorial membrane is hinged at the upper lip of the limbus. As a result, the axes of rotation are different for these two membranes so that their displacement causes them to move relative to one another. The result is a **shearing force** upon the stereocilia between them.

The essence of the notion just described appears to have been introduced by Kuile in 1900. The most widely accepted mechanism for this concept was proposed by Davis (1958) and is represented schematically in Fig. 4.10. Frame (a) in the figure shows the relative positions of the basilar membrane and tectorial membrane at rest, and frame (b) shows their relative positions when the scala media is deflected upward toward the scala vestibuli. Notice that the membranes are viewed as operating as stiff boards that pivot around the hinge points. The resulting motions shear the cilia so that they bend outward (away from the modiolus) when the membranes are deflected upward (toward scala vestibuli), resulting in depolarization of the hair cell. Interestingly, Manoussaki, Dimitriadis, and Chadwick (2006) recently found that the increasing curvature of the spiral-shaped cochlea acts to concentrate vibrations toward the outer wall of the duct, especially for the low frequencies.

Recall from Chapter 2 that the stereocilia of the **outer hair cells (OHCs)** are firmly attached to the overlying tectorial membrane, whereas the **inner hair cell (IHC)** stereocilia are in contact with the tectorial membrane but are not attached to it (e.g., Steel, 1983). This difference implies alternative means of communicating the movements of the membranes to the stereocilia of the two types of hair cells. To study this, Dallos and associates (1972a) compared the cochlear microphonics generated by the IHCs and OHCs in the guinea pig. (Cochlear microphonics are electrical potentials that reflect cochlear activity and are explained later in this chapter.) It is possible to differentiate the responses of the two cell groups because the normal cochlear microphonic is derived chiefly from the OHCs, and ototoxic drugs tend to obliterate these same cells. Thus, the cochlear microphonic responses of the two cell groups were separated by measuring the responses before and after the animals were injected with an ototoxic drug (kanamycin). The output of the OHCs was found to be proportional to the basilar membrane *displacement*. In contrast, the response of the IHCs was

proportional to the *velocity* of basilar membrane displacement. Subsequent studies have confirmed that the IHCs are activated by the *velocity* of basilar membrane movement (Sellick and Russell, 1980; Nuttall et al., 1981; Russell and Sellick, 1983; Dallos, 1984). In other words, the OHCs respond to the *amount* of basilar membrane displacement and the IHCs respond to the *rate* at which the displacement changes.

This difference in the mode of activation is consistent with the different relationships of the inner and outer hair cell stereocilia to the tectorial membrane. Since the OHC cilia attach to the tectorial membrane, an effective stimulus is provided by the relative movement of the reticular and tectorial membranes, which depends on basilar membrane displacement. The IHCs, on the other hand, stand free of the tectorial membrane. Their stimulus is thus provided by the *drag* imposed by the surrounding viscous fluid as the basilar membrane is displaced; the greater the velocity of basilar membrane displacement, the greater the drag exerted upon the cilia.

Suppose that all the necessary events have brought the signal to the relevant location along the organ of Corti, and that whatever relative appropriate movements of the reticular and tectorial membranes have operated in order to impart outward shearing forces upon the hair cells. We already know that the hair cells are activated by the ensuing deflections of their stereocilia away from the modiolus. How does this occur? In other words, what is the process by which the bending of the stereocilia translates into sensory transduction?

MECHANOELECTRICAL TRANSDUCTION

The **transduction process** has been described by Pickles and by Hudspeth and their collaborators (Hudspeth and Corey, 1977; Hudspeth and Jacobs, 1979; Hudspeth, 1982, 1985; Pickles et al., 1984; Roberts et al., 1988; Pickles and Corey, 1992). In addition, the interested student will find several detailed reviews (e.g., Dallos et al., 1996; Geisler, 1998; Robles and Ruggero, 2001; Corey, 2006; Fettiplace and Hackney, 2006; Vollrath, Kwan, and Corey, 2007). Recall from Chapter 2 that the stereocilia bundles are composed of rows of stiff cilia that are cross-linked by fine filaments. One general class of cross-linking fibers connects the stereocilia laterally within and between rows. The other general category involves **tip links**, which are filaments that go upward from the tip of a shorter stereocilium to the side of the adjacent taller stereocilium in the next row (Fig. 4.11).[2] Bending of the stereocilia toward their tallest row (i.e., toward the outer wall of

---

[2] Tip links are formed by the interaction of cadherin 23 and protocadherin 15 (Kazmierczak, Sakaguchi, Tokita, et al., 2007), but the properties of the transduction channels themselves are still being investigated (Corey, 2006; Vollrath et al., 2007). For a review of the molecular constituents involved in mechanoelectrical transduction, see Vollrath et al. (2007).

Excitation   Inhibition

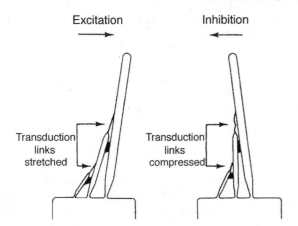

Transduction links stretched   Transduction links compressed

Figure 4.11 Tip links (identified as transduction links), which are upward-pointing (or tip-to-side) filaments between hair cell stereocilia, are shown in relation to the sensory transduction process (see text). *Source*: From *Hearing Research 15*, Pickles, Comis and Osborne (Cross-links between stereocilia in the guinea pig organ of Corti, and their possible relation to sensory transduction, 103–112, © 1984), with kind permission from Elsevier Science Publishers—NL, Sara Burgerhartstraat 25, 1055 KV Amsterdam, The Netherlands.

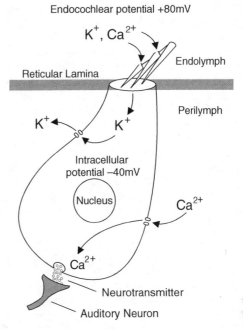

Figure 4.12 Bending of the stereocilia opens their transduction pores, leading to an inflow of potassium (K^+) and calcium (Ca^{2+}) ions. Changes in the receptor potential trigger the inflow of calcium ions (Ca^{2+}), which in turn activate the release of neurotransmitter to the afferent neurons attached to the hair cell.

the duct) is associated with *excitation*. This motion is illustrated in the left frame of Fig. 4.11, where we see that it *stretches* the tip links. Bending of the stereocilia in the opposite direction as in the right frame of the figure *compresses* the tip links and is associated with *inhibition*.

Stretching of the tip links causes **pores** known as **mechano-electrical transduction (MET) channels** to open on the tops of the shorter stereocilia, where the links are attached. In contrast, the pores would be closed when opposite bending of the stereocilia compresses the rows together. By analogy, the bending of the stereocilia in one direction or the other in effect pulls or pushes upon the tip link, which in turn opens or closes a "trap door" on the stereocilium. This opening of the MET channel grants access to a channel through which ions may flow. This mechanism may be thought of as being springy so that the pore alternates between being open and closed even when there is no stimulation. When stimulation deflects the stereocilia in the appropriate direction, the filaments are stretched so that the MET channel stays open for a longer proportion of the time, which in turn causes the ion current flow be greater and causes the hair cell to be activated. This mechanism constitutes the **mechanoelectrical transduction** process at the hair cells.

Figure 4.12 illustrates some of the basic electrochemical events associated with the electromechanical transduction process (see, e.g., Kros, 1996; Patuzzi, 1996; Wangemann and Schacht, 1996; Geisler, 1998; Fettiplace and Hackney, 2006; Vollrath et al., 2007). Notice that the endolymph is electrically positive (+80 mV) and the inside of the hair cell is electrically negative (−40 mV), constituting a polarity (voltage difference) of about 120 mV. (Cochlear electrical potentials are discussed further in the next section.) The mechanically gated opening of

the transduction channels at the apex of the hair cell leads to an inflow of potassium and calcium ions, constituting a **transduction current**. As a result, the hair cell becomes partially depolarized, and the transmembrane voltage triggers the inflow of calcium ions. In turn, the calcium ions trigger the release of a neurotransmitter from the hair cell to its associated auditory neurons. Thus, sound stimulation is transformed into basilar membrane vibrations, which lead to the opening and closing of MET channels on the stereocilia, and result in electrochemical responses, leading to the representation of the sound in the auditory nerve.

COCHLEAR ELECTRICAL POTENTIALS

Several electrical potentials may be recorded from various parts of the cochlea and its environs. References have already been made to the cochlear microphonic, which is one of these, and to the general conceptualization of the action of sensory receptors. **Resting potentials** are the positive and negative direct current (DC) polarizations of the various tissues and their surrounding fluids. **Receptor potentials** are electrical responses from a receptor cell (e.g., a cochlear hair cell) that result when the cell is stimulated. These may involve alternating current (AC) or DC. Note that the presence of a receptor potential does not necessarily mean that the nervous system is aware of the stimulus: it reflects the fact that the hair cell itself has responded. It is the transmission of a chemical mediator across the synapse and the resulting neural firing that indicate that the signal has now activated the nervous system. We may conceive of these potentials in terms of whether they are derived from a single cell or from many cells. Compound potentials include the contributions of many cells at various distances from the electrode and may include responses to different phases of the same stimulus (or to different stimuli) at different times and in different ways. Thus, the electrode "sees" a much different picture than it would if it were recording from a single cell.

The method of measurement chosen determines whether single-cell or compound (gross) potentials are recorded. The differences among methods boil down to a dichotomy between microelectrodes and gross electrodes. Basically, *microelectrodes* are electrodes small enough to impale an individual cell so that its activity can be monitored in relative isolation from other cells. Microelectrodes often have diameters much smaller than one micrometer. *Gross electrodes*, on the other hand, are not small enough to enter a cell. They include electrodes ranging in size from those that can be inserted into a nerve bundle (which are sometimes themselves called microelectrodes) to the large surface electrodes used in electroencephalography and other clinical applications. Electrodes are used in two general ways. One method uses a single *active electrode* to measure the electrical activity in an area (relative to a *ground electrode*). On the other hand, *differential electrodes* use two active electrodes, the signals of which are added, subtracted, or averaged, depending upon the specific need.

Resting Potentials

The unusual chemical situation in the cochlear duct was discussed in Chapter 2. Recall that endolymph is high in potassium, and that the proper ionic balance of the cochlear fluids has a profound effect upon the functioning of the organ of Corti.

Bekesy (1952) measured the cochlear resting potentials of the guinea pig by inserting an electrode into the perilymph of the scala vestibuli (which he set as a 0 mV reference), and then advancing it down through the scala media and the organ of Corti, and into the scala tympani. He found a positive 50 to 80 mV resting potential within the scala media. As the electrode was advanced through the organ of Corti, the voltage dropped from about +50 mV to about −50 mV, and then returned to near zero as the electrode passed through the basilar membrane into the perilymph of the scala tympani. Peake, Sohmer, and Weiss (1969) found the scala media potential to be about +100 mV. This *positive* resting potential is called the **endocochlear potential (EP)**, illustrated above the reticular lamina in Fig. 4.12. The stria vascularis is the source of the endocochlear potential (e.g., Tasaki et al., 1954; Tasaki and Spiropoulos, 1959; Konishi et al., 1961; Wangemann and Schacht, 1996).

Tasaki et al. (1954) measured a *negative* resting potential of about −60 to −70 mV in the organ of Corti, which is the **intracellular potential (IP)** of the hair cells (Dallos, 1973). Advances

in measurement techniques enabled subsequent studies to provide a more accurate picture of the resting potentials of the inner and outer hair cells (Russell and Sellick, 1978a, 1983; Dallos et al., 1982; Dallos, 1985, 1986; Wangemann and Schacht, 1996). For example, Dallos and colleagues measured the electrical potentials in the upper turns of the guinea pig cochlea by using a precisely controlled microelectrode that was advanced across the organ of Corti below and parallel to the reticular lamina (Dallos et al., 1982; Dallos, 1985, 1986). This approach enabled them to accurately establish intracellular potentials for both inner and outer hair cells, as well as to describe the details of both AC and DC intracellular receptor potentials, addressed below. Based on their data, it would appear that representative values are approximately −40 mV for the IHCs (as in Fig. 4.12) and −70 mV for the OHCs (Dallos, 1985, 1986). The net result of the positive endocochlear potential and negative intracellular potential is an electrical polarity difference of 120 mV or more across the reticular lamina.

Receptor Potentials

The measurement of electrical potentials that depend on the stimulation of the ear has impacted upon virtually all aspects of our understanding of auditory physiology. In this section, we will explore several aspects of the cochlear receptor potentials. The parameters of these potentials to a large extent also describe many other aspects of cochlear physiology, as well.

Cochlear Microphonics

In 1930, Wever and Bray reported that if the electrical activity picked up from the cat's auditory nerve is amplified and directed to a loudspeaker, then one can talk into the animal's ear and simultaneously hear himself over the speaker. This result demonstrated that the electrical potentials being monitored were a faithful representation of the stimulus waveform.

Wever and Bray originally thought that they were monitoring the auditory nerve alone. However, it was soon shown that the auditory nerve action potential was not the only signal being recorded. Instead, the *Wever–Bray effect* is actually due to an AC electrical potential being picked up by the electrodes placed near the nerve (Adrian, 1931; Davis et al., 1934). It was found, for example, that the response was stronger at the round window than at the nerve, and that it was still found even if the nerve was destroyed or anesthetized. Such findings demonstrated that the AC potential which reflects the stimulus with such remarkable fidelity is generated by the cochlea, and Adrian (1931) coined the term **cochlear microphonic (CM)** to describe it.

The relationship between the hair cells and the CM is firmly established (Wever, 1966; Dallos, 1973). Bekesy (1950) demonstrated that CMs are elicited by basilar membrane deflections. A classic study by Tasaki, Davis, and Eldridge (1954) revealed that the CM is generated at the cilia-bearing ends of the hair cells. To locate the generator of the CM, the polarity of the potential was monitored by an electrode that was advanced through

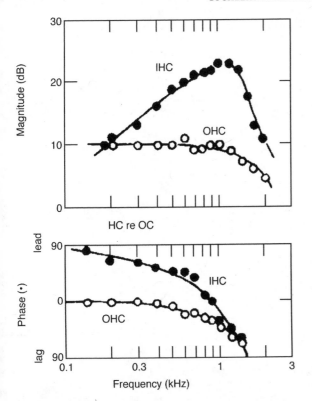

Figure 4.13 Comparison of the magnitudes (*upper graph*) and phases (*lower graph*) of intracellular AC reception potentials within the IHCs and OHCs to those in the organ of Corti outside of the hair cells (hence, HC re OC). Notice that the IHC values change as a function of frequency relative to those in the organ of Corti, whereas those for the OHCs remain relatively constant. *Source*: From *Hearing Research 14*, Dallos (Some electrical circuit properties of the organ of Corti. II. Analysis including reactive elements, 281–291, © 1984), with kind permission from Elsevier Science Publishers—NL, Sara Burgerhartstraat 25, 1055 KV Amsterdam, The Netherlands.

the cochlea from the scala tympani toward the scala vestibuli. The polarity of the CM reversed when the electrode crossed the reticular lamina, suggesting that this is the location of the CM generator. (The polarity of an electrical potential is out of phase when measured from opposite sides of its generator.) The site of CM polarity reversal was localized to the cilia-bearing ends of the hair cells (at the reticular lamina) because the DC resting potential changed dramatically to the positive EP at this point, indicating that the reticular membrane had been impaled.

Cochlear microphonics are produced by both the inner and outer hair cells, although there is evidence indicating that they reflect a greater contribution by the outer hair cells (Russell and Sellick, 1983; Dallos and Cheatham, 1976; Dallos, 1984, 1985, 1986). Figure 4.13 demonstrates one of the reasons for this conclusion. It shows the intracellular AC receptor potential relative to the AC potential outside of these cells, within the fluid of the organ of Corti. The latter is, of course, the cochlear microphonic. A value of zero implies no difference between what is

happening inside and outside of the cell, and any other value indicates the degree to which the intracellular activity differs from what is happening outside. The IHC values change as a function of frequency relative to those in the organ of Corti. However, even though the potentials are about 10 dB greater inside the OHC than outside, there is little change in magnitude or phase as a function of frequency for the AC potentials inside the OHCs compared to the fluids of the organ of Corti. The implication is that the OHCs must be making a principal contribution to the gross AC potential of the cochlea, namely, the cochlear microphonic.

How is the cochlear microphonic generated? The most widely accepted explanation is the **battery** or **variable resistance model** described by Davis (1957, 1965; see Kros, 1996; Wangemann and Schacht, 1996). Figure 4.14 shows a typical version of Davis' model. Think of the sources of the cochlear resting potentials as biological batteries generating a current flowing through the scala media, the basilar membrane, and the scala tympani. One pole of the biological battery goes to the cochlear blood supply, completing the circuit. (Recall at this point that opening of the transduction pores on the stereocilia results in a flow of ions into the cell, constituting a transduction current.) A sound stimulus would then be represented electrically (the CM) if it caused the resistance to current flow to change in accordance with the stimulus waveform. As Davis proposed, this variable resistance is provided by the movements of the hair cell stereocilia, which occur in response to basilar membrane displacement. (Recall now that the transduction pores open when bent one way and close when bent the other way, which modulates the transduction current.) In other words, the movements of the stereocilia modulate the resistance, which in turn sets up an alternating current (AC). This AC potential is monitored as the cochlear microphonic. The amount of current (CM magnitude) depends on the forces exerted upon the cilia, which is ultimately determined by the intensity of the sound stimulus.

The cochlear microphonic is a **graded potential**, which means that its magnitude changes as the stimulus level is raised or lowered. This is shown by the **input-output (I-O) function** of the cochlear microphonic. Figure 4.15 shows an idealized example of a cochlear microphonic I-O function abstracted from several classical sources. Notice that the magnitude of the cochlear microphonic increases linearly over a stimulus range of roughly 60 dB, as shown by the straight line segment of the I-O function (e.g., Wever and Lawrence, 1950, 1954). The hypothetical function in the figure shows the linear response extending down to about 0.4 μV, but CM magnitudes have actually been recorded as small as a few thousandths of a microvolt (Wever, 1966). Saturation occurs as the stimulus level is raised beyond the linear segment of the I-O function, as shown by the flattening of the curve. Increasing amounts of harmonic distortion occur in this region. Raising the intensity of the stimulus even further causes overloading, in which case the overall magnitude of the CM can actually decrease.

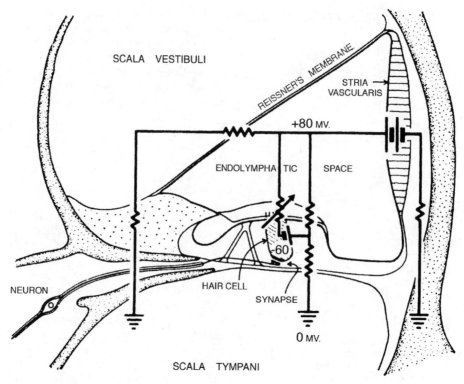

Figure 4.14 An electrical circuit representing the variable resistance model in relation to the major structures of the cochlea. *Source*: From Davis (1965), with permission.

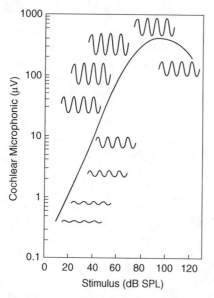

Figure 4.15 An idealized input-output function for cochlear microphonics in response to pure tone stimuli presented at increasing levels. The sine waves represent the cochlear microphonic responses at various points on the function (notice the distortion at high levels). *Source*: Based on various data and figures by Wever and Lawrence (1950, 1954) and Davis and Eldridge (1959).

The graded nature of the cochlear microphonic is also observed in terms of the intracellular AC reception potential, which is its equivalent measured within the hair cells. In fact, because these potentials are recorded *within* a given cell, they enable one to compare the relative thresholds of the inner versus outer hair cells. Using this approach, Dallos (1985) showed that the inner hair cells are on the order of 12 dB more sensitive than the outer hair cells. (This demonstration negated the previously held notion that the OHCs are more sensitive than the IHCs, which was largely based upon studies that measured thresholds following the destruction of OHCs with ototoxic drugs [Davis et al., 1958; Dallos et al., 1972a, 1972b].)

Figure 4.16 shows how the intracellular AC receptor potential changes in magnitude as a function of frequency in response to stimuli that are increased in 20-dB steps. The IHC–OHC sensitivity difference is marked by the comparison of their response magnitudes at the best frequency for the lowest stimulus level (0 dB). (The best, or characteristic, frequency is the one for which the hair cell has the lowest thresholds or the greatest magnitude of response.) The graded nature of the response is revealed by the increasing magnitude of the potential as the stimulus level increases. The slowing down of response growth at higher levels is easily seen in the figure: Even though any two successive stimuli are 20 dB apart, the resulting curves become closer and closer for the higher stimulus levels.

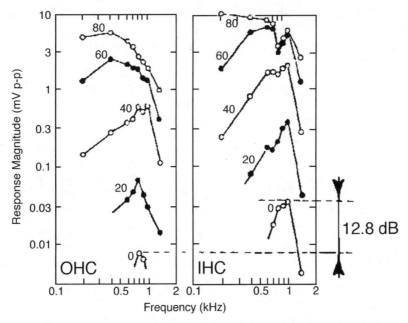

Figure 4.16 Effects of stimulus levels on the magnitude of the intracellular AC receptor potential as a function of frequency for an outer hair cell (*left frame*) and an inner hair cell (*right frame*). *Source*: From *Hearing Research 22*, Dallos (Neurobiology of cochlear inner and outer hair cells: Intracellular recordings, 185–198, © 1986), with kind permission of from Elsevier Science Publishers—NL, Sara Burgerhartstraat 25, 1055 KV Amsterdam, The Netherlands.

Distribution of the Cochlear Microphonic

Recall that large cochlear microphonic responses are recorded from the round window (Wever and Bray, 1930; Wever and Lawrence, 1954; Eggermont et al., 1974). In order to determine what contributes to the round window response, Misrahy et al. (1958) successively destroyed sections of the guinea pig's cochlea, beginning at the apex and working downward, while monitoring the CM in the basal turn. They found that the upper turns did not make significant contributions to the CM in the basal turn. It may thus be concluded that the CM recorded at the round window is for the most part derived from the activity of the basal turn.

Another approach to studying the distribution of the CM is to place electrodes along the cochlea to obtain CMs from more or less restricted locations. The distribution of the CM along the cochlear spiral was first reported with this method by Tasaki, Davis, and Legouix (1952). They inserted pairs of differential electrodes into the scalae tympani and vestibuli of the guinea pig. One electrode pair was placed in each of the four turns. This method allowed them to separate the CM, which is of opposite polarity in the two scalae, from the auditory nerve action potential (AP), which is always negative. (Addition of the out-of-phase signals cancels the CM and enhances the AP, whereas subtraction removes the AP and enhances the CM.) They found that the distribution of the CM was consistent with the propagation pattern of the traveling wave. Low-frequency signals had large CMs at the apical turn and minimal responses at the base, while high frequencies had maximal CMs at the base

and no response at the apex (Fig. 4.17). They also found that the velocity of the signal was very high in the first turn of the cochlea and smaller toward the apex.

Honrubia and Ward (1968) used microelectrodes in the scala media to measure the distribution of CM responses along the cochlear duct. The electrodes were precisely placed at intervals determined from place-frequency maps of the cochlear partition. Tones were then presented at fixed intensities, and CM magnitude was measured at various distances along the cochlear duct. For example, the CM was measured at each electrode site in response to a 1200-Hz tone at 78 dB, a 2500-Hz tone at 101 dB, etc. Figure 4.18 shows typical results, with stimulus level as the parameter. Consider first the distribution of CMs at the lowest stimulus levels (most sensitive curves). Consistent with the traveling wave envelope, the peaks of these curves occur closer to the apex as frequency decreases. However, the CM curves do not line up exactly with the basilar membrane displacement curve. This discrepancy is shown clearly in Fig. 4.19, in which the CM curve is wider and less peaked than the basilar membrane tuning curve. The difference occurs because the electrode "sees" CMs generated by thousands of hair cells in its general vicinity rather than by just those at its precise point of insertion (Dallos et al., 1974). In other words, the electrode really monitors a weighted average of many CMs, which has the effect of flattening the curve somewhat.

As shown in Fig. 4.15, CM magnitude increases with stimulus level for each frequency. Also, the place of maximum CM magnitude shifts downward toward the base as intensity increases.

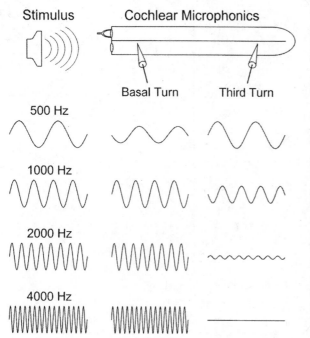

Figure 4.17 Artist's representation of the cochlear microphonics recorded with differential electrodes in the first and third turns of the guinea pig cochlea (*right*) in response to stimuli of various frequencies (*left*).

This may at first seem inconsistent with the place principle. However, the basal shift of maximum CM response is probably due to the wider range over which the more basal generators respond linearly (Dallos, 1973). In other words, as stimulus intensity increases, the CMs from the most sensitive place along the basilar membrane become saturated sooner than do the responses from more basal regions. Thus, CMs generated toward the base continue to increase in magnitude when those from the most sensitive place have already become saturated. The place of maximal CM response therefore shifts downward along the cochlear partition (upward in frequency).

The intracellular AC receptor potential also reveals a changing distribution with respect to frequency when the stimulus level increases, as shown in Fig. 4.16. Here, we see that the tuning of the AC potential is reasonably restricted around the best frequency when the stimulus level is low, and that it becomes wider, extending toward the low frequencies, when the stimulus level becomes greater. In other words, the intracellular AC receptor potential resembles a band-pass filter around the best frequency at low levels of stimulation and a low-pass filter at higher levels (Dallos, 1985).

Summating Potentials

The **summating potential (SP)** was first described by Davis, Fernandez, and McAuliffe (1950) and by Bekesy (1950). Unlike

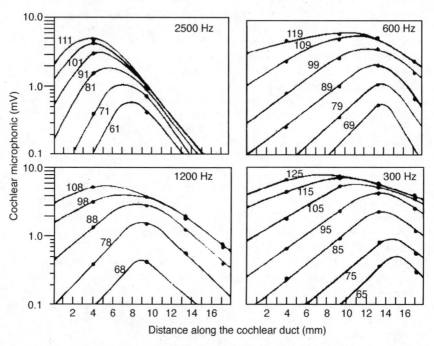

Figure 4.18 Cochlear microphonic magnitude as a function of distance along the basilar membrane for four frequencies presented at various intensities. *Source*: From Honrubia and Ward (1968), with permission of *J. Acoust. Soc. Am.*

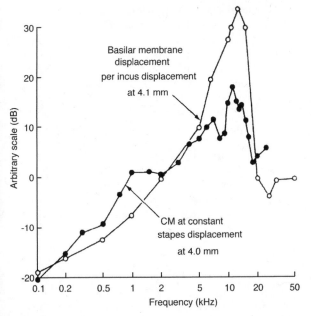

Figure 4.19 Comparison of basilar membrane tuning curves (based on Wilson and Johnstone, 1972) and the CM curve at similar locations in the guinea pig cochlea. *Source*: From Dallos et al. (1974), with permission of *J. Acoust. Soc. Am.*

the CM, which is an AC potential, the SP is a shift in the DC baseline in response to sound stimulation. In other words, the SP is a DC potential. Bekesy originally called this shift the "DC fall." Subsequent research revealed that it may be either a positive or a negative baseline shift (Davis et al., 1958). We will see that SP polarity is associated with the traveling wave envelope and how the potential is recorded. Like the cochlear microphonic, the SP is a graded potential that increases in magnitude as the stimulus level is raised (Davis et al., 1958). Although the origin of the SP was once a matter of debate, it is now well established that it is a *receptor potential* of the hair cells (Dallos and Cheatham 1976; Russell and Sellick, 1977a, 1977b, 1978a, 1978b, 1983; Dallos, 1985, 1986).

Honrubia and Ward (1969b) measured the SP and CM simultaneously in each turn of the guinea pig cochlea using electrodes located in scala media. We have already seen that the envelope of the distribution of CM amplitude along the length of the cochlear duct is a reasonable representation of the traveling wave envelope. Honrubia and Ward found that the SP was positive on the basal side of the CM envelope and negative on its apical side. This suggests that the SP is positive on the basal side of the traveling wave and becomes negative apical to the traveling wave peak.

Dallos and colleagues used a somewhat different recording approach (Dallos, 1973; Dallos et al., 1970, 1972b; Cheatham and Dallos, 1984). This method distinguishes between the average potential of both the scala vestibuli and the scala tympani on the one hand and the potential gradient (difference) across

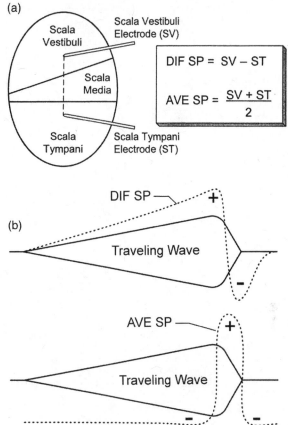

Figure 4.20 (a) Electrode arrangement and calculations used to obtain the DIF and AVE components of the summating potential. (b) Spatial relationships of the AVE SP and the DIF SP to the traveling wave envelope. *Source*: Modified from various drawings by Dallos, with permission.

the cochlear partition on the other. This at first complicated distinction is clarified in Fig. 4.20a. One electrode is in the scala vestibuli and the other is in the scala tympani. Each one registers the SP at the same cross-sectional plane along the cochlea, but from opposite sides of the scala media. Subtracting the SP in the scala tympani (ST) from the SP in the scala vestibuli (SV), (SV − ST), gives the potential difference of the SP across the cochlear partition. This difference is called the DIF component. The average (AVE) component is obtained by simply averaging the SPs from both scalae [(SV + ST)/2]. The AVE component thus expresses the common properties (common mode) of the SP on both sides of scala media.

The spatial arrangements of the DIF SP and AVE SP are shown superimposed upon the traveling wave envelope in Fig. 4.20b. Note that the DIF component becomes negative in the vicinity of the peak of the traveling wave envelope, a situation that resembles the spatial distribution of SP+ and SP− discussed above. The polarity of the AVE component is essentially the reverse, being positive around the traveling wave peak and negative

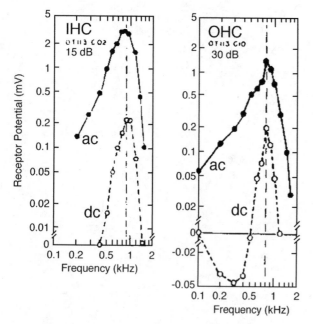

Figure 4.21 Intracellular AC and DC receptor potentials as a function of frequency at low levels of stimulation from an inner hair cell (*left frame*) and an outer hair cell (*right frame*) with comparable characteristic frequencies. *Source*: From *Hearing Research 22*, Dallos (Neurobiology of cochlear inner and outer hair cells: Intracellular recordings, 185–198, © 1986), with kind permission of from Elsevier Science Publishers—NL, Sara Burgerhartstraat 25, 1055 KV Amsterdam, The Netherlands.

elsewhere. The AVE SP and DIF SP components of the summating potential are probably produced by the same underlying processes (Cheatham and Dallos, 1984).

As we have seen for the cochlear microphonic, intracellular recordings also reveal that the summating potential is derived from the hair cells, with the principal contribution coming from the OHCs (Russell and Sellick, 1983; Dallos, 1985, 1986). Figure 4.21 provides insight into this relationship. It shows **tuning curves** obtained at low levels of stimulation for the AC and DC intracellular receptor potentials (the intracellular versions of the CM and SP, respectively) of an IHC and an OHC having comparable best frequencies. The figure reveals that the polarity of the outer hair cell's DC receptor potential changes in both the positive and negative directions. In contrast, the DC receptor potential of the inner hair cell is positive only. Thus, the distribution of the SP is consistent with that of the OHCs as opposed to the IHCs.

This negative–positive distribution of the intracellular DC receptor potential is in agreement with what we have just seen for the SP, which is the gross extracellular potential representing the contribution of many cells. (The negative–positive shape of the DC receptor potential as a function of frequency at low stimulus levels becomes positive only at higher levels.)

The effects of increasing stimulus level upon the intracellular DC potential are largely similar to those observed above for

the AC potential. Specifically, the magnitude of the potential increases with stimulus level, compressing once moderate levels are achieved. As a function of frequency, the response is sharply tuned and the band-pass around the best frequency at low levels of stimulation and becomes wider and low-pass at higher levels.

Several other observations might be made from Fig. 4.21. The data were obtained using the lowest stimulus levels, which allowed complete tuning curves to be generated. Note that this was 15 dB for the IHC and 30 dB for the OHC. This difference should not be surprising if one recalls that the IHCs are roughly 12 dB more sensitive than the OHCs. Second, notice that the tuning curves for the DC receptor potentials are sharper than those for the AC potentials. Finally, notice that these tuning curves obtained at low levels of stimulation are very sharp—much sharper than what we have seen for the traveling wave envelope.

COCHLEAR TUNING AND FREQUENCY SELECTIVITY

Basilar membrane displacement reaches a peak near the apex of the cochlea in response to low frequencies and near the base for higher frequencies. That is, the traveling wave causes a displacement pattern which is tuned as a function of distance along the basilar membrane. One may say that the cochlea is tuned to frequency as a function of distance along the cochlear partition. This relationship between the tuning of a location along the cochlear partition and the distance from the base to apex is depicted in Liberman's (1982) **cochlear frequency map** shown in Fig. 4.22. This map was derived by determining the **characteristic** or **best frequencies** of auditory neurons labeled with horseradish peroxidase (HRP), and then tracing these neurons back to their respective hair cells along the cochlear duct (see Chap. 5). This method made

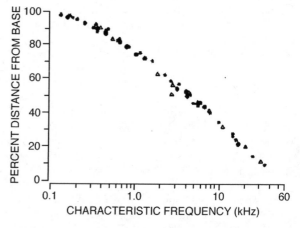

Figure 4.22 This cochlear map shows the relationship between frequency and distance in percent along the cochlear partition in the cat. *Source*: From Liberman (1982), with permission of *J. Acoust. Soc. Am.*

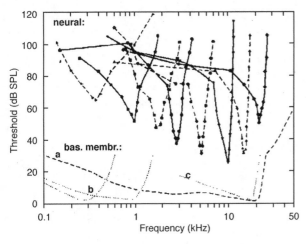

Figure 4.23 *Upper curves*: Neural tuning curves (guinea pig). *Lower curves*: Mechanical tuning (guinea pig) based on (a) Wilson and Johnstone, 1972, (b) Bekesy (1960/1989), and (c) Johnstone et al. (1970). *Source*: From Evans (1975), The sharpening of cochlear frequency selectivity. *Audiology*, 14, 419–442.

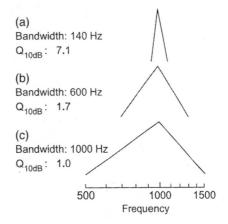

Figure 4.24 Q_{10dB} for three idealized "tuning curves" centered at 1000 Hz. These Q_{10dB} values were obtained as follows: (a) $1000/140 = 7.1$, (b) $1000/600 = 1.7$, and (c) $1000/1000 = 1.0$.

it possible to precisely locate the places along the cochlea that correspond to particular frequencies. This cochlear map expresses distance along the cochlea in terms of percentage, thereby accounting for differences in cochlear length across specimens.

In the following chapters, we shall see that fine frequency discriminations are made in psychoacoustic experiments, and that auditory nerve fibers are very sharply tuned. Can the mechanical displacement pattern in the cochlea account for this remarkable degree of frequency selectivity?

A key question is whether the *sharpness* of **cochlear tuning** approaches that of the auditory nerve. The upper curves in Fig. 4.23 show a set of **response areas** or **tuning curves** for auditory nerve fibers in the guinea pig. Neural tuning curves will be discussed in Chapter 5. For now, note their sharp peaks, which indicate that auditory nerve fibers respond best to a limited range of frequencies around a characteristic frequency. The low-frequency slopes of the neural tuning curves range from about 100 to 300 dB per octave, and the high-frequency slopes are approximately -100 to -600 dB per octave in a variety of species (e.g., Kiang, 1965; Evans and Wilson, 1971, 1973; Evans, 1972a, 1972b; Geisler et al., 1974).

The sharpness of tuning can be described by a value **Q**, which is the ratio of the center frequency to the bandwidth. For a particular center (characteristic) frequency, the narrower the bandwidth, the larger is the Q value. This relationship is illustrated in Fig. 4.24. Recall that the half-power points are the usual cutoff values used to define a bandwidth. Since it is difficult to determine the half-power points of physiological tuning curves, it has become standard practice to use the points on the curve that are 10 dB down from the peak. For this reason, we use the value Q_{10dB} to summarize the sharpness of physiologi-

cal tuning curves. Auditory neurons have Q_{10dB} values of about 2 to 10 for the midfrequencies (Evans and Wilson, 1973). With this in mind, let us proceed to examine the nature of frequency selectivity in the cochlea.

Bekesy (1949) was the first to describe **mechanical tuning** in the cochlea. He used a binocular microscope to observe **basilar membrane displacement patterns** in response to high-intensity signals. Figure 4.25 shows some of the basilar membrane tuning curves obtained by Bekesy. These curves are in terms of relative amplitude so that the peak is assigned a value of 1.0 and the displacements at other points along the curves are in proportions of the peak amplitude. The tuning curves tend to become sharper with increasing frequency, but the low-frequency slopes of about 6 dB per octave are far from the sharpness of neural tuning. This is illustrated in Fig. 4.23, in which Bekesy's curves (labeled b) are compared with neural tuning curves having similar characteristic frequencies.

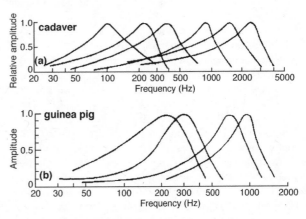

Figure 4.25 Basilar membrane tuning curves obtained in (a) cadaver (after Beksey, 1943/1949) and (b) guinea pig (after Bekesy, 1944).

Although Bekesy's data were of monumental significance, several experimental limitations make it difficult to compare these early findings with neural tuning data: Access to the cochlear partition was limited to the apical areas so that Bekesy's observations were restricted to relatively low frequencies. The observations were obtained visually. Absolute displacements were not specified (although they were in other contexts). Very high stimulus levels (roughly 120 dB SPL) were used, while neural data are available at much lower, including threshold, levels.

Subsequent studies investigated basilar membrane tuning using methods made possible by technological advances in the 1960s and 1970s (e.g., Johnstone et al., 1970; Rhode, 1971, 1978; Köhllofel, 1972; Wilson and Johnstone, 1972, 1975; Johnstone and Yates, 1974; Rhode and Robles, 1974). For example, Johnstone and Boyle (1967) measured tuning in the guinea pig cochlea by using the **Mössbauer technique**, which made it possible to use stimulus levels as low as 60 to 70 dB SPL. In this method, a radioactive source is placed on the basilar membrane and an absorber of the radiation is situated nearby. Vibration of the basilar membrane causes the amount of gamma rays absorbed to be modulated in a manner related to the vibration. Basilar membrane displacement is calculated based on these data. Mechanical tuning curves obtained with the Mössbauer method (e.g., curve *c* at the bottom of Fig. 4.23) were considerably sharper than what Bekesy found at low frequencies (e.g., curves labeled *b* in the figure).

Wilson and Johnstone (1972, 1975) measured basilar membrane tuning with a **capacitance probe**, which was a miniature version of the one used by Bekesy (1960/1989) (see Chap. 3). Their findings are of interest because they confirmed the Mössbauer data with another technique and also because the capacitance probe enabled them to measure basilar membrane vibrations for stimuli as low as 40 dB SPL (which is closer to the levels used to obtain neural tuning curves). Curve *a* in lower part of Fig. 4.23 shows an example. Comparing the upper and lower sections of Fig. 4.23 makes it clear that these measurements cannot account for the sharpness of the neural tuning data.

It was once thought that a **"second filter"** existing between the basilar membrane and neural responses might account for the sharpness of neural tuning. The main evidence for this idea was that neural tuning curves become wider when the metabolism of the cochlea is disturbed by interference with its oxygen supply or by chemical influences (Evans, 1972a, 1972b, 1974, 1975; Evans and Wilson, 1971, 1973). The appeal of the second filter concept to bridge the gap from broad mechanical to sharp neural tuning led to the proposal of several theories about its location and mechanism. One example involved **lateral inhibition**, which involves the suppression of activity in weakly stimulated neural units by more intense stimulation of adjoining units (e.g., Bekesy, 1960/1989), although other possible mechanisms were also proposed (e.g., Khanna et al., 1968; Duifhuis, 1976; Zwislocki, 1974, 1975, 1985; Manley, 1978; Crawford and

Fettiplace, 1981). An example of lateral inhibition from common experience is the sharply defined border that is seen between adjoining black and white bars known as Mach bands. However, we shall see that *active processes* are at work that provide for mechanical tuning just as sharp as neural tuning. Thus, a "second filter" is not necessary. Interested readers should refer to Pickles (1982) and Gelfand (1981) for reviews of second filter theories.

That sharp tuning already exists prior to the neural response was demonstrated by Russell and Sellick (1977a, 1977b, 1978a, 1978b). They measured the intracellular DC receptor potential (summating potential) in guinea pig IHCs as a function of stimulus frequency and level. Typical findings are shown in Fig. 4.26. Each curve shows the sound pressure level needed to reach a certain magnitude of DC potential within the IHC as a function of frequency. These curves are called *isoamplitude contours* because each point on a given curve represents the SPL needed to achieve the same amplitude of SP. The smallest intracellular SP response that could elicit a response from the auditory nerve was about 2.0 mV. At high stimulus levels (SPLs that result in larger SP amplitudes), the SP tuning is more or less like that of the mechanical data we have previously reviewed. However, as the stimulus level decreases, the reduction in SP amplitude (A in mV) comes with a clear increase in the frequency selectivity of IHC intracellular tuning curves. For example, when SP amplitude is 2.7 mV (within 10 dB of threshold), Q_{10dB} is 9.2. This is as sharp as neural tuning. Similarly sharp tuning of intracellular potentials has also been reported for the OHCs (e.g., Dallos et al., 1982). One might note in this context that Cheatham and Dallos (1984) showed that tuning curves for the SP are consistent with those of the basilar membrane and the auditory nerve action potential.

These findings demonstrate that frequency selectivity as sharp as what is found in the auditory neuron already exists within the hair cell and *before* it transmits to the nerve fiber. Clearly, the acuity of neural tuning does not require an intervening filter between the hair cell and the neuron.

What (and where), then, is the origin of the sharp tuning that is already seen in the hair cell? The answer comes from studies of the in vivo mechanical responses of virtually undamaged cochleas at stimulus levels as low as those used to generate neural tuning curves.

In 1982, Khanna and Leonard demonstrated sharp basilar membrane tuning in the cat by using **laser inferometry**. A detailed discussion of this technique and its applications may be found in an informative series of papers by Khanna and colleagues (Khanna and Leonard, 1982, 1986a, 1986b; Khanna, 1986; Khanna et al., 1986). The sharpness of mechanical tuning in the cochlea has been repeatedly corroborated (e.g., Sellick et al., 1982a; Robles et al., 1986; Ruggero et al., 1997).

Figure 4.27a shows three cat basilar membrane tuning curves. These curves show the sound pressure levels needed to yield a certain threshold amplitude of basilar membrane vibration as a function of frequency. The sharpest of these three curves is

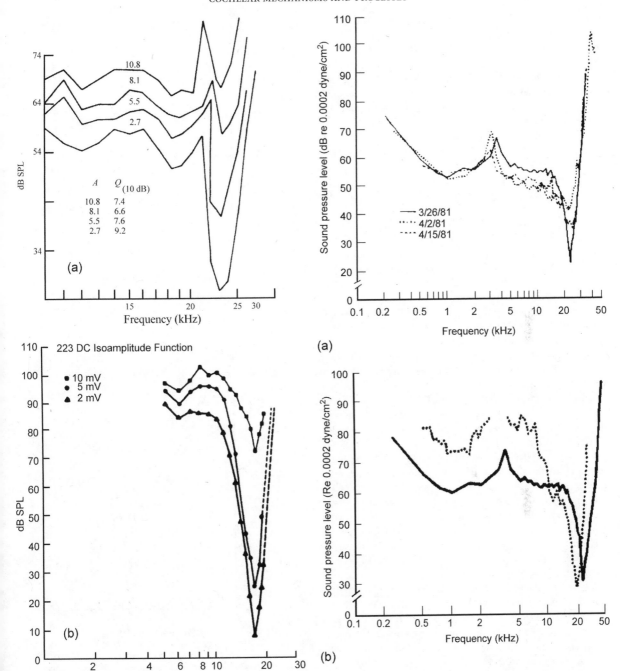

Figure 4.26 Intracellular DC receptor potentials (summating potentials) from guinea pig inner hair cells as a function of frequency: (a) Receptor potential amplitude (A in mV) is shown with corresponding values of Q_{10dB}. *Source*: From Russell and Sellick (1977a), courtesy of *Nature*. (b) Isoamplitude curves are shown for 2, 5, and 10 mV intracellular potentials. *Source*: From Russell and Sellick, Intracellular studies of cochlear hair cells: Filling the gap between basilar membrane mechanics and neural excitation, in *Evoked Electrical Activity in the Auditory Nervous System* (Naunton and Fernandez, eds.), © 1978 by Academic Press.

Figure 4.27 (a) The SPL necessary to achieve equal amplitudes of basilar membrane movements in three cats. (b) Comparison of the sharpest basilar membrane curve (3/26/81) with a neural tuning curve. *Source*: From Khanna and Leonard, Basilar membrane tuning in the cat cochlea, *Science*, 215, 305–306 (1982). Copyright © 1982. Reprinted with permission from American Association for the Advancement of Science.

shown redrawn in Fig. 4.27b along with a neural tuning curve. The basilar membrane curve is strikingly similar to that of the neuron in the sharply tuned tip of the tuning curve, but deviates from the neural response at lower frequencies. These graphs reveal that the basilar membrane's mechanical response is as sharp as that of the neural tuning curve in the region of the most sensitive response (where Q_{10dB} is 5.9 for both curves in this example).

Similar findings for the guinea pig cochlea were obtained by Sellick et al. (1982a, 1982b). Recall that the IHCs are activated by the velocity rather than the displacement of basilar membrane movement. As a consequence, they expressed the mechanical response of the basilar membrane in terms of the velocity of its motion. Figure 4.28a shows that the basilar membrane isovelocity curve (crosses) is remarkably similar to a representative neural tuning curve. Figure 4.28b shows the SPLs needed to yield an isoamplitude response of the basilar membrane. As in the previous figure, the isoamplitude response is similar to the neural response in the sharply tuned tip of the curve, but deviates at lower frequencies.

Sellick, Pauzzi, and Johnstone (1982a, 1982b) used the stimulus SPL needed to evoke an auditory nerve action potential (see Chap. 5) as a measure of the health of the cochlea over the course of their measurements. Examples of their results are shown in Fig. 4.29. They found that these thresholds worsened as time passed, revealing that the experimental invasion of the inner ear itself caused progressive damage to the cochlea. Khanna and Leonard (1982) also reported that trauma to the cochlea due to the experimental manipulations caused a loss of sharp mechanical tuning.

It is now clear that the mechanical tuning within the cochlea accounts for the sharpness of neural tuning; but what is the nature of this mechanical tuning process? We must recall at this juncture that the real concern is with the sharpness of the mechanical stimulus actually transmitted to the hair cells. The tuning of the cochlea involves more than just the passive traveling wave response of the basilar membrane. There also are **active processes** associated with the outer hair cells and their connections to surrounding structures.

Let us view the tuning curve somewhat differently in order to appreciate why the mechanical tuning of the cochlea involves active processes. The cochlea's mechanical response may be described as having two components (Khanna and Leonard, 1982, Leonard and Khanna, 1984; Kelly and Khanna, 1984a): One of these components has a broad low-pass response. The other is a sharply tuned band-pass filter. Together, the two components reveal the neural tuning curve's familiar sharp tip and broad tail. Injuries that affect the tip do not particularly affect the broad, low-pass component. In particular, injuries affecting the OHCs have been shown to affect the tip component but not the tail of the tuning curve, and the condition of the OHCs is correlated with the affect upon the tip of the tuning curve (Khanna and Leonard, 1986b; Leonard and Khanna, 1984; Liberman and Dodds, 1984). These changes in the tip of

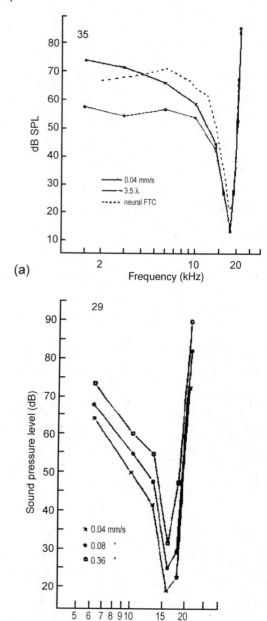

(a)

(b)

Figure 4.28 (a) The SPL necessary to achieve equal velocities (*crosses*) and amplitudes (*circles*) of basilar membrane vibration, and a comparable neural tuning curve (*dotted line*) in the guinea pig. (b) The SPL needed to achieve three velocities of basilar membrane vibration in the same guinea pig. *Source: From Sellick et al. (1982), with permission of J. Acoust. Soc. Am.*

the tuning curve are found in the absence of basilar membrane abnormalities (Kelly and Khanna, 1984a, 1984b). The tip component of the cochlea's mechanical tuning curve is associated with the outer hair cells.

One might note in this context the classic observation that thresholds become about 30 to 40 dB poorer when ototoxic

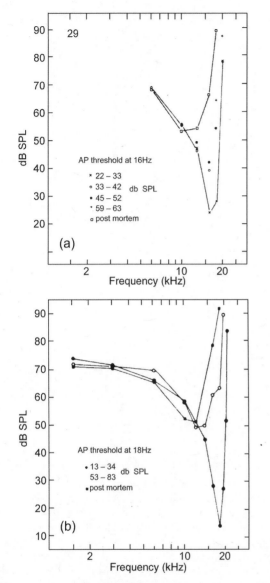

Figure 4.29 The loss of sharp mechanical tuning of the basilar membrane is observed as thresholds become elevated, revealing progressive damage to the cochlea over the course of the measurements, and post mortem, for two guinea pigs (a and b). From Sellick et al. (1982a, 1982b), with permission of *J. Acoust. Soc. Am.*

are on the order of 12 dB more sensitive than the OHCs (Dallos, 1985).

The two-component nature of cochlear tuning has also been demonstrated by Liberman and colleagues, who determined how various cochlear manipulations affected the associated auditory neurons' responses (Liberman, 1984; Liberman and Dodds, 1984; Liberman and Kiang, 1984; Kiang et al., 1986). They demonstrated that while both the IHCs and OHCs are needed to yield a normal neural tuning curve, the presence of the sharply tuned component of the response depends upon the presence and condition of the outer hair cells.

Smith et al. (1987) provided behavioral support for the contribution of the OHCs to the sensitivity and fine-tuning of the cochlea. They obtained **psychoacoustic tuning curves (PTCs)**, a behavioral measure of frequency selectivity (see Chap. 10), from patas monkeys before and after producing OHC damage with the drug dihydrostreptomycin. The drug caused elevations of threshold sensitivity of 50 dB or more, and the sharp tips of the PTCs to be obliterated, leaving only the broad, low-pass filter characteristic of the curves. Histological examination of the cochleas revealed that there was complete loss of OHCs but complete retention of the IHCs in the regions corresponding to the changes of the PTCs.

COCHLEAR NONLINEARITY

One of the seminal contributions to our knowledge of cochlear functioning was Rhode's (1971) demonstration that the mechanical response of the basilar membrane is **nonlinear**. The nonlinearity is seen in Fig. 4.30 as a lack of overlapping of the tuning curve peaks obtained at different stimulus levels. The three curves in the figure would have overlapped exactly if the basilar membrane's vibration was linear because the amplitude (in dB) is derived from the ratio of basilar membrane-to-malleus displacement. In a linear system, this ratio would stay the same for different stimulus levels. This nonlinearity, originally observed in the squirrel monkey, used to be the subject of controversy because other researchers at that time did not find it in the guinea pig. However, as we have seen for the sharpness of cochlear tuning, nonlinearity in the vicinity of the peak is the *normal* response (e.g., Rhode, 1971, 1978; Rhode and Robles, 1974; Sellick et al., 1982a, 1982b; Robles et al., 1986; Ruggero et al., 1997) (see Figs. 4.26, 4.28b, and 4.31).

Figure 4.31 provides a detailed illustration of this nonlinearity. Here, we see a set of tuning curves obtained from a healthy chinchilla cochlea by Ruggero et al. (1997), who used a wide range of stimulus levels and modern measurement techniques (a form of laser inferometry). Notice that the mechanical response is nonlinear around the characteristic frequency (tuning curve peak) and at higher frequencies, again indicated by the lack of overlapping. However, this does not occur at lower frequencies, where the curves are superimposed.

drugs have destroyed the *outer* hair cells (Dallos et al., 1972a, 1972b). The long-held interpretation of this observation was that the *inner* hair cells, which survived the ototoxic assault, are not as sensitive as the outer hair cells. However, we now know that the drop in thresholds is due to the loss of the sensitizing effects of the OHCs (Dallos and Harris, 1978). In fact, as previously noted and in contrast to previously held notions, intracellular recordings have established that the IHCs

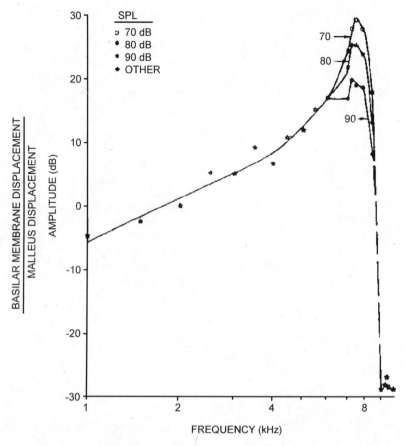

Figure 4.30 Basilar membrane tuning curves obtained in the squirrel monkey using stimulus levels of 70, 80, and 90 dB SPL. Notice that the peaks obtained at different stimulus levels do not overlap, indicating that the response is nonlinear. *Source*: From Rhode (1971), with permission of *J. Acoust. Soc. Am.*

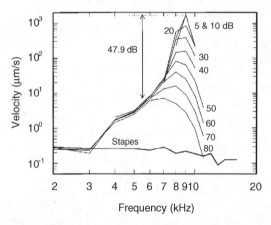

Figure 4.31 Basilar membrane tuning curves (gain in response velocity divided by stimulus level as a function of frequency) in the chinchilla cochlea, using a wide range of stimulus levels (indicated by the numbers next to each curve). The response is nonlinear for frequencies in the vicinity of the peak and above (revealed by the lack of overlapping), but is linear for lower frequencies (where the curves overlap). *Source*: Adapted from Ruggero et al. (1997), by permission of *J. Acoust. Soc. Am.*

The *compressive* nature of the nonlinear response of the basilar membrane is clearly seen in Fig. 4.32, which shows data from six essentially healthy chinchilla cochleas. Each curve shows how the magnitude of the basilar membrane response at the tuning curve peak is related to the sound pressure level of the stimulus. The straight line in the graph illustrates linear growth. The tipping-over of these curves shows that the growth of response magnitude slows down as the stimulus level rises. The nonlinear nature of these curves is highlighted by comparing them with the straight line representing linear growth.

As for sharp tuning, the sensitivity and nonlinear nature of the basilar membrane response depend on the health and integrity of the cochlea (e.g., LePage and Johnstone, 1980; Sellick et al., 1982a, 1982b; Yates et al., 1990). For example, Sellick et al. (1982a, 1982b) showed that sharp turning and the nonlinear response deteriorated as thresholds worsened, and that they were present early during experimental testing when the cochlea was still reasonably healthy, but were lost as the experiment proceeded and at postmortem (Fig. 4.29).

The nonlinearity of the cochlea also can be observed in the production of distortion products and by two-tone suppression.

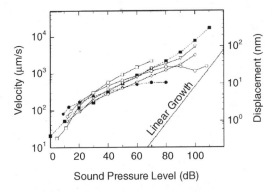

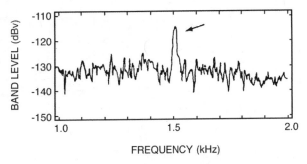

Figure 4.33 Example of a spontaneous otoacoustic emission at approximately 1500 Hz (*arrow*) detected above the noise floor in an occluded ear canal. Its level corresponds to about 11 dB SPL. *Source*: From Zurek, 1985, with permission of *J. Acoust. Soc. Am.*

Figure 4.32 Magnitude of the basilar membrane response at the characteristic frequency (tuning curve peak) as a function of stimulus level from six chinchillas with essentially healthy cochleas. The compressive nature of the basilar membrane response is seen by comparing these curved lines with the straight line representing linear growth. (Filled circles indicate the function for the animal whose tuning curves are shown in Fig. 4.31.) *Source*: Adapted from Ruggero et al. (1997), by permission of *J. Acoust. Soc. Am.*

Distortion products occur when the output of a system includes components that were not present at the input. For example, if two tones with frequencies f_1 and f_2 are presented to the ear (input), the basilar membrane's vibratory response (output) might include the *primaries* f_1 and f_2 plus *distortion products* such as f_2-f_1 and $2f_1-f_2$ (e.g., Nuttall et al., 1990; Nuttall and Dolan, 1993; Robles et al., 1991, 1997; Rhode and Cooper, 1993; Cooper and Rhode, 1997; Robles and Ruggero, 2001). The first example, f_2-f_1, is sometimes called the **quadratic difference tone** and is produced when f_1 and f_2 are presented at high levels. On the other hand, the **cubic difference tone** $2f_1-f_2$ occurs when f_1 and f_2 are presented at low levels and is rather sensitive to the proximity of the primary tones. We will return to f_2-f_1 and $2f_1-f_2$ in the context of otoacoustic emissions below, and will discuss their perception in Chapter 12.

Two-tone suppression in the cochlea occurs when the response of the basilar membrane produced by one tone (at the characteristic frequency) is weakened by the presence of a second (suppressor) tone at a different frequency, and is the most likely origin of two-tone suppression in the auditory nerve, discussed in Chapter 6 (see, e.g., Ruggero et al., 1992; Cooper, 1996; Geisler, 1998; Robles and Ruggero, 2001). The effect is greatest when the characteristic frequency and suppressor tones are very close in frequency and decreases as their frequencies become further apart.

OTOACOUSTIC EMISSIONS

Kemp (1978, 1979) demonstrated that the cochlea can *produce* sounds as well as receive them. He found that when a click is directed into the ear, it is followed by an echo that is emitted back from the cochlea. This *cochlear echo* can be detected roughly 5 ms or more after the click, typically peaking at latencies in the vicin-

ity of approximately 5 to 15 ms. This phenomenon was originally referred to as the *Kemp echo* and has come to be known as the **evoked or stimulated otoacoustic emission. Spontaneous otoacoustic emissions** occur as well (Kemp, 1979; Zurek, 1981; Strickland et al., 1985). These signals generated in the cochlea are measurable with a probe microphone in the ear canal. Figure 4.33 shows an example of a spontaneous otoacoustic emission at about 1500 Hz. However, we will concentrate upon evoked otoacoustic emissions here. The interested student will find a growing number of informative reviews and discussions about the nature, parameters, and applications of otoacoustic emissions in the literature (e.g., McFadden and Wightman, 1983; Zurek, 1985; Lonsbury-Martin et al., 1991; Probst et al., 1991; Dekker, 1992; Berlin, 1998; Robinette and Glattke, 2002).

It is worthwhile to review how the stimulated or evoked otoacoustic emission is obtained. Suppose a probe device like the one represented in Fig. 4.34a is inserted into someone's ear. This probe contains both a sound source (an earphone) and a microphone, and it occludes the ear when inserted. A click is presented to the ear and the sound pressure in the occluded ear is measured over time.

Before putting the probe into a human ear, let's first see what happens when it is inserted into a *Zwislocki coupler*, which is a metal cavity that has the same impedance characteristics as the human ear. In this case, there would be a damped oscillation like the one shown in the *upper* tracing of Fig. 4.34b. Now let's put the coupler into a human ear. In this case, the resulting waveform will resemble the *middle* tracing in Fig. 4.34b. Here we see an initial damped oscillation lasting about 6 ms and also a much smaller oscillation occurring after a latency of roughly 6 to 7 ms. The *initial* oscillations are the *impulse response* of the ear and are similar to what we just saw in the metal coupler. The *later* and smaller oscillations constitute the *cochlear echo*, or the evoked otoacoustic emission. The lower tracing in Fig. 4.34b shows just the evoked otoacoustic emission after the response has been amplified and displaced by 5 ms to remove the initial part of the response.

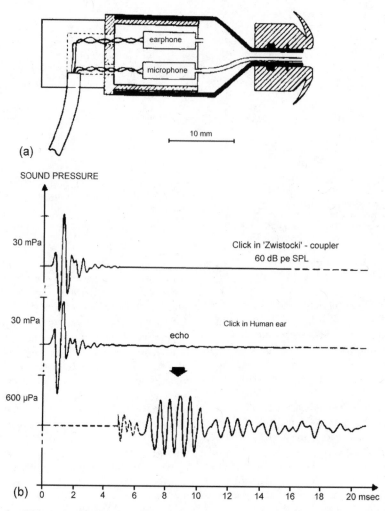

Figure 4.34 (a) The probe for eliciting and measuring otoacoustic emissions is inserted into the ear canal. The sound source is provided by the earphone and the microphone measures the sound pressure in the ear canal, which is occluded by the ear tip. (b) Responses to a click stimulus: *Upper tracing*: Damped oscillation in a metal cavity (Zwislocki coupler). *Middle tracing*: Responses in a human ear consisting of initial damped oscillations followed by the evoked otoacoustic emission (echo). *Lower tracing*: Amplified echo response displaced by 5 ms. *Source*: From Johnsen and Elberling (1982), with permission of *Scandinavian Audiology*.

Many studies of evoked otoacoustic emissions were undertaken within a short period after its original description and it continues to be the topic of extensive investigation (see, e.g., reviews by Wit and Ritsma, 1979, 1980; McFadden and Wightman, 1983; Zurek, 1985; Lonsbury-Martin et al., 1991; Probst et al., 1991; Dekker, 1992; Robinette and Glattke, 2002). A number of generalities have been derived from these and other studies. To begin with, virtually all normal hearing humans appear to have a stimulated acoustic emission in response to clicks and/or tone bursts. A given ear's emission is extraordinarily reproducible; however, the details of evoked emissions differ widely from ear to ear, just as we have seen with respect to the sharpness and nonlinearity of the cochlea's mechanical tuning. The evoked acoustic emission is also vulnerable to such insults as ototoxicity

and noise exposure and is obliterated by any substantive degree of sensorineural hearing loss.

The latency and magnitude of the echo depend on the level of the stimulus. Latency tends to decrease as the stimulus levels become greater. Although the magnitude of the evoked emission gets larger with increasing stimulus level, this relationship is linear only for low stimulus levels, above which the input-output curve becomes compressed, and saturates by the time the emission reaches about 20 dB SPL.

The latency of the emission decreases with increasing frequency. This association is important because it is consistent with the idea that the location within the cochlea from which the echo originates moves closer to the base with increasing frequency, as one would expect. An apparent problem with this

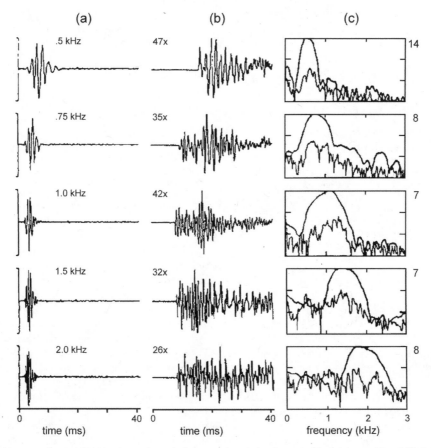

Figure 4.35 Effect of frequency from 500 to 2000 Hz on the evoked otoacoustic emission for one subject. Columns (a) and (b) show evoked otoacoustic emission waveforms before and after processing. Column (c) compares the spectra of the stimuli (*smoother curves*) to those of the otoacoustic emissions. *Source*: From Norton and Neeley (1987), by permission of *J. Acoust. Soc. Am.*

point has been the observation that the actual latencies of the echo seem to be two or three times longer than the estimated time it would take for the signal to reach and then return from a given place along the cochlear duct. However, it has been pointed out that otoacoustic emission latencies fall within the expected round-trip travel time when the latter is based upon data obtained at low stimulus levels, similar to those employed in acoustic emissions work (e.g., Neeley et al., 1986; Norton and Neeley, 1987).

The spectral characteristics of click-evoked otoacoustic emissions do not exactly match those of the click used to elicit them. Instead, they tend to show energy concentrations in fairly narrow frequency ranges. Norton and Neeley (1987) using tone-bursts showed that the frequency concentrations in the spectra of otoacoustic emissions follow those of the stimuli, as exemplified in Fig. 4.35. The third column of the figure compares the spectra of the otoacoustic emissions to those of the stimuli (represented by the smooth lines). Notice that there is an orderly change in the spectra of the otoacoustic emissions with the changes in the stimulus spectra.

Distortion product otoacoustic emissions (DPOAEs) occur at frequencies corresponding to the f_2-f_1 **difference tone** and the $2f_1$-f_2 **cubic difference tone**. Here f_1 and f_2 are the frequencies of the lower and higher **primary tones**, respectively. The level of f_1 is L_1, and L_2 is the level of f_2. The cubic difference tone otoacoustic emission is the most interesting and widely studied of the DPOAEs. Its level tends to be about 60 dB weaker than the levels of the primary tones. Several examples of DPOAEs are provided in Fig. 4.36 from an experiment by Bums et al. (1984). In the *lower* tracing, we see *spontaneous* otoacoustic emissions (SOAEs) at 1723 and 2049 Hz. These behave as primary tones to produce a cubic difference tone ($2f_1$-f_2) SOAE of 1397 Hz. In the *upper* tracing of the figure, we see that the introduction of an external tone masks (see Chap. 10) the higher primary. As a result, this leaves only the lower primary SOAE, and the cubic difference tone, which previously resulted from the interaction of f_1 and f_2, is now obliterated. These findings provide further evidence of active processes in the cochlea.

It is generally accepted that DPOAEs are best observed when (1) the primaries are in the 1000- to 4000-Hz region with an f_2/f_1

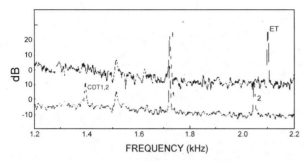

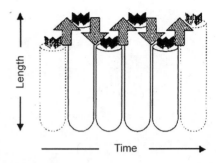

Figure 4.36 *Lower tracing*: Primary (1, 2) spontaneous otoacoustic emissions (SOAEs) at 1723 and 2049 Hz yield a cubic difference tone SOAE at 1397 Hz (CDT1,2). *Upper tracing*: Adding an external tone (ET) masks tone 2, leaving only tone 1, thus obliterating the distortion product. *Source*: From *Hearing Research 24*, Burns, Strickland, Tubis, and Jones (Interactions among spontaneous otoacoustic emissions. I. Distortion products and linked emissions, 271–278, ©1984), with kind permission of from Elsevier Science Publishers—NL, Sara Burgerhartstraat 25, 1055 KV Amsterdam, The Netherlands.

Figure 4.37 The electromotile response of an outer hair cell (changing length over time) acts as a positive-feedback mechanism, providing the force for active cochlear processes. The magnitude of the length change, which is actually on the order of about 1% to 4%, is highly exaggerated in the drawing for illustrative purposes.

frequency ratio approximating 1.2, and (2) the L_1 is the same as L_2 for low stimulus levels, and L_1 is 10 to 15 dB greater than L_2 for high stimulus levels. However, more complicated relationships among the frequencies and levels of the primaries have been shown to optimize DPOAE levels (e.g., Johnson, Neely, Garner, and Gorga, 2006).[3]

When continuous tones are presented to the ear, the acoustic emission has the same frequency as the stimulus but is delayed by its latency. The stimulus and emission will interact, resulting in peaks and valleys at frequencies where they are in and out of phase. This effect is seen at low levels of the stimulus, becoming less apparent and finally disappearing when the stimulus level exceeds 40 to 50 dB SPL. This level dependency is expected because of the emission's very low amplitude. That is, interference between the stimulus and emission can only occur when their levels are relatively similar; the low level of the emission means that this condition can only be met at lower levels of the stimulus.

These phenomena are consistent with the concept that the evoked acoustic emissions monitored in the ear canal are cochlear in origin. It is apparent that active processes enable the cochlea to produce as well as receive acoustical signals.

ACTIVE PROCESSES AND THE COCHLEAR AMPLIFIER

We have seen that the outer hair cells have a significant impact upon the sharpness and nonlinearity of cochlear processes.

This influence involves **active processes** that contribute to the cochlear response above and beyond the passive vibratory response of the basilar membrane (the traveling wave) and transmission of the transduced signals to the nervous system. This **cochlear amplifier** enhances the vibratory stimulus delivered to the inner hair cells, results in the cochlea's sharply tuned and nonlinear response, and generates otoacoustic emissions. The active mechanism relies on **outer hair cell electromotility**, which is the unique ability of the OHCs to rapidly contract and expand (by up to about 4%) in response to the sound stimulus, and thereby to affect cochlear micromechanics (e.g., Brownell et al., 1985; Brownell, 1990; Kalinec and Kachar, 1995; Holley, 1996; Patuzzi, 1996; Brownell and Popel, 1998; Geisler, 1998; Santos-Sacchi, 2003).

The prevalent explanation of OHC electromotility may be summarized as follows: Recall from Chapter 2 that there is positive hydrostatic pressure (turgor) within the OHC due to its cytoplasm, while its test tube–like shape is maintained by the tension of the matrix of structures in its lateral "walls" (see Figs. 2.29 and 2.30). The arrangement of these forces is such that changing the cell's surface area will change its length and girth. The surface area of the OHC is altered by conformational changes of components in the cell membrane, which, in turn, is controlled by the cell's polarization. Depolarization causes the OHCs to contract and hyperpolarization causes them to expand. As we have already seen, sound stimulation eventuates the bending of the OHC stereocilia, varying the ion currents through the opening and closing transduction channels, and thus varying the receptor potential. The changing polarization activates the cycle-by-cycle electromotile responses of the OHCs, which is able to occur fast enough to operate at all audible frequencies. Recalling that the OHCs are "mounted" between the Deiter's cells below and the reticular lamina above, this pushing-and-pulling motile response (Fig. 4.37) operates like a positive-feedback mechanism, which provides the forces that drive the cochlear amplifier.

Outer hair cell electromotility, which drives the cochlear amplifier, appears to be generated by the interaction of two

---

[3] Specifically, Johnson et al. (2006) found that, on average, normal DPOAEs were largest when

(a) $f_2/f_1 = 1.22 + \log_2(9.6/f_2) \cdot (L_2/415)^2$, and
(b) $L_1 = 80 + 0.137 \cdot \log_2(18/f_2) \cdot (L_2 - 80)$.

mechanisms or "motors" (Dallos, Zheng, and Cheatham, 2006; Kennedy, Evans, Crawford, and Fettiplace, 2006; Fettiplace and Hackney, 2006). The **somatic motor** relies on **prestin**, which has been identified as the *motor protein* of the OHC (Zheng et al., 2000; Oliver et al., 2001; Santos-Sacchi et al., 2001; Dallos and Fakler, 2002; Liberman et al., 2002; Dallos et al., 2006). The prestin motor is believed to operate by shuttling chloride ions back and forth between the inner and outer parts of the cell membrane (Fig. 4.38). Shortening is triggered by depolarization, which causes the prestin molecule to transport the chloride ion toward its inner side (Fig. 4.38a), and lengthening is triggered by hyperpolarization, which causes the prestin molecule to move the chloride ion toward its outer side (Fig. 4.38b). The **hair bundle motor** relies on the force generated by the changing compliance of the stereocilia bundle that occurs with the opening and closing of the transduction pores (Fettiplace, 2006; Fettiplace and Hackney, 2006; Kennedy et al., 2006).

In addition to the fast electromotile response just discussed, slower motile responses are also produced when OHCs are exposed to chemical agents and the efferent neurotransmitter acetylcholine and electrical stimulation (e.g., Brownell et al., 1985; Zenner et al., 1985; Flock et al., 1986; Kachar et al., 1986; Ashmore, 1987; Ulfendahl, 1987; Slepecky et al., 1988a, 1988b; Zajic and Schacht, 1991; Holley, 1996). Figure 4.39 shows an example for a guinea pig OHC, which was removed from the

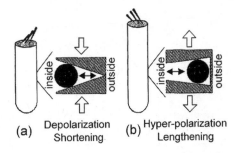

(a) Depolarization Shortening   **(b)** Hyper-polarization Lengthening

Figure 4.38 Artist's conceptualization of the somatic (prestin) motor of OHC electromotility. (a) Depolarization causes the prestin molecule to transport the chloride ion toward the inner side (shortening). (b) Hyperpolarization causes the prestin molecule to transport the chloride ion toward the outer side (lengthening).

cochlea and exposed to potassium gluconate (Slepecky et al., 1988b).

The central nervous system influences the active processes of the cochlea via the efferent innervation of the OHCs from the medial efferent (olivocochlear) system (e.g., Guinan, 1996, 2006; Robles and Ruggero, 2001; see Chaps. 2 and 6). For example, activation of the medial efferent system has been found to reduce the magnitude and nonlinearity of basilar membrane vibrations in the vicinity of the characteristic frequency (e.g., Murugasu and Russell, 1996; Dolan et al., 1997; Russell and Murugasu, 1997; see Chap. 6).

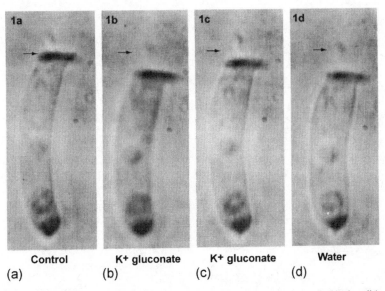

1a	1b	1c	1d
Control	K+ gluconate	K+ gluconate	Water
(a)	(b)	(c)	(d)

Figure 4.39 Effects of potassium gluconate on an isolated outer hair cell. (a) Original length of the hair cell. (b) The cell is shortened when exposed to potassium gluconate for 1 minute. (c) Cell returned to its original length after 4 minutes of contact. (d) The cell became swollen and shorter when the chemical medium was diluted with water (indicating that the cell membrane stayed intact during the experiment because it retained its normal osmotic characteristics). Arrows show the original length of the cell for comparison. *Source*: From *Hearing Research 24*, Slepecky, Ulfendahl, and Flock (Shortening and elongation of isolated outer hair cells in response to application of potassium gluconate, acetylcholine, and cationed ferritin, 119–126, © 1988), with kind permission of from Elsevier Science Publishers—NL, Sara Burgerhartstraat 25, 1055 KV Amsterdam, The Netherlands. Photograph courtesy of Dr. Norma Slepecky.

REFERENCES

Adrian, ED. 1931. The microphonic action of the cochlea: An interpretation of Wever and Bray's experiments. *J Physiol* 71, 28–29.

Ashmore, JE. 1987. A fast motile response in guinea-pig outer hair cells: The cellular basis of the cochlear amplifier. *J Physiol* 388, 323–347.

Bekesy, G. 1928. Zur Theorie des Hörens: Die Schwingungsform der Basilarmembran. *Physik Zeitschrchr* 29, 793–810.

Bekesy, G. 1944. Über die mechanische Frequenzanalyse in der Schnecke verschiedener Tiere. *Akust Zeitschr* 9, 3–11.

Bekesy, G. 1947. The variations of phase along the basilar membrane with sinusoidal vibrations. *J Acoust Soc Am* 19, 452–460.

Bekesy, G. 1948. On the elasticity of the cochlear partition. *J Acoust Soc Am* 20, 227–241. [Original in German: *Akust Zeitschr* 6: 265–278, 1941.]

Bekesy, G. 1949. On the resonance curve and the decay period at various points on the cochlear partition. *J Acoust Soc Am* 21, 245–254. [Original in German: *Akust Zeitschr*, 8: 66–76, 1943.]

Bekesy, G. 1950. D-C potentials and energy balance of the cochlear partition. *J Acoust Soc Am* 22, 576–582.

Bekesy, G. 1952. D-C resting potentials inside the cochlear partition. *J Acoust Soc Am* 24, 72–76.

Bekesy, G. 1953. Description of some mechanical properties of the organ of Corti. *J Acoust Soc Am* 25, 770–785.

Bekesy, G. 1960/1989. *Experiments in Hearing.* New York, NY: McGraw-Hill. [Republished by the Acoustical Society of America].

Berlin, CI (ed). 1998. *Otoacoustic Emissions: Basic Science and Clinical Applications.* San Diego, CA: Singular.

Brownell, WE. 1990. Outer hair cell electromotility and otoacoustic emissions. *Ear Hear* 11, 82–92.

Brownell, WE, Bader, CR, Bertrand, D, deRibaupierre, Y. 1985. Evoked mechanical response of isolated cochlear outer hair cells. *Science* 227, 194–196.

Brownell, WE, Popel, AS. 1998. Electrical and mechanical anatomy of the outer hair cell. In: AR Palmer, A Rees, AQ Summerfield, R Meddis (eds.), *Psychophysical and Physiological Advances in Hearing.* London, UK: Whurr, 89–96.

Burns, EM, Strickland, EA, Tubis, A, Jones, K. 1984. Interactions among spontaneous otoacoustic emissions. I. Distortion products and linked emissions. *Hear Res* 16, 271–278.

Cheatham, MA, Dallos, P. 1984. Summating potential (SP) tuning curves. *Hear Res* 16, 189–200.

Cooper, NP. 1996. Two-tone suppression in cochlear mechanics. *J Acoust Soc Am* 99, 3087–3098.

Cooper, NP, Rhode, WS. 1997. Mechanical responses to two-tone distortion products in the apical and basal turns of the mammalian cochlea. *J Neurophysiol* 78, 261–270.

Corey, DP. 2006. What is the hair cell transduction channel? *J Physiol* 576, 23–28.

Crawford, AC, Fettiplace, R. 1981. An electrical tuning mechanism in turtle cochlear hair cells. *J Laryngol* 312, 377–422.

Dallos, P. 1973. *The Auditory Periphery.* New York, NY: Academic Press.

Dallos, P. 1984. Some electrical circuit properties of the organ of Corti. II. Analysis including reactive elements. *Hear Res* 14, 281–291.

Dallos, P. 1985. Response characteristics of mammalian cochlear hair cells. *J Neurosci* 5, 1591–1608.

Dallos, P. 1986. Neurobiology of cochlear inner and outer hair cells: Intracellular recordings. *Hear Res* 22, 185–198.

Dallos, P, Billone, MC, Durrant, JD, Wang, C-Y, Raynor, S. 1972a. Cochlear inner and outer hair cells: Functional differences. *Science* 177, 356–358.

Dallos, P, Cheatham, MA. 1976. Production of cochlear potentials by inner and outer hair cells. *J Acoust Soc Am* 60, 510–512.

Dallos, P, Cheatham, MS, Ferraro, J. 1974. Cochlear mechanics, nonlinearities, and cochlear potentials. *J Acoust Soc Am* 55, 597–605.

Dallos, P, Fakler, B. 2002. Prestin, a new type of motor protein. *Nat Rev Mol Cell Biol* 3, 104–111.

Dallos, P, Harris, D. 1978. Properties of auditory-nerve responses in the absence of outer hair cells. *J Neurophys* 41, 365–383.

Dallos, P, Popper, AN, Fay, RR. (eds.), 1996. *The Cochlea.* New York, NY: Springer-Verlag.

Dallos, PJ, Santos-Sacchi, J, Flock, A. 1982. Intracellular recordings from cochlear outer hair cells. *Science* 218, 582–584.

Dallos, P, Shoeny, ZG, Cheatham, MA. 1970. Cochlear summating potentials: Composition. *Science* 170, 641–644.

Dallos, P, Shoeny, ZG, Cheatham, MA. 1972b. Cochlear summating potentials: Descriptive aspects. *Acta Otol Suppl* 302, 1–46.

Dallos, D, Zheng, J, Cheatham, MA. 2006. Prestin and the cochlear implifier. *J Physiol* 576(1), 37–42.

Davis, H. 1957. Biophysics and physiology of the inner ear. *Physiol Rev* 37, 1–49.

Davis, H. 1958. A mechano-electrical theory of cochlear action. *Ann Otol* 67, 789–801.

Davis, H. 1961. Some principles of sensory receptor action. *Physiol Rev* 4, 391–416.

Davis, H. 1965. A model for transducer action in the cochlea. *Cold Spring Harb Symp Quant Biol* 30, 181–190.

Davis, H, Deatherage, BH, Eldredge, DH, Smith, CA. 1958. Summating potentials of the cochlea. *Am J Physiol* 195, 251–261.

Davis, H, Deatherage, B, Rosenblut, B, Fernandez, C, Kimura, R, Smith, CA. 1958. Modificatiaon of cochlear potentials by streptomycin poisoning and by extensive venous obstruction. *Laryngoscope* 68, 596–627.

Davis, H, Derbyshire, A, Lurie, M, Saul, L. 1934. The electric response of the cochlea. *Ann Otol* 68, 665–674.

Davis, H, Eldridge, DH. 1959. An interpretation of the mechanical detector action of the cochlea. *Ann Otol Rhinol Laryngol* 68, 665–674.

Davis, H, Fernandez, C, McAuliffe, DR. 1950. The excitatory process in the cochlea. *Proc Natl Acad Sci U S A* 36, 580–587.

Dekker, TN, (ed). 1992. Otoacoustic emissions. *Sem Hear* 13(1), 1–104.

Dolan, DF, Guo, MH, Nuttall, AL. 1997. Frequency-dependent enhancement of basilar membrane velocity during olivocochlear bundle stimulation. *J Acoust Soc Am* 102, 3587–3596.

Duifhuis, H. 1976. Cochlear nonlinearity and second filter: Possible mechanisms and implications. *J Acoust Soc Am* 59, 408–423.

Eggermont, JJ, Odenthal, DW, Schmidt, PN, Spoor, A. 1974. Electrocochleography: Basic principles and clinical application. *Acta Otol Suppl* 316, 1–84.

Evans, EF. 1972a. The frequency response and other properties of single nerve fibers in the guinea pig cochlea. *J Physiol* 226, 263–287.

Evans, EF. 1972b. *Does frequency sharpening occur in the cochlea?* In: Symposium on Hearing Theory. Eindhoven, The Netherlands: Institute for Perception Research.

Evans, EF. 1974. The effects of hypoxia on tuning of single fibers in the cochlear nerve. *J Physiol* 238, 65–67.

Evans, EF. 1975. The sharpening of cochlear frequency selectivity in the normal and abnormal cochlea. *Audiology* 14, 419–442.

Evans, EF, Wilson, JP. 1971. *Frequency resolving power of the cochlea: The effective bandwidth of cochlear nerve fibers.* In: Proceedings of the 7th International Congress on Acoustics, Vol. 3. Budapest, Hungary: Akademiai Kiado, 453–456.

Evans, EF, Wilson, JP. 1973. Frequency selectivity of the cochlea. In: AR Møller (ed.), *Basic Mechanisms in Hearing.* New York, NY: Academic Press, 519–554.

Eybalin, M. 1993. Neurotransmitters and neuromodulators of the mammalian cochlea. *Physiol Rev* 73, 309–373.

Fettiplace, R. 2006. Active hair bundle movements in auditory hair cells. *J Physiol* 576 (1), 29–36.

Fettiplace, R, Hackney, CM. 2006. The sensory and motor roles of auditory hair cells. *Nat Rev Neurosci* 7(1), 19–29.

Flock, A. 1971. Sensory transduction in hair cells. In: WR Lowenstein (ed.), *Principles of Receptor Physiology*, Vol. I. New York, NY: Springer-Verlag, 396–441.

Flock, A, Flock, B, Ulfendahl, M. 1986. Mechanisms of movement in outer hair cells and a possible structural basis. *Arch Otorhinolaryugol* 243, 83–90.

Geisler, CD. 1998. *From Sound to Synapse: Physiology of the Mammalian Ear.* New York, NY: Oxford University Press.

Geisler, CD, Rhode, WS, Kenedy, DT. 1974. Responses to tonal stimuli of single auditory nerve fibers and their relationship to basilar membrane motion in the squirrel monkey. *J Neurophysiol* 37, 1156–1172.

Gelfand, SA. 1981. *Hearing: An Introduction to Phychological and Physiological Acoustics.* New York, NY: Marcel Dekker.

Grundfest, H. 1971. The general electrophysiology of input membrane in electrogenic excitable cells. In: WR Lowenstein (ed.), *Handbook of Sensory Physiology. Vol. 1: Principles of Receptor Physiology.* New York, NY: Springer-Verlag, 136–165.

Guinan, JJ Jr. 1996. Physiology of olivocochlear efferents. In: P Dallos, AN Popper, RR Fay (eds.), *The Cochlea.* New York, NY: Springer-Verlag, 435–502.

Guinan, JJ Jr. 2006. Olivocochlear efferents: Anatomy, physiology, function, and the measurement of efferent effects in humans. *Ear Hear* 27, 589–607.

Helmholtz, H. von. 1870. *Die Lehre von den Tonempfindungen als physiologische Grundlage für die Theorie der Musik. Dritte umgearbeitete Ausgabe.* Braunschweig: Vieweg.

Holley, MC. 1996. Cochlear mechanics and micromechanics. In: P Dallos, AN Popper, RR Fay (eds.), *The Cochlea.* New York, NY: Springer-Verlag, 386–434.

Honrubia, V, Ward, PH. 1968. Longitudinal distribution of the cochlear microphonics inside the cochlear duct (guinea pig). *J Acoust Soc Am* 44, 951–958.

Honrubia, V, Ward, PH. 1969a. Dependence of the cochlear microphonic and summating potential on the endocochlear potential. *J Acoust Soc Am* 46, 388–392.

Honrubia, V, Ward, PH. 1969b. Properties of the summating potential of the guinea pig's cochlea. *J Acoust Soc Am* 45, 1443–1449.

Hudspeth, AJ. 1982. Extracellular current flow and the site of transduction by vertibrate hair cells. *J Neurosci* 2, 1–10.

Hudspeth, AJ. 1985. The cellular basis of hearing: The biophysics of hair cells. *Science* 230, 745–752.

Hudspeth, AJ, Corey, DP. 1977. Sensitivity, polarity, and conductance change in the response of vertibrate hair cells to controlled mechanical stimulation. *Proc Natl Acad Sci U S A* 74, 2407–2411.

Hudspeth, AJ, Jacobs, R 1979. Stereocilia mediate transduction in vertibrate cells. *Proc Natl Acad Sci U S A* 76, 1506–1509.

Johnsen, NJ, Elberling, C. 1982b. Evoked acoustic emissions from the human ear I. Equipment and response parameters. *Scand Audiol* 11, 3–12.

Johnson, TA, Neely, ST, Garner, CA, Gorga, MP. 2006. Influence of primary-level and primary-frequency ratios on human distortion product otoacoustic emissions. *J Acoust Soc Am* 119, 418–428.

Johnstone, BM, Boyle, JE. 1967. Basilar membrane vibration examined with the Mossbauer technique. *Science* 15S, 389–390.

Johnstone, BM, Taylor, KJ, Boyle, AJ. 1970. Mechanics of the guinea pig cochlea. *J Acoust Soc Am* 47, 504–509.

Johnstone, BM, Yates, GK 1974. Basilar membrane tuning curves in the guinea pig. *J Acoust Soc Am* 55, 584–587.

Kachar, B, Brownell, WE, Altschuler, R, Fex, J. 1986. Electrokinetic shape changes of cochlear outer hair cells. *Nature* 322, 365–368.

Kalinec, F, Kachar, B. 1995. Structure of the electromechanical transduction mechanism in mammalian outer hair cells. In: A Flock, D Ottoson, M Ulfendahl (eds.), *Active Hearing*. Kidlington, UK: Pergamon, 181–193.

Kazmierczak, P, Sakaguchi, H, Tokita, J, Wilson-Kubalek, EM, Ronald, A, Milligan, RA, Muller, U, Bechara Kachar, B. 2007. Cadherin 23 and protocadherin 15 interact to form tip-link filaments in sensory hair cells. *Nature* 449(7158), 87–92.

Kelly, JP, Khanna, SM. 1984a. Ultrastructural damage in cochleae used for studies of basilar membrane mechanics. *Hear Res* 14, 59–78.

Kelly, JP, Khanna, SM. 1984b. The distribution of darnage in the cochlea after removal of the round window membrane. *Hear Res* 16, 109–126.

Kemp, DT. 1978. Stimulated acoustic emissions from within the human auditory system. *J Acoust Soc Am* 64, 1386–1391.

Kemp, DT. 1979. Evidence of mechanical nonlinearity and frequency selective wave amplification in the cochlea. *Arch Otol Rhinol Laryngol* 224, 37–45.

Kennedy, HJ, Evans, MG, Crawford, AC, Fettiplace, R. 2006. Depolarization of cochlear outer hair cells evoked active hair bundle motion by two mechanisms. *J Neurosci* 26, 2757–2766.

Khanna, SM. 1986. Homodyne interferometer for basilar membrane measurements. *Hear Res* 23, 9–26.

Khanna, SM, Johnson, GW, Jacobs, J. 1986. Homodyne interferometer for basilar membrane vibration measurements. II. Hardware and techniques. *Hear Res* 23, 27–36.

Khanna, SM, Leonard, DGB. 1982. Basilar membrane tuning in the cat cochlea. *Science* 215, 305–306.

Khanna, SM, Leonard, DGB. 1986a. Measurement of basilar membrane vibrations and evaluation of the cochlear condition. *Hear Res* 23, 37–53.

Khanna, SM, Leonard, DGB. 1986b. Relationship between basilar membrane tuning and hair cell condition. *Hear Res* 23, 55–70.

Khanna, SM, Sears, RE, Tonndorf, J. 1968. Some properties of longitudinal shear waves: A study by computer simulation. *J Acoust Soc Am* 43, 1077–1084.

Kiang, NYS. 1965. *Discharge Patterns of Single Nerve Fibers in the Cat's Auditory Nerve*. Cambridge, MA: MIT Press.

Kiang, NYS, Liberman, NC, Sewell, WF, Guinan, JJ. 1986. Single unit clues to cochlear mechanisms. *Hear Res* 22, 171–182.

Kim, DO. 1986. Active and nonlinear cochlear biomechanics and the role of outer-hair-cell subsystem in the mammalian auditory system. *Hear Res* 22, 105–114.

Klink, R. 1986. Neurotransmission in the inner ear. *Hear Res* 22, 235–243.

Kohllofel, LUE. 1972. A study of basilar membrane vibrations. *Acustica* 27, 49–89.

Konishi, T, Butler, RA, Fernandez, C. 1961. Effect of anoxia on cochlear potentials. *J Acoust Soc Am* 33, 349–356.

Kros, CJ. 1996. Physiology of mammalian cochlear hair cells. In: P Dallos, AN Popper, RR Fay (eds.), *The Cochlea*. New York, NY: Springer-Verlag, 318–385.

Leonard, DGB, Khanna, SM. 1984. Histological evaluation of damage m cat cochleae used for measurement of basilar membrane mechanics. *J Acoust Soc Am* 75, 515–527.

LePage, EL, Johnstone, BM. 1980. Nonlinear mechanical behavior of the basilar membrane in the basal turn of the guinea pig cochlea. *Hear Res* 2, 183–192.

Liberman, MC. 1982. The cochlear frequency map for the cat: Labeling auditory-nerve fibers of known characteristic frequency. *J Acoust Soc Am* 72, 1441–1449.

Liberman, MC. 1984. Single-neuron labeling and chronic cochlear pathology. I. Threshold shift and characteristic-frequency shift. *Hear Res* 16, 33–41.

Liberman, MC, Dodds, LW. 1984. Single-neuron labeling and chronic cochlear pathology. II. Stereocilia damage and alterations of spontaneous discharge rates. *Hear Res* 16, 43–53.

Liberman, MC, Gao, J, He, DZZ, Wu, X, Jia, S, Zuo, J. 2002. Prestin is required for electromotility of the outer hair cell and for the cochlear amplifier. *Nature* 419, 300–304.

Liberman, MC, Kiang, NYS. 1984. Single-neuron labeling and chronic cochlear pathology. IV. Stereocilia damage and alterations in rate- and phase-level functions. *Hear Res* 16, 75–90.

Lim, DJ. 1986. Cochlear micromechanics in understanding otoacoustic emission. *Scand Audiol* 25, 17–25.

Lonsbury-Martin, BL, Whitehead, ML, Martin, GK. 1991. Clinical applications of otoacoustic emissions. *J Speech Hear Res,* 34, 964–981.

Manley, GA. 1978. Cochlear frequency sharpening—A new synthesis. *Acta Otol* 85, 167–176.

Manoussaki, D, Dimitriadis, EK, Chadwick, RS. 2006. Cochlea's graded curvature effect on low frequency waves. *Phys Rev Lett* 96, 088701.

McFadden, D, Wightman, EL. 1983. Audition: Some relations between normal and pathological hearing. *Ann Rev Psychol* 34, 95–128.

Misrahy, GS, Hildreth, KM, Shinabarger, EW, Gannon, WJ. 1958. Electrical properties of the wall of endolymphatic space of the cochlea (guinea pig). *Am J Physiol* 194, 396–402.

Murugasu, E, Russell, IJ. 1996. The effect of basilar membrane displacement in the basal cochlea. *J Neurosci* 16, 325–332.

Naidu, RC, Mountain, DC. 1998. Measurements of the stiffness map challenge a basic tenet of cochlear theories. *Hear Res* 124, 124–31.

Neeley, ST, Norton, SJ, Gorga, MP, Jesteadt, W. 1986. Latency of otoacoustic emissions and ABR wave V using tone-burst stimuli. *J Acoust Soc Am* 79(suppl. 1), S5.

Norton, SJ, Neeley, ST. 1987. Tone-burst-evoked otoacoustic emissions from normal-hearing subjects. *J Acoust Soc Am* 81, 1860–1872.

Nuttall, AL, Brown, MC, Masta, RI, Lawrence, M. 1981. Inner hair-cell responses to velocity of basilar membrane motion in the guinea pig. *Brain Res* 211, 171–174.

Nuttall, AL, Dolan, DF. 1993. Intermodulation distortion (f2-f1) in inner hair cell and basilar membrane responses. *J Acoust Soc Am* 93, 2061–2068.

Nuttall, AL, Dolan, DF, Avinash, G. 1990. Measurements of basilar membrane tuning and distortion with laser velocimetry. In: P Dallos, JW Matthews, CD Geisler, MA Ruggero, CR Steele, (eds.), *The Mechanics and Biophysics of Hearing*. Berlin, Germany: Springer-Verlag, 288–295.

Oliver, D, He, DZZ, Klöcker, N, Ludwig, J, Schulte, U, Waldegger, S, Ruppersberg, JP, Dallos, P, Fakler, B. 2001. Intracellular anions as the voltage sensor of prestin, the outer hair cell motor protein. *Science* 292, 2340–2343.

Patuzzi, R. 1996. Cochlear mechanics and micromechanics. In: P Dallos, AN Popper, RR Fay (eds.), *The Cochlea*. New York, NY: Springer-Verlag, 186–257.

Peake, WT, Sohmer, HS, Weiss, TE. 1969. Microelectrode recordings of intracochlear potentials. *MIT Res Lab Electron Quart Prog Rep* 94, 293–304.

Pickles, JO. 1982. *An Introduction to the Physiology of Hearing*. London, U.K.: Academic Press.

Pickles, JO, Corey, DP. 1992. Microelectrical transduction by hair cells. *Trends Neurosci* 15(7), 254–259.

Pickles, JO, Comis, SD, Osborne, MP. 1984. Cross-links between stereocilia in the guinea pig organ of Corti, and their possible relation to sensory transduction. *Hear Res* 15, 103–112.

Probst, R, Lonsbury-Martin, BL, Martin, GK. 1991. A review of otoacoustic emissions. *J Acoust Soc Am* 89, 2027–2067.

Rhode, WS. 1971. Observations of the vibration of the basilar membrane in squirrel monkey using the Mossbauer technique. *J Acoust Soc Am* 49, 1218–1231.

Rhode, WS. 1978. Some observations on cochlear mechanics. *J Acoust Soc Am* 64, 158–176.

Rhode, WS, Cooper, NP. 1993. Two-tone suppression and distortion production on the basilar membrane in the hook region of cat and guinea pig cochleae. *Hear Res* 66, 31–45.

Rhode, WS, Robles, L. 1974. Evidence from Mossbauer experiments for nonlinear vibration in the cochlea. *J Acoust Soc Am* 55, 588–596.

Roberts, WM, Howard, J, Hudspeth, AJ. 1988. Hair cells: Transduction, tuning, and transmission in the inner ear. *Ann Rev Cell Biol* 4, 63–92.

Robinette, MS, Glattke, TJ, (eds.). 2002. *Otoacoustic Emissions: Clinical Applications*, 2nd ed. New York, NY: Thieme Medical Publishers.

Robles, L, Ruggero, MA. 2001. Mechanics of the mammalian cochlea. *Physiol Rev* 81, 1305–1352.

Robles, L, Ruggero, MA, Rich, NC. 1986. Basilar membrane mechanics at the base of the chinchilla cochlea: I. Input-output functions, tuning curves, and response phase. *J Acoust Soc Am* 80, 1363–1374.

Robles, L, Ruggero, MA, Rich, NC. 1991. Two-tone distortion in the basilar membrane of the cochlea. *Nature* 349, 413–414.

Robles, L, Ruggero, MA, Rich, NC. 1997. Two-tone distortion on the basilar membrane of the chinchilla cochlea. *J Neurophysiol* 77, 2385–2399.

Ruggero, MA, Rich, NC, Recio, A, Narayan, SS, Robles, L. 1997. Basilar membrane responses to tones at the base of the chinchilla cochlea. *J Acoust Soc Am* 101, 2151–2163.

Ruggero, MA, Robles, L, Rich, NC. 1992. Two-tone suppression in the basilar membrane of the cochlea: Mechanical basis of auditory nerve rate suppression. *J Neurophysiol* 68, 1087–1099.

Russell, IJ, Murugasu, E. 1997. Medial efferent inhibition suppresses basilar membrane responses to near characteristic frequency tones of moderate to high intensities. *J Acoust Soc Am* 102, 1734–1738.

Russell, IJ, Sellick, PM. 1977a. Tuning properties of cochlear hair cells. *Nature* 267, 858–860.

Russell, IJ, Sellick, PM. 1977b. The tuning properties of cochlear hair cells. In: EF Evans, JP Wilson (eds.), *Psychophysics and Physiology of Hearing*. London, UK: Academic Press, 71–87.

Russell, IJ, Sellick, PM. 1978a. Intracellular studies of hair cells in the mammalian cochlea. *J Physiol* 284, 261–290.

Russell, IJ, Sellick, PM. 1978b. Intracellular studies of cochlear hair cells: Filling the gap between basilar membrane mechanics and neural excitation. In: RF Naunton, C Fernandez (eds.), *Evoked Electrical Activity in the Auditory Nervous System*. London, UK: Academic Press, 113–139.

Russell, IJ, Sellick, PM. 1983. Low frequency characteristics of intracellularly recorded potentials in guinea pig cochlear hair cells. *J Physiol* 338, 179–206.

Rutherford, W. 1886. A new theory of hearing. *J Anat Physiol* 21, 166–168.

Santos-Sacchi, J. 2003. New tunes from Corti's organ: The outer hair cell boogie rules. *Cur Opin Neurobiol* 13, 1–10.

Santos-Sacchi, J, Shen, W, Zheng, J, Dallos, P. 2001. Effects of membrane potential and tension on prestin, the outer hair cell lateral membrane motor protein. *J Physiol* 531, 661–666.

Sellick, PM, Patuzzi, R, Johnstone, BM. 1982a. Measurement of basilar membrane motion in the guinea pig using the Mossbauer technique. *J Acoust Soc Am* 72, 131–141.

Sellick, PM, Patuzzi, R, Johnstone, BM. 1982b. Modulation of responses of spiral ganglion cells in the guinea pig by low frequency sound. *Hear Res* 7, 199–221.

Sellick, PM, Russell, IJ. 1980. The responses of inner hair cells to basilar membrane velocity during low frequency auditory stimulation in the guinea pig cochlea. *Hear Res* 2, 439–445.

Sewell, WF. 1996. Neurotransmitters and synaptic transmission. In: P Dallos, AN Popper, RR Fay (eds.), *The Cochlea*. New York, NY: Springer-Verlag, 503–533.

Slepecky, N, Ulfendahl, M, Flock, A. 1988a. Effects of caffeine and tetracaine on outer hair cell shortening suggest intracellular calcium involvement. *Hear Res* 32, 11–32.

Slepecky, N, Ulfendahl, M, Flock, A. 1988b. Shortening and elongation of isolated outer hair cells in response to application of potassium gluconate, acetylcholine and cationized ferritin. *Hear Res* 34, 119–126.

Smith, DW, Moody, DB, Stebbins, WC, Norat, MA. 1987. Effects of outer hair cell loss on the frequency selectivity of the patas monkey auditory system. *Hear Res* 29, 125–138.

Steel, KR. 1983. The tectorial membrane of mammals. *Hear Res* 9, 327–359.

Strickland, EA, Burns, EM, Tubis, A. 1985. Incidence of spontaneous otoacoustic emissions in children and infants. *J Acoust Soc Am* 78, 931–935.

Tasaki, I, Davis, H, Eldredge, DH. 1954. Exploration of cochlear potentials in guinea pig with a microelectrode. *J Acoust Soc Am* 26, 765–773.

Tasaki, I, Davis, H, Legouix, JP. 1952. The space–time pattern of the cochlear microphonic (guinea pig) as recorded by differential electrodes. *J Acoust Soc Am* 24, 502–518.

Tasaki, I, Spiropoulos, CS. 1959. Stria vascularis as a source of endocochlear potential. *J Neurophysiol* 22, 149–155.

Tonndorf, J. 1960. Shearing motion in scale media of cochlear models. *J Acoust Soc Am* 32, 238–244.

Tonndorf, J. 1975. Davis-1961 revisited: Signal transmission in the cochlear hair cell-nerve junction. *Arch Otol* 101, 528–535.

Ulfendahl, M. 1987. Motility in auditory sensory cells. *Acta Physiol Scand* 13Q, 521–527.

Vollrath, MA, Kwan, KY, Corey, DP. 2007. The micromachinery of mechanotransduction in hair cells. *Ann Rev Neurosci* 30, 339–365.

von Helmholtz, H. 1870. *Die Lehre von den Tonempfindugen als physiologische Grundlage fur die Theorie der Musik. Dritte umgearbeitete Ausgabe.* Braunschweig, Germany: Vieweg.

Wangemann, P, Schacht, J. 1996. Homeostatic mechanisms in the cochlea. In: P Dallos, AN Popper, RR Fay (eds.), *The Cochlea.* New York, NY: Springer-Verlag, 130–185.

Wever, EG. 1949. *Theory of Hearing.* New York. NY: Dover.

Wever, EG. 1966. Electrical potentials of the cochlea. *Physiol Rev* 46, 102–126.

Wever, EG, Bray, CW. 1930. Action currents in the auditory nerve in response to acoustic stimulation. *Proc Natl Acad Sci U S A* 16, 344–350.

Wever, EG, Lawrence, M. 1950. The acoustic pathways to the cochlea. *J Acoust Soc Am* 22, 460–467.

Wever, EG, Lawrence, M. 1954. *Physiological Acoustics.* Princeton, NJ: Princeton University Press.

Wilson, JP, Johnstone, JR. 1972. *Capacitive probe measures of basilar membrane vibration.* In: Symposium on Hearing Theory. Eindhoven, The Netherlands: Institute for Perception Research, 172–181.

Wilson, JP, Johnstone, JR. 1975. Basilar membrane and middle ear vibration in guinea pig measured by capacitive probe. *J Acoust Soc Am* 57, 705–723.

Wit, HP, Ritsma, RJ. 1979. Stimulated acoustic emissions from the human ear. *J Acoust Soc Am* 66, 911–913.

Wit, HP, Ritsma, RJ. 1980. Evoked acoustical emissions from the human ear: Some experimental results. *Hear Res* 2, 253–261.

Yates, GK, Winter, IM, Robertson, D. 1990. Basilar membrane nonlinearity determines auditory nerve rate-intensity functions and cochlear dynamic range. *Hear Res* 45, 203–220.

Zajic, G, Schacht, J. 1991. Shape changes in isolated outer hair cells: Measurements with attached microspheres. *Hear Res* 407–411.

Zenner, HP, Zimmerman, U, Schmitt, U. 1985. Reversible contraction of isolated mammalian cochlear hair cells. *Hear Res* 18, 127–133.

Zheng, J, Shen, W, He, DZZ, Long, K, Madison, LD, Dallos, P. 2000. Prestin is the motor protein of cochlear outer hair cells. *Nature* 405, 149–155.

Zurek, PM. 1981. Spontaneous narrow-band acoustic signals emitted by human ears. *J Acoust Soc Am* 69, 514–523.

Zurek, PM. 1985. Acoustic emissions from the ear: A summary of results from humans and animals. *J Acoust Soc Am* 78, 340–344.

Zwislocki, J. 1974. A possible neuro-mechanical sound analysis in the cochlea. *Acustica* 31, 354–359.

Zwislocki, J. 1975. Phase opposition between inner and outer hair cells and auditory sound analysis. *Audiology* 14, 443–455.

Zwislocki, J. 1985. Cochlear function—An analysis. *Acta Otol* 100, 201–209.

5 Auditory Nerve

This chapter deals with the coding of information in the auditory nerve. This is usually measured by monitoring the electrical responses of individual neurons or the compound output of the nerve "as a whole" during the presentation of various (usually acoustic) stimuli. The resulting observations suggest how various parameters of sound are represented in this primary stage of the auditory nervous system. Moreover, as we have already seen in previous chapters, responses from the auditory nerve have also been used as a window for observing cochlear processes.

Major advances in this area have been made possible by the use of intracellular recordings from individual auditory neurons labeled with **horseradish peroxidase (HRP)**, which was introduced by Liberman (1982a). This approach makes it possible to definitively identify the neuron from which recordings have been made, as well as to trace its course to other neurons or to the hair cells. Two fundamental and interrelated findings based upon this method must of necessity be highlighted at the outset of this chapter. First, recall from Chapter 2 that Kiang et al. (1982) established the correspondence of the **type I auditory neurons** (marked intracellularly) and **inner radial fibers**, which synapse with the inner hair cells, and that the **type II auditory neurons** (marked extracellularly) continue as the **outer spiral fibers** to the outer hair cells. Second, it is now accepted that all individual auditory nerve fiber responses of the type discussed here have actually been derived from the type I auditory neurons that innervate the inner hair cells (Liberman and Simmons, 1985; Kiang et al., 1986).

Let us briefly review a number of simple definitions and concepts about neural activity before we proceed. Nerve fibers elicit *all-or-none* electrical discharges called **action potentials**, which are picked up by electrodes and typically appear on recording devices as "spikes" at certain points in time (Fig. 5.1). For obvious reasons, action potentials are often called **spikes** or spike potentials and the discharging of a spike potential is also called firing. Similarly, the number of action potentials discharged per second is known as the **firing rate** or **discharge rate**, and the manner in which spikes are elicited over time is known as the **discharge pattern** or **firing pattern**. Figure 5.1 shows a number of idealized auditory nerve firing patterns. The rate at which a neuron fires "on its own" when there is no stimulation is called its **spontaneous rate** and is illustrated in frame a of the figure. Activation of the neuron by a stimulus is associated with an increase in its firing rate above its spontaneous rate (frames b and c). Finally, an increase in the level of a stimulus is typically associated with an increase in the firing rate (frame b vs. frame c), at least within certain limits.

FREQUENCY CODING

Tuning Curves

The responses of single auditory nerve fibers to acoustic stimulation at various frequencies were reported by Galambos and Davis (1943), and their results were confirmed and expanded upon by many others. The response areas of single neurons as a function of frequency are shown by their **tuning curves**, as illustrated in Fig. 5.2. A narrowly tuned cell responds to a very limited range of frequencies, whereas a broadly tuned cell responds to a much wider frequency range. Since an unstimulated neuron maintains an ongoing spontaneous discharge rate even in the absence of any apparent stimulation, its threshold may be determined by varying the stimulus level until the lowest intensity is reached, at which the neuron responds above its spontaneous rate. An alternative approach is to present the stimulus at a fixed intensity and to measure the number of spike potentials with which the unit responds at different stimulus frequencies. The former method measures the neuron's sensitivity, and the latter its firing rate, as functions of frequency. The frequency with the lowest threshold (or the greatest firing rate) is the **characteristic frequency (CF)** or **best frequency** of the neuron.

The tuning curves of various single fibers in the auditory nerve of the cat are shown in Fig. 5.2. Frequency is along the x-axis and the level needed to reach the neuron's threshold is on the y-axis. Notice that each fiber will respond to a range of frequencies if the stimulus level is high enough. This frequency range extends considerably below the CF, but is quite restricted above it. In other words, a fiber responds readily to intense stimulation below its CF, but is only minimally responsive to stimulation above it. At lower intensity levels, the fibers are quite narrowly tuned to a particular frequency, as is shown by the V-shaped troughs around each characteristic frequency (Kiang, 1965, 1968; Kiang et al., 1967; Kiang and Moxon, 1972, 1974).

The sensitivity of a particular neuron generally falls at a rate of more than 25 dB per octave below the CF and well over 100 dB per octave above it. The *low-frequency "tails"* of higher-CF fibers actually extend very far below the CF, and **phase-locked responses** for low-frequency stimuli at high levels have been demonstrated for these fibers (Kiang and Moxon, 1974). **Phase locking** refers to a clear and fixed relationship between some aspect of the response and the phase (or time) of some aspect of the stimulus. The importance of this phenomenon will become clear in the following sections dealing with firing patterns. (The low-frequency tails in the figure should not be surprising, since we know that much of the cochlear partition is affected at high intensities.)

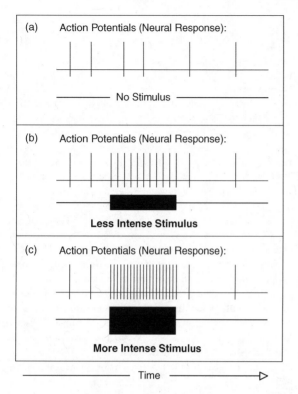

Figure 5.1 Idealized all-or-none action potentials or "spikes" generated by auditory nerve fibers (a) in the absence of a stimulus (the spontaneous firing rate), (b) in response to a relatively low intensity stimulus, and (c) in response to a relatively high intensity stimulus.

The tuning of the auditory nerve fibers thus appears to reflect the frequency analysis of the cochlea. Figure 5.2 also shows that there tends to be a gradation in the sharpness of neural tuning with increasing frequency. In other words, the high-frequency neural tuning curves tend to have sharper tips (as well as the above-noted low-frequency tails) than do the lower-frequency tuning curves (which do not possess low-frequency tails). The same general relationships occur in the cochlea and are demonstrated by comparing the tuning curves for the intracellular receptor potentials of the hair cells in the first (higher-frequency) and third (lower-frequency) turns (Dallos, 1985).

One might recall here that the characteristic frequencies of individual auditory nerve fibers are related to distance along the length of the cochlea by Liberman's (1982b) **cochlear frequency map** (see Fig. 4.22). This relationship was developed by determining the CFs of individual auditory neurons, which were labeled with HRP, and then tracing these fibers back to where they innervated various inner hair cells along the cochlear partition. Keithley and Schreiber (1987) developed a spiral ganglion frequency map for the cat in which CF is related to percentage distance from the base of Rosenthal's canal.

Firing Patterns
The firing patterns of fibers can suggest how information is coded and transmitted in the auditory nervous system. The firing patterns of auditory nerve fibers also provide corroborative information about cochlear mechanics.

Various stimuli are used to provide different kinds of information about neural coding. Clicks (at least ideally) are discrete

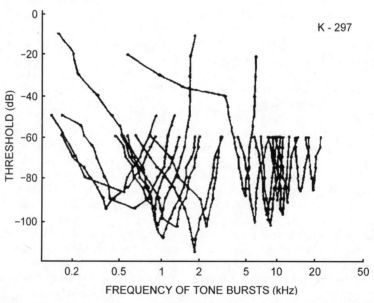

Figure 5.2 Tuning curves showing the response areas of single auditory nerve fibers in the cat. *Source*: Reprinted from *Discharge Patterns of Single Fibers in the Cat's Auditory Nerve* by NYS Kiang with permission of the M.I.T. Press, Cambridge, MA, Copyright © 1965, p. 87.

and instantaneous in time, with energy distributed equally throughout the frequency range. On the other hand, pure tones (also ideally) extend indefinitely in time, but are discrete in frequency. Thus, click stimuli lend themselves to the study of the temporal characteristics of the discharge pattern, while sinusoids can be used to study frequency-related aspects. Tone bursts can be used to investigate both frequency and temporal characteristics, as they are similar to clicks in their duration and to tones in their frequency specificity (Kiang, 1975). One should remember, however, that a tone burst is a compromise between the two extremes so that it is really less discrete in time than a click and less discrete in frequency than a pure tone.

Responses to Clicks

One way to study the response of an auditory nerve fiber is to determine the probability that it will discharge under given circumstances. This is not as complicated as it sounds. Assume that we have placed a microelectrode into an auditory nerve fiber. We then present a click to the animal's ear and record the time between the click onset and the discharge of any spike potential that it may elicit. In other words, we record the time delay or latency of each spike from the start of the click. This procedure is repeated many times for the same fiber, and the number of spikes that occurred after each latency is counted. These data are plotted on a graph called a **post-stimulus time (PST) histogram**, in which the latencies are shown on the abscissa and the number of spikes on the ordinate (Fig. 5.3). If many spikes occurred at a latency of 2 ms, for example, then we can say that there is a high probability that the fiber will respond at 2 ms. If concentrations of spikes (modes) also occur at other latencies, we can say that there is a good probability that the fiber will respond at these other latencies as well as at the first one.

Figure 5.3 shows the PST histograms obtained by Kiang (1965) for 18 auditory nerve fibers in one cat. The CF of each fiber is given to the left of its histogram. Note that fibers with lower CFs have multiple peaks, while those with higher CFs have single peaks. Three other observations are important. First, the latency to the first peak decreases as the CF increases. Second, the interpeak intervals (the time between successive modes) get smaller as the CF increases. Closer scrutiny reveals that the interpeak interval corresponds to the period of the characteristic frequency of a fiber (i.e., to 1/CF) in a relationship that constitutes a linear function. Lastly, baseline activity is actually reduced between the peaks. Kiang found that these time-locked multiple peaks and the reduced baseline activity were maintained even at very low levels of stimulation. Decreased baseline activity was, in fact, the initial response noted at the lowest stimulus levels.

If the PST histograms are compared for clicks of opposite polarity, the peaks resulting from rarefaction clicks are found to occur between those in response to condensation clicks (Kiang, 1965). That is, when the click's polarity is reversed (which

means that drum, and eventually basilar membrane, deflection is reversed; see Chap. 4), then so are the times at which the peaks and dips occur in the PST histogram. Furthermore, the rarefaction phase is related to increased neural activity, in agreement with the earlier findings of Davis et al. (1950) for stimuli up to 2000 Hz.

The traveling wave response to an impulsive stimulus such as a click travels up the cochlea at a speed that is quite fast at the basal end and slows down toward the apex (Bekesy, 1960/1989). We would therefore expect the PST histogram to reflect rapid and synchronous discharges of higher-frequency fibers originating from the basal turn. This effect is shown by the short latencies of the first peak for higher CFs. The longer latencies for successively lower CFs reflect the propagation time of the traveling wave up the cochlear partition to the places from which the fibers arise. Thus, the latency to the first peak represents a neural coding of the mechanical activity in the cochlea.

The interpeak interval also reflects the activity of the cochlea, as it is a function of the period of the frequency (1/f) of the click stimulus to which the fiber responds. Because the latencies of the peaks do not change with click level, Kiang suggested that deflections of the cochlear partition in one direction result in increased neural activity, while neural activity is reduced relative to the baseline rate when the basilar membrane is deflected in the opposite direction. This interpretation is further supported by the reversal of peaks and dips for clicks of opposite polarity.

Responses to Tones and Tonal Complexes

The PST histograms in Fig. 5.4 illustrate the typical firing patterns of auditory neurons in response to tone bursts (e.g., Kiang, 1965; Westerman and Smith, 1984). Notice that each firing pattern has an initial peak (**onset response**). The size of this peak is a function of the tone burst level. The peak is followed by a gradual decrease in the discharge rate (**adaptation**) over a period of about 10 to 20 ms, beyond which a stable level is attained. The stable rate continues until the tone burst is turned off, at which time activity drops sharply to a level below the spontaneous discharge rate. The spontaneous rate is then gradually reattained. The neural discharges are time-locked to individual cycles of the tone burst for fibers up to about 5000 Hz. (This effect is not seen in the figure because of the restricted time scale.)

Kiang (1965) found that the discharges of auditory nerve fibers are time-locked to tonal stimuli up to 4000 to 5000 Hz. This relationship was demonstrated by the presence on the PST histogram of single peaks corresponding to individual cycles of the stimulus, and it is consistent with other evidence that auditory nerve fibers respond to the particular phase of the stimulus within this frequency range (Hind et al., 1967; Rose et al., 1967). Furthermore, there is impressive evidence that auditory nerve fibers respond only to deflections of the basilar membrane in one direction (which is consistent with the click data), and that the timing of the firings corresponds to

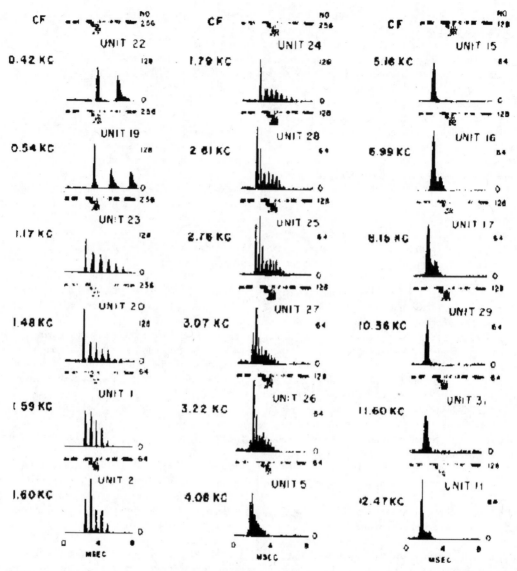

Figure 5.3 PST histograms for 18 auditory nerve fibers of a single cat in response to clicks. *Source*: Reprinted from *Discharge Patterns of Single Fibers in the Cat's Auditory Nerve* by NYS. Kiang with permission of the M.I.T. Press, Cambridge, MA, Copyright © 1965, p. 28.

elevations of the partition (Brugge et al., 1969; Rose et al., 1969; see Chap. 4).

The relationship of the responses of single auditory nerve fibers to stimulus phase is illustrated in Fig. 5.5. These graphs are not PST histograms, instead they show the number of spikes discharged at various time intervals in response to 1-s pure tones from 412 to 1600 Hz. The tones were presented at 80 dB SPL. A single fiber was monitored. It responded to frequencies between 412 and 1800 Hz, with its best responses between 1000 and 1200 Hz.

The dots under each histogram correspond to integral multiples of the period of the stimulus tone. Thus, in the upper left-hand graph of Fig. 5.5, with a frequency of 412 Hz and a period of 2427 μs, the dots indicate 2427 μs time intervals (2427, 4854, 7281 μs, etc.). The spikes in each histogram cluster at a number of relatively discrete latencies, with fewer spikes at successively higher multiples of the period. Of primary significance is that the locations of the peaks closely correspond to integral multiples of the period for each stimulus frequency up to and including 1100 Hz. At higher frequencies, the period of the peaks become as low as 625 μs (for 1600 Hz), although the latencies of the first peak stay in the range of 800 to 900 μs. This minimum period reflects the fiber's refractory period.

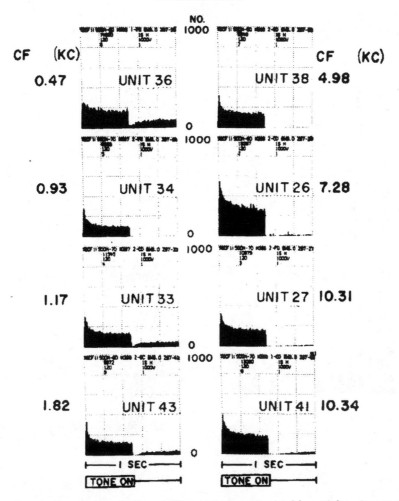

Figure 5.4 PST histograms in response to tone burst for fibers of different CFs. *Source*: Reprinted from *Discharge Patterns of Single Fibers in the Cat's Auditory Nerve* by NYS Kiang with permission of the M.I.T. Press, Cambridge, MA, Copyright © 1965, p. 69.

These findings suggest that, at least for pure tones, a period-time code is used to transmit frequency information in auditory nerve fibers: The discharge pattern of the neuron is in cadence with the period of the stimulus. The locking of the response pattern to the period of the sinusoid is maintained even if the stimulus frequency is not the CF of the fiber, and regardless of stimulus intensity. When the spike discharges were studied relative to a fixed point on the stimulus cycle, phase locking of the discharge pattern was found for frequencies as high as 5000 Hz. This result is not to suggest that place coding is unfounded. On the contrary, the importance of place coding is demonstrated by the tuning curves in Fig. 5.2. Both mechanisms contribute to frequency coding.

When an auditory nerve fiber is stimulated simultaneously by two relatively low-frequency tones, the resulting firing pattern will be phase-locked to either (1) the cycles of the first sinusoid, (2) the cycles of the second sinusoid, or (3) the cycles of both

stimuli (Hind et al., 1967). When the response pattern is to only one of the two original tones, the phase-locked response is the same as it would have been if that tone were presented alone. Which of the three response modes occurs is determined by the intensities of the two tones and by whether their frequencies lie within the fiber's response area.

Brugge et al. (1969) reported the discharge patterns in response to complex periodic sounds. Their stimuli were made up of two relatively low-frequency primary tones combined in various ways, as shown in Fig. 5.6. The firing patterns are shown in **period histograms**, in which discharges are represented as a function of the period of the stimulus (i.e., as though they all occurred during one period of the complex wave). Again, we see clear-cut phase locking of the discharge pattern to the stimulus, reflecting neural coding of the mechanical activity along the cochlear partition in a straightforward manner. Note that the neural activity shown by the period histogram follows the

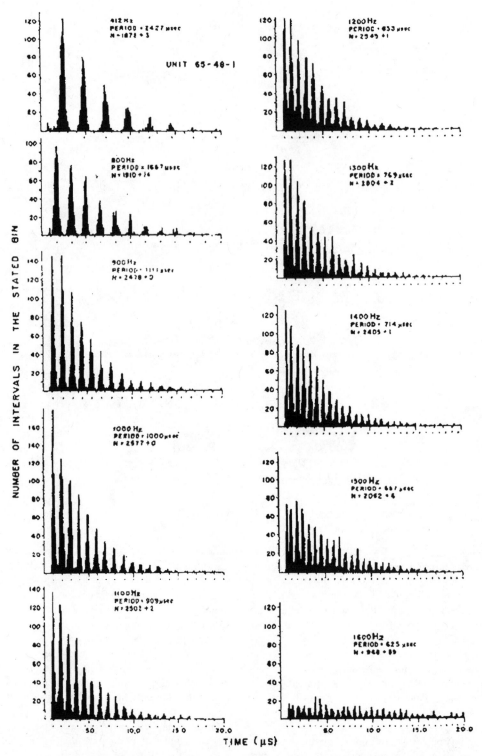

Figure 5.5 Interspike intervals for a single auditory neuron of a squirrel monkey in response to 1 s tones at 80 dB SPL. Stimulus frequency is shown above each graph. The dots below the abscissa are integral multiples of the period of the stimulus. (N is the number of intervals plotted plus the number of intervals with values greater than shown on the abscissa.) *Source*: From Rose, Brugge, Anderson, and Hind (1969) with permission of *J. Neurophysiol.*

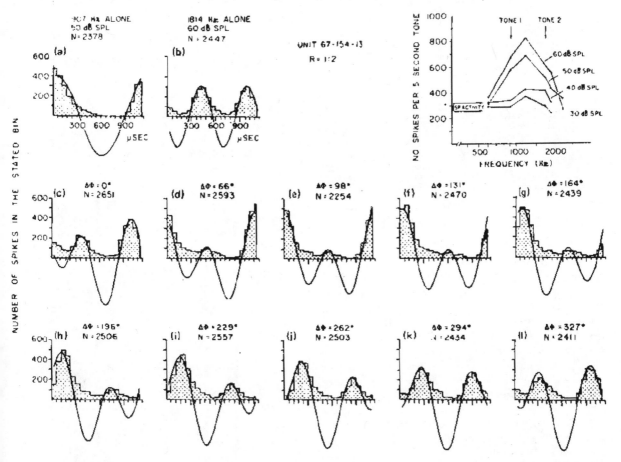

Figure 5.6   Complex tonal stimuli and period histograms of resulting discharge patterns: (a) and (b), primary tones; (c) to (l), complex tones; φ is the phase shift between the primaries; upper right-hand graph shows the response areas for various SPLs. *Source*: From Rose, Brugge, Anderson, and Hind (1969) with permission of *J. Neurophysiol.*)

shape of the stimulus waveform above and below the origin of the y-axis. These observations were associated with the concept that nerve fiber activation is linked to the upward deflections of the basilar membrane (Brugge et al., 1969). However, several studies have revealed that neural activation is also associated with downward deflections of the cochlear partition (Konishi and Nielsen, 1973; Sokolich et al., 1976; Sellick et al., 1982; Ruggero and Rich, 1983; Zwislocki, 1984, 1985, 1986). This reflects a more complicated state of affairs and has been the subject of some controversy.

The neural firing patterns reported by Brugge et al. were corroborated by Rose et al. (1969). They found that when two tones resulted in a complex wave whose peaks are not equidistant, then the spikes cluster about integral multiples of the period of the complex wave. The complex wave's period corresponds to its fundamental frequency, which, in turn, is the greatest common denominator of the two original tones. Note in this regard that when the ratio of the low to the high primary has a numerator of 1 less than the denominator, as for 1000 and 1100 Hz

(1000/1100 = 10/11), the fundamental is the difference tone (1100 − 1000 = 100 Hz). In this case, the spike discharges correspond to a period of 100 Hz, and the listener would perceive a tone corresponding to a pitch of 100 Hz. This provides one basis for the missing fundamental phenomenon discussed in Chapter 12.

Two-Tone Suppression

Two-tone suppression (or **inhibition**) occurs when the response of an auditory neuron produced by one tone is reduced by the presence of a second tone (the suppressor) at a different frequency (e.g., Nomoto et al., 1964; Kiang, 1965; Hind et al., 1967; Sachs and Kiang, 1968). Assume that an auditory nerve fiber is firing in response to a continuous tone presented at its characteristic frequency (Fig. 5.7a). A second tone at a slightly different frequency is then added to the first. The presence of the second tone will actually cause a decrease in the firing rate (Fig. 5.7b)—this is two-tone suppression. Many studies of two-tone suppression have used tone bursts to inhibit a unit's

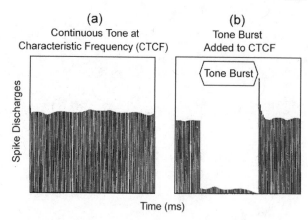

(a)
Continuous Tone at
Characteristic Frequency (CTCF)

(b)
Tone Burst
Added to CTCF

Figure 5.7 Idealized example of two-tone suppression (see text).

response to a continuous tone at its CF, as shown schematically in Fig. 5.7b.

Two-tone suppression can be produced by suppressor tone frequencies that are higher or lower than the CF. The former is often called *high-side suppression* and the latter is known as *low-side suppression*. It would be very cumbersome to "map out" the **inhibitory area(s)** of a neuron using discrete tone bursts because of the enormous number of frequencies and intensities that would have to be tested one at a time. Instead of tone bursts, Sachs and Kiang (1968) used a *sweep-frequency tone* to suppress the fiber's response to a *continuous tone at its characteristic frequency (CTCF)*. (A sweep-frequency tone is one that changes frequency continuously over time.) Figure 5.8 shows a series of PST histograms for a fiber with a CF of 22.2 kHz. The left column shows the firing patterns (as a function of log frequency) for the sweep-frequency (inhibiting) tone alone. The frequency of the sweep-frequency tone was changed from 6 to 60 kHz and then back down to 6 kHz. Thus, the sweep-frequency tone approached the CF first from below and then from above. The histograms in the right-hand column of the figure are for the ongoing CTCF combined with the sweep-frequency tone. Observe that the sweep-frequency tone causes a reduction in the firing rate at frequencies near the CF. Comparing the histograms in the right-hand column shows that a wider range of frequencies suppressed the discharge rate as the level of the sweep-frequency tone increased from −75 to −20 dB.

The results obtained using various sweep-frequency tone frequencies and levels can be compiled and then plotted in a manner similar to a tuning curve. An idealized representation is given in Fig. 5.9, where the cross-hatched areas show the combinations of frequencies and intensities that inhibit the firing of a fiber for a CTCF. This figure illustrates several aspects of two-tone suppression.

Two-tone suppression can be elicited by a suppressing (sweep-frequency) tone either higher or lower than the CF, as long as its intensity and frequency are appropriate. In general, the greatest

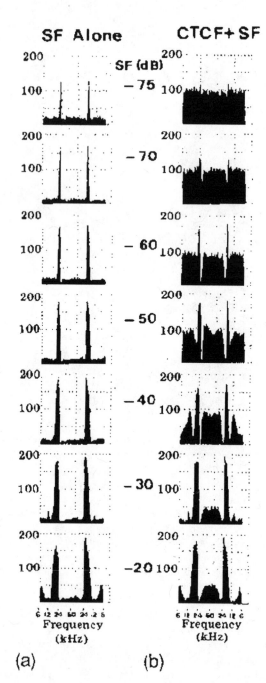

Figure 5.8 Discharge rates for (a) a sweep frequency (SF) tone presented alone and (b) the SF tone added to a continuous tone at its characteristic frequency (CTCF) at various levels of the SF tone. The CTCF is 22.2 kHz at −75 dB. Duration is 72 s going from 6 to 60 kHz and back to 6 kHz. *Abscissa*: log frequency for the SF tone; *ordinate*: spike rate. *Source*: Adapted from Sachs and Kiang (1968), with permission of *J. Acoust. Soc. Am.*

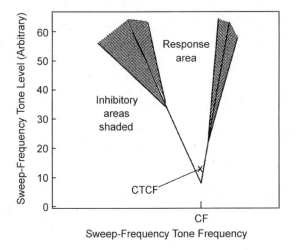

Figure 5.9 Idealized response and inhibitory areas in a two-tone suppression experiment. *Source*: Adapted from Sachs and Kiang (1968), with permission of *J. Acoust. Soc. Am.*

amount of suppression occurs when the suppressor tone is close to the CF, and less suppression occurs as the frequency difference widens. In Fig. 5.9, the high-frequency inhibitory area (*high-side suppression*) extends to within 10 dB of the level of the CTCF, whereas the low-frequency inhibitory area (*low-side suppression*) does not. In other words, inhibitory tones higher in frequency than the CF are more effective at lower intensities than tones whose frequencies are below the CF. Other intensity and frequency dependencies in two-tone suppression have been described, but are beyond the current scope (see Geisler, 1998 for a review). One might also note in this context that two-tone inhibition can affect auditory neuron tuning curves, although these effects are different depending upon whether the inhibitory tone is in close proximity to the CF or considerably below it (Kiang and Moxon, 1974; Javell et al., 1983; Patuzzi and Sellick, 1984). For example, the sharpness of tuning is hardly affected in the former case, whereas broader tuning results from the latter.

A considerable body of evidence reveals that two-tone suppression is the result of nonlinear processes in the cochlea (e.g., Geisler, 1998; Robles and Ruggero, 2001) (see Chap. 4). For example, two-tone suppression has been shown to occur for the vibratory response of the basilar membrane (Rhode, 1977; Ruggero et al., 1992; Cooper, 1996), cochlear microphonics and intracellular receptor potentials (e.g., Pfeiffer and Molnar, 1970; Legouix et al., 1973; Dallos and Cheatham, 1974; Sellick and Russell, 1979) and otoacoustic emissions (e. g., Kemp and Chum, 1980).

INTENSITY CODING

Determining how intensity is coded by the auditory neural system is a formidable problem. The most difficult aspect is to explain how the auditory nerve is able to subserve an intensity continuum covering 120+ dB.

The first neural responses at barely threshold intensities appear to be a decrease in spontaneous activity (Kiang, 1965), and phase locking of spike discharges to the stimulus cycle (Rose et al., 1967). This is not to say that the fiber will fire in response to every cycle of a near-threshold stimulus. Rather, even though the overall discharge rate may not be significantly greater than the spontaneous level, those spikes that do occur will tend to be locked in phase with the stimulus cycle (Hind, 1972). Effects such as this might provide some degree of intensity coding, since it has been known for some time that fibers with higher spontaneous rates have lower thresholds (Kiang, 1965; Salvi et al., 1983). We will return to the latter relationship below.

While threshold differences are unquestionably important, it makes sense to also consider the neuron's **dynamic range**, which is the intensity range over which the auditory nerve fiber continues to respond with increasing magnitude. **Saturation** is said to have occurred when the neuron's response no longer increases as the stimulus level is raised. In order to make this concept clear, Fig. 5.10 shows an example of the growth and saturation of an auditory neuron's firing pattern with increasing stimulus intensity. In their classic experiment, Galambos and Davis (1943) found that the dynamic range of auditory nerve fibers is only about 20 to 40 dB. In other words, the discharge rate increases with stimulus intensity from threshold up to a level 20 to 40 dB above it. At higher intensities the spike rate either levels off or decreases. Obviously, a single fiber cannot accommodate the 120+ dB range from minimal audibility to the upper usable limits of hearing. However, if there were a set of units with graded thresholds, they could cooperate to produce the dynamic range of the ear (Rose et al., 1971). For example, if there were four fibers with similar CF having dynamic ranges 0–40, 30–70, 60–100, and 90–130 dB, respectively, then they could conceivably accommodate the ear's dynamic range.

Subsequent findings reveal a wider dynamic range in fibers with similar CFs than was previously thought, and it is now established that auditory neurons can have dynamic ranges of as much as 40 dB or more (Davis, 1961; Rose et al., 1971; Evans and Palmer, 1980; Schalk and Sachs, 1980; Kiang, 1984; Liberman and Kiang, 1984; Liberman, 1988). The relationship between stimulus level and firing rate is shown by the **rate-level function**. Several examples of rate-level functions for various fibers with similar CFs in the same cat are shown in Fig. 5.11 from the study by Sachs and Abbas (1974). In each case, the arrow indicates the fiber's threshold. Notice that whereas the lower threshold fibers tend to saturate about 20 dB above threshold, the units with higher thresholds tend to have dynamic ranges that can be roughly 40 dB wide.

Considerable insight into this area was provided by the identification of three relatively distinct groups of auditory nerve fibers with respect to their spontaneous rates and thresholds by

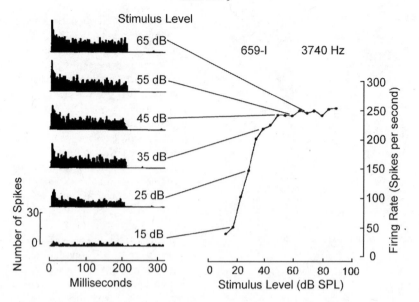

Figure 5.10 The input-output (rate-level) function on the right shows the effect of stimulus intensity on the firing rate of an auditory nerve fiber. The PST histograms on the left correspond to various points indicated on the input/output function. *Source*: From Salvi, Henderson, and Hamernik, Physiological bases of sensorineural hearing loss, in *Hearing Research and Theory*, Vol. 2, Tobias and Shuber (eds.), Copyright © 1983 by Academic Press.

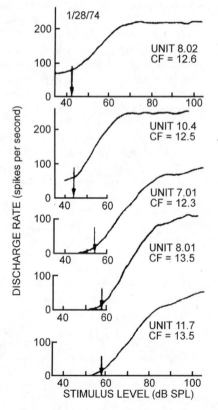

Figure 5.11 Discharge rate as a function of stimulus level for five auditory nerve fibers with similar CFs in the same cat. Arrows are fiber thresholds. *Source*: From Sachs and Abbas (1974), with permission of *J. Acoust. Soc. Am.*

Liberman (1978). The groups described by Liberman included units covering an overall threshold range as great as about 80 dB for fibers with similar CFs in the same cat. The relationship between auditory neuron thresholds and spontaneous rates has also been reported by Kim and Molnar (1979). Figure 5.12 shows the three groups of auditory nerve fibers in terms of the relationship between their spontaneous firing rates and their relative threshold sensitivities. The fibers that had high spontaneous rates (over 18 spikes/s) had the lowest thresholds of the three groups. These are indicated as group c in the figure. Within this high spontaneous rate (SR) group, the thresholds were essentially the same regardless of the actual spontaneous rate. That is, thresholds were within 5 dB whether the SR was 20 spikes/s or 100 spikes/s. These high-SR fibers made up about 61% of those sampled.

The second group included fibers with medium spontaneous rates (between 0.5 and 18 spikes/s). These medium-SR units comprised approximately 23% of the fibers and are shown as group b in Fig. 5.12. The remaining 16% had low SRs (under 0.5 spikes/s). Not only did these low-SR units have the highest thresholds of the three groups, but they also had a threshold range covering about 50 dB (group a).

It is now established that they are all inner radial units innervating the inner hair cells, and that each inner hair cell receives all three types of fibers (Liberman, 1982a). They are also distinguished on the basis of size, morphology, and where they attach to the inner hair cells (Liberman, 1978, 1980a, 1980b, 1982a, 1982b, 1988; Kim and Molnar, 1979; Kiang et al., 1982; Liberman and Oliver, 1984; Liberman and Brown, 1986). The high-SR fibers have the largest diameters and the greatest

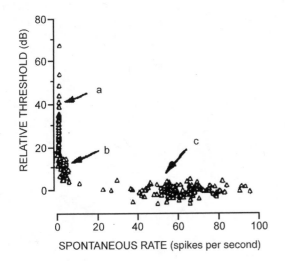

Figure 5.12 Relationship between spontaneous rate and relative thresh-olds for fibers with (a) low, (b) medium, and (c) high spontaneous fir-ing rates. *Source*: From Liberman, 1978, with permission of *J. Acoust. Soc. Am.*

number of mitochondria. On the other hand, the low-SR units have the smallest diameters and relatively fewest mitochondria. Figure 2.35 shows the attachments of the three types of fibers to a typical inner hair cell. Notice that the thick, high-SR fiber synapses on the side of the hair cell which faces toward the tunnel and outer hair cells (toward the right in the figure). In contrast, low-SR and medium-SR fibers attach on the surfaces facing the modiolus (toward the left). Of the three groups, the low-SR fibers appear to have the greatest association with the efferent neurons.

The individual rate-level functions of a larger number of high-, medium-, and low-SR fibers obtained by Liberman (1988) are shown in Fig. 5.13. Because these rate-level func-tions have been normalized in terms of both spike rates and stimulus levels, it is possible to directly compare the dynamic ranges. These functions revealed that high-SR and medium-SR auditory nerve fibers reached saturation about 25 dB above their thresholds; however, this did not occur for any of the fibers with low SRs. Instead, the spike rates of the low-SR units continued to increase with stimulus level through 40 dB above threshold, and some achieved continuing growth of magnitude as high as 60 dB above threshold.

To recapitulate, it appears that type I auditory nerve fibers with similar best frequencies have a considerable range of thresholds and dynamic ranges, and both of these parameters are correlated with the SRs of the fibers. In turn, these SR char-acteristics tend to categorize themselves in three groups, which are also distinguishable on the bases of their size, morphology, and the locations of their synapses. Moreover, each inner hair cell synapses with all three types of fibers. It would thus appear that there is a reasonable basis for the coding of intensity on the

basis of the auditory nerve fibers and their responses, at least to a first approximation.

A complementary if not alternative explanation that is based on several things we already know is also consistent with the factors already covered. For example, we know that auditory nerve fiber activity reflects the pattern of cochlear excitation in a rather straightforward manner. Figure 5.14 shows the effect of stimulus intensity on the response area of a single auditory neuron whose CF is 2100 Hz. Note that as intensity is increased, the number of spikes per second also increases, as does the frequency range to which the fiber responds. Also, the frequency range over which the fiber responds tends to increase more below than above the characteristic frequency.

Keeping this in mind, also recall that the basilar membrane may be conceived of as an array of elements that are selec-tively responsive to successively lower frequencies going from the base to the apex. Now refer to Fig. 5.15 by Whitfield (1967). Here, frequency is represented along the horizontal axis from left to right, and the ordinate represents spike rate. The hypoth-esis for neural coding illustrated in this figure is as follows: Fig. 5.15a represents the response area resulting from stimula-tion at a given frequency and intensity. Figure 5.15b shows the discharge pattern for an equivalent amount of stimulation at a higher frequency. The frequency change is represented by a simple displacement of the hypothetical response area (or exci-tation pattern) along the frequency axis and is analogous to the movement of the traveling wave envelope along the basi-lar membrane. Figure 5.15c represents the effect of increasing the stimulus level at the same frequency as in Fig. 5.15a. As the stimulus level increases, the fibers increase their spike rates (until saturation is reached). Although some fibers saturate, other fibers with similar CFs but different thresholds continue to increase their discharge rates as the level increases. As inten-sity continues to increase, the stimulus enters the excitatory areas of other fibers, which respond to that frequency only at higher intensities. The overall effect, then, is for the intensity increment to be coded by increased overall firing rates among more fibers and over a wider frequency range. We shall see in the next section that increasing the stimulus level also results in greater synchrony of the individual neural discharges, so that the whole-nerve action potential has a shorter latency and greater magnitude.

Such a model could employ all of the preceding factors in arriving at the overall change in the excitation pattern between Fig. 5.15a and 5.15 5.15c, and could account for the wide dynamic range of the ear. It does not, however, account for the observation in Fig. 5.14 that the peak of a fiber's response curve shifts in frequency as the stimulus level is increased (Rose et al., 1971). The implication is that phase-locking to the stimulus cycle would be particularly important in maintaining frequency coding when the intensity increment is encoded by increases in density of discharges per unit time and by widening of the array of active fibers.

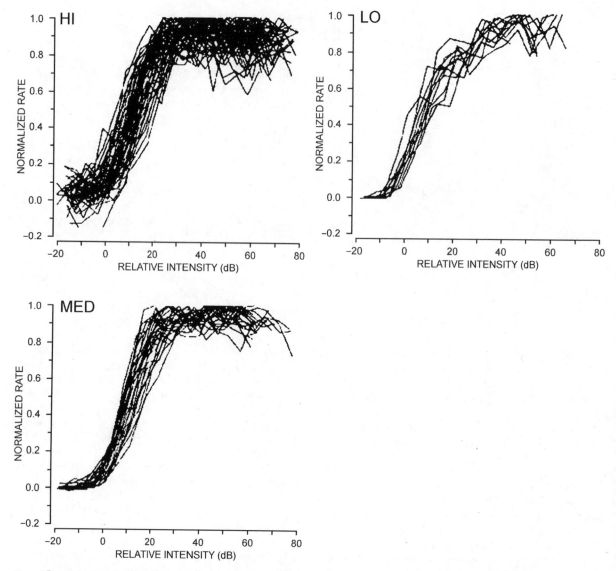

Figure 5.13 Normalized rate-level functions for various individual high-SR, medium-SR, and low-SR auditory nerve fibers (cat). *Source*: From *Hearing Research* 34, Liberman (Physiology of cochlear efferent and afferent neurons: Direct comparisons in the same animal, 179–192, ⓒ 1988) with kind permission from Elsevier Science Publishers, NL, Sara Burgerhartstraat 25, 1055 KV Amsterdam, The Netherlands.

SPEECH CODING

As is the case for other sounds, considerable attention has also been given to representation of speech signals in the auditory nerve. The coding of vowels has received considerable attention. For example, it has been shown that auditory neurons phase-lock to **formants** (vocal tract resonances; see Chap. 14) close to their characteristics frequencies and can represent the spectrum of a vowel (e.g., Sachs and Young, 1979, 1980; Young and Sachs, 1979; Sachs, 1984; Delgutte and Kiang, 1984a; Palmer, Winter, and Darwin, 1986; Palmer, 1990). Although space and scope limit our attention to the coding of vowels, one should be aware that studies have also addressed the neural representation of consonant characteristics (e.g., Miller and Sachs, 1983; Sinex and Geisler, 1983; Carney and Geisler, 1986, Delgutte and Kiang, 1984b; Deng and Geisler, 1987; Sinex, McDonald, and Mott, 1991), as well as other issues, such as the neural coding of speech in noise (e.g., Delgutte and Kiang, 1984c; Geisler and Gamble, 1989; Silkes and Geisler, 1991). The interested student will find several reviews that provide a nice starting point for further study (e.g., Delgutte, 1997; Geisler, 1998; Palmer and Shamma, 2004).

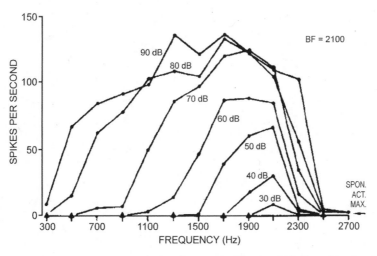

Figure 5.14 Effect of stimulus intensity on the response area of a single auditory neuron (CF = 2100 Hz). *Source*: From Rose, Hind, Anderson, and Brugge (1971), with permission of *J. Neurophysiol*.

Figure 5.16a shows the spectrum of the synthesized vowel /ɛ/, which was one of the stimuli used in experiments by Sachs and Young (1979). The spectral peaks shown here are the formants that correspond to this vowel. The curves in Fig. 5.16b to 5.16d show examples of how the spectrum of the vowel was represented by the firing rate (*normalized rate*) of a *population* of neural fibers (rather than a single neuron) as a function of the characteristic frequencies of the neurons. In other words, these curves show the normalized firing rate produced by the vowel /ɛ/ for each of many fibers having different characteristic frequencies. (The arrows in Fig. 5.16b show the locations of the vowel formants with respect to the frequency scale used in frames b to d). The three curves show the patterns of firing rates that resulted when the vowel is presented at different intensities, indicated by the decibel values in each frame. Notice that the formants were clearly delineated when the vowel was presented at relatively low and moderate levels (28 and 48 dB in frames b and c), but that the details of the spectrum were lost when the vowel was presented at higher intensities (78 dB as in frame d). This is not surprising because neural firing rates saturate at high levels. However, it does pose a problem because we can identify and discriminate among vowels over a very wide range of intensities, including the high levels where the discharge rates fail to preserve the spectral peaks. Hence, the ability of the auditory nerve to represent the speech spectrum must rely on more than just the firing rates. It appears that this goal may be accomplished by combining the firing-rate information with a measure of the *phase-locking* or *synchrony* of the neural firings, known as the **averaged localized synchronized rate (ALSR)**. As shown in Fig. 5.17, the ALSR is able to preserve the configuration of the vowel's spectral peaks even at high intensities (Young and Sachs, 1979).

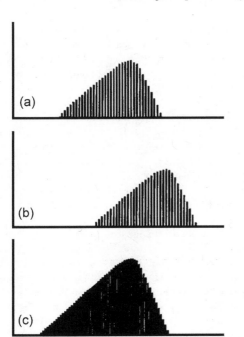

Figure 5.15 Hypothetical changes in the array of auditory nerve responses (Whitfield, 1967). See text. *Source*: Courtesy of IC Whitfield.

WHOLE-NERVE ACTION POTENTIALS

So far we have examined individual auditory nerve fibers. In this section we shall review some aspects of the **whole-nerve** or **compound action potential (AP)** of the auditory nerve. The whole-nerve AP, as its name suggests, is a composite of many individual fiber discharges. These more or less synchronous discharges are recorded by an extracellular electrode as a negative deflection. Recall from Chapter 4 that the AP must be separated from the

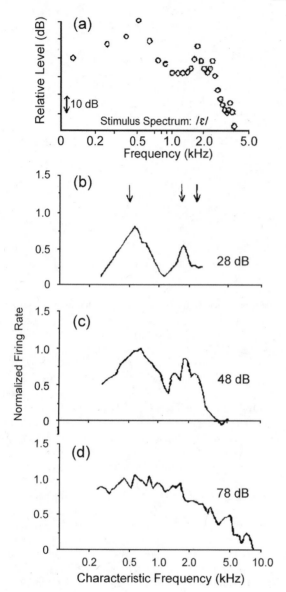

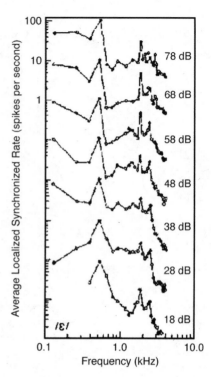

Figure 5.17 The degree of synchrony of neural discharges (averaged localized synchronized rate) as a function of frequency in response to steady-state presentations of /ɛ/ at various levels. Stimulus levels are indicated next to the curves. *Source*: Adapted from Young and Sachs (1979), with permission of the *J. Acoust. Soc. Am.*

Figure 5.16 (a) The spectrum of the vowel /ɛ/ stimulus. (b–d) Normalized firing rates as a function of characteristic frequency in a population of auditory neurons in response to steady-state presentations of /ɛ/ at 28, 48, and 78 dB. *Source*: Adapted from Sachs and Young (1979), with permission of *J. Acoust. Soc. Am.*

cochlear microphonic, which is generally accomplished by an averaging procedure. (Recall that the cochlear microphonic is in opposite phase in the scalae vestibuli and tympani, whereas the AP is always negative. Thus, averaging the responses from the two scalae cancels the cochlear microphonic and enhances the AP.)

The AP is also frequently recorded from locations other than the inside of the cochlea, for example, at the round window in animals, and at the promontory and even from the ear canal in humans. In these cases, averaging the responses has the important effect of enhancing the AP and reducing the random background noise. (See Chap. 6 for a discussion of signal averaging.)

As shown in Fig. 5.18, the AP appears as a negative amplitude peak identified as **N1**, at some latency following stimulus onset, which is followed by one or more smaller peaks, known as **N2** and **N3**. Whole-nerve APs are elicited by transient stimuli with fast rise times, such as clicks or tone bursts. It has been known for a long time that the transient stimulus leads to the *synchronous firing* of many fibers from the basal turn of the cochlea (Tasaki, 1954; Goldstein and Kiang, 1958). The AP is attributed to the basal turn because the high speed of the traveling wave in this part of the cochlea causes a large number of receptors to be stimulated almost simultaneously, leading to the synchrony of the neural discharges. More apical parts of the cochlea are not thought to contribute because the longer travel time up the partition would cause firings from these regions to be nonsynchronous. However, there is some evidence that other parts of the cochlea may also contribute to the response (e.g., Legouix and Pierson, 1974).

The first peak of the compound AP is generated by the synchronous firings of many auditory nerve fibers. This also appears to be the case for N2, although its origin has been

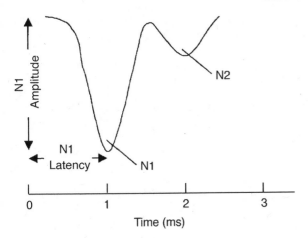

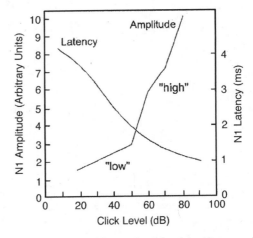

Figure 5.18 Hypothetical whole-nerve action potential (AP).

Figure 5.19 Amplitude and latency functions of the AP response based on Yoshie's (1968) data. Amplitude is in arbitrary units where 10 is the amplitude of the response to a click at 80 dB SPL.

the subject of some controversy. Some of the suggested origins of N2 have included a diphasic waveform (a negative deflection followed by a positive one) resulting in two peaks (Teas et al., 1962), discharges coming from the more apical areas of the cochlea (Pugh et al., 1973), repeated firings of the auditory nerve fibers (Tasaki, 1954), and discharges from second-order neurons in the cochlear nucleus (Tasaki et al., 1952). Eggermont (1975) found distinct N2 peaks in guinea pigs but not in the human response and suggested that N2 might be due to cochlear nucleus discharges which are more readily recorded in the guinea pig than in humans. Experimental data, however, have shown that N2 is the positive deflection of the diphasic response that separates the AP into N1 and N2 peaks, and that this separation occurs within the internal auditory meatus (Legouix and Pierson, 1974; Legouix et al., 1978). These studies showed that when the central end of the auditory nerve (in the internal auditory canal) was deactivated chemically or mechanically, the result was a change in the AP wave so that the N2 peak was absent. This loss is apparently due to the removal of the positive deflection of the diphasic response, which normally separates the N1 and N2 peaks.

Figure 5.19 shows that both the magnitude and latency of the AP depend on stimulus intensity (Goldstein et al., 1958; Yoshie, 1968). Increasing the level of the stimulus increases the amplitude of the response and decreases its latency. This relationship is actually not a simple one-to-one correspondence between stimulus level and AP amplitude and latency. Notice that the amplitude curve in Fig. 5.19 is made up of two rather distinct line segments rather than of a single straight line. There is a portion with a shallow or "low" slope at lower stimulus levels, and a segment that becomes abruptly steep or "high" in slope as stimulus intensity continues to increase. Furthermore, the function is not necessarily monotonic, that is, the relationship between stimulus level and AP amplitude is not always in the same direction for all parts of the curve. A small dip in AP amplitude has been reported to occur at about the place where

the low and high segments meet, before the curve resumes increasing with stimulus level (Kiang et al., 1962).

In the past, it has been proposed that the source of the two-part amplitude function might be the two populations of receptor cells in the cochlea (e.g., Davis, 1961; Eggermont, 1976a, 1976b). That is, the low segment was interpreted as reflecting the output of the outer hair cells and the high portion was seen as derived from the inner hair cells. This concept was based upon contemporary interpretations of the different innervation patterns of the two hair cell populations, and the subsequently disproven notion that the outer hair cells are more sensitive than the inner hair cells. As discussed in Chapters 2 and 4, these suppositions are now known to be erroneous. There are other experimental data that also contradict the previously held idea that the different sets of receptor cells cause the two segments of the AP amplitude function. In particular, the amplitude function has been found to have a single slope over its entire length when the central end of the nerve within the internal auditory meatus is deactivated (Legouix et al., 1978). Deactivation of this part of the auditory nerve changes the shape of the AP waveform by removing the positive deflection that separates the N1 and N2 peaks.

Alternative models to explain the two segments of the AP amplitude function, which have obvious implications for intensity coding in general, have been proposed by Evans (1975, 1976, 1978) and by Ozdamar and Dallos (1976). These similar models explain the shape of the amplitude function on the basis of single-fiber tuning curves. Recall that the typical tuning curve has two parts: a narrowly tuned area around the CF at low levels, and a more widely tuned area extending downward in frequency as stimulus intensity is raised. This shape is shown in Fig. 5.20a. The important point is that the low-frequency tails make a neuron responsive to a wide frequency range provided the intensity is great enough. Consider the responses of various

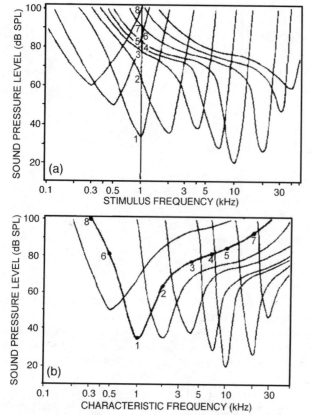

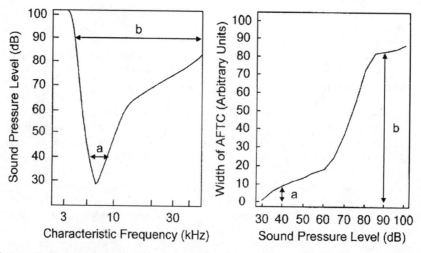

Figure 5.20 (a) Auditory-nerve fiber tuning curves. (b) Across-fiber tuning curves. *Source*: From Ozdamar and Dallos (1976), with permission of *J. Acoust. Soc. Am.*

fibers to a 1000-Hz tone, represented by the vertical line at 1000 Hz in the figure. Point 1 represents the lowest level at which a 1000-Hz CF fiber responds. The remaining points (2–8) show the levels at which the 1000-Hz tone activates fibers with other characteristic frequencies.

The 1000-Hz tone primarily crosses the low-frequency tails of the higher-CF tuning curves, but it also crosses the higher-frequency portions of some lower CF tuning curves (e.g., point 6). Thus, a 1000-Hz tone activates more and more fibers with different CFs as its level increases. This situation is plotted in Fig. 5.20b, which shows **across-fiber tuning curves**. The numbers correspond to those in Fig. 5.20a. Across-fiber tuning curves show the levels at which fibers with various CFs respond to a particular frequency (1000 Hz here). The tip of the across-fiber tuning curve represents the lowest level at which any fiber responds to that frequency. The width of the across-fiber tuning curve shows the *range* of neurons with different CFs that respond at a given stimulus level. For example, only the 1000-Hz CF fiber responds to 1000 Hz at 35 dB SPL, but fibers with CFs between about 500 and 10,000 Hz may respond when the same tone is presented at 80 dB SPL (i.e., between points 6 and 5).

Across-fiber tuning curves have high-frequency tails instead of the low-frequency tails of individual fiber tuning curves. This situation occurs because the low-frequency tails of an increasing number of high-frequency fibers respond as the intensity is raised (Fig. 5.20a).

How might this effect account for the two segments of the AP amplitude function? The left panel in Fig. 5.21 shows the width of a hypothetical across-fiber tuning curve. Line **a** shows the width of the across-fiber tuning curve within the narrowly

Figure 5.21 *Left panel*: Across-fiber tuning curve. *Right panel*: Width of an across-fiber tuning curve (AFTC) as a function of SPL. Lines **a** and **b** correspond on both panels. *Source*: Adapted from Ozdamar and Dallos (1976), with permission of *J. Acoust. Soc. Am.*

tuned segment. The width of the tuning curve at 90 dB SPL is shown by line **b**, which is in the widely tuned part of the curve. The right panel shows the width of the across-fiber tuning curve on the y-axis as a function of SPL. Lines a and b correspond in both panels. Only a small population of fibers with CFs close to the stimulus frequency responds at low intensity levels. At higher levels there is a dramatic increase in the number of responding fibers, as the stimulus level reaches the low-frequency tails of the other neurons. There is thus a slow increase in the width of the across-fiber tuning curve followed by a sharp increase as intensity rises. Comparison of Fig. 5.21 with Fig. 5.19 shows that this curve is remarkably similar to the AP amplitude function. The portion of the curve in the vicinity of line a corresponds to the low portion of the AP amplitude function, while the part around line b corresponds to the steeper high segment. This correspondence provides a mechanism that might underlie the two segments of the compound AP amplitude function. (One might also consider this mechanism with respect to excitation models like the one in Fig. 5.15.) Physiological findings by Ozdamar and Dallos (1978) support this mechanism.

REFERENCES

Abbas, RJ, Sachs, MB. 1976. Two-tone suppression in auditory-nerve fibers: Extension of a stimulus–response relationship. *J Acoust Soc Am* 59, 112–122.

Bekesy, G. 1960/1989. *Experiments in Hearing.* New York, NY: McGraw-Hill. [Republished by the Acoustical Society of America].

Brugge, JE, Anderson, DJ, Hind, JE, Rose, JE. 1969. Time structure of discharges in single auditory nerve fibers of the squirrel monkey in response to complex periodic sounds. *J Neurophysiol* 32, 386–401.

Carney, LH, Geisler, CD. 1986. A temporal analysis of auditory-nerve fiber responses to spoken stop-consonant syllables. *J Acoust Soc Am* 79, 1896–1914.

Cooper, NP. 1996. Two-tone suppression in cochlear mechanics. *J Acoust Soc Am* 99, 3087–3098.

Dallos, P. 1985. Response characteristics of mammalian cochlear hair cells. *J Neurosci* 5, 1591–1608.

Dallos, P, Cheatham, MA. 1974. Cochlear microphonic correlates of cubic difference tones. In: E Z wicker, E Terhardt (eds.), *Facts and Models in Hearing.* New York, NY: Springer-Verlag.

Davis, H. 1961. Peripheral coding of auditory information. In: WA Rosenblith (ed.), *Sensory Communication.* Cambridge, MA: M.I.T. Press, 119–141.

Davis, H, Fernandez, C, McAuliffe, DR. 1950. The excitatory process in the cochlea. *Proc Natl Acad Sci USA,* 36, 580–587.

Delgutte, B. 1997. Auditory neural processing of speech. In: WJ Hardcastle, J Laver (eds.), *The Handbook of Phonetic Sciences.* Oxford, UK: Blackwell, 507–538.

Delgutte, B, Kiang, NYS. 1984a. Speech coding the auditory nerve: I. Vowel-like sounds. *J Acoust Soc Am* 75, 866–878.

Delgutte, B, Kiang, NYS. 1984b. Speech coding the auditory nerve: III. Voiceless fricative consonants. *J Acoust Soc Am* 75, 887–896.

Delgutte, B, Kiang, NYS. 1984c. Speech coding the auditory nerve: V. Vowels in background noise. *J Acoust Soc Am* 75, 908–918.

Deng, L, Geisler, CD. 1987. Responses of auditory-nerve fibers to nasal consonant-vowel syllables. *J Acoust Soc Am* 82, 1977–1988.

Eggermont, JJ. 1976a. Analysis of compound action potential responses to tone bursts in the human and guinea pig cochlea. *J Acoust Soc Am* 60, 1132–1139.

Eggermont, JJ. 1976b. Electrocochleography. In: WD Keidel, WD Neff (eds.), *Handbook of Sensory Physiology, Vol. 3.* Berlin, Germany: Springer-Verlag, 625–705.

Evans, EF. 1975. The sharpening of cochlear frequency selectivity in the normal and abnormal cochlea. *Audiology* 14, 419–442.

Evans, EF. 1976. The effects of bandwidths of individual cochlear nerve fibers from pathological cochleae in the cat. In: SDG Stephens (ed.), *Disorders of Auditory Function.* London, UK: Academic Press, 99–110.

Evans, EF. 1978. Peripheral auditory processing in normal and abnormal ears: Physiological considerations for attempts to compensate for auditory deficits by acoustic or electrical prostheses. *Scand Audiol Suppl* 6, 9–47.

Evans, EE, Palmer, AA. 1980. Relationship between the dynamic range of cochlear nerve fibers and their spontaneous activity. *Exp Brain Res* 240, 115–118.

Galambos, R, Davis, H. 1943. The response of single auditory nerve fibers to acoustic stimulation. *J Neurophysiol* 6, 39–57.

Geisler, CD. 1998. *From Sound to Synapse: Physiology of the Mammalian Ear.* New York, NY: Oxford University Press.

Geisler, CD, Gamble, T. 1989. Responses of "high-spontaneous" auditory-nerve fibers to consonant–vowel syllables in noise. *J Acoust Soc Am* 85, 1639–1652.

Goldstein, MH, Kiang, NYS. 1958. Synchrony of neural activity in electrical responses evoked by transient acoustic clicks. *J Acoust Soc Am* 30, 107–114.

Hind, JE. 1972. Physiological correlates of auditory stimulus periodicity. *Audiology* 11, 42–57.

Hind, JE, Anderson, DJ, Brugge, JE, Rose, JE. 1967. Coding of information pertaining to paired low-frequency tones in single auditory nerve fibers of the squirrel monkey. *J Neurophysiol* 30, 794–816.

Javell, E, McGee, J, Walsh, EJ, Farley, GR; Gorga, MR. 1983. Suppression of auditory nerve responses. II. Suppression threshold and growth, isosuppression contours. *J Acoust Soc Am* 74, 801–813.

Keithley, EM, Schreiber, RC. 1987. Frequency map of the spiral ganglion in the cat. *J Acoust Soc Am* 81, 1036–1042.

Kemp, DT, Chum, RA. 1980. Observations on the generator mechanism of stimulus frequency acoustic emissions-two tone suppression. In: G van den Brink, EA Bilsen (eds.),

Physiological and Behavioral Studies in Hearing. Delft, The Netherlands: Delft University Press, 34–42.

Kiang, NYS. 1965. *Discharge Patterns of Single Fibers in the Cat's Auditory Nerve*. Cambridge, MA: M.I.T. Press.

Kiang, NYS. 1968. A survey of recent developments in the study of auditory physiology. *Ann Otol* 77, 656–675.

Kiang, NYS. 1975. Stimulus representation in the discharge patterns of auditory neurons. In: DB Tower, EL Eagles (eds.), *The Nervous System. Vol. 3: Human Communication and Its Disorders*. New York, NY: Raven, 81–96.

Kiang, NYS. 1984. Peripheral neural processing of auditory information. In: JM Brookhart, VB Mountcastle (eds.), *Handbook of Physiology: The Nervous System, Vol. III*, Part 2. Bethesda, MD: American Physiological Society, 639–674.

Kiang, NYS, Goldstein, MH, Peake, WT. 1962. Temporal coding of neural responses to acoustic stimuli. *Inst Radio Eng Trans Inform Theory* IT-8, 113–119.

Kiang, NYS, Liberman, MC, Sewell, WE, Guinan, JJ. 1986. Single unit clues to cochlear mechanisms. *Hear Res* 22, 171–182.

Kiang, NYS, Moxon, EC. 1972. Physiological considerations in artificial stimulation of the inner ear. *Ann Otol* 81, 714–731.

Kiang, NYS, Moxon, EC. 1974. Tails of tuning curves of auditory-nerve fibers. *J Acoust Soc Am* 55, 620–630.

Kiang, NYS, Rho, JM, Northrop, CC, Liberman, MC, Ryugo, DK. 1982. Hair-cell innervation by spiral ganglion cells in adult cats. *Science* 217, 175–177.

Kiang, NYS, Sachs, MB, Peake, WT. 1967. Shapes of tuning curves for single auditory-nerve fibers. *J Acoust Soc Am* 42, 1341–1342.

Kim, DO, Molnar, CE. 1979. A population study of cochlear nerve fibers: Comparison of special distributions of average-rate and phase-locking measures of responses to single tones. *J Neurophysiol* 48, 16–30.

Konishi, T, Nielsen, DW. 1973. The temporal relationship between basilar membrane motion and nerve impulse inhibition in auditory nerve fibers of guinea pigs. *Jpn J Physiol* 28, 291–307.

Legouix, JP, Pierson, A. 1974. Investigations on the source of whole-nerve action potentials from various places in the guinea pig cochlea. *J Acoust Soc Am* 56, 1222–1225.

Legouix, JP, Remond, MC, Greenbaum, HB. 1973. Interference and two tone inhibition. *J Acoust Soc Am* 53, 409–419.

Legouix, JP, Teas, DC, Beagley, HC, Remond, MC. 1978. Relation between the waveform of the cochlear whole nerve action potential and its intensity function. *Acta Otol* 85, 177–183.

Liberman, MC. 1978. Auditory-nerve response from cats raised in a low-noise chamber. *J Acoust Soc Am* 63, 442–455.

Liberman, MC. 1980a. Morphological differences among radial afferent fibers in the cat cochlea: An electron microscopic study of serial sections. *Hear Res* 3, 45–63.

Liberman, MC. 1980b. Efferent synapses in the inner hair cell area of the cat cochlea: An electron microscopic study of serial sections. *Hear Res* 3, 189–204.

Liberman, MC. 1982a. Single-neuron labeling in cat auditory nerve. *Science* 216, 1239–1241.

Liberman, MC. 1982b. The cochlear frequency map for the cat: Labeling auditory nerve fibers of known characteristic frequency. *J Acoust Soc Am* 72, 1441–1449.

Liberman, MC. 1988. Physiology of cochlear efferent and afferent neurons: Direct comparisons in the same animal. *Hear Res* 34, 179–192.

Liberman, MC, Brown, MC. 1986. Physiology and anatomy of single olivocochlear neurons in the cat. *Hear Res* 24, 17–36.

Liberman, MC, Kiang, NYS. 1984. Single-neuron labeling and chronic cochlear pathology. IV. Stereocilia damage and alterations in rate- and phase-level functions. *Hear Res* 16, 75–90.

Liberman, MC, Oliver, ME. 1984. Morphometry of intracellularly labeled neurons of the auditory nerve: Correlations with functional properties. *J Comp Neurol* 223, 163–176.

Liberman, MC, Simmons, DD. 1985. Applications of neuronal labeling techniques to the study of the peripheral auditory system. *J Acoust Soc Am* 78, 312–319.

Miller, MI, Sachs, MB 1983. Representation of stop consonants in the discharge patterns of auditory-nerve fibers. *J Acoust Soc Am* 74, 502–517.

Nomoto, M, Suga, N, Katsuki, Y. 1964. Discharge pattern and inhibition of primary auditory nerve fibers in the monkey. *J Neurophysiol* 27, 768–787.

Ozdamar, O, Dallos, P. 1976. Input-output function of cochlear whole-nerve action potentials: Interpretation in terms of one population of neurons. *J Acoust Soc Am* 59, 143–147.

Ozdamar, O, Dallos, P. 1978. Synchronous responses of the primary auditory fibers to the onset of tone burst and their relation to compound action potentials. *Brain Res* 155, 169–175.

Palmer, AR. 1990. The representation of the spectra and fundamental frequencies of steady-state single and double vowel sounds in the temporal discharge patterns of guinea-pig cochlear nerve fibers. *J Acoust Soc Am* 88, 1412–1426.

Palmer, A, Shamma, S. 2004. Physiological representations of speech. In: S Greenberg, WA Ainsworth, AN Popper, RR Fay (eds.), *Speech Processing in the Auditory System*. New York, NY: Springer, 163–230.

Palmer, AR, Winter, IM, Darwin, CJ. 1986. The representation steady-state vowel sounds in the temporal discharge patterns of guinea-pig cochlear nerve and primarylike cochlear nucleus neurones. *J Acoust Soc Am* 79, 100–113.

Patuzzi, R, Sellick, RM. 1984. The modulation of the sensitivity of mammalian cochlea by low frequency tones. II. Inner hair cell receptor potentials. *Hear Res* 13, 9–18.

Pfeiffer, RR, Molnar, CE. 1970. Cochlear nerve fiber discharge patterns: Relationship to cochlear microphonic. *Science* 167, 1614–1616.

Pugh, JE Jr, Anderson, DJ, Burgio, PA. 1973. The origin of N2 of the cochlear whole-nerve action potential. *J Acoust Soc Am* 53, 325(A).

Rhode, WS. 1977. Some observations on two-tone interaction measured with the Mossbauer effect. In: EE Evans, JR Wilson (eds.), *Psychophysics and Physiology of Hearing*. London, UK: Academic Press, 27–38.

Robles, L, Ruggero, MA. 2001. Mechanics of the mammalian cochlea. *Physiol Rev* 81, 1305–1352.

Rose, JE, Brugge, JF, Anderson, DJ, Hind, JE. 1967. Phase-locked response to low-frequency tones in single auditory nerve fibers of the squirrel monkey. *J Neurophysiol* 30, 769–793.

Rose, JE, Brugge, JE, Anderson, DJ, Hind, JE. 1969. Some possible neural correlates of combination tones. *J Neurophysiol* 32, 402–423.

Rose, JE, Hind, JE, Anderson, DJ, Brugge, JF. 1971. Some effects of stimulus intensity on response of auditory nerve fibers in the squirrel monkey. *J Neurophysiol* 34, 685–699.

Ruggero, MA, Rich, NC. 1983. Chinchilla auditory-nerve responses to low frequency tones. *J Acoust Soc Am* 73, 2096–2108.

Ruggero, MA, Robles, L, Rich, NC. 1992. Two-tone suppression in the basilar membrane of the cochlea: Mechanical basis of auditory nerve rate suppression. *J Neurophysiol* 68, 1087–1099.

Sachs, MB. 1984. Neural coding of complex sounds: Speech. *Annu Rev Physiol* 46, 261–273.

Sachs, MB, Abbas, PJ. 1974. Rate versus level functions for auditory-nerve fibers in cats: Tone-burst stimuli. *J Acoust Soc Am* 56, 1835–1847.

Sachs, MB, Abbas, PJ. 1976. Phenomenological model for two-tone inhibition. *J Acoust Soc Am* 60, 1157–1163.

Sachs, MB, Kiang, NYS. 1968. Two-tone inhibition in auditory nerve fibers. *J Acoust Soc Am* 43, 1120–1128.

Sachs, MB, Young, ED. 1979. Encoding of steady-state vowels in the auditory nerve: Representation in terms of discharge rate. *J Acoust Soc Am* 66, 470–479.

Sachs, MB, Young, ED. 1980. Effects of nonlinearities on speech encoding in the auditory nerve. *J Acoust Soc Am* 68, 858–875.

Salvi, R, Henderson, D, Hamernick, R. 1983. Physiological bases of sensorineural hearing loss. In: JV Tobias, ED Schubert (eds.), *Hearing Research and Theory, Vol. 2*. New York, NY: Academic Press, 173–231.

Schalk, TB, Sachs, MB. 1980. Nonlinearities in auditory-nerve fiber responses to bandlimited noise. *J Acoust Soc Am* 67, 903–913.

Sellick, PM, Patuzzi, R, Johnstone, BM. 1982. Modulation of responses of spiral ganglion cells in the guinea pig by low frequency sound. *Hear Res* 7, 199–221.

Sellick, RM, Russell, IJ. 1979. Two-tone suppression in cochlear hair cells. *Hear Res* 1, 227–236.

Silkes, SM, Geisler, CD. 1991. Responses of lower-spontaneous-rate auditory-nerve fibers to speech syllables presented in noise. 1. General characteristics. *J Acoust Soc Am* 90, 3122–3139.

Sinex, DG, Geisler, CD. 1983. Responses of auditory-nerve fibers to consonant-vowel syllables. *J Acoust Soc Am* 73, 602–615.

Sinex, DG, McDonald, LP, Mott, JB. 1991. Neural correlated of nonmonotonic temporal acuity for voice onset time. *J Acoust Soc Am* 90, 2441–2449.

Sokolich, WG, Hamernick, RP, Zwislocki, JJ, Schmiedt, RA. 1976. Inferred response polarities of cochlear hair cells. *J Acoust Soc Am* 59, 963–974.

Tasaki, I. 1954. Nerve impulses in individual auditory nerve fibers. *J Neurophysiol* 17, 97–122.

Tasaki, I, Davis, H, Goldstein, R. 1952. The peripheral organization of activity, with reference to the ear. *Cold Spring Harb Symp Quant Biol* 17, 143–154.

Teas, DC, Eldridge, DH, Davis, H. 1962. Cochlear responses to acoustic transients: An interpretation of whole nerve action potentials. *J Acoust Soc Am* 34, 1438–1459.

Westerman, LA, Smith, RL. 1984. Rapid and short-term adaptation in auditory nerve responses. *Hear Res* 15, 249–260.

Whitfield, IC. 1967. *The Auditory Pathway*. London, UK: Arnold.

Yoshie, N. 1968. Auditory nerve action potential responses to clicks in man. *Laryngoscope* 78, 198–213.

Young, ED, Sachs, MB. 1979. Representation of steady-state vowels in the temporal aspects of discharge patterns of populations of auditory-nerve fibers. *J Acoust Soc Am* 66, 1381–1403.

Zwislocki, J. 1984. How OHC lesions can lead to neural cochlear hypersensitivity. *Acta Otol* 97, 529–534.

Zwislocki, J. 1985. Cochlear function—An analysis. *Acta Otol* 100, 201–209.

Zwislocki, J. 1986. Analysis of cochlear mechanics. *Hear Res* 22, 155–169.

6 Auditory Pathways

The previous chapter discussed the coding of information in the auditory nerve, the peripheral segment of the auditory nervous system. This chapter continues our coverage by addressing several fundamental topics pertaining to the representation of information at various levels in the central auditory nervous system, from the cochlear nuclei through the cortex. Students wishing to pursue their study of the central auditory nervous system and related issues will find many extensive reviews that will facilitate their efforts (e.g., Popper and Fay, 1992; Webster et al., 1992; Ehret and Romand, 1997; Irvine, 1986, 1992; Møller, 2000; Palmer and Shamma, 2004; Musiek and Baran, 2007).

RESPONSES OF THE AUDITORY NERVOUS SYSTEM

In this section, we will look at several examples of the types of responses that occur at various levels in the central auditory nervous system, after which we will consider how binaural stimulation is represented.

Recall from Chapter 5 that the responses of auditory nerve fibers (often referred to as **primary auditory neurons**) are exclusively *excitatory*. In other words, their mode of operation is to fire in response to incoming signals. As we shall see, this and other characteristics of the responses of auditory nerve fibers are not seen in all neurons at higher levels. In fact, discharge patterns dramatically different from those of auditory nerve units are seen as low as the cochlear nuclei.

The nature of stimulus coding in the cochlear nuclei has been described in great detail for several animals, such as the cat (e.g., Rose et al., 1959; Kiang et al., 1965; Godfrey et al., 1975a, 1975b; Rhode, 1985). A variety of discharge patterns occur, which are in turn associated with neurons differing in terms of their morphologies, and which are variously distributed within the cochlear nuclei. It is interesting to note in this context that greater degrees of phase-locking (Joris, Carney, Smith, and Yin, 1994a, 1994b) and synchronized responses to modulation (Frisina, Smith, and Chamberlain, 1990; Wang and Sachs, 1994; Rhode and Greenberg, 1994) have been found in the cochlear nucleus compared to the auditory nerve.

Several examples of the descriptively named neural firing patterns observed in central auditory pathways are illustrated in Fig. 6.1. These kinds of discharge patterns are often called **peri-stimulus time histograms (PSTHs)** because they indicate spike rates (vertically) as a function of the time while a stimulus is on. Figure 6.2 shows examples of several of the cells associated with these firing patterns.

Primary-like units have firing patterns that are like those of auditory nerve fibers. This firing pattern is associated with

bushy cells found in the anterior ventral cochlear nucleus (AVCN) and in the posterior ventral cochlear nucleus (PVCN).

Onset units respond to the onset of a tone burst with a momentary discharge of spikes, but do not respond during the remainder of the tone burst or to continuous tones. These response patterns have been associated with **octopus** cells, as well as with small **stellate** and large **monopolar** cells, and are found in the PVCN and the dorsal cochlear nucleus (DCN), as well as in the AVCN.

Choppers get their name from the chopped appearance of their PSTHs, which look as though segments have been chopped out. The chopping is probably due to the presence of preferred discharge times, which are regularly spaced over time; the rate of chopping is related to the tone burst's level, duration, and rate. The response is greatest at onset of the tone burst and decreases over the time that the stimulus is left on. This firing pattern is associated with **stellate** cells found in the AVCN, PVCN, and DCN.

Pausers and **buildup units** are associated with **fusiform cells** encountered in the DCN.

The pausers are so named because they respond after longer latencies than the other cells. At higher stimulus levels pausers have an initial discharge peak, then a silent interval followed by discharges that last for the rest of the tone burst. Buildup units are characterized by a graduated increase in their firing rates until they achieve a steady-state discharge rate for the remainder of the tone burst.

These five discharge patterns are by no means the only types encountered, nor are they mutually exclusive. There are other types, such as discharge patterns that decay at an exponential rate, as well as combined patterns. For example, some superior olivary complex fibers respond to clicks with a single discharge, others with two, and still others with a train of firings (e.g., Galambos et al., 1959; Rupert et al., 1966). Moreover, onset units, pausers, and fibers responding to the duration are found in the inferior colliculus (e.g., Rose et al., 1959; Faure, Fremouw, Casseday, and Covey, 2003). The central point is that the responses of neurons in the central auditory nervous system are more diverse than the exclusively excitatory firing patterns we have seen in auditory nerve fibers. Informative reviews of SOC functioning are provided by Helfert and Aschoff (1997) and Rouiller (1997).

Many fibers in the medial geniculate body (MGB) are onset units, while others are pausers, cells that fire upon stimulus offset, and cells that respond as long as the stimulus is present (e.g., Galambos, 1952; Katsuki et al., 1959; Aitkin et al., 1966). Moreover, many cells in the MGB respond to trains of clicks by firing synchronously with the clicks, at the onset of the click train, or through the duration of the train rather than synchronously with the clicks (Rouiller et al., 1981; Rouiller and de Ribaupierre, 1982). Responses are also elicited by frequency

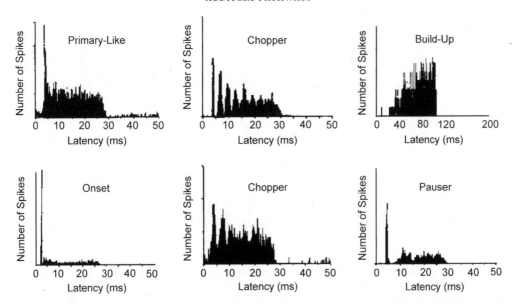

Figure 6.1 Peristimulus time histograms (spike rate as a function of time from stimulus onset) showing representative firing patterns obtained from neurons in the cochlear nuclei. *Source*: Adapted from Rhode (1985), with permission of *J. Acoust. Soc. Am.*

and/or amplitude modulation (e.g., Creutzfeldt et al., 1980; Allon et al., 1981; Mendelson and Cynader, 1985; Preuss and Müller-Preuss, 1990).

Neurons in the auditory cortex are more interested in stimulus *novelty* or change than in ongoing stimulation. Thus, while auditory cortical neurons are not particularly responsive to steady-state tones or continuous noises, they do respond to a host of stimulus changes, such as onsets and offsets (e.g., Hind, 1960; Katsuki et al., 1962) as well as frequency and amplitude

modulation (e.g., Whitfield and Evans, 1965; Creutzfeldt et al., 1980; Mendelson and Cynader, 1985; Schreiner and Urbas, 1986; Phillips and Hall, 1987; Bieser and Müller-Preuss, 1996; Liang et al., 2002). Other examples include responses to click-trains in a similar fashion as just described for MGB neurons (e.g., de Ribaupierre et al., 1972), as well as to differences between the ears and movements of a sound source around the head (discussed below).

BINAURAL CODING

A variety of auditory functions depend upon information from both ears, or **binaural hearing**. For example, the ability to localize a sound source depends on the differences in the time of arrival and level of the sound at the two ears, known as **interaural time differences (ITDs)** and **interaural level differences (ILDs)**, as well as monaural **spectral cues** introduced by the pinna. These issues are discussed further in Chapter 13. The current question deals with how this information from the two ears is represented within the auditory system.

Superior Olivary Complex

Recall from Chapter 2 that the superior olivary complex is the lowest level at which binaural information is available. This binaural input is illustrated schematically in Fig. 6.3a, which shows cells in the medial superior olive receiving inputs from both the ipsilateral and contralateral cochlear nuclei. Neurons in the SOC code binaural information through an interaction of excitatory and inhibitory inputs, which are the results of intensity and time (phase) differences in the stimuli at the

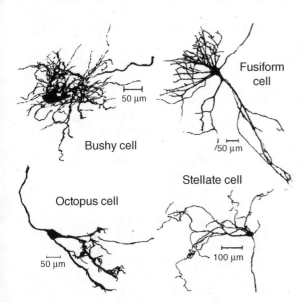

Figure 6.2 Examples of bushy, octopus, fusiform, and stellate cells. *Source*: Adapted from Rhode (1985), with permission of *J. Acoust. Soc. Am.*

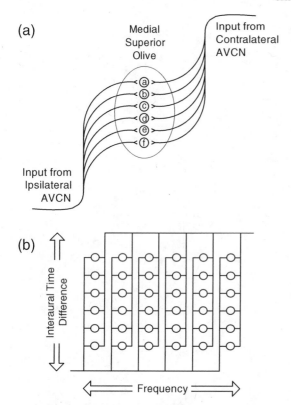

(a)

Medial
Superior
Olive

Input from
Contralateral
AVCN

ⓐ
ⓑ
ⓒ
ⓓ
ⓔ
ⓕ

Input from
Ipsilateral
AVCN

(b)

Interaural Time Difference

Frequency

Figure 6.3 Artist's conceptualizations of (**a**) the basic Jeffress (1948) model, and (**b**) the spatial mapping of ITDs across neurons with different characteristic frequencies.

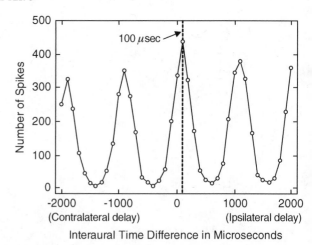

Figure 6.4 Firing rate as a function of interaural time difference for a neuron in the medial superior olive with a characteristic delay of 100 μs. The stimulus is a 1000-Hz tone presented to both ears, with a delay of 100 μs at the ipsilateral ear compared to the contralateral ear. The periodic peaks indicate that the cell is phase-locked to the period of the 1000-Hz tone. *Source*: Adapted from Yin and Chan (1990), with permission of *J. Neurophysiol.*

two ears. The majority of SOC neurons are excited by either contralateral or ipsilateral stimulation, about one-quarter are excited by stimulation from one side and inhibited by stimulation from the other side, and about 10% respond to only contralateral stimulation (see, e.g., Rouiller, 1997).

The lateral superior olive is principally receptive to higher frequencies and interaural level differences, whereas the medial superior olive is predominantly responsive to lower frequencies and interaural time differences. Lateral superior olivary neurons sensitive to ILDs tend to receive ipsilateral inputs that are excitatory and contralateral inputs that are inhibitory, and various cells respond to different ILDs (e.g., Boudreau and Tsuchitani, 1968; Caird and Klinke, 1983; Glendenning et al., 1985; Cant and Casseday, 1986; Tsuchitani, 1988a, 1988b; Smith et al., 1993, 1998; Park, 1998). Moreover, several investigators have identified neurons in the LSO that respond to ITDs in the envelopes of high-frequency signals and the fine structures of low-frequency sounds (e.g. Caird and Kinlke, 1983; Finlayson and Caspary, 1991; Joris and Yin, 1995; Joris, 1996).

Cells sensitive to ITDs in the MSO receive excitatory inputs from the cochlear nuclei on both sides (e.g., Warr, 1966; Goldberg and Brown, 1969; Yin and Chan, 1988, 1990). Medial superior olivary neurons fire maximally in response to a certain

ITD, or **characteristic delay** (e.g., Goldberg and Brown, 1969; Yin and Chan, 1990). An example is shown in Fig. 6.4, which shows firing rate as a function of ITD for an MSO neuron in response to a pure tone presented to both ears at its best frequency of 1000 Hz. Notice that this cell responds maximally when the ITD is 100 μs (highlighted by the dashed line in the figure), indicating that this is its characteristic delay. (Peaks occur periodically because the cell's response is phase-locked to the period of the tone.) Neurons in the MSO appear to be arranged according to their characteristic delays along the anterioposterior axis of the nucleus (Yin and Chan, 1990).

The principal model explaining the coding of binaural signals in the SOC was introduced by Jeffress (1948), although modifications have been proposed over the years (see, e.g., Stern and Trahiotis, 1997; Joris et al., 1998). The fundamental concept is illustrated in Fig. 6.3a, which shows ipsilateral and contralateral inputs to neurons in the MSO. Recall that the direction of the sound source (azimuth) produces a certain ITD, which is zero when the source is in the midline (equidistant between the ears), and favors the closer ear when it is off to one side. Now, notice in the figure how the paths from the two sides are arranged so that they constitute *neural delay lines*, causing a signal coming from the contralateral side to arrive soonest at cell **a**, and progressively later at cells **b** through **f**. In addition, a signal coming from the ipsilateral side arrives soonest at cell **f**, and progressively later at cells **e** through **a**. Because of these delay lines, there will be a set of neural delays that compensates for the ITDs that are between the two ears, resulting in maximum excitation of the MSO cell(s) receiving these coincident signals. The orderly arrangement of these cells receiving the coincident

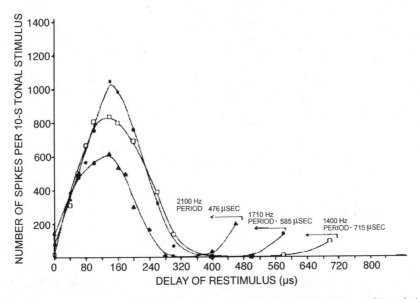

Figure 6.5 Responses of a single neuron in the inferior colliculus with a characteristic delay of approximately 140 μs to binaural stimulation at various low frequencies. Note that the peak occurs at the characteristic delay regardless of frequency. *Source*: From Rose et al. (1966), with permission of *J. Neurophysiol.*

signals causes a spatial mapping of ITDs, as suggested by the figure. Figure 6.3b illustrates how this spatial mapping of ITDs is maintained across neurons with different characteristic frequencies, which we have seen are arranged tonotopically.

Responses to ILD and ITDs have also been found in the **dorsal nucleus of the lateral lemniscus (DNLL)** (Brugge et al., 1970), where the findings have been similar to those for the superior olivary complex.

Inferior Colliculus

The inferior colliculus also responds to interaural differences, receiving its principal inputs for ITDs from the ipsilateral MSO and for ILDs from the contralateral LSO. In general, cells sensitive to ILDs in the **central nucleus of the inferior colliculus (ICC)** receive ipsilateral inputs that are inhibitory and contralateral inputs that are excitatory (Brugge et al., 1970; Roth et al., 1978; Semple and Aitkin, 1979; Semple and Kitzes, 1987; Caird and Klinke, 1987; Irvine and Gago, 1990). The changeover from ipsilateral-excitation/contralateral-inhibition in the LSO to the opposite arrangement in the ICC may occur because projections from the LSO go to the opposite ICC (Glendenning and Masterson, 1983).

As in the MSO, cells in the ICC also respond to ITDs with characteristic delays (e.g., Rose et al., 1966; Geisler et al., 1969; Benevento and Coleman, 1970; Kuwada et al., 1979; Spitzer and Semple, 1993; Fitzpatrick et al., 1997). For example, Fig. 6.5 shows spike counts as a function of ITD for an inferior colliculus neuron in response to various stimulus frequencies. Notice that the number of discharges is greatest when the ITD is about 140 μs (the characteristic delay) regardless of

the frequency. If the time scale were extended, one would see additional peaks repeated at intervals equal to the periods of the stimulus tones (e.g., at 476 μs intervals for the 2100-Hz tone and 715-μs intervals for 1400 Hz). In addition to ILD- and ITD-sensitive cells, Benevento and Coleman (1970) found inferior colliculus neurons sensitive to both ILD and ITD, as well as units not sensitive to either one.

Medial Geniculate Body

Sensitivity to binaural information continues beyond the inferior colliculus to the auditory thalamus and cortex. Neurons in the medial geniculate body respond to ILDs or ITDs, both ILDs and ITDs, and to the locations (azimuths) of sound sources (e.g., Aitkin and Dunlop, 1968; Aitkin and Webster, 1972; Aitkin, 1973; Ivarsson et al., 1988; Stanford et al., 1992; Samson et al., 2000). It is interesting to note that the degree of tuning to ITDs appears to become increasingly selective (i.e., tuned to narrower ranges of ITDs) going from the SOC to the inferior colliculus and then to the auditory thalamus (Fitzpatrick et al., 1997). This is clearly seen in Fig. 6.6, which shows that normalized responses are narrower as a function of ITD for cells in the auditory thalamus compared to those in the SOC.

Auditory Cortex

Cells responsive to ILDS or ITDs are found in the auditory cortex (Brugge et al., 1969; Brugge and Merzenich, 1973; Reale and Kettner, 1986; Benson and Teas, 1976; Phillips and Irvine, 1981; Reale and Brugge, 1990; Mendelson and Grasse, 2000), and some auditory cortical neurons are responsive to interaural differences in both level and time (Benson and Teas, 1976; Kitzes et al., 1980).[1] While many auditory cortical cells respond to characteristic interaural delays, there are also others that do not (Benson and Teas, 1976). Auditory cortical neurons also respond to the locations (azimuths) of sound sources and to the direction of sound source movement (Sovijäri and Hyvärinen, 1974; Rajan et al., 1990; Imig et al., 1990). For a comprehensive review of auditory cortical responses to monaural and binaural stimulation, see Clarey et al. (1992).

In summary, the processing of binaural information exists at all levels for which binaural inputs are represented, from the superior olivary complex up to and including the cortex.

TONOTOPIC ORGANIZATION

Tuning curves providing **best** or **characteristic frequencies (CFs)** have been reported for the all levels of the auditory system from the cochlear nuclei through the auditory cortex (e.g., Hind, 1960; Katsuki, 1961; Katsuki et al., 1962; Rose et al., 1963; Kiang, 1965; Boudreau and Tsuchitani, 1970; Guinan et al., 1972; Kiang et al., 1973).

One of the most interesting aspects of the auditory pathways is the relatively systematic representation of frequency at each level. That is, there is a virtual "mapping" of the audible frequency range within each nuclear mass—neurons most sensitive to high frequencies are in one area, those sensitive to lows are in another part, and those sensitive to intermediate frequencies are located successively between them. This orderly representation of frequency according to place is called **tonotopic organization**. In addition, one should be aware that accumulating evidence is revealing that the "*what*" (e.g., spectral) and "*where*" (spatial location) characteristics of a sound object appear to be separately represented in different parts of the auditory cortex (e.g., Ahveninen, Jääskeläinen, Raij, et al., 2006; Hall and Barrett, 2006; Lomber and Malhotra, 2008).

High frequencies are represented basally in the cochlea, tapering down to low frequencies at the apex. This tonotopic arrangement is continued in the auditory nerve, where apical fibers are found toward the core of the nerve trunk and basal fibers on the outside and of the inferior margin (Sando, 1965), as shown in Fig. 6.7. Moreover, as pointed out in Chapters 4 and 5, frequency maps have been developed that relate auditory nerve fiber characteristic frequencies to distance along the cochlear duct and to distance from the base of Rosenthal's canal (Liberman, 1982; Keithley and Schreiber, 1987). Keithley and Schreiber (1987) used these two sets of data to establish the relationship of the relative distances (from the base to apex) along the organ of Corti and Rosenthal's canal (Fig. 6.8).

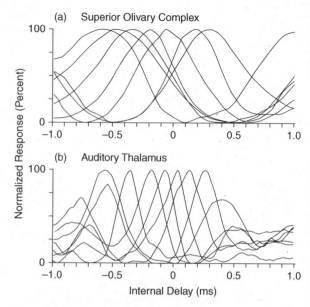

Figure 6.6 Normalized responses of neurons, as a function of interaural time differences become narrower (more selective) going from the (a) superior olivary complex to the (b) auditory thalamus. *Source*: Adapted from Fitzpatrick, Batra, Stanford, and Kuwada (1997) with permission of *Nature*.

Cochlear Nuclei

Lewy and Kobrak (1936) found that basal axons enter the dorsal part of the dorsal cochlear nucleus, and apical fibers enter the **ventral cochlear nucleus (VCN)** as well as part of the DCN. As illustrated in Fig. 6.7, Sando (1965) found that eighth nerve axons bifurcate into an anterior branch to the VCN and a posterior branch to the DCN. Fibers from the basal turn distribute dorsomedially in the CN, while fibers with more apical origins in the cochlea distribute ventrolaterally. Furthermore, the apical fibers of the posterior branch were found more inferiorly in the DCN than the corresponding fibers of the anterior branch of the VCN. On the other hand, the basally derived fibers in the posterior branch are distributed more superiorly in the DCN than the corresponding anterior branch fibers in the VCN. Overall, auditory nerve fibers originating from the more basal (high-frequency) areas of the cochlea terminate in the dorsomedial portions of the cochlear nuclei, and the ventrolateral portions of the cochlear nuclei receive neurons originating from the more apical (low-frequency) parts of the cochlea (Cant, 1992).

Rose and colleagues (Rose et al., 1959; Rose, 1960) advanced microelectrodes through the cochlear nuclei of anesthetized cats to measure the number of neural discharges in response to tone pips of various frequencies. At a given intensity, a neuron responds with the greatest number of spikes at its characteristic frequency. As illustrated in Fig. 6.9, they found that each of the nuclei of the cochlear nuclear complex has a complete frequency mapping in a dorsoventral direction; that is, low frequencies map ventrally and high frequencies dorsally in each division of the cat's cochlear nuclei.

---

[1] We will not address **echolocation** in bats, but interested students will find several informative reviews of this topic (e.g., Suga, 1990; Popper and Fay, 1995).

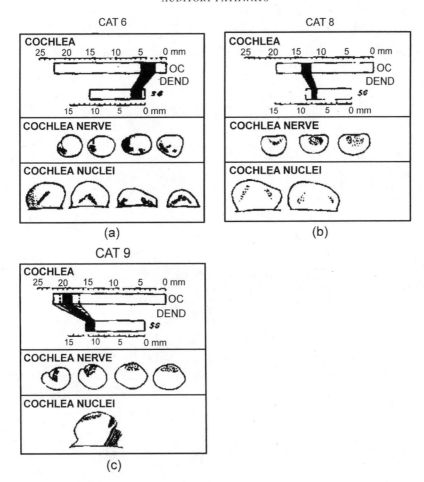

Figure 6.7 Tonotopic relations between the organ of Corti (OC), spiral ganglia (SG), auditory nerve, and cochlear nuclei based on degeneration observed after selective lesions of the organ of Corti and spiral ganglia. Solid lines indicate the induced lesions; crosshatched and dotted areas are resulting degenerations: (a) basal, (b) middle, and (c) apical turns of different cats. *Source*: From Sando (1965), with permission of *Acta Otol*.

Superior Olivary Complex

Tonotopic organization continues in the **superior olivary complex (SOC)**, although the representation of frequency is disproportional, favoring the low frequencies in the **medial superior olive (MSO) and** the highs in the **lateral superior olive (LSO)** (e.g., Tsuchitani and Boudreau, 1966; Guinan et al., 1972).

Tsuchitani and Boudreau (1966) studied the responses of single neurons in the S-shaped LSO in cats. This structure appears as a backward S, as shown in Fig. 6.10**a**. The higher CFs were found in the curve lying downward toward the dorsomedial curve of the S. Goldberg and Brown (1968) studied the distribution of CFs in the MSO of dogs. By advancing a microelectrode through the U-shaped nucleus, they found that the neurons with higher CFs are in the ventral leg of the structure and those with lower CFs are in the dorsal leg (Fig. 6.10**b**).

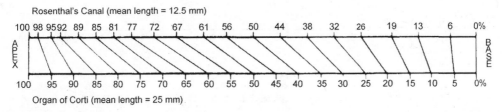

Figure 6.8 Relationship of distances (in percent) along the organ of Corti and Rosenthal's canal. *Source*: From Keithley and Schreiber (1987), with permission of *J. Acoust. Soc. Am*.

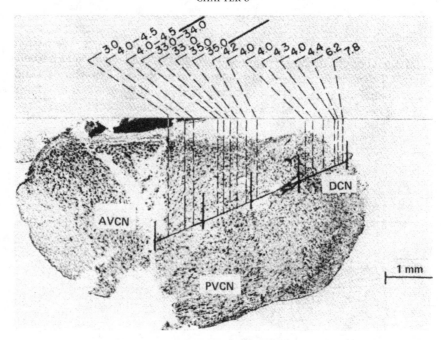

Figure 6.9 Tonotopic arrangement of anteroventral (AV), posteroventral (PV), and dorsal (DC) cochlear nuclei of a cat (saggital section on left side). Each nuclear group has its own sequence from low- to high-frequency representation. *Source*: Used with permission from Rose, Galambos, and Hughes. Microelectrode studies of the cochlear nuclear nuclei of the cat, *Bull. Johns Hopkins Hosp.* 104, 211–251, © 1959. Johns Hopkins University Press.

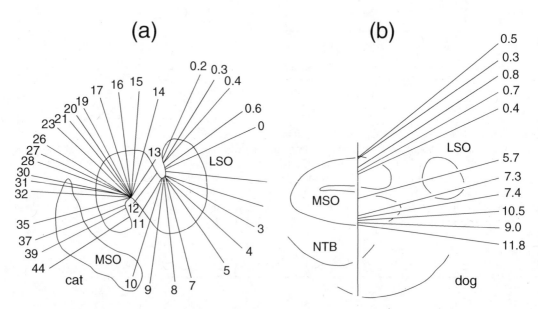

Figure 6.10 Tonotopic arrangement of the cells in (**a**) the lateral superior olivary nucleus of the cat (Tsuchitani and Boudreau, 1966), and (**b**) the medial superior olivary nucleus of the dog (Goldberg and Brown, 1968). Numbers show characteristic frequencies in kHz. *Abbreviations*: LSO, lateral superior olive; MSO, medial superior olive; NTB, nucleus of trapezoid body. *Source*: From Tsuchitani and Boudreau (1966) and Goldberg and Brown (1968), with permission of *J. Neurophsiol.*

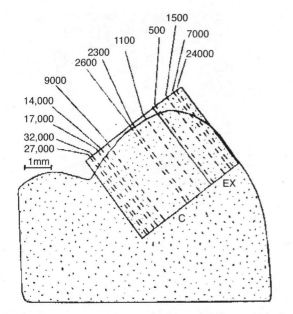

Figure 6.11 Tonotopic representation of characteristic frequencies in the central nucleus (C) and external nucleus (EX) of the inferior colliculus of the cat. *Source*: Based on Rose et al. (1963).

Lateral Lemniscus

Early studies found tonotopic organization in the ventral and dorsal nuclei of the **lateral lemniscus**, with neurons having high CFs found ventrally and those with low CFs found dorsally in both nuclei (Aitkin et al., 1970; Brugge and Geisler, 1978). This relationship has been confirmed for the dorsal nucleus, but it now appears that tonotonicity in the lateral nucleus is less clear or has a more complicated arrangement (see, e.g., Helfert, Snead, and Altschuler, 1991; Merchán and Berbel, 1996; Glendenning and Hutson, 1998).

Inferior Colliculus

The tonotopic arrangement of the cat's **inferior colliculus** was studied by Rose et al. (1963). They inserted a microelectrode into the dorsomedial surface of the inferior colliculus and advanced it in a ventromedial direction (Fig. 6.11). The electrode thus passed through the external nucleus and into the central nucleus. Within the central nucleus, cells with increasing CFs were encountered as the electrode proceeded ventromedially into the nucleus. The opposite arrangement was observed in the external nucleus, that is, the CFs went from high to low as the electrode was advanced ventromedially. A high-to-low frequency organization was found in the external nucleus, but it was not as consistent as in the central nucleus of the inferior colliculus.

Medial Geniculate Body

The existence of tonotopic organization in the **medial geniculate body** (MGB) was confirmed by Aitkin and Webster (1971).

They found that lateral units in the pars principalis of the cat responded to low frequencies, while medial neurons were responsive to high. This was a significant finding because there was little to support tonotonicity in the MGB prior to their report (Whitfield, 1967).

Tonotopic Organization of the Cortex

In their classic study, Woolsey and Walzl (1942) found two auditory areas in each hemisphere of the cat, each with its own projection of the auditory nerve. A primary auditory area (AI) was identified in the middle ectosylvian area, and a secondary auditory area (AII) was found just ventral to AI. Stimulating the basal (low-frequency) auditory nerve fibers resulted in responses in the rostral part of AI, and stimulating apical (low-frequency) fibers yielded responses from the caudal part. The opposite arrangement was observed in AII; that is, the basal fibers projected caudally and the apical fibers rostrally. A similar arrangement was found in the dog by Tunturi (1944), who later reported a third auditory area (AIII) under the anterior part of the suprasylvian gyrus. Working with cats, Abeles and Goldstein (1970) showed that tonotonicity in the auditory cortex is not organized by depth; that is, cells in a given vertical column of cortex show the same CFs as a microelectrode is advanced deeper into the cortex. Thus, the tonotopic organization of AI has cells with essentially similar CFs arranged in vertical columns and in bands horizontally. These isofrequency bands widen as stimulus intensity is increased (Brugge, 1975), that is, as a stimulus gets more intense a wider band of cortex responds to it.

Figure 6.12 is a slightly modified version of Woolsey's (1960) classical summary of the tonotopic organization of the animal cortex. It shows tonotopic organization in several areas, with locations responsive to low frequencies labeled *a*, and areas responsive to high frequencies labeled *b*. Area AI is arranged from high frequencies rostrally to lows caudally. Area AII is organized in the opposite direction, although other studies found a wide range of CFs among the cells in the same part of AII (Reale and Imig, 1980; Schreiner and Cynader, 1984). Merzenich and Brugge (1973) found high frequencies represented caudomedially and lows rostrally in the monkey AI, and a secondary auditory belt around area AI. In the ectosylvian area, highs are represented above and lows are below. Separately identifiable areas have been found on the posterior margin of AII and in the posterior ectosylvian sulcus on the anterior aspect of Ep (Knight, 1977; Reale and Imig, 1980). Tunturi's area AIII is situated in the head subdivision of somatic sensory area II (SII). Some degree of frequency representation has been identified in the insular area (INS) (Loeffler, 1958; Desmedt and Michelse, 1959). The sylvian fringe area (SF) has a high frequencies represented posteriorly and lows anteriorly. The anterior auditory field (AAF) is a separate tonotopically organized area (Knight, 1977; Reale and Imig, 1980) that was previously considered the lower-frequency section of SF.

Contemporary findings have revealed that there are several tonotopic arrangements in the human auditory cortex

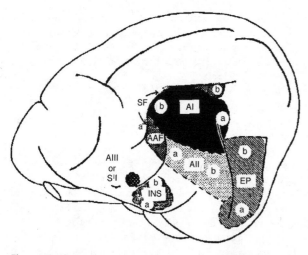

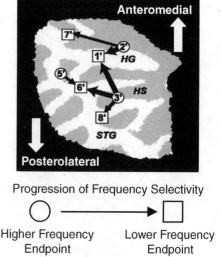

Progression of Frequency Selectivity

Higher Frequency
Endpoint

Lower Frequency
Endpoint

Figure 6.12 Composite summary of the tonotopic organization of the animal cortex based on Woolsey (1960), with some modifications based on more recent findings. Regions identified by Woolsey as responsive to lower frequencies are designated by the letter **a**, and those responsive to higher frequencies are labeled **b**. See text for details. *Source*: Adapted from Woolsey, CN (1960). Organization of the cortical auditory system: A review and synthesis. In: GL Rasmussen, WF Windle (eds.), *Neural Mechanisms of the Auditory and Vestibular Systems*. Courtesy of Charles C. Thomas, Publisher.

Figure 6.13 Tonotopic organization in the human auditory cortex showing six numbered tonotopic progressions with frequencies represented from high (*circles*) to low (*squares*). *Abbreviations*: HG, Heschl's gyrus; HS, Heschl's sulcus; STG, superior temporal gyrus. The unfamiliar appearance of the anatomy is the result of projecting the folded, three-dimensional layout of the actual anatomy onto a flat, two-dimensional picture. *Source*: From Talavage, Sereno, Melcher, Ledden, Rosen, Dale (2004). *Journal of Neurophysiology*, Vol 91, used with permission from the American Physiological Society.

(e.g., Thomas, Talavage, Ledden, et al., 2000; Talavage, Sereno, Melcher, et al., 2004). For example, Fig. 6.13 shows six tonotopic progressions identified by Talavage et al. (2004). These are shown as arrows, with a circle indicating the high-frequency end of each tonotopic arrangement and a square representing its low-frequency end.

It has been known for some time that most of the auditory areas are interconnected within each cerebral hemisphere and are connected via commissural pathways with their counterparts on the other side in both cats and monkeys (Diamond et al., 1968a, 1968b; Hall and Goldstein, 1968; Pandya et al., 1969). These findings have been extended by more recent anatomical studies in the cat, which demonstrated tonotopically organized projections among the thalamus and cortex, and the auditory cortex and several frontal lobe areas on the same side and between hemispheres via commissural connections (e.g., Lee, Imaizumi, Schreiner, and Winer, 2004; Lee and Winer, 2005).

Before leaving the topic of frequency representation in the auditory system, it is interesting to be aware that functional magnetic resonance studies by Janata et al. (2002) have identified cortically active areas related to tonality in listeners with musical experience. Most notably, responses were obtained from the superior temporal gyri on both sides, although more extensively in the right hemisphere, and topographical representations related to musical tonality were identified in the rostromedial prefrontal cortex. Their findings may provide physiological correlates to several aspects of musical perception like those discussed in Chapter 12.

AUDITORY EVOKED POTENTIALS

Until now we have been primarily concerned with the responses of single cells, measured by inserting microelectrodes directly into the neural material. It is also possible to measure the neural responses evoked by sound stimulation by using electrodes placed on the surface of the brain or, more often, on the scalp. Although this approach does not allow one to focus upon the activity of single neurons, it does permit the study of aggregate responses of various nuclei. The major advantage is that surface electrodes allow noninvasive study, and hence may readily be applied to diagnostic audiology as well as a wide range of research applications. This section provides a brief description of these **evoked potentials**.

Two problems need to be addressed when evoked responses are measured. One is the very low intensity of any single response, and the other is the excessive noise in the form of ongoing neural activity. Both problems are overcome by obtaining an **averaged response** from many stimulus repetitions.

Suppose we measure the ongoing electrical response of the brain, or the **electroencephalographic response (EEG)**. In the absence of stimulation, the EEG will be random at any particular moment. That is, if we randomly select and line up a large number of segments from an ongoing EEG, there will be about as many positive as negative values at the points being compared. The algebraic sum of these random values will be zero. Alternatively, suppose a group of cells fire at a given time (latency) after

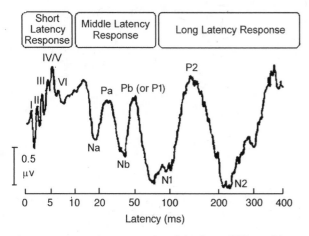

Figure 6.14 Composite representation of the short, middle-, and long-latency responses of the major auditory evoked potentials (note the logarithmic time scale). *Source:* Adapted from *ASHA* (1987), with permission of American Speech-Language-Hearing Association.

the onset of a click. If we always measure the activity at the same latency, then we would find that the responses at that point are always positive (or negative) going. Instead of averaging these responses out, algebraic summation will exaggerate them, since positives are always added to positives and negatives to negatives. Thus, the averaging (or summation) process improves the signal-to-noise ratio by averaging out the background activity (noise) and summating the real responses, which are locked in time to the stimulus.

Auditory evoked potentials are described with regard to their response latencies, as illustrated by the composite diagram in Fig. 6.14. The earliest set of response waves were originally described by Sohmer and Feinmesser (1967) and by Jewett, Romano, and Williston (1970). They are collectively known as the **short latency response**, **auditory brainstem response**, or **brainstem auditory evoked response**, and occasionally referred to as "*Jewett bumps*" in some of the earlier literature. The short latency response occurs within the first 8 ms of stimulus onset (e.g., Jewett, 1970; Jewett et al., 1970; Jewett and Williston, 1971; Buchwald and Huang, 1975). They appear as about seven successive peaks, the largest and most stable of which is the fifth one, known as **wave V**. Comprehensive reviews are provided by Hall (2007) and Burkhard and Don (2007).

On the basis of their latencies, there has been a tendency to associate the various waves with successive nuclei in the auditory pathways. **Waves I** and **II** are generated by the auditory nerve, and correspond to the negative peaks (N1 and N2) of the auditory nerve compound action potential discussed in the prior chapter. **Wave III** has been attributed to the superior olive, **wave IV** with the lateral lemniscus and/or inferior colliculus, **wave V** with the inferior colliculus and possible higher centers, and **wave VI** with the medial geniculate. However, one should not attribute specific peaks beyond waves I and II to individual

neural centers. On the contrary, they are actually due to the combined activity of *multiple generators* in the auditory brainstem (Jewett and Williston, 1971; Møller and Jannetta, 1985; Scherg and vonCramon, 1985; Moore, 1987, 2000; Rudell, 1987; Hall, 2007; Møller, 2007).

The **middle latency response** occurs at latencies of roughly 10 to 60 ms (e.g., Geisler et al., 1958; Ruhm et al., 1967; Hall, 2007; Pratt, 2007), as is shown in Fig. 6.14 as a succession of positive (P) and negative (N) waves labeled **Na, Pa, Nb,** and **Pb**. Wave Pb is generally considered part of the middle latency response, but it is also identified as **P1** in the figure because it is sometimes considered the first positive peak of the long latency response. The middle latency response appears to be produced by the neural activity of the auditory cortex, as well as subcortical sites involving the midbrain, thalamocortical pathways, and reticular system.

Long latency responses, also known as auditory **cortical evoked potentials**, are observed at latencies between about 70 and 300 ms (e.g., Davis, 1964; McCandless and Best, 1964, 1966; Hall, 2007; Martin, Tremblay, and Stapells, 2007; Martin, Tremblay, and Korezak, 2008), and have been the subject of extensive study. Its components are identified as **N1, P2,** and **N2** in Fig. 6.14. The long latency response (particularly waves P2 and N2) is largely due to the activity in the temporal and frontal lobes of the cortex, as well as due to some contributions from the limbic system.

Another group of evoked auditory responses may be referred to as **event-related potentials**. A large positive wave called **P300** or **P3** occurs at a latency of about 300 ms when the subject must listen for and make a cognitive response to infrequently occurring "oddball" stimuli that are randomly interspersed among a much larger number of frequently occurring signals (Sutton et al., 1965; Hall, 2007; Starr and Golob, 2007). The frequent signals are all the same, and the oddball signals differ from them in some way (e.g., frequency). When the listener *ignores* the stimuli, the resulting long latency responses are similar regardless of whether or not the oddballs are included among the signals used to obtain the averaged response (Fig. 6.15a). However, a P3 wave is generated when oddballs are included among the signals and the subject *listens for them* (Fig. 6.15b).

The **contingent negative variation** is a slow shift in the DC baseline after a latency of about 300 ms that occurs when the subject is required to perform a mental or motor task in response to a stimulus (Davis, 1964; McCandless and Best, 1964, 1966).

Mismatch negativity (Näätänen, 1995; Hall, 2007; Starr and Golob, 2007; Martin et al., 2008) is a negative deflection at latencies of about 150 to 275 ms, which occurs when a subject detects a signal that differs from the ones that came before it. This electrophysiological discrimination measure occurs even if the subject is not attending to the stimuli. It should not be surprising that the event-related potentials are reflecting cortical activity that involves more than just the auditory areas.

A given potential, such as the P300 wave, can be monitored simultaneously at many different sites on the surface of the head.

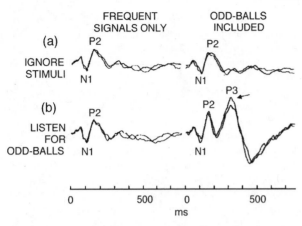

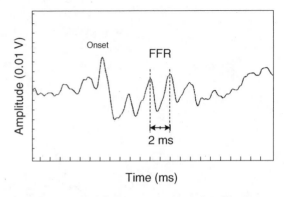

Figure 6.15 (a) The long latency response is not changed by the presence of oddball signals when the listener *ignores* the stimuli. (b) The long latency response includes a P3 wave (*arrow*) when the oddballs are present and the subject listens for them. *Source:* Adapted from Squires and Hecox (1983), "Electrophysiological evaluation of higher level auditory function," with permission.

Figure 6.16 Frequency-following response (FFR) elicited by 500-Hz tone bursts. *Source:* From Ananthanarayan and Durrant (1992). The frequency-following response and the onset response. *Ear Hear,* Vol 13, p. 229, ©1992, used with permission from Lippincott Williams and Wilkins.

The amplitudes of the potentials picked up by the electrodes will depend on their locations, being greatest where there is the most underlying neural activity, and least over inactive sites. These simultaneously recorded potentials can then be analyzed to generate a set of differently shaded (or colored) areas or contour lines that indicate equally active locations on the head. Similar to the color coded weather maps commonly seen on television weather reports, the resulting **topographic brain map** reveals brain locations that are more or less active ("hot") or inactive ("cold") with respect to the neurological activity that is associated with a particular perceptual event, response, or activity.

Frequency-Following Response

In contrast to responses we have considered so far, the frequency-following response and the auditory steady-state response are evoked potentials that occur during a period of ongoing (albeit short duration) stimulation. The **frequency-following response (FFR)** is a steady-state evoked potential that is elicited by periodic signals. In the case of tonal signals, the FFR is synchronized (i.e., phase-locked) to the period of the stimulus. For example, Fig. 6.16 shows the FFR produced by 25-ms, 500-Hz tone bursts. Notice that the FFR waveform has a 2-ms period, corresponding to the period of the 500-Hz stimulus (t = 1/f = 1/500 Hz = 0.002 s, or 2 ms). When measured using surface electrodes on the scalp, the FFR is most robust in response to lower frequency tones like 500 Hz but can elicited by tone bursts up to about 2000 Hz (Moushegian, Rupert, Stillman, 1973; Glaser, Suter, Dasheiff, and Goldberg, 1976).

The FFR is likely the result of multiple generators, with various lines of evidence implicating the brainstem nuclei (e.g., Moushegian and Rupert, 1970; Huis in't Veldt, Osterhammel,

and Terkildsen, 1977; Sohmer and Pratt, 1977; Stillman, Crow, and Moushegian, 1978; Gardi and Merzenich, 1979; Galbraith, Bagasan, and Sulahian, 2001), the auditory nerve (e.g., Huis in't Veld et al., 1977; Galbraith et al., 2001), and contributions from the cochlear microphonic (e.g., Huis in't Veld et al., 1977; Sohmer and Pratt, 1977; Gardi and Merzenich, 1979). For a comprehensive discussion of the FFR, see Krishnan (2007).

Auditory Steady-State Response

The **auditory steady-state response (ASSR)** is evoked by signals that modulate periodically. As an example, we will assume that the stimulus is a sinusoidally amplitude modulated (SAM or just AM) tone.[2] Figure 6.17a shows the envelope of the amplitude-modulated waveform; the inset in the figure distinguishes between the *carrier frequency* of the tone and the *modulation rate* (or *frequency*), which is the rate at which the amplitude of the carrier tone fluctuates over time. Let us suppose that the carrier frequency is 2000 Hz and that the modulation rate is 100 times per second, or 100 Hz. In this case, 2000 Hz is the *carrier frequency* and 100 Hz is the *modulation rate* or *frequency*. The spectrum of this stimulus is shown on the right side of Fig. 6.17c. Notice that this kind of signal has considerable frequency specificity, containing just the carrier frequency (2000 Hz) and components at frequencies equal to the carrier frequency plus-and-minus the modulation rate (i.e., 2000−100 = 1900 Hz and 2000 + 100 = 2100 Hz).

Modulated signals like the one in Fig. 6.17a elicit neural activity that is phase-locked to the modulation pattern, as in Fig. 6.17b. In other words, the period of the ASSR waveform corresponds to the period of the modulating signal. Notice, too,

---

[2] We are using an SAM tone for clarity and to highlight the frequency-specificity provided by this kind of stimulus. However, the ASSR can also be evoked by other kinds of modulation, such as frequency modulation (FM) or a combination of both AM and FM, as well as using noise instead of a tonal signal.

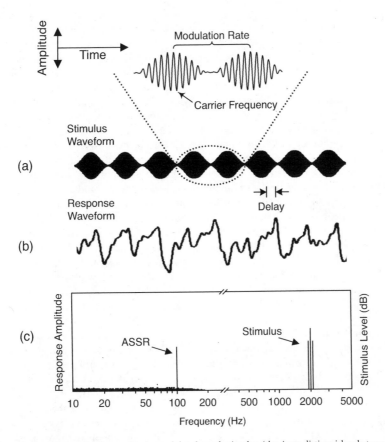

Figure 6.17   (a) Idealized envelope of a sinusoidally amplitude-modulated tonal stimulus (the *inset* distinguishes between the carrier frequency and modulation rate). (b) ASSR (response) waveform [adapted from Grason-Stadler, Inc. (2001) with permission] synchronized to the stimulus modulation rate with slight delay indicated by arrows. (c) Idealized spectra of a 2000-Hz AM tone with a 100-Hz modulation rate (*right*) and the resulting 100-Hz ASSR response (*left*).

that the ASSR waveform is delayed (phase shifted) relative to the stimulus (highlighted in the figure by the arrows marked "delay" between frames a and b). In the frequency domain, the spectrum of the ASSR has a distinct peak at the frequency corresponding to the modulation rate (100 Hz in our example), illustrated on the left side of Fig. 6.17c. Unlike most AEPs, which are evaluated by inspection of the waveform, the presence of an ASSR is determined by a statistical analysis of the amplitude and/or phase of the response (e.g., Rance, Rickards, Cohen, et al., 1995; Dimitrijevic, John, Van Roon, et al., 2002). This is typically accomplished by using automated procedures programmed into the measurement instrumentation.

The ASSR has been studied in considerable detail and has been incorporated into clinical practice (see Hall, 2007; Picton, 2007). The ASSR can be elicited in infants, children, and adults (Lins, Picton, Boucher, et al., 1996; Cone-Wesson, Parker, Swiderski, and Richards, 2002; Rance, Tomlin, and Rickards, 2006). On average, ASSR thresholds are found within about 15 dB of behavioral thresholds (Lins et al., 1996; Herdman and Stapells, 2001, 2003; Dimitrijevic et al., 2002; Picton, Dimitri-

jevic, Perez-Abalo, and Van Roon, 2005; Van der Werff and Brown, 2005). However, amplitudes are small in neonates, and ASSR thresholds improve over the course of the infant's first 12 months (Savio, Cárdenas, Pérez Abalo, et al., 2001; John, Brown, Muir, and Picton, 2004; Rance and Tomlin, 2004).

The ASSR includes contributions from brainstem and auditory cortex generators, with the brainstem contribution dominating the response at higher modulation rates and the cortical contribution dominating at lower modulation rates (e.g., Herdman, Lins, Van Roon, et al., 2002; Szalda and Burkard, 2005). Consistent with these contributions, state of arousal does not have a substantial effect on the ASSR when obtained with high (roughly ≥80 Hz) modulation rates (Cohen, Rickards, and Clark, 1991; Levi, Folsom, and Dobie, 1993; Aoyagi, Kiren, Kim, et al., 1993), similar to what we saw for the ABR. In contrast, the ASSR obtained with lower modulation rates (e.g., 40 Hz) is greatly affected by sleep and anesthesia (Jerger, Chmiel, Frost, and Coker, 1986; Picton, John, Purcell, and Plourde, 2003), similar to what we saw for the longer-latency potentials.

EFFECTS OF CORTICAL ABLATION

Which auditory functions are subserved at a cortical level? Equivalent to this question is the more testable one of which functions can still be accomplished (or relearned) after the auditory cortex has been removed, and which ones can be carried out only when the cortex is intact. This question has been investigated extensively in laboratory animals, particularly cats. The fundamental approach has been fairly consistent. This approach has been to bilaterally ablate the auditory cortex, and then to test the animal's ability to perform (or relearn) various sound discrimination tasks. The assumption is that discriminations unaffected by the ablations are subserved by subcortical and/or nonauditory cortical centers, whereas discriminations impaired after ablation must require processing in the auditory cortices.

It is well established that certain sound discriminations can be accomplished after *bilateral* ablation of the auditory cortices, while others cannot. The bilaterally ablated animal *can* discriminate: (1) the onset of a sound (Kryter and Ades, 1943; Meyer and Woolsey, 1952), (2) changes in tonal intensity (Raab and Ades, 1946; Rosenzweig, 1946; Neff, 1960), and (3) changes in the frequency of a tonal stimulus (Meyer and Woolsey, 1952; Butler and Diamond, 1957; Goldberg and Neff, 1961). However, the type of frequency discrimination is critical, especially when the discrimination is between sequences of tones. Diamond et al. (1962) presented bilaterally ablated animals with discrimination tasks between two sequences of three tones each. One sequence contained three low-frequency tones (LO-LO-LO), and the other group had two low tones separated by a higher frequency (LO-HI-LO). The LO-HI-LO sequence could be discriminated from the LO-LO-LO group, but the discrimination could no longer be performed when the task was reversed (i.e., when all low tones was the positive stimulus to be discriminated from the LO-HI-LO sequence).

Bilaterally ablated animals *cannot* discriminate: (1) changes in tonal duration (Scharlock et al., 1965), (2) changes in the temporal pattern of a tonal sequence (Diamond and Neff, 1957), or (3) sound localizations in space (Neff et al., 1956). Surgically induced lesions and ablation of the auditory cortex also affect temporal resolution, revealed by lengthened gap detection thresholds (GDTs) in rodents (Kelly, Rooney, and Phillips, 1996; Syka, Rybalko, Mazelová, and Druga, 2002). However, Syka et al. (2002) found that GDTs did improve with time after surgery, eventually becoming slightly longer than those in normal (control) animals.

Masterton and Diamond (1964) presented bilaterally ablated cats with a series of pairs of clicks separated by 0.5 ms, in which the first click of each pair went to one ear and the second click went to the other ear. If the first click is directed to the right ear (R-L), then the clicks are lateralized to the right; if the first click goes to the left ear (L-R), they are lateralized left (see Chap. 13). These workers found that bilaterally ablated cats could not discriminate the change from a series of L-R click pairs to R-L click pairs. In this regard, Neff (1967) suggested

that the auditory cortex plays an important role in the accurate localization of sounds in space.

Cats with bilateral ablations of the auditory cortex evidence a startle response to sound, but do not exhibit the orientation response of reflexive head turning in the direction of the sound source found in normal cats (Neff, 1967). Also, bilaterally ablated animals do appear to be able to push a response lever indicating whether a sound came from the right or left, but cannot approach the sound source to get a reward (Heffner and Masterton, 1975; Neff et al., 1975). Neff and Casseday (1977) suggested that the right-left distinction may be based upon different perceptual cues than spatial location. However, they explained that the auditory cortex is essential if the animal is to perceive spatial orientations and the relationships of its own body to the environment. Heffner and Heffner (1990) found that monkeys with bilateral ablations of the auditory cortex experienced deficits in a variety of tasks involving sound location in space, such as discriminating signals presented from the same side, making right-left discriminations, and the ability to approach the sound source.

There is evidence that localization ability is impaired by *unilateral* ablation of the auditory cortex (Whitfield et al., 1972). An experiment by Neff and Casseday (1977) is especially interesting in this regard. They surgically destroyed one cochlea each in a group of cats, and then trained these unilaterally hearing animals to make sound localizations. Following this procedure, half of the animals were subjected to unilateral ablations of the auditory cortex opposite the good ear, and half were ablated ipsilateral to the good ear (opposite the deaf ear). Those with cortical ablations on the same side as the hearing ear were essentially unaffected in localization ability. The animals whose cortical ablations were contralateral to the good ear could not relearn the localization task. These findings demonstrate that localization behavior is affected by destruction of the auditory cortex opposite to a functioning ear. They also suggest that excitation of the auditory cortex on one side serves as a cue that the opposite ear is stimulated. These results are consistent with single-cell data suggesting that contralateral stimulation is excitatory to cells in the auditory cortex.

Most studies on humans with central auditory lesions have employed speech tests. However, tests using nonverbal materials are also valuable since they are directly comparable with the results of animal studies (Neff, 1977). Bilateral temporal lobe damage in humans has been shown to result in impaired ability to make temporal pattern discriminations (Jerger et al., 1969; Lhermitte et al., 1971; Karaseva, 1972). Temporal lobe damage in humans has also been reported to result in impaired sound localization in space (Jerger et al., 1969; Neff et al., 1975). These results essentially confirm the animal studies. Clinical data also tend to support Neff and Casseday's (1977) position that neural activity at the contralateral cortex provides a "sign" of the stimulated ear. For example, patients who underwent unilateral temporal lobectomies have reported localization difficulties on the side opposite to the removed cortex (Penfield and Evans, 1934), and electrical stimulation of the auditory cortex has resulted in hallucinations of sounds or hearing loss at the ear opposite to the stimulated cortex (Penfield and Rasmussen, 1950; Penfield and Jasper, 1954).

Neff (1960, 1967) has proposed that in order for sound discriminations to be accomplished after *bilateral* ablation of the auditory cortex, it is necessary for the positive stimulus to excite neural units that were not excited by the previous (neutral) stimulus. Thus, stimulus onset, as well as intensity and frequency changes, is discriminated because new neural units are excited by the changes in each case. The same is true when the sequence LO-HI-LO is discriminated from LO-LO-LO. However, LO-LO-LO is not discriminated from LO-HI-LO, because there is nothing new in the LO-LO-LO sequence that was not already present in LO-HI-LO, so no new neural units are excited by the change. These functions may be processed below the level of the auditory cortex, or by other cortical areas. On the other hand, discriminations that involve the processing of serial orders or time sequences (i.e., discriminations in the temporal domain) are subserved by the auditory cortex. Thus, they are obliterated when the auditory cortex is bilaterally removed.

OLIVOCOCHLEAR EFFERENT SYSTEM

Recall that the olivocochlear pathways are composed of both a medial system terminating directly on the outer hair cells and a lateral system terminating on the afferent nerve fibers of the inner hair cells rather than on the IHCs themselves (Chap. 2). However, this section concentrates on the medial olivocochlear system because little is currently known about effects of the lateral system (see, e.g., Guinan, 1996, 2006; Groff and Liberman, 2003).

The medial olivocochlear system (MOC) is activated with electricity or sound, its effects are generally studied by comparing measurements made with and without activation. Electrical stimulation usually involves the crossed olivocochlear bundle (COCB) where it crosses the floor of the fourth ventricle, and sound activation typically involves presenting a noise to the opposite ear. The effects of sound stimulation are often called the **medial efferent acoustic reflex** or **medial olivocochlear reflex** that involves activating the medial olivocochlear system by sound stimulation. This reduces the gain of the cochlear amplifier, and provides a reduction of masking effects, suppression of otoacoustic emissions, and a degree of protection to the cochlea from overstimulation due to loud sounds (e.g., Guinan, 1996, 2006; Brown, DeVenecia, and Guinan, 2003; DeVenecia, Liberman, Guinan, et al., 2005). Let us briefly look at examples of a few of these effects.

Activation of the medial olivocochlear system results in a lowering in the magnitude and nonlinearity of basilar membrane vibrations in the vicinity of the characteristic frequency, a reduction in auditory nerve action potentials, endocochlear potentials and summating potentials, and increases in cochlear microphonics (Fex, 1959, 1967; Galambos, 1959; Wiederhold

and Peake, 1966; Konishi and Slepian, 1971; Gifford and Guinan, 1987; Mountain et al., 1980; Gifford and Guinan, 1987; Guinan, 1996, 2006; Dolan et al., 1997; Russell and Murugasu, 1997). It appears that the efferent system evokes these effects by affecting the outer hair cells (Guinan, 1996, 2006).

The resulting loss of sensitivity is seen in Fig. 6.18, which shows basilar membrane displacement as a function of stimulus level with and without electrical activation of the medial olivocochlear system. The rightward shift of the curves indicates that higher stimulus levels are needed to obtain a particular magnitude of response when the MOC is activated. Also notice that the functions become more linear (especially in frames c, e, and f) with stimulation of the medial efferent system, indicating its affect on the compressive nonlinearity of the basilar membrane response. (Dolan et al. (1997) also found that activation of the medial efferent system caused an increase in response magnitude for high stimulus levels.)

The inhibitory effect of medial olivocochlear system activation is also seen as a reduction in the firing rate of the afferent auditory neurons (Kiang et al., 1970; Brown and Nuttall, 1984; Guinan and Gifford, 1988a; Warren and Liberman, 1989). If firing rate is expressed as a function of the sound pressure level of the stimulus, then the inhibitory effect of MOC activation is observed as a shift to the right of this function, as illustrated in Fig. 6.19. The primary effects occur at the sharply tuned tip of the auditory neuron's tuning curve. This phenomenon is depicted in Fig. 6.20, where we see that it is tantamount to a reduction in sensitivity in the vicinity of the tip of the tuning curve.

Studies using various approaches to activate the MOC have suggested that auditory neuron firing rates are suppressed after latencies of about 15 ms or more, and it is often found that there is a greater effect on the afferent responses to higher-frequency sounds than to lower ones (e.g., Wiederhold, 1970; Wiederhold and Kiang, 1970; Teas et al., 1972; Gifford and Guinan, 1987). The rightward movement of the rate-level function and the sensitivity decrement at the tip of the tuning curve are often on the order of approximately 20 dB. Consistent with its effect on afferent auditory neurons are a reduction of intracellular receptor potential magnitudes and a drop of sensitivity at the tip of the tuning curves for the *inner* hair cells (Brown et al., 1983; Brown and Nuttall, 1984).

Stimulating the medial efferent system also has a suppressive effect on click-evoked, tone-burst-evoked and distortion product otoacoustic emissions (e.g., Mountain, 1980; Siegel and Kim, 1982; Collet et al., 1990; Ryan et al., 1991; Moulin et al., 1993; Killan and Kapadia, 2006; Wagner, Heppelmann, Müller, et al., 2007), and also causes spontaneous OAEs to shift upward in frequency (but up or down in amplitudes) (e.g., Mott et al., 1983; Harrison and Burns, 1993). These observations, along with those already mentioned, provide compelling evidence that the medial efferent system influences the active processes in the cochlea associated with its nonlinear responses, amplification, and tuning.

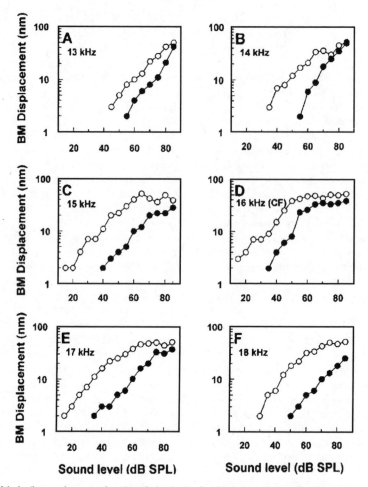

Figure 6.18 Displacement of the basilar membrane as a function of stimulus level with (*closed symbols*) and without (*open symbols*) electrical activation of the medial olivocochlear system (guinea pig). The characteristic frequency (CF) for the basilar membrane location involved was 16 kHz, and the stimulus frequencies are shown in each frame. *Source*: From Russell and Murugasu (1997), by permission of *J. Acoust. Soc. Am.*

Further insight into the nature and potential practical implications of the efferent system is gained when one examines the effects of medial olivocochlear system stimulation in the presence of masking noise (Nieder and Nieder, 1970a, 1970b; Winslow and Sachs, 1987; Dolan and Nuttall, 1988; Guinan and Gifford, 1988b; Kawase et al., 1993). For example, Dolan and Nuttall (1988) studied how MOC stimulation affects the responses to the different levels of a stimulus presented with and without various levels of masking noise. Their results are shown in Fig. 6.21. Notice first that the effect upon the magnitude of the auditory nerve compound action potential (CAP) of medial olivocochlear system stimulation alone is very much like

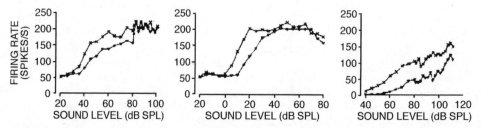

Figure 6.19 Rate-level functions of individual cat auditory neurons showing the rightward shift of the functions during stimulation of the COCB. (Xs, without COCB stimulation; triangles, with COCB stimulation). *Source*: From Gifford and Guinan (1983), with permission of *J. Acoust. Soc. Am.*

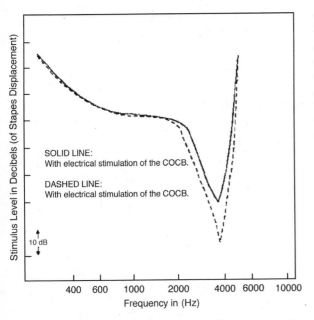

Figure 6.20 Effect of COCB stimulation on the auditory neuron tuning curve. *Source*: Based on the findings of Kiang, Moxon, and Levine (1970), used with the authors' permission.

what we have already seen for individual neuron rate-level functions: The response magnitude is reduced considerably at lower stimulus levels and less so (or not at all) at the highest levels of the tone burst. This effect (seen by comparing the "control" and "COCB" curves) is the same in each frame of the figure. Also, see how CAP magnitude is reduced more and more as the masker is increased from 30 dB (frame a) to 42 dB (frame b) to 53 dB (frame c).

The unmasking effect of medial olivocochlear system stimulation can be seen by comparing the curves for the masker alone ("BBN") with those for MOC combined with the noise ("BBN and COCB"). Combining MOC stimulation with the low-level masker (frame a) causes a smaller response (compared to the masker alone) at low stimulus levels and a slight improvement at high levels. For the higher-level maskers (frames b and c), adding MOC stimulation to the masker increases the response magnitude over what it was for the masker alone for all conditions where the comparison is made.

REFERENCES

Abeles, M, Goldstein, MH. 1970. Functional architecture in cat primary auditory cortex: Columnar organization and organization according to depth. *J Neurophysiol* 33, 172–187.

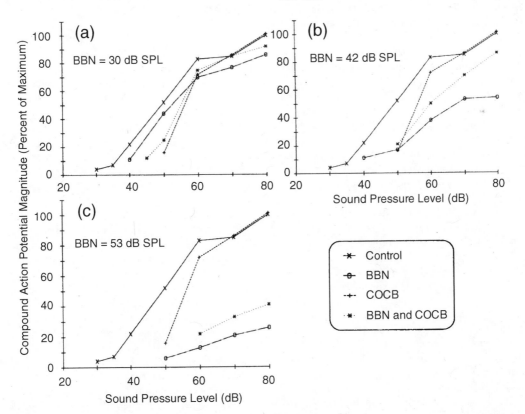

Figure 6.21 Effects of combining COCB stimulation with various masking noise (BBN) levels upon the compound action potential response to 10 kHz tone bursts presented at low to high sound pressure levels. *Source*: Adapted from Dolan and Nuttall (1988), with permission of *J. Acoust. Soc. Am.*

Ahveninen, J, Jääskeläinen, IP, Raij, T, Bonmassar, G, Devore, S, Hämäläinen, M, Levänen, S, Lin, FH, Sams, M, shinn-Cunningham, BG, Witzel, T, Belliveau, JW. 2006. Task-modulated "what" and "where" pathways in human auditory cortex. *Proc Natl Acad Sci USA* 103, 14608–14613.

Aitkin, IM, Anderson, DJ, Brugge, JE. 1970. Tonotopic organization and discharge characteristics of single neurons in nuclei of the lateral lemniscus of the cat. *J Neurophysiol* 33, 421–440.

Aitkin, IM, Dunlop, CW. 1968. Interplay of excitation and inhibition in the cat medial geniculate body. *J Neurophysiol* 31, 44–61.

Aitkin, IM, Dunlop, CW, Webster, WR. 1966. Click evoked response patterns in single units in the medial geniculate body of the cat. *J Neurophysiol* 29, 109–123.

Aitkin, IM, Webster, WR. 1971. Tonotopic organization in the medial geniculate body of the cat. *Brain Res* 26, 402–405.

Aitkin, LM, Webster, WR. 1972. Medial geniculate body of the cat: Organization and responses to tonal stimuli of neurons in the ventral division. *J Neurophysiol* 35, 356–380.

Aitkin, LM. 1973. Medial geniculate body of the cat: Responses to tonal stimuli of neurons in the medial division. *J Neurophysiol* 36, 275–283.

Allon, N, Yeshurun, Y, Wolberg, Z. 1981. Responses of single cells in the medial geniculate body of awake squirrel monkeys. *Exp Brain Res* 41, 222–232.

American Speech-Language-Hearing Association (ASHA). 1987. *The Short Latency Auditory Evoked Potentials*. Rockville Pike, MD: ASHA.

Ananthanarayan, AK, Durrant, JD. 1992. The frequency-following response and the onset response: Evaluation of frequency specificity using a forward-masking paradigm. *Ear Hear* 13, 228–232.

Aoyagi, M, Kiren, T, Kim, Y, Suzuki Y, Fuse, T, Koike, Y. 1993. Optimal modulation frequency for amplitude-modulation following response in young children during sleep. *Hear Res* 65, 253–261.

Benevento, LA, Coleman, PD. 1970. Responses of single cells in cat inferior colliculus to binaural click stimuli: Combinations of intensity levels, time differences and intensity differences. *Brain Res* 17, 387–405.

Benson, DA, Teas, DC. 1976. Single unit study of binaural interaction in the auditory cortex of the chinchilla. *Brain Res* 103, 313–338.

Bieser, A, Müller-Preuss, P. 1996. Auditory responsive cortex in the squirrel monkey: Neural responses to amplitude-modulated sounds. *Exp Brain Res* 108, 273–284.

Boudreau, JC, Tsuchitani, C. 1968. Binaural interaction in the cat superior olive S segment. *J Neurophysiol* 31, 442–454.

Boudreau, JD, Tsuchitani, CC. 1970. Cat superior olivary S segment cell discharge to tonal stimulation. In: WD Neff (ed.), *Contributions to Sensory Physiology*. New York, NY: Academic Press, 143–213.

Brown, MC, DeVenecia, RK, Guinan, JJ Jr. 2003. Responses of medial olivocochlear neurons. Specifying the central pathways of the medial olivocochlear reflex. *Exp Brain Res* 153, 491–498.

Brown, MC, Nuttall, AL. 1984. Efferent control of cochlear inner hair cell responses in the guinea pig. *J Physiol* 354, 625–646.

Brown, MC, Nuttall, AL, Masta, RI. 1983. Intracellular recordings from cochlear inner hair cells: Effects of the crossed olivocochlear efferents. *Science* 222, 69–72.

Brugge, JF. 1975. Progress in neuroanatomy and neurophysiology of auditory cortex. In: DB Tower (ed.), *The Nervous System. Vol. 3: Human Communication and Its Disorders*. New York, NY: Raven, 97–111.

Brugge, JF, Anderson, DJ, Aitkin, LM. 1970. Responses of neurons in the dorsal nucleus of the lateral lemniscus of cat to binaural tonal stimulation. *J Neurophysiol* 33, 441–458.

Brugge, JF, Dubrovsky, NA, Aitkin, LM, Anderson, DJ. 1969. Sensitivity of single neurons in auditory cortex of cat to binaural tonal stimulation: Effects of varying interaural time and intensity. *J Neurophysiol* 32, 1005–1024.

Brugge, JF, Geisler, CD. 1978. Auditory mechanisms of the lower brainstem. *Annu Rev Neurosci* l, 363–394

Brugge, JF, Merzenich, MM. 1973. Patterns of activity of single neurons of the auditory cortex in monkey. In: AR Møller (ed.), *Basic Mechanisms in Hearing*. New York, NY: Academic Press.

Buchwald, JS, Huang, CM. 1975. Far-field acoustic response: Origins in the cat. *Science* 189, 382–384.

Burkhard, RF, Don, M, Eggermont, JJ (eds.). 2007. *Auditory Evoked Potentials: Basic Principles and Clinical Applications*. Philadelphia, PA: Lippincott Williams & Wilkins.

Burkhard, RF, Don, M. 2007. The auditory brainstem response. In: RF Burkhard, M Don, JJ Eggermont (eds.), *Auditory Evoked Potentials: Basic Principles and Clinical Applications*. Philadelphia, PA: Lippincott Williams & Wilkins, 229–253.

Butler, RA, Diamond, IT, Neff, WD. 1957. Role of auditory cortex in discrimination of changes in frequency. *J Neurophysiol* 20, 108–120.

Caird, D, Klinke, R. 1983. Processing of binaural stimuli by cat superior olivary complex neurons. *Exp Brain Res* 52, 385–399.

Caird, D, Klinke, R. 1987. Processing of interaural time and intensity differences in the cat inferior colliculus. *Exp Brain Res* 68, 379–392.

Cant, NB. 1992. The cochlear nucleus: Neronal types and their synaptic organization. In: WB Webster, AN Popper, RR Fay (eds.), *The Mammalian Auditory Pathway: Neuroanatomy*. New York, NY: Springer-Verlag, 66–116.

Cant, NB, Casseday, JH. 1986. Projections from the anteroventral cochlear nucleus to the lateral and medial superior olivary nuclei. *J Comp Neurol* 247, 457–476.

Clarey, JC, Barone, P, Imig, TJ. 1992. Physiology of the thalamus and cortex. In: AN Popper, RR Fay (eds.), *The Mammalian Auditory Pathway: Neurophysiology*. New York, NY: Springer-Verlag, 232–334.

Cohen, L, Rickards, F, Clark, G. 1991. A comparison of steady-state evoked potentials to modulated tones in awake and sleeping humans. *J Acoust Soc Am* 90, 2467–2479.

Collet, L, Kemp, DT, Veuillet, E, Duclaux, R, Moulin, A, Morgon, A. 1990. Effect of contralateral auditory stimuli on active cochlear micro-mechanical properties in human subjects. *Hear Res* 43, 251–262.

Cone-Wesson, B, Parker, J, Swiderski, N, Richards, F. 2002. The auditory steady-state response: Full-term and premature neonates. *J Am Acad Audiol* 13, 260–269.

Creutzfeldt, O, Hellweg, FC, Schreiner, C. 1980. Thalamocortical transformation of responses to complex auditory stimuli. *Exp Brain Res* 39, 87–104.

Davis, H. 1964. Some properties of the slow cortical response in humans. *Science* 146, 434.

de Ribaupierre, F, Goldstein, MH Jr, Yeni-Komshian, GH. 1972. Cortical coding of repetitive acoustic pulses. *Brain Res* 48, 205–225.

Desmedt, JE, Michelse, K. 1959. Corticofugal projections from temporal lobe in cat and their possible role in acoustic discrimination. *J Physiol* (London) 147, 17–18.

DeVenecia, RK, Liberman, MC, Guinan, JJ Jr, Brown, MC. 2005. Medial olivocochlear reflex interneurons are located in the posteroventral cochlear nucleus: A kainic acid lesion study in guinea pigs. *J Comp Neurol* 487, 345–360.

Diamond, IT, Goldberg, JM, Neff, WD. 1962. Tonal discrimination after ablation of auditory cortex. *J Neurophysiol* 25, 223–235.

Diamond, IT, Jones, EG, Powell, TPS. 1968a. Interhemispheric fiber connections of the auditory cortex of the cat. *Brain Res* 11, 177–193.

Diamond, IT, Jones, EG, Powell, TPS. 1968b. The association connections of the auditory cortex of the cat. *Brain Res* 11, 560–579.

Diamond, IT, Neff, WD. 1957. Ablation of temporal cortex and discrimination of auditory patterns. *J Neurophysiol* 20, 300–315.

Dimitrijevic, A, John, M, Van Roon, P, Purcell, D, Adamonis, J, Ostroff, J, Nedzelski, J, Picton T. 2002. Estimating the audiogram using multiple auditory steady-state responses. *J Am Acad Audiol* 13, 205–224.

Dolan, DF, Guo, MH, Nuttall, AL. 1997. Frequency-dependent enhancement of basilar membrane velocity during olivocochlear bundle stimulation. *J Acoust Soc Am* 102, 3587–3596.

Dolan, DF, Nuttall, AL. 1988. Masked cochlear whole-nerve response intensity functions "altered by electrical stimulation of the crossed olivocochlear bundle. *J Acoust Soc Am* 83, 1081–1086.

Faure, PA, Fremouw, T, Casseday, JH, Covey, E. 2003. Temporal masking reveals properties of sound-evoked inhibition in duration-tuned neurons of the inferior colliculus. *J Neurosci* 23, 3052–3065.

Fex, J. 1959. Augmentation of the cochlear microphonics by stimulation of efferent fibers to the cochlea. *Acta Otolaryngol* 50, 540–541.

Fex, J. 1967. Efferent inhibition in the cochlea related to hair-cell dc activity: Study of postsynaptic activity of the crossed olivocochlear fibers in the cat. *J Acoust Soc Am* 41, 666–675.

Finlayson, PG, Caspary, DM. 1991. Low-frequency neurons in the lateral superior olive exhibit phase-sensitive binaural inhibition. *J Neurophysiol* 65, 598–605.

Fitzpatrick, DC, Batra, R, Stanford, TR, Kuwada, S. 1997. A neuronal population code for sound localization. *Nature* 388, 871–874.

Frisina, RD, Smith, RL, Chamberlain, SC. 1990. Encoding of amplitude modulation in the gerbil cochlear nucleus: I. A hierarchy of enhancement. *Hear Res* 44, 99–122.

Galambos, R. 1952. Microelectrode studies on medial geniculate body of cat. III. Response to pure tones. *J Neurophysiol* 15, 381–400.

Galambos, R, Schwartzkopff, J, Rupert, AL. 1959. Microelectrode study of superior olivary nuclei. *Am J Physiol* 197, 527–536.

Galambos, R. 1959. Suppression of auditory activity by stimulation of efferent fibers to cochlea. *J Neurophysiol* 19, 424–437.

Galbraith, G, Bagasan, B, Sulahian, J. 2001. Brainstem frequency-following response recorded from one vertical and three horizontal electrode derivations. *Percept Mot Skills* 92, 99–106.

Gardi, J, Merzenich, M. 1979. The effect of high-pass noise on the scalp-recorded frequency-following response (FFR) in humans and cats. *J Acoust Soc Am* 65, 1491–1500.

Geisler, C, Frishkopf, L, Rosenblith, W. 1958. Extracranial responses to acoustic clicks in man. *Science* 128, 1210–1211.

Geisler, CD, Rhode, WS, Hazelton, DW. 1969. Responses of inferior colliculus neurons in the cat to binaural acoustic stimuli having wide-band spectra. *J Neurophysiol* 32, 960–974.

Gifford, ML, Guinan, JJ. 1983. Effects of crossed-olivocochlear-bundle stimulation on cat auditory nerve fiber responses to tones. *J Acoust Soc Am* 74, 115–123.

Gifford, ML, Guinan, JJ. 1987. Effects of cross-olivocochlear-bundle stimulation on cat auditory nerve fiber responses to tone. *J Acoust Soc Am* 74, 115–123.

Glaser, EM, Suter, CM, Dasheiff, R, Goldberg, A. 1976. The human frequency-following response: Its behavior during continuous tone and tone burst stimulation. *Electroencephalogr Clin Neurophysiol* 40, 25–32.

Glendenning, KK, Hutson, KA. 1998. Lack of topography in the ventral nucleus of the lateral lemniscus. *Microsc Res Tech* 41, 298–312.

Glendenning, KK, Hutson, KA, Nudo, RJ, Masterton, RB. 1985. Acoustic chiasm II: Anatomical basis of binaurality in lateral superior olive of cat. *J Comp Neurol* 232, 261–285.

Glendenning, KK, Masterson, RB. 1983. Acoustic chiasm: Efferent projections of the lateral superior olive. *J Neurosci* 3, 1521–1537.

Godfrey, DA, Kiang, NYS, Norris, BE. 1975a. Single unit activity in the posteroventral cochlear nucleus of the cat. *J Comp Neurol* 162, 247–268.

Godfrey, DA, Kiang, NYS, Norris, BE. 1975b. Single unit activity in the dorsal cochlear nucleus of the cat. *J Comp Neurol* 162, 269–284.

Goldberg, JM, Brown, RB. 1968. Functional organization of the dog superior olivary complex: An anatomical and physiological study. *J Neurophysiol* 31, 639–656.

Goldberg, JM, Brown, RB. 1969. Response of binaural neurons of dog superior olivary complex to dichotic tonal stimuli: Some physiological mechanisms of sound localization. *J Neurophysiol* 32, 613–636.

Goldberg, JM, Neff, WD. 1961. Frequency discrimination after bilateral ablation of auditory cortical areas. *J Neurophysiol* 24, 119–128.

Grason-Stadler, Inc. (GSI). 2001. *Auditory Steady-state response: A new tool for frequency-specific hearing assessment in infants and children.* Madison, WI: Viasys NeuroCare/GSI.

Groff, JA, Liberman, MC. 2003. Modulation of the cochlear afferent response by the lateral olivocochlear system: Activation via electrical stimulation of the inferior colliculus. *J Neurophysiol* 90, 3178–3200.

Guinan, JJ Jr. 1996. Physiology of the olivocochlear efferents. In: P Dallos, AN Popper, RR Fay (eds.). *The Cochlea.* New York, NY: Springer-Verlag, 435–502.

Guinan, JJ Jr. 2006. Olivocochlear efferents: Anatomy, physiology, function, and the measurement of efferent effects in humans. *Ear Hear* 27, 589–607.

Guinan, JJ Jr, Gifford, ML. 1988a. Effects of electrical stimulation of efferent olivocochlear neurons on cat auditory-nerve fibers. III. Tuning curves and thresholds at CF. *Hear Res* 37, 29–46.

Guinan, JJ Jr, Gifford, ML. 1988b. Effects of electrical stimulation of efferent olivocochlear neurons on cat auditory-nerve fibers. II. Spontaneous rate. *Hear Res* 33, 115–128.

Guinan, JJ Jr, Norris, BE, Guinan, SS. 1972. Single auditory units in the superior olivary complex II. Locations of unit categories and tonotopic organization. *Int J Neurosci* 4, 147–166.

Hall, DA, Barrett, DJK. 2006. Response preferences for "what" and "where" in human. *Neuroimage* 32, 968–977.

Hall, JL, Goldstein, MH. 1968. Representation of binaural stimuli by single units in primary auditory cortex of unanesthesized cats. *J Acoust Soc Am* 43, 456–461.

Hall, JW. 2007. *New Handbook For Auditory Evoked Responses.* Boston, MA: Allyn and Bacon.

Harrison, WA, Burns, EM. 1993. Effects of contralateral acoustic stimulation on spontaneous otoacoustic emissions. *J Acoust Soc Am* 94, 2649–2658.

Heffner, HE, Heffner, RS. 1990. Effect of bilateral auditory cortex lesions on sound localization in Japanese macaques. *J Neurophysiol* 64, 915–931.

Heffner, HE, Masterton, RB. 1975. The contributions of auditory cortex to sound localization in the monkey. *J Neurophysiol* 38, 1340–1358.

Helfert, RH, Aschoff, A. 1997. Superior olivary complex and nuclei of the lateral lemniscus. In: G Ehret, R Romand (eds.), *The Central Auditory System.* New York, NY: Oxford University Press, 193–258.

Helfert, RH, Snead, CR, Altschuler, RA. 1991. The ascending auditory pathways. In: RA Altschuler, RP Bobbin, DW Hoffman, BM Clopton (eds.), *Neurobiology of Hearing: The Auditory System.* New York, NY: Raven Press, 1–21.

Herdman, AT, Lins, O, Van Roon, P, Stapells, DR, Scherg, M, Picton, TW. 2002. Intracerebral sources of human auditory steady-state responses. *Brain Topogr* 15, 69–86

Herdman, AT, Stapells, DR. 2001. Thresholds determined using the monotic and dichotic multiple auditory steady-state response technique in normal-hearing subjects. *Scand Audiol* 30, 41–49.

Herdman, AT, Stapells, DR. 2003. Auditory steady-state response thresholds of adults with sensorineural hearing impairment. *Int J Audiol* 42, 237–248.

Hind, JE. 1960. Unit activity in the auditory cortex. In: GL Rasmussen, WE Windle (eds.), *Neural Mechanisms of the Auditory and Vestibular Systems.* Springfield, IL: Charles C. Thomas, 201–210.

Huis in't Veld, F, Osterhammel, P, Terkildsen, K. 1977. Frequency following auditory brain stem responses in man. *Scand Audiol* 6, 27–34.

Imig, TJ, Irons, WA, Samson, FR. 1990. Single-unit selectivity to azimuthal direction and sound pressure level of noise bursts in cat high-frequency primary auditory cortex. *J Neurophysiol* 63, 1448–1466.

Irvine, DRF, Gago, G. 1990. Binaural interaction in high-frequency neurons in inferior colliculus of cat: Effects of variations in sound pressure level on sensitivity to interaural intensity differences. *J Neurophysiol* 63, 570–591.

Irvine, DRF. 1986. The auditory brainstem: A review of structure and function of auditory brainstem processing mechanisms. In: D Ottoson (ed.), *Progress in Sensory Physiology, Vol. 7.* Berlin, Germany: Spriger-Verlag, 1–279.

Irvine, DRF. 1992. Physiology of the auditory brainstem. In: AN Popper, RR Fay (eds.), *The Mammalian Auditory Pathway: Neurophysiology.* New York, NY: Springer-Verlag, 153–231.

Ivarsson, C, DeRibaupierre, Y, DeRibaupierre, E. 1988. Influence of auditory localization cues on neuronal activity in the auditory thalamus of the cat. *J Neurophysiol* 59, 586–606.

Janata, P, Birk, JL, Van Horn, JD, Leman, M, Tillmann, B, Bharucha, JJ. 2002. The cortical topography of tonal structures underlying western music. *Science* 298, 2167–2170.

Jeffress, LA. 1948. A place code theory of sound localization. *J Comp Physiol Psychol* 41, 35–39.

Jerger, J, Chmiel, R, Frost, J, Coker, N. 1986. Effect of sleep on the auditory steady state evoked potential. *Ear Hear* 7, 240–245.

Jerger, J, Weikers, NJ, Sharbrough, F, Jerger, S. 1969. Bilateral lesions of the temporal lobe: A case study. *Acta Otolaryngol Suppl* 258, 1–51.

Jewett, DL. 1970. Volume-conducted potentials in response to auditory stimuli as detected by averaging in the cat. *Electroencephalogr Clin Neurophysiol* 28, 609–618.

Jewett, DL, Romano, MN, Williston, JS. 1970. Human auditory evoked potentials: Possible brainstem components detected on the scalp. *Science* 167, 1517–1518.

Jewett, DL, Williston, JS. 1971. Auditory-evoked far fields averaged from the scalp of humans. *Brain* 94, 681–696.

John, MS, Brown, DK, Muir, PJ, Picton, TW. 2004. Recording auditory steady-state responses in young infants. *Ear Hear* 25, 539–553.

Joris, PX. 1996. Envelope coding in the lateral superior olive. II. Characteristic delays and comparison with responses in the medial superior olive. *J Neurophysiol* 76, 2137–2156.

Joris, PX, Carney, LH, Smith, PH, Yin, TCT. 1994a. Enhancement of neural synchronation in the anteroventral cochlear nucleus. I. Responses to tones at the characteristic frequency. *J Neurophysiol* 71, 1022–1036.

Joris, PX, Smith, PH, Yin, TCT. 1994b. Enhancement of neural synchronation in the anteroventral cochlear nucleus. II. Responses in the tuning curve tail. *J Neurophysiol* 71, 1037–1051.

Joris, PX, Smith, PH, Yin, TCT. 1998. Coincidence detection in the auditory system: 50 years after Jeffress. *Neuron* 21, 1235–1238.

Joris, PX, Yin, TCT. 1995. Envelope coding in the lateral superior olive. I. Sensitivity to interaural time differences. *J Neurophysiol* 73, 1043–1062.

Karaseva, TA. 1972. The role of the temporal lobe in human auditory perception. *Neuropsychology* 10, 227–231.

Katsuki, Y. 1961. Neural mechanisms of auditory sensation in cats. In: WA Rosenblith (ed.), *Sensory Communication.* Cambridge, MA: MIT Press, 561–583.

Katsuki, Y, Suga, N, Kanno, Y. 1962. Neural mechanisms of the peripheral and central auditory systems in monkeys. *J Acoust Soc Am* 32, 1396–1410.

Katsuki, Y, Watanabe, T, Maruyama, N. 1959. Activity of auditory neurons in upper levels of brain of cat. *J Neurophysiol* 22, 343–359.

Kawase, T, Degutte, B, Liberman, MC. 1993. Anti-masking effects of the olivocochlear reflex, II. Enhancement of auditory-nerve response to masked tones. *J Neurophysiol* 70, 2533–2549.

Keithley, EM, Schreiber, RC. 1987. Frequency map of the spiral ganglion in the cat. *J Acoust Soc Am* 81, 1036–1042.

Kelly, JB, Rooney, BJ, Phillips, DP. 1996. Effects of bilateral auditory cortical lesions on gap-detection thresholds in the ferret (*Mustela putorius*). *Behav Neurosci* 110, 542–550.

Kiang, NYS, Morest, DK, Godfrey, DA, Guinan, JJ, Kane, EC. 1973. Stimulus coding at caudal levels of the cat's auditory nervous system: I. Response characteristics of single units. In: AR Møller (ed.), *Basic Mechanisms in Hearing.* New York, NY: Academic Press, 455–478.

Kiang, NYS, Moxon, EC, Levine, RA. 1970. Auditory-nerve activity in cats with normal and abnormal cochleae. In: GEW Wolstenholme, J Knight (eds.), *Sensorineural Hearing Loss, (CIBA Foundation Symposium).* London, UK: Churchill, 241–273.

Kiang, NYS, Pfeiffer, RR, Warr, WB, Backus, AS. 1965. Stimulus coding in the cochlear nucleus. *Ann Otol* 74, 463–485.

Killan, EC, Kapadia, S. 2006. Simultaneous suppression of tone burst-evoked otoacoustic emissions–Effect of level and presentation paradigm. *Hear Res* 212(1–2), 65–73

Kitzes, LM, Wrege, KS, Cassady, M. 1980. Patterns of responses of cortical cells to binaural stimulation. *J Comp Neurol* 192, 455–472.

Knight, PL. 1977. Representation of the cochlea within the anterior field (AAF) of the cat. *Brain Res* 130, 447–467.

Konishi, T, Slepian, JZ. 1971. Effects of electrical stimulation of the crossed olivocochlear bundle on cochlear potentials recorded with intracochlear electrodes in guinea pigs. *J Acoust Soc Am* 49, 1762–1769.

Krishnan, A. 2007. Frequency-following response. In: RF Burkhard, M Don, JJ Eggermont (eds.), *Auditory Evoked Potentials: Basic Principles and Clinical Applications.* Philadelphia, PA: Lippincott Williams & Wilkins, 313–333.

Kryter, KD, Ades, HW. 1943. Studies on the function of the higher acoustic nerve centers. *Am J Psychol* 56, 501–536.

Kuwada, S, Yin, TCT, Wickesberg, RE. 1979. Response of cat inferior colliculus to binaural best frequency: Possible mechanisms for sound localization. *Science* 206, 586–588.

Lee, CC, Imaizumi, K, Schreiner, CE, Winer, JA. 2004. Principles governing auditory cortex connections. *Cereb Cortex* 15, 1804–1814.

Lee, CC, Winer, JA. 2005. Principles governing auditory cortex connections. *Cereb Cortex* 15, 1804–1814.

Levi, E, Folsom, R, Dobie, R. 1993. Amplitude-modulated following response (AMFR): Effects of modulation rate carrier frequency age and state. *Hear Res* 68, 42–52.

Lewy, EH, Kobrak, H. 1936. The neural projection of the cochlear spirals of primary acoustic centers. *Schweiz Arch Neurol Psychiat* 35, 839–852.

Lhermitte F, Chain, F, Escourolle, R, Ducarne, B, Pillon, B, Chendru, F. 1971. Etude de troubles perceptifs auditifs dans les lesions temporales bilaterales. *Rev Neurol* 124, 329–351.

Liang, L, Lu, T, Wang, X. 2002. Neural representations of sinusoidal amplitude and frequency modulations in the primary auditory cortex of awake primates. *J Neurophysiol* 87, 2237–2261.

Liberman, MC. 1982. The cochlear frequency map for the cat: Labeling auditory nerve fibers of known characteristic frequency. *J Acoust Soc Am* 72, 1441–1449.

Lins, OG, Picton, TW, Boucher, BL, Durieux-Smith, A, Champagne, SC, Moran, LM, Perez-Abalo, MC, Martin, V, Savio, G. 1996. Frequency-specific audiometry using steady-state responses. *Ear Hear* 17, 81–96.

Loeffler, JD. 1958. *An investigation of auditory responses in insular cortex of cat and dog.* Unpublished Thesis. Madison, WI: University of Wisconsin.

Lomber, SG, Malhotra, S. 2008. Double dissociation of "what" and "where" processing in auditory cortex. *Nat Neurosci* 11(5), 609–616.

Martin, BA, Tremblay, KL, Korezak, P. 2008. Speech evoked potentials: From the laboratory to the clinic. *Ear Hear* 29, 285–313

Martin, BA, Tremblay, KL, Stapells, DR. 2007. Principles and applications of cortical auditory evoked potentials. In: RF Burkhard, M Don, JJ Eggermont (eds.), *Auditory Evoked Potentials: Basic Principles and Clinical Applications.* Philadelphia, PA: Lippincott Williams & Wilkins, 482–507.

Masterton, RB, Diamond, IT. 1964. Effects of auditory cortex ablation on discrimination of small binaural time differences. *J Neurophysiol* 27, 15–36.

McCandless, G, Best, L. 1964. Evoked response to auditory stimulation in man using a summating computer. *J Speech Hear Res* 7, 193–202.

McCandless, G, Best, L. 1966. Summed evoked responses using pure tone stimuli. *J Speech Hear Res* 9, 266–272.

Mendelson, JR, Cynader, MS. 1985. Sensitivity of cat primary auditory cortex (AI) neurons to direction and rate of frequency modulation. *Brain Res* 327, 331–335.

Mendelson, JR, Grasse, KL. 2000. Auditory cortical responses to the interactive effects of interaural intensity disparities and frequency. *Cerebral Cortex* 10, 32–39.

Merchán, MA, Berbel, P. 1996. Anatomy of the ventral nucleus of the lateral lemniscus in rats: A nucleus with a concentric laminar organization. *J Comp Neurol* 372, 245–263.

Merzenich, MM, Brugge, JE. 1973. Representation of the cochlear partition on the superior temporal plane of the macaque monkey. *Brain Res* 50, 275–296.

Meyer, DR, Woolsey, CN. 1952. Effects of localized cortical destruction on auditory discriminative conditioning in cat. *J Neurophysiol* 15, 149–162.

Møller, AR. 2000. *Hearing: Its Physiology and Pathophysiology.* San Diego, CA: Academic Press.

Møller, AR. 2007. Neural generators for auditory brainstem evoked potentials. In: RF Burkhard, M Don, JJ Eggermont (eds.), *Auditory Evoked Potentials: Basic Principles and Clinical Applications.* Philadelphia, PA: Lippincott Williams & Wilkins, 336–354.

Møller, AR, Jannetta, PJ. 1985. Neural generators of the auditory brainstem response. In: JT Jacobson (ed.), *The Auditory Brainstem Response.* San Diego, CA: College Hill, 13–31.

Moore, JK. 1987. The human auditory brainstem as a generator of auditory evoked potentials. *Hear Res* 29, 33–43.

Moore, JK. 2000. Organization of the human superior olivary complex. *Microsc Res Tech* 51, 403–412.

Mott, JT, Norton, SJ, Neely, ST, Warr, WB. 1983. Changes in spontaneous otoacoustic emissions produced by acoustic stimulation of the contralateral ear. *Hear Res* 38, 229–242.

Moulin, A, Collet, L, Duclaux, R. 1993. Contralateral auditory stimulation alters distortion products in humans. *Hear Res* 65, 193–210.

Mountain, DC. 1980. Changes in endolymphatic potential and crossed olivocochlear bundle stimulation alter cochlear mechanics. *Science* 210, 71–72.

Mountain, DC, Geisler, CD, Hubbard, AE. 1980. Stimulation of efferents alters the cochlear microphonic and the sound induced resistance changes measured in scala media of the guinea pig. *Hear Res* 3, 231–240.

Moushegian, G, Rupert, AL, Stillman, RD. 1973. Scalp-recorded early responses in man to frequencies in the speech range. *Electroencephalogr Clin Neurophysiol* 35, 665–667.

Moushegian, G, Rupert, AL. 1970. Response diversity of neurons in ventral cochlear nucleus of kangaroo rat to low-frequency tones. *Electroencephalogr Clin Neurophysiol* 33, 351–364.

Musiek, FE, Baran, JA. 2007. *The Auditory System: Anatomy, Physiology, and Clinical Correlates.* Boston, MA: Allyn & Bacon.

Näätänen, R (ed.). 1995. Special issue: Mismatch negativity as an index of central auditory function. *Ear Hear* 16, 1–146.

Neff, WD. 1960. Role of the auditory cortex in sound discrimination. In: GL Rasmussen, WE Windle (eds.), *Neural Mechanisms of the Auditory and Vestibular Systems.* Springfield, IL: Charles C. Thomas, 221–216.

Neff, WD. 1967. Auditory discriminations affected by cortical ablation. In: AB Graham (ed.), *Sensorineural Hearing Processes and Disorders.* Boston, MA: Little, Brown, 201–210.

Neff, WD. 1977. The brain and hearing: Auditory discriminations affected by brain lesions. *Ann Otol* 86, 500–506.

Neff, WD, Casseday, JH. 1977. Effects of unilateral ablation of auditory cortex on monaural cat's ability to localize sounds. *J Neurophysiol* 40, 44–52.

Neff, WD, Diamond, IT, Casseday, JH. 1975. Behavioral studies of auditory discrimination: Central nervous system. In: WD Keiday, WD Neff (eds.), *Handbook of Sensory Physiology. Vol. 5: Auditory System.* New York, NY: Springer-Verlag, 307–400.

Neff, WD, Fisher, JF, Diamond, IT, Yela, M. 1956. Role of auditory cortex in discrimination requiring localization of sound in space. *J Neurophysiol* 19, 500–512.

Nieder, P, Nieder, I. 1970a. Antimasking effect of crossed olivocochlear bundle stimulation with loud clicks in guinea pig. *Exp Neurol* 28, 179–188.

Nieder, P, Nieder, I. 1970b. Stimulation of efferent olivocochlear bundle causes release from low level masking. *Nature* 227, 184–185.

Palmer, A, Shamma, S. 2004. Physiological representations of speech. In: S Greenberg, WA Ainsworth, AN Popper, RR Fay (eds.), *Speech Processing in the Auditory System*. New York, NY: Springer, 163–230.

Pandya, DN, Hallett, M, Mukherjee, SK. 1969. Intra- and inter-hemispheric connections of the neocortical auditory system in the rhesus monkey. *Brain Res* 14, 49–65.

Park, TJ. 1998. IID sensitivity differs between two principal centers in the interaural intensity difference pathway: the LSO and the IC. *J Neurophysiol* 79, 2416–2431.

Penfield, W, Evans, J. 1934. Functional deficits produced by cerebral lobectomies. *A Res Nerv Ment Dis Proc* 13, 352–377.

Penfield, W, Jasper, H. 1954. *Epilepsy and the Functional Anatomy of the Human Brain*. Boston, MA: Little, Brown.

Penfield, W, Rasmussen, T. 1950. *The Cerebral Cortex: A Clinical Study of Localization of Function*. New York, NY: MacMillan.

Phillips, DP, Hall, SE. 1987. Responses of single neurons in cat auditory cortex to time-varying stimuli: Linear amplitude modulations. *Exp Brain Res* 67, 479–492.

Phillips, DP, Irvine, DRF. 1981. Responses of single neurons in physiologically defined area AI of cat cerebral cortex: Sensitivity to interaural intensity differences. *Hear Res* 4, 299–307.

Picton, TW. 2007. Audiometry using auditory steady-state responses. In: RF Burkhard, M Don, JJ Eggermont (eds.), *Auditory Evoked Potentials: Basic Principles and Clinical Applications*. Philadelphia, PA: Lippincott Williams & Wilkins, 441–462.

Picton, TW, Dimitrijevic, A, Perez-Abalo, MC, Van Roon, P. 2005. Estimating audiometric thresholds using auditory steady-state responses. *J Am Acad Audiol* 16, 140–156.

Picton, TW, John, MS, Purcell, DW, Plourde, G. 2003. Human auditory steady-state responses: The effects of recording technique and state of arousal. *Anesth Analg* 97, 1396–1402.

Popper, N, Fay, RR (eds.). 1992. *The Mammalian Auditory Pathway: Neurophysiology*. New York, NY: Springer-Verlag.

Popper, N, Fay, RR (eds.). 1995. *Hearing by Bats*. New York, NY: Springer-Verlag.

Pratt, H. 2007. Middle-latency responses. In: RF Burkhard, M Don, JJ Eggermont (eds.), *Auditory Evoked Potentials: Basic Principles and Clinical Applications*. Philadelphia, PA: Lippincott Williams & Wilkins, 463–481.

Preuss, AP, Müller-Preuss, P. 1990. Processing of amplitude modulated sounds in the medial geniculate body of squirrel monkeys. *Exp Brain Res* 79, 207–211.

Raab, DH, Ades, HW. 1946. Cortical and midbrain mediation of a conditioned discrimination of acoustic intensities. *Am J Psychol* 59, 59–83.

Rajan, R, Aitkin, LM, Irvine, DRF, McKay, J. 1990. Azimuthal sensitivity of neurons in primary auditory cortex of cats. I. Types of sensitivity and the effects of variations in stimulus parameters. *J Neurophysiol* 64, 872–887.

Rance, G, Rickards, F, Cohen, L, DeVidi S, Clark G. 1995. The automated prediction of hearing thresholds in sleeping subjects using auditory steady state evoked potentials. *Ear Hear* 16, 499–507.

Rance, G, Tomlin, D. 2004. Maturation of auditory steady-state responses in normal babies. *Ear Hear* 27, 20–29.

Rance, G, Tomlin, D, Rickards, FW. 2006. Comparison of auditory steady-state responses and tone-burst auditory brainstem responses in normal babies. *Ear Hear* 27, 751–762.

Reale, RA, Brugge, JF. 1990. Auditory cortical neurons are sensitive to static and continuously changing interaural phase cues. *J Neurophysiol* 64, 1247–1260.

Reale, RA, Imig, TJ. 1980. Tonotopic organization in cortex of the cat. *J Comp Neurol* 192, 265–291.

Reale, RA, Kettner, RE. 1986. Topograpy of binaural organization in primary auditory cortex of the cat: Effects of changing interaural intensity. *J Neurophysiol* 56, 663–682.

Rhode, WS. 1985. The use of intracellular techniques in the study of the cochlear nucleus. *J Acoust Soc Am* 78, 320–327.

Rhode, WS, Greenberg, S. 1992. Physiology of the cochlear nuclei. In: AN Popper, RR Fay (eds.), *The Mammalian Auditory Pathway: Neurophysiology*. New York, NY: Springer-Verlag, 94–152.

Rhode, WS, Greenberg, S. 1994. Encoding of amplitude modulation in the cochlear nucleus of the cat. *J Neurophysiol* 71, 1797–1825.

Rhode, WS, Smith, RH, Oertel, D. 1983a. Physiological response properties of cells labeled intracellularly with horseradish peroxidase in cat dorsal cochlear nucleus. *J Comp Neurol* 213, 426–447.

Rhode, WS, Smith, RH, Oertel, D. 1983b. Physiological response properties of cells labeled intracellularly with horseradish peroxidase in cat ventral cochlear nucleus. *J Comp Neurol* 213, 448–463.

Romand, R, Avan, P. 1997. Anatomical and functional aspects of the cochlear nucleus. In: G Ehret, R Romand (eds.), *The Central Auditory System*. New York, NY: Oxford University Press, 97–192.

Rose, JE. 1960. Organization of frequency sensitive neurons in the cochlear nuclear complex of the cat. In: GL Rasmussen, WE Windle (eds.), *Neural Mechanisms of the Auditory and Vestibular Systems*. Springfield, IL: Charles C. Thomas, 116–136.

Rose, JE, Galambos, R, Hughes, JR. 1959. Microelectrode studies of the cochlear nuclei of the cat. *Bull Johns Hopkins Hosp* 104, 211–251.

Rose, JE, Greenwood, DD, Goldberg, JM, Hind. JE. 1963. Some discharge characteristics of single neurons in the inferior colliculus of the cat. I. Tonotopical organization, relation of spike-counts to tone intensity, and firing patterns of single elements. *J Neurophysiol* 26, 294–320.

Rose, JE, Gross, NB, Geisler, CD, Hind, JE. 1966. Some neural mechanisms in the inferior colliculus of the cat which may be relevant to localization of a sound source. *J Neurophysiol* 29, 288–314.

Rosenzweig, MR. 1946. Discrimination of auditory intensities in the cat. *Am J Psychol* 59, 127–136.

Roth, GL, Aitkin, LM, Andersen, RA, Merzenich, MM. 1978. Some features of the spatial organization of the central nucleus of the inferior colliculus of the cat. *J Comp Neurol* 182, 661–680.

Rouiller, E, de Ribaupierre, F. 1982. Neurons sensitive to narrow ranges of repetitive acoustic transients in the medial geniculate body of the cat. *Exp Brain Res* 48, 323–326.

Rouiller, E, de Ribaupierre, Y, Toros-Morel, A, de Ribaupierre, F. 1981. Neural coding of repetitive clicks in the medial geniculate body of cat. *Hear Res* 5, 81–100.

Rouiller, EM. 1997. Functional organization of the auditory pathways. In: G Ehret, R Romand (eds.), *The Central Auditory System*. New York, NY: Oxford University Press, 3–65.

Rudell, AP. 1987. A fiber tract model of auditory brainstem responses. *Electroencephalogr Clin Neurophysiol* 62, 53–62.

Ruhm, H, Walker, E, Flanigin, H. 1967. Acoustically evoked potentials in man: Mediation of early components. *Laryngoscope* 77, 806–822.

Rupert, AL, Moushegian, GM, Whitcomb, MA. 1966. Superior olivary complex response patterns to monaural and binaural clicks. *J Acoust Soc Am* 39, 1069–1076.

Russell, IJ, Murugasu, E. 1997. Medial efferent inhibition suppresses basilar membrane responses to near characteristic frequency tones of moderate to high intensities. *J Acoust Soc Am* 102, 1734–1738.

Ryan, S, Kemp, DT, Hinchcliffe, R. 1991. The influence of contralateral acoustic stimulation on click-evoked otoacoustic emissions in humans. *Br J Audiol* 25, 391–397.

Samson, FK, Barone, P, Irons, WA, Clarey, JC, Poirier, P, Imig, TJ. 2000. Directionality derived from differential sensitivity to monaural and binaural cues in the cat's medial geniculate body. *J Neurophysiol* 84, 1330–1345.

Sando, I. 1965. The anatomical interrelationships of the cochlear nerve fibers. *Acta Otolaryngol* 59, 417–436.

Savio, G, Cárdenas, J, Pérez Abalo, M, González, A, Valdés, J. 2001. The low and high frequency auditory steady state responses mature at different rates. *Audiol Neurootol* 6, 279–287.

Scharlock, DP, Neff, WD, Strominger, NL. 1965. Discrimination of tonal duration after ablation of cortical auditory areas. *J Neurophysiol* 28, 673–681.

Scherg, M, vonCramon, D. 1985. A new interpretation of generators of BAEP waves I–V: Results of a spatio-temporal dipole model. *Electroencephalogr Clin Neurophysiol* 62, 290–299.

Schreiner, CE, Cynader, MS. 1984. Basic functional organization of second auditory cortical field (AII) of the cat. *J Neurophysiol* 51, 1284–1305.

Schreiner, CE, Urbas, JV. 1986. Representation of amplitude modulation in the auditory cortex of the cat: I. The anterior auditory field (AAF). *Hear Res* 21, 227–341.

Semple, MN, Aitkin, LM. 1979. Representation of sound frequency and laterality by units in central nucleus of cat inferior colliculus. *J Neurophysiol* 42, 1626–1639.

Semple, MN, Kitzes, LM. 1987. Binaural processing of sound pressure level in the inferior colliculus. *J Neurophysiol* 57, 1130–1147.

Siegel, JH, Kim, DO. 1982. Efferent neural control of cochlear mechanics? Olivocochlear bundle stimulation affects cochlear biomechanical nonlinearity. *Hear Res* 6, 171–182.

Smith, PH, Joris, PX, Yin, TCT. 1993. Projections of physiologically characterized spherical bushy cell axons from the cochlear nucleus of the cat: Evidence for delay lines to the medial superior olive. *J Comp Neurol* 331, 245–260.

Smith, PH, Joris, PX, Yin, TCT. 1998. Anatomy and physiology of principal cells of the medial nucleus of the trapezoid body (MNTB) of the cat. *J Neurophysiol* 79, 3127–3142.

Sohmer, H, Feinmesser, M. 1967. Cochlear action potentials recorded from the external ear in man. *Ann Otol Rhinol Laryngol* 76, 427–435.

Sohmer, H, Pratt, H. 1977. Identification and separation of the frequency following responses (FFR) in man. *Electroencephalogr Clin Neurophysiol* 42, 493–500.

Sovijarvi, ARA, Hyvarinen, J. 1974. Auditory cortical neurons in the cat sensitive to the direction of sound source movement. *Brain Res* 73, 455–471.

Spitzer, MW, Semple, MN. 1993. Responses of inferior colliculus neurons to time-varying interaural phase disparity: Effects of shifting the locus of virtual motion. *J Neurophysiol* 69, 1245–1263.

Squires, KC, Hecox, KE. 1983. Electrophysiological evaluation of higher level auditory processing. *Sem Hear* 4, 415–433.

Stanford, TR, Kuwada, S, Batra, R. 1992. A comparison of the interaural time sensitivity of neurons in the inferior colliculus and thalamus of the unanesthetized rabbit. *J Neurosci* 12, 3200–3216.

Starr, A, Golob, EJ. 2007. Cognitive factors modulating auditory cortical potentials. In: RF Burkhard, M Don, JJ Eggermont (eds.), *Auditory Evoked Potentials: Basic Principles and Clinical Applications*. Philadelphia, PA: Lippincott Williams & Wilkins, 508–524.

Stern, RM, Trahiotis, C. 1997. Models of binaural perception. In: R Gilkey, T Anderson (eds.), *Binaural and Spatial Hearing in Real and Virtual Environments*. Hillsdale, NJ: Erlbaum, 499–531.

Stillman, RD, Crow, G, Moushegian, G. 1978. Components of the frequency-following potential in man. *Electroencephalogr Clin Neurophysiol* 44, 438–446.

Suga, N. 1990. Bisonar and neural computation in bats. *Sci Am* 262, 60–68.

Sutton, S, Barren, M, Zubin, J, John, JE. 1965. Evoked-potential correlates of stimulus uncertainty. *Science* 150, 1187–1188.

Syka, J, Rybalko, N, Mazelová, J, Druga, R. 2002. Gap detection threshold in the rat before and after auditory cortex ablation. *Hear Res* 172, 151–159.

Szalda, K, Burkard, R. 2005. The effects of nembutal anesthesia on the auditory steady-state response (ASSR) from the inferior colliculus and auditory cortex of the chinchilla. *Hear Res* 203, 32–44.

Talavage, TM, Sereno, MI, Melcher, JR, Ledden, PJ, Rosen, BR, Dale, AM. 2004. Tonotopic organization in human auditory cortex revealed by progressions of frequency sensitivity. *J Neurophysiol* 91, 1282–1996.

Teas, DC, Konishi, T, Neilsen, DW. 1972. Electrophysiological studies on the special distribution of the crossed olivocochlear bundle along the guinea pig cochlea. *J Acoust Soc Am* 51, 1256–1264.

Thomas, M, Talavage, TM, Ledden, PJ, Benson, RR, Rosen, BR, Melcher, JR. 2000. Frequency-dependent responses exhibited by multiple regions in human auditory cortex. *Hear Res* 150, 225–244.

Tsuchitani, C. 1988a. The inhibition of cat lateral superior olive unit excitatory responses to binaural tone-bursts. I. The transient chopper response. *J Neurophysiol* 59, 164–183.

Tsuchitani, C. 1988b. The inhibition of cat lateral superior olive unit excitatory responses to binaural tone-bursts. II. The sustained discharges. *J Neurophysiol* 59, 184–211.

Tsuchitani, C, Boudreau, JC. 1966. Single unit analysis of stimulus frequency and intgensity by cat superior olive S-segment cell discharge. *J Neurophysiol* 42, 794–805.

Tunturi, AR. 1944. Audio frequency localization in the acoustic cortex of the dog. *Am J Physiol* 141, 397–403.

Van Der Werff, KR, Brown, CF. 2005. Effect of audiometric configuration on threshold and suprathreshold auditory steady-state responses. *Ear Hear* 26, 310–326.

Wagner, W, Heppelmann, G, Müller, J, Janssen, T, Zenner, H-P. 2007. Olivocochlear reflex effect on human distortion product otoacoustic emissions is largest at frequencies with distinct fine structure dips. *Hear Res* 223, 83–92.

Wang, XQ, Sachs, MB. 1994. Neural encoding of single-formant stimuli in the cat: II. Responses of anteroventral cochlear nucleus units. *J Neurophysiol* 71, 59–78.

Warr, WB. 1966. Fiber degeneration following lesions in the anteroventral cochlear nucleus of the cat. *Exp Neurol* 14, 453–474.

Warren, ML, Liberman, MC. 1989. Effects of contralateral sound on auditory-nerve response: I. Contributions of cochlear efferents. *Hear Res* 37, 89–104.

Webster, DB, Popper, N, Fay, RR, (eds.). 1992. *The Mammalian Auditory Pathway: Neuroanatomy*. New York, NY: Springer-Verlag.

Whitfield, IC. 1967. *The Auditory Pathway*. London, UK: Arnold.

Whitfield, IC, Cranford, J, Ravizza, R, Diamond, IT. 1972. Effects of unilateral ablation of auditory cortex in cat on complex sound localization. *J Neurophysiol* 35, 718–731.

Whitfield, IC, Evans, EE. 1965. Responses of auditory cortical neurons to stimuli of changing frequency. *J Neurophysiol* 28, 655–672.

Wiederhold, ML. 1970. Variations in the effects of electrical stimulation of the crossed olivo-cochlear bundle on cat single auditory nerve fiber responses to tone bursts. *J Acoust Soc Am* 48, 966–977.

Wiederhold, ML, Kiang, NYS. 1970. Effects of electrical stimulation of the crossed olivo-cochlear bundle on single auditory nerve fibers in the cat. *J Acoust Soc Am* 48, 950–965.

Wiederhold, ML, Peake, WT. 1966. Efferent inhibition of auditory nerve responses: Dependence on acoustic stimulus parameters. *J Acoust Soc Am* 40, 1427–1430.

Winslow, RL, Sachs, MB. 1987. Effect of electrical stimulation of the crossed olivocochlear bundle on auditory nerve responses to tones in noise. *J Neurophysiol* 57, 1002–1021.

Woolsey, CN. 1960. Organization of cortical auditory system: A review and a synthesis. In: GL Rasmussen, WF Windle (eds.), *Neural Mechanisms of the Auditory and Vestibular Systems*. Springfield, IL: Charles C. Thomas, 165–180.

Woolsey, CN, Walzl, EM. 1942. Topical projection of nerve fibers from local regions of the cochlea to the cerebral cortex of the cat. *Bull Johns Hopkins Hosp* 71, 315–344.

Yin, TCT, Chan, JCK. 1988. Neural mechanisms underlying interaural time sensitivity to tones and noise. In: GM Edelman, WE Gall, WM Cowan (eds.), *Auditory Function*. New York: Wiley, 385–430.

Yin, TCT, Chan, JC. 1990. Interaural time sensitivity in medial superior olive of cat. *J Neurophysiol* 64, 465–488.

Psychophysics is concerned with how we perceive the physical stimuli impinging upon our senses. The branch of psychophysics that deals with the perception of sound is **psychoacoustics**. In defining this term we make a sharp distinction between the physical **stimulus** and the psychological **response** to it. We may think of the sound presented to our ears as the stimulus and of what we hear as the response. For example, what we hear as *loudness* is the perceptual correlate of *intensity*: Other things being equal, a rise in intensity is perceived as an increase in loudness. Similarly, *pitch* is the *perception* related to sound *frequency*: Other things being equal, pitch gets higher as frequency increases.

If there were a simple one-to-one correspondence between the physical parameters of sound and how they are perceived, then we could quantify what we hear directly in terms of the attributes of the sound. That would mean that all physically existing sounds could be heard, that all changes in them would be discriminable, and that any change in stimulus magnitude would result in a perceptual change of the same magnitude. This is not the case. It is thus necessary to describe the manner in which sound is perceived, and to attempt to explain the underlying mechanisms of the auditory system. This is the province of psychoacoustics.

SCALES OF MEASUREMENT

The study of auditory perception almost always involves measurements, the assignment of numbers that reflect the phenomena being investigated. Our ability to properly analyze what we find and to arrive at valid interpretations depends on knowing the properties of the measurements made and the qualities of the resulting data. Stevens' (1951, 1958, 1961, 1975) four scales of measurement provide us with this foundation.

Nominal scales are the least restrictive, in the sense that the observations are simply assigned to groups. This is the lowest order of scaling because the nominal label does not tell us anything about the relationship among the groups other than that they are different with respect to some parameter. For example, the nominal scale "gender" enables us to separate people into two categories, "male" and "female." All we know is that the two categories are differentiable, and that we can count how many cases fall into each one. The same would apply to the number of subcompact cars made by different manufacturers. We know that there are so many Fords, Toyotas, etc., but we have no idea of their relative attributes. A nominal scale, then, makes no assumptions about the order among the classes; thus, it is the least restrictive and least informative of the levels of scaling.

Ordinal scales imply that the observations have values, which can be rank-ordered so that one class is greater or lesser than another with respect to the parameter of interest. However, an ordinal scale does not tell us how far apart they are. Consider the relative quality of artistic reproductions. Painter A may produce a better reproduction of the Mona Lisa than painter B, who in turn makes a better copy than painter C, and so on. However, there may be one magnitude of distance between A and B, a second distance between B and C, and still a third distance between C and D. An ordinal scale thus gives the rank order of the categories ($A > B > C...$), but does not specify the distances between them. Whereas the nominal scale allows us to express the **mode** of the data (which category contains more cases than any other), ordinal scales permit the use of the **median** (the value with the same number of observations above and below it). However, the lack of equal distances between values precludes the use of most mathematical operations. Sometimes the nature of the categories enables some of them to be rank-ordered, but not others. This constitutes a *partially ordered scale* (Coomb, 1953), which lies between the nominal and ordinal scales.

An **interval scale** specifies both the order among categories and the fixed distances among them. In other words, the distance between any two successive categories is equal to the distance between any other successive pair. Interval scales, however, do not imply a true zero reference point. Examples are temperature (in degrees Celsius or Fahrenheit) and the dates on a calendar. In contrast to nominal and ordinal data, equal distances between category values make it possible to use most mathematical operations with interval data. For example, the central tendency of interval data may be expressed as a *mean* (average). However, interval data cannot be expressed as proportions (ratios) of one another, because a true zero point is not assumed. It is also possible to rank the categories in such a way that there is an ordering of the distances between them. For example, the distances between successive categories may become progressively longer, as follows:

$$A - B - - C - - - D - - - - E - - - - - F - - - - - - G ...$$

This is an *ordered metric scale* (Coomb, 1953). An ordered metric scale actually falls between the definitions of ordinal and interval scales, but may be treated as an interval scale (Abelson and Tukey, 1959).

Ratio scales include all the properties of interval scales as well as an inherent zero point. The existence of a *true zero* point permits values to be expressed as ratios or in decibels, and the use of all mathematical operations. As the most restrictive level, ratio scales give the most information about the data and their interrelationships. Examples are length, time intervals, and temperature (in kelvins), as well as loudness (sone) and pitch (mel) scales.

MEASUREMENT METHODS

Establishing relationships between the sound presented and how the subject perceives it is a primary goal. To accomplish this goal, the investigator contrives a special situation designed to home in on the relation of interest. An experimental situation is used to avoid the ambiguities of presenting a stimulus and, in effect, asking the open-ended question "What did you hear?" Instead, the stimulus and response are clearly specified, and then some aspect of the stimulus (intensity, frequency, etc.) is manipulated. The subject's task is to respond in a predetermined manner so that the investigator can get an unambiguous idea of what was heard. For example, one may vary the intensity of a tone and ask the subject whether it was heard during each presentation. The lowest level at which the sound is heard (the transition between audibility and inaudibility) might be considered an estimate of **absolute sensitivity**. Alternatively, two tones might be presented, one of which is varied in frequency. The subject is asked whether the varied tone is higher (or lower) in pitch, and the smallest perceivable frequency difference—the just noticeable difference (jnd)—might be considered an estimate of **differential sensitivity**.

We must also distinguish between what the subject actually hears and the manner in which he responds. The former is **sensory capability** or **sensitivity**, and the latter is **response proclivity**. For the most part, we are interested in sensory capability. Response proclivity reflects not only the subject's sensitivity, but also the biases and criteria that affect how he responds. We therefore try to select measurement methods and techniques that minimize the effects of response bias. An excellent discussion of the many details to be considered in psychoacoustic experiments is given in Robinson and Watson (1973). In

this chapter, we shall be concerned with classical psychophysical methods, adaptive techniques, and some aspects of scaling. Chapter 8 covers the theory of signal detection.

CLASSICAL METHODS OF MEASUREMENT

There are three classical psychophysical methods: limits, adjustment, and constant stimuli.

Method of Limits

In the **method of limits**, the stimulus is under the investigator's control and the subject simply responds after each presentation. Suppose we are interested in the **absolute sensitivity** or **threshold** for a particular sound. The sound is presented at a level expected to be well above threshold. Since it is clearly audible, the subject responds by saying that he heard the sound (+ in Fig. 7.1). The level of the sound is then decreased by a discrete amount (2 dB in Fig. 7.1) and presented again. This process is repeated until the subject no longer perceives the sound (−), at which point the series (or run) is terminated. This example involves a descending run. In an ascending series, the sound is first presented at a level known to be below the threshold and is increased in magnitude until a positive (+) response is obtained. The odd-numbered runs in Fig. 7.1 are descending series and the even-numbered runs are ascending. Since the crossover between "hearing" and "not hearing" lies somewhere

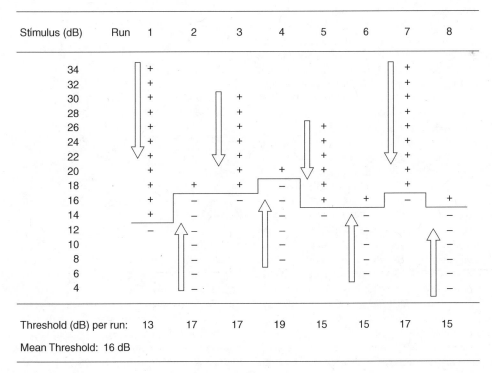

Figure 7.1 An example of the method of limits in hypothetical threshold experiments.

between the lowest audible level and the highest inaudible one, the "threshold" for each series may be taken as the halfway point between them. The subject's threshold is obtained by averaging the threshold levels across runs. This average is 16 dB for the data in Fig. 7.1.

Several forms of **response bias** are associated with the method of limits. Since a series either ascends or descends, and is terminated by a change in response, the subject may anticipate the level at which his response should change from "no" to "yes" in an ascending run and from "yes" to "no" in a descending series. **Anticipation** thus results in a lower (better) ascending threshold because the subject anticipates hearing the stimulus, and a higher (poorer) descending threshold since he anticipates not hearing it. An opposite affect is caused by **habituation**. Here, the subject does not change his response from "no" to "yes" during an ascending run until the actual threshold is exceeded by a few trials (raising the measured threshold level), and he continues to respond "yes" for one or more descending trials after the sound has actually become inaudible (lowering the measured threshold level). These biases may be minimized by using an equal number of ascending and descending test runs in each threshold determination. These runs may be presented alternatively (as in the figure) or randomly. A second way to minimize these biases is to vary the starting levels for the runs. Both tactics are illustrated in Fig. 7.1.

The method of limits is also limited in terms of step size and inefficiently placed trials. Too large a step size reduces accuracy because the actual threshold may lie anywhere between two discrete stimulus levels. For example, a 10-dB step is far less precise than a 2-dB increment; and the larger the increment between the steps, the more approximate the result. Too large a step size may place the highest inaudible presentation at a level with a 0% probability of response, and the lowest audible presentation at a level with a 100% probability of response. The 50% point (threshold) may be anywhere between them! To make this point clear, consider the psychometric functions in Fig. 7.2. A **psychometric function** shows the probability (percentage) of responses for different stimulus levels. Figure 7.2a shows the psychometric function for a particular sound. It is inaudible (0% responses) at 13 dB and is always heard (100% responses) at 21 dB. It is customary to define the **threshold** as the level at which the sound is heard 50% of the time (0.5 probability). The threshold in Fig. 7.2a is thus 17 dB. Suppose we try to find this threshold by using a 10-dB step size, with increments corresponding to 14 dB, 24 dB, etc. Notice that this step size essentially includes the whole psychometric function, so that we do not know where the responses change from 0% to 100%, nor do we know whether they do so in a rapid jump (a step function) or along a function where gradual changes in the proportion of "yes" responses correspond to gradual changes in stimulus level. The result is low precision in estimating the location of the 50% point. However, a large step size is convenient in that it involves fewer presentations (and thus shorter test time), since responses go from "yes" to "no" in

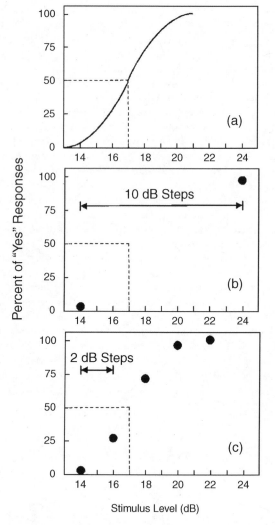

Figure 7.2 (a) Psychometric function showing the 50% threshold at 17 dB. (b) Responses obtained at near 0% at 14 dB and 100% at 24 dB with a 10-dB step size. (c) Percent responses at various levels with a 2-dB step size. The 50% threshold is shown on each graph. The 2-dB and 10-dB step sizes are illustrated in frames (b) and (c).

very few trials, each of which is either well above or well below threshold.

A smaller step size permits a more precise estimate of threshold because the reversals from "yes" to "no" (and vice versa) are better placed (closer) in relation to the 50% point. The relationship of a 2-dB step to the psychometric function is shown in Fig. 7.2c, which gives the probability of a response in 2-dB intervals. Notice that these points are better placed than those for the 10 dB step size in Fig. 7.2b. For this reason, even though there may be "wasted" presentations due to test levels well above or below the threshold, the method of limits with an appropriate step size is still popular. This is particularly true in pilot experiments and in clinical evaluations, both of which take advantage

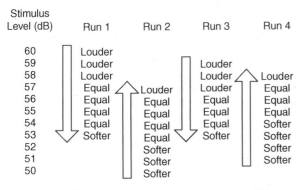

Stimulus Level (dB)	Run 1	Run 2	Run 3	Run 4

Figure 7.3 An example of the method of limits in a hypothetical discrimination experiment.

of the speed with which thresholds are estimated by the method of limits. The clinical method of limits (e.g., ASHA, 2005), however, is actually a hybrid technique with characteristics of the staircase method, discussed below.

The method of limits may also be used to determine **differential thresholds**. In this case, two stimuli are presented in each trial, and the subject is asked whether the second is greater than, less than, or equal to the first with respect to some parameter. The first stimulus is held constant, and the second is varied by the investigator in discrete steps. The procedure is otherwise the same as for determining thresholds, although the findings are different. Suppose the subject is to make an equal loudness judgment. The method of limits would result in a range of intensities in which the second stimulus is louder than the first, a range in which the second is softer, and a range in which the two sounds appear equal. In Fig. 7.3, the average **upper limen** (halfway between "higher" and "equal") is 57 dB, and the average **lower limen** (halfway between "equal" and "lower") is 53.5 dB. The range between these values is the **interval of uncertainty**, which is 57 − 53.5 = 3.5 dB wide in this example. Although there is a range of "equal" judgments, we may estimate the "equal level" to lie halfway between the upper and lower limens, at 55.25 dB in this example. This point is commonly referred to as the **point of subjective equality (PSE)**. The **just noticeable difference (jnd)** or **difference limen (DL)** is generally estimated as one-half of the uncertainty interval, or 1.75 dB for the data in Fig. 7.3.

Method of Adjustment

The **method of adjustment** differs from the method of limits in two ways. First, the stimulus is controlled by the subject instead of by the investigator. In addition, the level of the stimulus is varied continuously rather than in discrete steps. As in the method of limits, the level is adjusted downward from above threshold until it is just inaudible, or increased from below threshold until it is just audible. Threshold is taken as the average of the just audible and just inaudible levels. To obtain an estimate of differential sensitivity, the subject adjusts the level of one sound until it is as loud as a standard sound, or

adjusts the frequency of one sound until it has the same pitch as the other.

The stimulus control (generally a continuous dial) must be unlabeled and should have no detents that might provide tactile cues that could bias the results. Furthermore, a second control is sometimes inserted between the subject's dial and the instrumentation, allowing the investigator to vary the starting point of a test series by an amount unknown to the subject. This strategy avoids biases based on the positioning of the response dial and the use of dial settings as "anchors" from one series to the next. Even with these precautions, however, it is difficult for the investigator to exercise the same degree of control over the procedure as in the method of limits. Furthermore, the subject may change his criterion of audibility during test runs, introducing another hard-to-control bias into the method of adjustment.

Just as anticipation and habituation affect the results obtained with the method of limits, stimulus persistence (perseveration) biases the results from the method of adjustment. Persistence of the stimulus means that a lower threshold is obtained on a descending run because the subject continues to turn the level down below threshold as though the sound were still audible. Thus, we may think of this phenomenon as **persistence of the stimulus**, or as **perseveration of the response**. In an ascending trial, the absence of audibility persists so that the subject keeps turning the level up until the true threshold is passed by some amount, which has the opposite effect of raising the measured threshold level. These biases may be minimized by using both ascending and descending series in each measurement. Another variation is to have the subject **bracket** his threshold by varying the level up and down until a just audible sound is perceived. After the ending point is recorded, the investigator may use the second stimulus control discussed above to change the starting level by an amount unknown to the subject, in preparation for the next trial.

Method of Constant Stimuli

The **method of constant stimuli** (or **constants**) involves the presentation of various stimulus levels to the subject in random order. Unlike the methods of limits and adjustments, the method of constants is a nonsequential procedure. In other words, the stimuli are not presented in an ascending or descending manner. A range of intensities is selected which, based upon previous experience or a pilot experiment, encompasses the threshold level. A step size is selected, and the stimuli are then presented to the subject in random order. In an absolute sensitivity (threshold) experiment, an equal number of stimuli are presented at each level. The subject indicates whether the stimulus presentation has been perceived during each test trial. In a differential sensitivity (DL) experiment, the subject's task would be to say whether two items are the same or different.

In an experiment to determine the threshold for a tone by using the method of constant stimuli, one might randomly present tones in 1-dB increments between 4 and 11 dB, for a total of 50 trials at each level. Sample results are tabulated

Table 7.1   Threshold of a Tone Using the Method of Constant Stimuli

Stimulus level (dB)	Number of responses	Percent of responses
11	50	100
10	50	100
9	47	94
8	35	70
7	17	34
6	3	6
5	0	0
4	0	0

Table 7.2   Data from an Experiment on Differential Sensitivity for Intensity Using the Method of Constant Stimuli

Level of second tone (dB)	Percentage of louder judgments
70	100
68	95
66	85
64	70
62	55
60	35
58	20
56	10
54	8
52	5
50	0

in Table 7.1. When these data are graphed in the form of a psychometric function (Fig. 7.4), the 50% point corresponds to 7.5 dB, which is taken as the threshold.

Table 7.2 shows the results of an experiment using the method of constants to find differential sensitivity for intensity. Two tones are presented and the subject is asked whether the second tone is louder or softer than the first. The intensity of the second tone is changed so that the various stimulus levels are presented randomly. Table 7.2 shows the percentage of presentations in which the subject judged the second tone to be louder than the first tone at each of the levels used. (The percentage of "softer" judgments is simply obtained by subtracting the percentage of "louder" judgments from 100%. Thus, the 60-dB presentations of the second tone were "softer" 100% − 35% = 65% of the time.) Figure 7.5 shows the psychometric function for these data. Because the intensity at which the second tone is judged louder 50% of the time is also the tone for which it was judged softer half of the time, the 50% point is where the two tones were perceived as equal in loudness. This is the PSE. In experiments of this kind, the 75% point is generally accepted as the threshold for "louder" judgments. (If we had also plotted "softer" judgments, then the 75% point on that psychometric function

would constitute the "softer" threshold.) The DL is taken as the difference in stimulus values between the PSE and the "louder" threshold. For the data in Fig. 7.5, this difference is 64.8 dB − 61.5 dB = 3.3 dB.

The method of constant stimuli enables the investigator to include "catch" trials over the course of the experiment. These are intervals during which the subject is asked whether a tone was heard, when no tone was really presented. Performance on catch trials provides an estimate of guessing, and performance on real trials is often corrected to account for this effect (see Chap. 8). This correction reduces, but does not completely remove, response biases from the results.

The method of constants has the advantage over the methods of limits and adjustments of greater precision of measurement, and, as just mentioned, has the advantage of allowing direct estimation of guessing behavior. However, it has the disadvantage of inefficiency, because a very large number of trials are needed

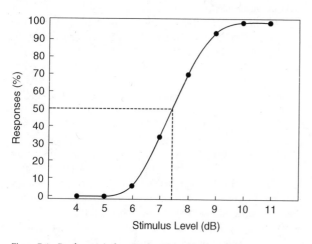

Figure 7.4   Psychometric function based on data from Table 7.1 obtained by using the method of constant stimuli. The threshold corresponds to 7.5 dB.

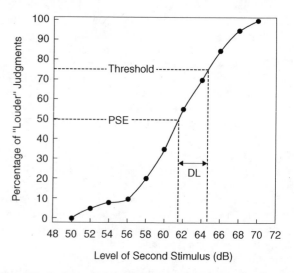

Figure 7.5   Psychometric function for a differential sensitivity experiment showing the point of subjective equality (PSE), "higher" threshold, and difference limen (DL). The data are from Table 7.2.

to obtain the data. Most of these trial points are poorly placed relative to the points of interest (generally the 50% and 75% points), so that the method of constants costs heavily in time and effort for its accuracy. The prolonged test time increases the effects of subject fatigue and the difficulty of maintaining motivation to respond.

FORCED CHOICE METHODS

Until now, we have focused for the most part on a "yes/no" testing approach. However, other formats are used as well and are actually more commonly employed in actual experiments. These approaches involve forced choice paradigms in which the subject is presented with two or more alternatives from which he must choose a response. Suppose, for example, that we want to find out whether a subject can hear a tone in the presence of a noise. In a "yes/no" experiment the subject hears one stimulus presentation, which might be a just a tone, or perhaps a noise alone versus a tone-plus-noise combination. In either case, the subject's task is to indicate whether the tone was there or not ("yes" or "no"). In a **two-alternative forced choice (2AFC) method**, the subject is presented with two stimuli in succession, only one of which contains the tone. After listening to both stimuli, he must decide whether the tone was present in the first one or the second. Similarly, in a 4AFC experiment, the subject must decide which of four successive stimuli includes the tone. Because the two or more presentations occur as successive *intervals*, we could also say that the subject must decide which interval contained the stimulus. Therefore, these experiments are often called 2- **(or more) interval forced choice methods** (hence, 2-IFC, 3-IFC, etc.). These topics are covered further in the context of the theory of signal detection in the next chapter.

ADAPTIVE PROCEDURES

In an **adaptive procedure**, the level at which a particular stimulus is presented to the subject depends upon how the subject responded to the previous stimuli (Wetherill and Levitt, 1965; Levitt, 1971; Bode and Carhart, 1973). Broadly defined, even the classical method of limits can be considered an adaptive method because of its sequential character and the rule that stimuli are presented until there is a reversal in the subject's responses from "yes" to "no" or vice versa. However, use of the term "adaptive procedures" has come to be associated with methods that tend to converge upon the threshold level (or some other target point), and then place most of the observations around it. This approach, of course, maximizes the efficiency of the method because most of the test trials are close to the threshold rather than being "wasted" at some distance from it. It also has the advantage of not requiring prior knowledge of where the threshold level is located, since adaptive methods tend to home in on the threshold regardless of the starting point, and often include step sizes which are large at first and then become smaller as the threshold level is approached. As a result, both efficiency and precision are maximized.

Bekesy's Tracking Method

Bekesy (1960/1989) devised a **tracking method** which shares features with both the classical methods of adjustment and limits and with adaptive procedures. The level of the stimulus changes at a fixed rate (e.g., 2.5 dB/s) under the control of a motor-driven attenuator, and the direction of level change is controlled by the subject via a pushbutton switch. The motor is also connected to a recorder, which shows the sound level as a function of time (Fig. 7.6) or frequency. The pushbutton causes the motor to decrease the sound level when it is depressed and to increase the level when it is up. The subject is asked to press the button whenever he hears the tone and to release it whenever the tone is inaudible. Thus, the sound level is increased toward threshold from below when the tone is inaudible and decreased toward threshold from above when the sound is heard. The threshold is thus tracked by the subject, and its value is the average of the midpoints of the excursions on the recording (once they are stabilized).

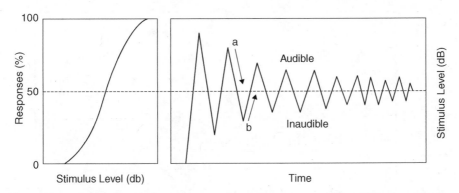

Figure 7.6 Bekesy's tracking method. (a) Intensity decreases as the subject depresses the response button when he hears the sound. (b) Intensity increases as the subject releases the button when he cannot hear the sound. The midpoints of the excursions correspond to the 50% point on the psychometric function shown to the left of the tracing.

Tracking has the advantages of speed and reasonable precision. It is, of course, subject to several sources of response bias. At fast attenuation rates (intensity change speeds), the subject's reaction time can substantially affect the width of the tracking excursions and the precision of measurement. For example, if the tone increases and decreases in level at 5 dB/s and a subject has a 2-s reaction time, then the motor will have advanced the stimulus level (and pen position on the recorder) 10 dB above threshold before the button is finally depressed. Precision is improved and reaction time becomes less critical at reasonably slower attenuation rates, although the tracking may meander somewhat on the recording as the subject's criterion for threshold varies.

Simple Up-Down or Staircase Method

The **simple up-down (or staircase) method** involves increasing the stimulus when the subject did not respond to the previous stimulus presentation and decreasing the intensity when there was a response to the prior stimulus (Dixon and Mood, 1948; Levitt, 1971). It differs from the method of limits in that testing does not stop when the responses change from "yes" to "no" or from "no" to "yes." Similar to the method of limits, the stimuli are changed in discrete steps.

Figure 7.7 shows the first six runs of a staircase procedure to find the threshold of a tone using a 2-dB step size. Here, a run is a group of stimulus presentations between two response reversals. In other words, a descending run starts with a positive response and continues downward until there is a negative response, while an ascending run begins with a negative response and ends with a positive one. Because stimulus intensity is always increased after a negative (−) response and decreased after a positive (+) response, the staircase method converges upon the 50% point on the psychometric function. The procedure is continued through at least six to eight reversals (excluding the first one), and the threshold value is then calculated as the average of the midpoints of the runs, or as the average of their peaks and troughs (Wetherill, 1963; Wetherill and Levitt,

1965). The latter method appears to give a somewhat better estimate. The precision of the method can be increased by first estimating the threshold with a larger step size, and then using a smaller step size (generally half that of the previous one) to locate the threshold in the vicinity of the first estimate (Wetherill, 1963). For example, if the average of six runs using a 4-dB step is 10 dB, a second group of runs using a 2-dB step might begin at 10 dB in order to obtain a more precise estimate of the threshold.

The simple up-down method has several advantages and limitations (Levitt, 1971). It quickly converges upon the 50% point so that most trials are efficiently placed close to the point of interest. It also has the advantage of being able to follow changes (drifts) in the subject's responses. On the other hand, the subject may bias his responses if he realizes that the stimuli are being presented according to a sequential rule, which depends on the way he responds. As with the method of limits, if the step size is too small, a large number of trials are wasted, and if the step is too large, they are badly placed for estimating the 50% point. Another limitation is that only the 50% point can be converged upon with the simple up-down rule.

Parameter Estimation by Sequential Testing

Parameter estimation by sequential testing (PEST) is an adaptive procedure which uses changes in both the direction and step size of the stimulus to home in on a targeted level of performance (Taylor and Creelman, 1967; Taylor, Forbes, and Creelman, 1983). The investigator may set the target value to any location on the psychometric function he chooses (for example, 50% or 80%). However, we will concentrate here only on the 50% point in order to make clear the salient features which distinguish the PEST procedure. As in the simple up-down method, positive responses are followed by decreases in stimulus level because the threshold is probably lower, and negative responses are followed by increases in intensity because the threshold is probably higher. The difference is that PEST includes a series of *rules for doubling and halving the stimulus level* depending upon the previous sequence of responses.

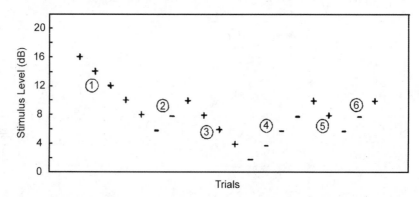

Figure 7.7   The first six runs of a threshold search using the simple up-down or staircase method. Each (+) indicates a positive response and each (−) indicates a negative response. Odd numbers are descending runs and even numbers are ascending runs. The first reversal is generally omitted from the threshold calculation.

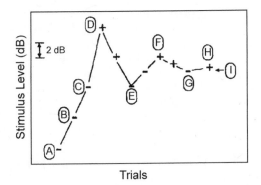

Figure 7.8   An example of how the threshold is obtained with the PEST procedure. Points identified by letters are discussed in the text. Point I is the estimate of threshold.

At each stimulus level, PEST in effect asks whether the threshold has been exceeded. The level is then changed so that the maximum amount of information is obtained from the next trial. To do this, the step size is varied in the manner specified in Fig. 7.8. Although it is most efficient to know the approximate location of the threshold range in advance, it is not essential. Suppose we begin testing at some value below threshold corresponding to point A in Fig. 7.8. Since the subject gives a negative response, the stimulus is presented at a higher level (B). This level also produces no response and the stimulus is raised by the same amount as previously and is presented again (C). Since there is still no response, the stimulus level is again increased. However, PEST has a rule which states that if there is a negative response on two successive presentations in the same direction, then the step size is doubled for the next presentation. Thus, the next stimulus is presented at level D. The doubling rule ensures that a minimal number of trials are wasted in finding the range of interest.

A positive response at level D indicates that the threshold has been exceeded. As in the staircase method, the direction of the trials is changed after a response reversal. However, the PEST procedure also halves the step size at this point. The halving rule causes the stimuli to be presented closer to the threshold value. Thus, precision is improved as the threshold is converged upon. Since D is followed by another positive

response, the stimulus is then presented at a lower level (E). A negative response at E causes the direction of stimulus change to be changed again, and the step size is halved compared to the previous one. The stimulus is heard again at the next higher level (F), so the direction is changed again and the step size is again halved. Stimuli are now presented in a descending run until there is a negative response (G). Halving the step size and changing direction results in a positive response at H, indicating that the threshold lies somewhere between points G and H. Since this interval represents an acceptable degree of precision, the procedure is terminated. The level at which the next stimulus would have been presented is taken as the threshold. This level is point I, which lies halfway between levels G and H. Note on the scale for Fig. 7.8 that the step size between E and F is 2 dB, between F and G is 1 dB, and between G and H is 0.5 dB. This observation highlights the rapidity with which PEST results in a precise threshold estimate.

Block Up-Down Methods

Suppose we are interested in the 75% point on the psychometric function. One way to converge upon the point is to modify the simple up-down procedure by replacing the single trial per stimulus level with a block of several trials per level. Then, by adopting three out of four positive responses (75%) as the criterion per level, the strategy will home in on the 75% point. If blocks of five were used with a four out of five criterion, then the 80% point would be converged upon. The procedure may be further modified by changing the response from *yes-no* to a *two-alternative* (*interval*) *forced choice*. In other words, the subject is presented with two stimulus intervals during each trial and must indicate which of the intervals contains the stimulus. This is the **block up-down temporal interval forced-choice (BUDTIF) procedure** (Campbell 1963). Using the two-interval forced choice method allows the investigator to determine the proportion of responses to the no-stimulus interval—the "false alarm" rate. We shall see when the theory of signal detection is discussed in the next chapter that this distinction is important in separating sensitivity from bias effects.

The BUDTIF procedure is illustrated in Fig. 7.9. Note that each block is treated as though it were one trial in a staircase procedure. Since the target point has been preselected as 75%,

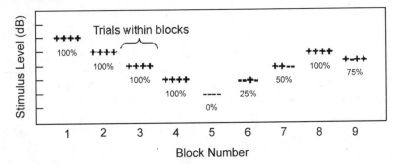

Figure 7.9   An example of convergence upon the 75% point of the psychometric function using BUDTIF.

stimulus intensity is raised whenever there are less than three out of four correct responses in a block and is decreased when all four are correct. Testing is terminated when three out of four correct responses are obtained. The last level is the target level (75% in this case). Notice that since blocks of trials are presented at each level, poor placement of the initial test level will cause many wasted trials in converging upon the target range.

A modification of BUDTIF replaces the two-alternative forced-choice paradigm with the familiar yes-no response. This adaptation is called the **block up-down yes-no (BUDYEN)** method (Campbell and Counter, 1969). However, the BUDYEN paradigm is less advantageous than its forced-choice predecessor because an estimate of false alarms is not obtained (Creelman and Taylor, 1969).

Transformed Up-Down or Staircase Procedures

The simple up-down method converges on the 50% point of the psychometric function because each positive response leads to a decrease in stimulus level and each negative response leads to an intensity increase. If the up-down rule is modified so that stimulus level is changed only after certain sequences have occurred, then the procedure will home in on other points on the psychometric function (Wetherill and Levitt, 1965; Levitt and Rabiner, 1967; Levitt, 1971, 1978). These other target points depend upon the particular set of sequences chosen by the investigator.

We will go over the fundamental principles of transformed up-down methods because they are ubiquitous in hearing science research. When the target is 50% on the psychometric function, as in the simple up-down method, the chances of a positive response to stimuli well below the 50% point are very small. Similarly, it is likely that stimuli presented at levels well above the 50% point will frequently be heard. However, as the intensity corresponding to 50% is approached, the chances of positive and negative responses become closer and closer. At the 50% point, the probability of a positive response is the same as of a negative one. This is, of course, exactly what we mean by 50%. Now, suppose that the total probability of all responses is 1.00. If we call the probability of a positive response (p), then the probability of a negative response would be $(1 - p)$. At the 50% point

$$p = (1 - p) = 0.5 \tag{7.1}$$

In other words, the probability of a positive response at the 50% point is 0.5, which is also the probability of a negative response. In effect, the simple up-down rule forces the intensity to the point on the psychometric function where the probabilities of positive and negative responses are equal (0.5 each).

Other target levels can be converged upon by changing the up-down rule so that the probabilities of increasing and decreasing stimulus intensity are unequal. This is done by setting the criteria for increasing stimulus level (the "up rule") to be a certain response sequence, and those for decreasing stimulus level (the "down rule") to be other response sequences. An example will demonstrate how the transformed up-down method works.

Suppose we are interested in estimating a point above 50% on the psychometric function, say 70%. To accomplish this, we would increase the stimulus level after a negative response $(-)$ or a positive response followed by a negative one $(+, -)$, and lower the stimulus level after two successive positives $(+, +)$. In other words, we have established the following rules for changing stimulus level:

$$\begin{aligned} \text{Up rule}: & \quad (-) \text{ or } (+, -) \\ \text{Down rule}: & \quad (+, +) \end{aligned} \tag{7.2}$$

As with the simple staircase rule, levels well above the target will often yield $(+, +)$ responses, and those well below will tend to have $(-)$ or $(+, -)$ responses. However, at the target level, the probability of increasing the stimulus level will be

$$(1 - p) + p(1 - p) \tag{7.3}$$

and the probability of two successive positive responses $(+, +)$ will be

$$p \times p \text{ or } p^2 \tag{7.4}$$

The up-down strategy will converge on the point where the up and down rules have the same probabilities (0.5). In other words, the probability of the transformed positive response $(+, +)$ at the target is

$$p^2 = 0.5 \tag{7.5}$$

Since we are interested in the probability (p) of a single positive response, which is the square root of p^2, we simply find the square root of $p^2 = 0.5$, and we obtain

$$p = 0.707 \tag{7.6}$$

Converting to percent, the transformed procedure just outlined homes in on the 70.7% point of the psychometric function, which is a quite acceptable estimate of the 70% point.

To converge on the 29.3% of the psychometric function (which is a reasonable estimate of the 30% point), we might choose to increase the stimulus after a sequence of two successive negative responses $(-, -)$, and to decrease stimulus level after a positive response $(+)$ or a negative response followed by a positive one $(-, +)$.

The 70.7% and 29.3% **transformed up-down strategies** are illustrated in Fig. 7.10. As with the simple up-down method, each transformed strategy would be continued through six to eight reversals, and the average of the peaks and valleys would be taken as the target level. Because these two points are on the rising portion of the psychometric function and are equidistant from 50%, a reasonably good estimate of the 50% point can be obtained by averaging the levels from 70.7% to 29.3%. To increase efficiency, one might start with a large step size, and then halve it in the target range for increased precision.

Other target points can be converged upon by various sequences of positive and negative responses, and different sequences may be used to converge upon the same target points

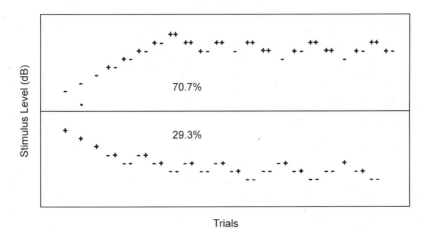

Figure 7.10 Examples of how the transformed up-down procedure converges upon the 70.7% point (*upper frame*) and the 29.3% point (*lower frame*) of the psychometric function.

(Levitt and Rabiner, 1967; Levitt, 1971, 1973). Transformed up-down procedures can also be used in the measurement of subjective judgments, such as for loudness balances (Jesteadt, 1980). In addition, both simple and transformed up-down procedures are particularly adaptable to testing various aspects of speech recognition functions under a variety of conditions (e.g., Levitt, 1971; Bode and Carhart, 1974; Plomp and Mimpen, 1979; Duquesnoy, 1983; Dubno, Morgan, and Dirks, 1984; Gelfand, Ross, and Miller, 1988).

A useful approach to minimizing biases is to interleave different testing strategies (Levitt, 1968). In other words, two points on the psychometric function are converged upon during the same test session. This is done by switching in an approximately random manner between the two test strategies. For example, two reversals on the 29.3% strategy might be followed by a few reversals on the 70.7% strategy, then the investigator would return to where he left off on the 29.3% sequence, and so forth. Such interleaving can also be applied to other psychoacoustic methods. Of course, greater flexibility and ease of measurement is made possible when the procedure is automated, and, almost needless to say, computerized administrations of these procedures are the norm.

Modifications, Other Procedures, and Comparisons

Numerous approaches have been introduced that modify the methods already discussed and/or combine adaptive procedures with maximum likelihood, Bayesian, or other techniques (Hall, 1968, 1981, 1983; Pentland, 1980; Watson and Pelli, 1983; Emmerson, 1984; Findlay, 1978; Simpson, 1989; Kaernbach, 1991; King-Smith, Grigsby, Vingrys, et al., 1994; Kontsevich and Tyler, 1999; Remus and Collins, 2008). The *maximum likelihood methods* use the history of the subject's responses combined with certain assumptions about the nature of the psychometric function to estimate where the threshold (actually the midpoint of the function) lies after each response. This estimated value then becomes the level of the next stimulus presentation.

For example, Hall's (1981, 1983) hybrid procedure combines aspects of maximum likelihood methods with features of PEST. In the *Bayesian adaptive procedures*, the step size is adaptive rather than fixed and each stimulus value is calculated based on a running update of the probability distribution.[1]

Many studies have compared the various adaptive methods and between adaptive and more traditional approaches (Pentland, 1980; Shelton et al., 1983; Shelton and Scarrow (1984); Taylor et al., 1983; Hesse, 1986; Marshall and Jesteadt, 1986; Madigan and Williams, 1987; Kollmeier, Gilkey and Sieben, 1988; Simpson, 1988, 1989; Leek, 2001; Marvit, Florentine, and Buus, 2003; Amitay, Irwin, Hawkey, et al., 2006; Rowan, Hinton, and Mackenzie, 2006; Remus and Collins, 2008). Generally speaking, thresholds obtained with the various adaptive approaches tend to be relatively close to each other. For example, Shelton et al. (1983) found that thresholds were nearly the same when obtained using the transformed up-down, PEST, and maximum likelihood procedures. However, it does appear that somewhat better performance is obtained with forced choice compared to nonforced choice paradigms (Taylor et al., 1983; Hesse, 1986; Marshall and Jesteadt, 1986; Kollmeier et al., 1988), and with adaptive step sizes and Bayesian approaches than with fixed step size methods (Pentland, 1980; Leek, 2001; Marvit et al., 2003; Remus and Collins, 2008). One should consult these papers when deciding upon the most appropriate approach for a given experiment.

DIRECT SCALING

The methods discussed so far in this chapter, in which the subject's task is to detect the presence of or small differences between

---

[1] For readily available explanations of Bayesian probabilities and methods see, e.g., http://www.bayesian.org/bayesexp/bayesexp.html, or http://drambuie.lanl.gov/~bayes/tutorial.htm.

stimuli, are often referred to as **discriminability** or **confusion scales**. In contrast, **direct scaling** involves having the subject establish perceptual relationships among stimuli (**magnitude and ratio scales**) or to divide a range of stimuli into equally spaced or sized perceptual categories (**category or partition scales**). In other words, the subject must specify a perceptual continuum that corresponds to a physical continuum. Two types of continua may be defined (Stevens, 1961). **Prothetic continua**, such as loudness, have the characteristic of *amount*. They are *additive* in that the excitation due to an increase in stimulus level is added to the excitation caused by the intensity which was already present. On the other hand, pitch has the characteristic of *kind* and azimuth has the characteristic of *location*. These are **metathetic continua** and are *substantive* rather than additive. In other words, a change in the pitch corresponds to a substitution of one excitation pattern, as it were, for another.

Ratio Estimation and Production

In **ratio estimation**, the subject is presented with two stimuli differing in terms of some parameter and is asked to express the subjective magnitude of one stimulus as a ratio of the other. Subjective values are thus scaled as a function of the physical magnitudes. Suppose two 1000-Hz tones with different intensities are presented to a subject, who must judge the loudness of the second tone as a ratio of the first. He might report that the intensity of the second tone sounds one-half, one-quarter, twice, or five times as loud as the first tone.

Ratio production, or **fractionalization**, is the opposite of ratio estimation in that the subject's task is to adjust the magnitude of a variable stimulus so that it sounds like a particular ratio (or fraction) of the magnitude of a standard stimulus. For example, the subject might adjust the intensity of a comparison tone so that it sounds half as loud as the standard, twice as loud, etc. Fractionalization has been used in the development of scales relating loudness to intensity (Stevens, 1936) and pitch to frequency (Stevens, Volkmann, and Newman, 1937; Stevens and Volkmann, 1940).

Magnitude Estimation and Production

In **magnitude estimation**, the subject assigns to physical intensities numbers that correspond to their subjective magnitudes. This may be done in two general ways (Stevens, 1956, 1975). In the first method, the subject is given a standard or reference stimulus and is told that its intensity has a particular value. This reference point is called a **modulus**. He is then presented with other intensities and must assign numbers to these, which are ratios of the modulus. Consider a loudness scaling experiment in which the subject compares the loudness of variable tones to a standard tone of 80 dB. If the 80-dB standard is called 10 (modulus), then a magnitude estimate of 1 would be assigned to the intensity 1/10 as loud, 60 would be assigned to the one that is 6 times as loud, etc. The relationship between these magnitude estimates and intensity is shown by the closed circles in Fig. 7.11.

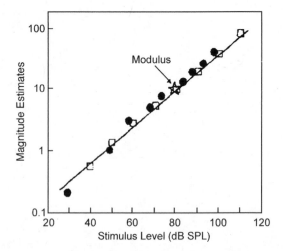

Figure 7.11 Magnitude estimations of loudness obtained with a modulus (*closed circles*) and without a modulus (*open squares*) as a function of stimulus intensity based on data from Stevens (1956).

An alternative approach is to omit the modulus. Here, the subject is presented with a series of stimuli and is asked to assign numbers to them reflecting their subjective levels. The results of such an experiment are shown by the open squares in Fig. 7.11. As the figure shows, magnitude estimates obtained with and without a modulus result in similar findings.

The reverse of magnitude estimation is **magnitude production**. In this approach, the subject is presented with numbers representing the perceptual values and must adjust the physical magnitude of the stimulus to correspond to the numbers.

Absolute magnitude estimation (AME) and absolute **magnitude production (AMP)** involve the performance of magnitude estimates (or productions) without any specified or implied reference value, and with each estimate (or production) made without regard to the judgments made for previous stimuli (Hellman and Zwislocki, 1961, 1963, 1968; Hellman, 1976, 1981; Zwislocki and Goodman, 1980; Zwislocki, 1983a; Hellman and Meiselman, 1988). There has been some discussion regarding this approach (e.g., Mellers, 1983a, 1983b; Zwislocki, 1983b). However, the convincing preponderance of evidence reveals that it is valid, reliable, and efficient, and that AMEs and AMPs are readily performed by naive clinical patients as well as laboratory subjects (Hellman and Zwislocki, 1961, 1963, 1968; Hellman, 1976, 1981; Zwislocki and Goodman, 1980; Zwislocki, 1983a; Hellman and Meiselman, 1988).

Subject bias causes magnitude estimation and production to yield somewhat different results, especially at high and low stimulus levels. Specifically, subjects tend not to assign extreme values in magnitude estimation, or to make extreme level adjustments in magnitude production. These bias effects are in opposite directions so that the "real" function lies somewhere between the ones obtained from magnitude estimations and productions. This is illustrated in Fig. 7.12 by the

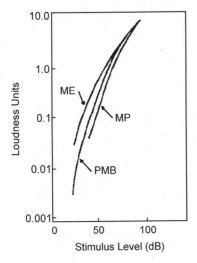

Figure 7.12 Bias effects in magnitude estimation (ME) and magnitude production (MP) are minimized by geometric averaging in the method of psychological magnitude balance (PMB). *Source*: Adapted from Hellman and Zwislocki (1968) with permission of *J. Acoust. Soc. Am.*

divergence of the magnitude estimation and magnitude production functions. An unbiased function may be obtained by using the method of **psychological magnitude balance** (Hellman and Zwislocki, 1963, 1968). This is done by calculating the geometric mean of the corresponding magnitude estimations and magnitude productions along the intensity axis or the loudness axis. An example is illustrated by the curve labeled PMB in Fig. 7.12.

Cross-Modality Matches

A scaling approach related to magnitude estimation and production is called **cross-modality matching** (Stevens and Guirao, 1963; Stevens and Marks, 1965, 1980; Stevens, 1975; Hellman and Meiselman, 1988, 1993). In this technique, the subject is asked to express the perceived magnitude for one sense in terms of another sensory modality. For example, *loudness* (an auditory perception) might be expressed in terms of *apparent line length* (a visual perception). A very useful variation of this approach has been developed and applied by Hellman and Meiselman (1988, 1993). In this method, the slope of the power function for loudness is derived from that for line length combined with the cross-modality match between loudness and line length.

Category Rating of Loudness

Category rating methods are often used in loudness measurements, particularly in clinical assessments related to hearing aids. These methods involve presenting sounds to the listener at various levels, who gives a loudness rating to each of them based on a list of descriptive loudness categories (e.g., Allen, Hall, Jeng, 1990; Hawkins, Walden, Montgomery, and Prosek, 1987; Cox, Alexander, Taylor, and Gray, 1997). For example, in the Contour Test developed by Cox et al. (1997), the listener

assigns numerical loudness ratings to pulsed warble tone stimuli using a seven-point scale from *1* for "very soft," to *7* for "uncomfortably loud." Sherlock and Formby (2005) found no significant differences between sound levels rated "uncomfortably loud" using this approach and directly measured loudness discomfort levels (Sherlock and Formby, 2005).

REFERENCES

Abelson, RP, Tukey, JW. 1959. Efficient conversion of nonmetric information into metric information. In: ER Tufte (ed.), *The Quantitative Analysis of Social Problems*. Reading, MA: Addison Wesley, 407–417.

Allen, JB, Hall, JL, Jeng, PS. 1990. Loudness growth in ½-octave bands (LGOB)—A procedure for the assessment of loudness. *J Acoust Soc Am* 88, 745–753.

American Speech-Language-Hearing Association (ASHA). 2005. *Guidelines for manual pure-tone threshold audiometry*. Rockville, MD: ASHA.

Amitay, S, Irwin, A, Hawkey, DJC, Cowan, JA, Moore, DR. 2006. A comparison of adaptive procedures for rapid and reliable threshold assessment and training in naive listeners. *J Acoust Soc Am* 119, 1616–1625.

Bekesy, G. 1960/1989. *Experiments in Hearing*. New York, NY: McGraw-Hill. [Republished by the Acoustical Society of America].

Bode, DL, Carhart, R. 1973. Measurements of articulation functions using adaptive test procedures. *IEEE Trans Audiol Electroacoust* AU-21, 196–201.

Bode, DL, Carhart, R. 1974. Stability and accuracy of adaptive tests of speech discrimination. *J Acoust Soc Am* 56, 963–970.

Campbell, RA. 1963. Detection of a noise signal of varying duration. *J Acoust Soc Am* 35, 1732–1737.

Campbell, R.A, Counter, SA. 1969. Temporal energy integration and periodicity pitch. *J Acoust Soc Am* 45, 691–693.

Coomb, CH. 1953. Theory and methods of measurement. In: L Festinger, D Katz (eds.), *Research Methods in the Behavioral Sciences*. New York, NY: Holt, Rinehart, and Winston, 471–535.

Cox, RM, Alexander, GC, Taylor, IM, Gray, GA. 1997. The Contour Test of loudness perception. *Ear Hear* 18, 388–400.

Creelman, CD, Taylor, MM. 1969. Some pitfalls in adaptive testing: Comments on "Temporal integration and periodicity pitch". *J Acoust Soc Am* 46, 1581–1582.

Dixon, WJ, Mood, AM. 1948. A method for obtaining and analyzing sensitivity data. *J Am Stat Assn* 43, 109–126.

Dubno, JR, Dirks, DD, Morgan, DE. 1984. Effects of age and mild hearing loss on speech recognition in noise. *J Acoust Soc Am* 76, 87–96.

Duquesnoy, AJ. 1983. Effect of a single interfering noise or speech sound upon the binaural sentence intelligibility of aged persons, *J Acoust Soc Am* 74, 739–743.

Emmerson, PL. 1984. Observations on a maximum likelihood method of sequential threshold estimation and a simplified approximation. *Percept Psychophys* 36, 199–203.

Findlay, JM. 1978. Estimates on probability functions: A more virulent PEST. *Percept Psychophys* 23, 181–185.

Gelfand, SA, Ross, L, Miller, S. 1988. Sentence reception in noise from one versus two sources: Effects of aging and hearing loss. *J Acoust Soc Am* 83, 248–256.

Hall, JL. 1968. Maximum-likelihood sequential procedure for estimation of psychometric functions. *J Acoust Soc Am* 44, 370.

Hall, JL. 1981. Hybrid adaptive procedure for estimation of psychometric functions. *J Acoust Soc Am* 69, 1763–1769.

Hall, JL. 1983. A procedure for detecting variability of psychophysical thresholds. *J Acoust Soc Am* 73, 663–669.

Hawkins, DB, Walden, BE, Montgomery, A, Prosek, RA. 1987. Description and validation of an LDL procedure designed to select SSPL-90. *Ear Hear* 8, 162–169.

Hellman, RP. 1976. Growth of loudness at 1000 and 3000 Hz. *J Acoust Soc Am* 60, 672–679.

Hellman, RP. 1981. Stability of individual loudness functions obtained by magnitude estimation and production. *Percept Psychophys* 29, 63–78.

Hellman, RP, Meiselman, CH. 1988. Prediction of individual loudness exponents from cross-modality matching. *J Speech Hear Res* 31, 605–615.

Hellman, RP, Meiselman, CH. 1993. Rate of loudness growth for pure tones in normal and impaired hearing. *J Acoust Soc Am* 93, 966–975.

Hellman, RP, Zwislocki, JJ. 1961. Some factors affecting the estimation of loudness. *J Acoust Soc Am* 33, 687–694.

Hellman, RP, Zwislocki, J. 1963. Monaural loudness function of a 1000-cps tone and interaural summation. *J Acoust Soc Am* 35, 856–865.

Hellman, R.P, Zwislocki, J. 1968. Loudness summation at low sound frequencies. *J Acoust Soc Am* 43, 60–63.

Hesse, A. 1986. Comparison of several psychophysical procedures with respect to threshold estimates, reproducibility, and efficiency. *Acustica* 59, 263–266.

Jesteadt, W. 1980. An adaptive procedure for subjective judgments. *Percept Psychophys* 2S, 85–88.

Kaernbach, C. 1991. Simple adaptive testing with the weighted up-down method. *Percept Psychophys* 49, 227–229.

King-Smith, PE, Grigsby, SS, Vingrys, AJ, Benes, SC, Supowit, A. 1994. Efficient and unbiased modifications of the QUEST threshold method: Theory, simulations, experimental evaluation and practical implementation. *Vision Res* 34, 885–912.

Kollmeier, B, Gilkey, RH, Sieben, UK. 1988. Adaptive staircase techniques in psychoacoustics: A comparison of human data and a mathematical model. *J Acoust Soc Am* 83, 1852–1862.

Kontsevich, LL, Tyler, CW. 1999. Bayesian adaptive estimation of psychometric slope and threshold. *Vision Res* 39, 2729–2737.

Leek, MR. 2001. Adaptive procedures in psychophysical research. *Percept Psychophys* 63, 1279–1292.

Levitt, H. 1968. Testing for sequential dependencies. *J Acoust Soc Am* 43, 65–69.

Levitt, H. 1971. Transformed up-down methods in psychoacoustics. *J Acoust Soc Am* 49, 467–477.

Levitt, H. 1978. Adaptive testing in audiology. *Scand Audiol* Suppl 6, 241–291.

Levitt, H, Rabiner, LR. 1967. Use of a sequential strategy in intelligibility testing. *J Acoust Soc Am* 42, 609–612.

Madigan, R, Williams, D. 1987. Maximum-likelihood procedures in two alternative forced-choice: evaluation and recommendations. *Percept Psychophys* 42, 240–249.

Marshall, L, Jesteadt, W. 1986. Comparison of pure-tone audibility thresholds obtained with audiological and two-interval forced-choice procedures. *J Speech Hear Res* 29, 82–91.

Marvit, P, Florentine, M, Buus, S. 2003. A comparison of psychophysical procedures for level-discrimination thresholds. *J Acoust Soc Am* 113, 3348–3361.

Mellers, BA. 1983a. Evidence against "absolute" scaling. *Percept Psychophys* 33, 523–526.

Mellers, BA. 1983b. Reply to Zwislocki's views on "absolute" scaling. *Percept Psychophys* 34, 405–408.

Pentland, A. 1980. Maximum likelihood estimation: The best PEST. *Percept Psychophys* 28, 377–379.

Plomp, R, Mimpen, AM. 1979. Speech-reception threshold for sentences as a function of age and noise. *J Acoust Soc Am* 66, 1333–1342.

Remus, JJ, Collins, LM. 2008. Comparison of adaptive psychometric procedures motivated by the Theory of Optimal Experiments: Simulated and experimental results. *J Acoust Soc Am* 123, 315–326.

Robinson, DE, Watson, CS. 1973. Psychophysical methods in modern psychoacoustics. In: JV Tobias (ed.), *Foundations of Modern Auditory Theory, Vol. 2.* New York, NY: Academic Press, 99–131.

Rowan, D, Hinton, K, Mackenzie, E. 2006. Comparison of Levitt- and Zwislocki-type adaptive procedures for stimulus placement in human listeners. *J Acoust Soc Am* 119, 3538–3541.

Shelton, BR, Scarrow, I. 1984. Two-alternative versus three-alternative procedures for threshold estimation. *Percept Psychophys* 35, 385–392.

Shelton, BR, Picardi, MC, Green, DM. 1983. Comparison of three adaptive psychophysical procedures. *J Acoust Soc Am* 71, 1527–1532.

Sherlock, P, Formby, C. 2005. Estimates of loudness, Loudness discomfort, and the auditory dynamic range: Normative estimates, comparison of procedures, and test-retest reliability. *J Am Acad Audiol* 16, 85–100.

Simpson, WA. 1988. The method of constant stimuli is efficient. *Percept Psychophys* 44, 433–436.

Simpson, WA. 1989. The step method: A new adaptive psychophysical procedure. *Percept Psychophys* 45, 572–576.

Stevens, SS. 1936. A scale for the measurement of a psychological magnitude: Loudness. *Psychol Rev* 43, 405–416.

Stevens, SS. 1951. Mathematics, measurement, and psychophysics. In: SS Stevens (ed.), *Handbook of Experimental Psychology*. New York, NY: Wiley.

Stevens, SS. 1958. Problems and methods in psychophysics. *Psychol Bull* 55, 177–196.

Stevens, SS. 1956. The direct estimation of sensory magnitudes—loudness. *Am J Psychol* 69, 1–25.

Stevens, SS. 1961. The psychophysics of sensory function. In: WA Rosenblith (ed.), *Sensory Communication*. Cambridge, MA: MIT Press.

Stevens, SS. 1975. *Psychophysics*. New York, NY: Wiley.

Stevens, SS, Guirao, M. 1963. Subjective scaling of length and area and the matching of length to loudness and brightness. *J Exp Psychol* 66, 177–186.

Stevens, JC, Marks, LM. 1965. Cross-modality matching of brightness and loudness. *Proc Natl Acad Sci U S A* 54, 407–411.

Stevens, JC, Marks, LM. 1980. Cross-modality matching functions generated by magnitude estimation. *Precept Psychophys* 27, 379–389.

Stevens, SS, Volkmann, J. 1940. The relation of pitch to frequency: A revised scale. *Am J Psychol* 53, 329–353.

Stevens, SS, Volkmann, J, Newman, EB. 1937. A scale for the measurement of the psychological magnitude pitch. *J Acoust Soc Am* 8, 185–190.

Taylor, MM, Creelman, CD. 1967. PEST: Efficient estimates on probability functions. *J Acoust Soc Am* 41, 782–787.

Taylor, MM, Forbes, SM, Creelman, CD. 1983. PEST reduces bias in forced choice psychophysics. *J Acoust Soc Am* 74, 1367–1374.

Watson, AB, Pelli, DG. 1983. QUEST: A Bayesian adaptive psychometric method. *Percept Psychophys* 33, 113–120.

Wetherill, GB. 1963. Sequential estimation of quantal responses. *J R Stat Soc* 25, 1–48.

Wetherill, GB, Levitt, H. 1965. Sequential estimation of points on a psychometric function. *Br J Math Stat Psychol* 18, 1–10.

Zwislocki, JJ. 1983a. Group and individual relations between sensation magnitudes and their numerical estimates. *Percept Psychophys* 33, 460–468.

Zwislocki, JJ. 1983b. Absolute and other scales: The question of validity views on "absolute" scaling. *Percept Psychophys* 33, 593–594.

Zwislocki, JJ, Goodman, DA. 1980. Absolute scaling of sensory magnitudes: A validation. *Percept Psychophys* 28, 28–38.

The previous chapter addressed itself to the classical and modern psychoacoustical methods and the direct scaling of sensory magnitudes with respect to hearing. It left essentially unresolved, however, the problem of how to effectively separate sensitivity from response proclivity. In this chapter, we shall approach this problem from the standpoint of the theory of signal detection.

FACTORS AFFECTING RESPONSES

The theory of signal detection (Swets, 1965; Greene and Swets, 1974; Egan, 1975) provides the best approach to separate the effects of sensitivity from those of response bias. We might think of the **theory of signal detection (TSD)** as asking the question, "what led to a "yes" (or "no") decision?" as opposed to "what did the subject hear (or not hear)?"

Suppose a subject were asked to say "yes" when he hears a tone during a test trial and "no" when a tone is not heard. A large number of trials are used for each of several stimulus levels, and half of those at each level are "catch trials" during which signals are not actually presented. There are thus four possible outcomes for each test trial. Two of them are correct:

1. A **hit** occurs when the signal is present and the subject says "yes."
2. A **correct rejection** occurs when the signal is absent and the subject says "no." The other two alternatives are wrong:
3. The signal is present but the subject says "no." This is called a **miss**.
4. The signal is absent but the subject says "yes". Here a **false alarm** has occurred.

A convenient way to show these possible stimulus and response combinations is to tabulate them in a stimulus–response matrix, which is illustrated in Fig. 8.1.

The stimulus–response table is generally used to summarize the results of all trials at a particular test level; there would thus be such a table for each stimulus level used in an experiment. For example, Fig. 8.2 shows the results of 100 trials containing a signal and 100 catch trials. The subject responded to 78 of the signal trials (so that the probability of a hit was 0.78), did not respond to 22 signals (the probability of a miss is 0.22), said "yes" for 17 out of 100 catch trials (the probability of a false alarm is 0.17), and said "no" for the remaining absent-stimulus trials (the probability of a correct rejection is 0.83). One is tempted to say that the percent correct at this stimulus level is 78% (the hit rate), but the fact that the subject also responded 17 times when there was no stimulus present tells us that even the 78% correct includes some degree of chance success or guessing. One way to account for this error is to use the proportion of false alarms as an estimate of the overall guessing rate and to correct the hit

rate accordingly. The traditional formula to correct the hit rate for chance success is

$$p(\text{hit})_{\text{corrected}} = \frac{p(\text{hit}) - p(\text{false alarm})}{1 - p(\text{false alarm})}$$

In other words, the probability p of a hit corrected for chance success is obtained by dividing the difference between the hit rate and the false alarm rate by 1 minus the false alarm rate. [If this seems odd, recall that the total probability of all catch trials is 1.0, so that $1 - p(\text{false alarm})$ is the same as the probability of a correct rejection.] Thus, for this example:

$$p(\text{hit})_{\text{corrected}} = \frac{0.78 - 0.17}{1.0 - 0.17} = \frac{0.61}{0.83} = 0.735$$

The original 78% correct thus falls to 73.5% when we account for the proportion of the "yes" responses due to chance.

Correcting for chance success is surely an improvement over approaches that do not account for guessing, but it still does not really separate the effects of auditory factors (sensitivity) and nonauditory factors. In essence, this process highlights the importance of nonauditory factors in determining the response, because the very fact that the subject said "yes" to catch trials and "no" to stimulus trials indicates that his decision to respond was affected by more than just sensitivity to the stimulus. The theory of signal detection is concerned with the factors that enter into this decision.

Let us, at least for the moment, drop the assumption that there is some clear-cut threshold that separates audibility from inaudibility and replace it with the following assumptions of TSD. First, we assume that there is always some degree of noise present. This may be noise in the environment, instrumentation noise, or noise due to the subject's moving around and fidgeting. Even if all of these noises were miraculously removed, there would still remain the subject's unavoidable physiological noises (heartbeat, pulse, breathing, blood rushing through vessels, stomach gurgles, etc.). Indeed, the noise is itself often presented as part of the experiments. For example, the task may be to detect a tone in the presence of a noise. Since there is always noise, which is by nature random, we also assume that the stimulation of the auditory system varies continuously. Finally, we shall assume that all of the stimulation occurs (or is at least measurable) along a single continuum. In other words, the subject must decide whether the stimulation in the auditory system (e.g., energy) is due to **noise alone (N)** or to **signal-plus-noise (SN)**. This process may be represented by distributions along a **decision axis** like the one in Fig. 8.3. Here, the abscissa may be conceived of as representing the energy contained in the noise and in the noise-plus-signal. The x-axis may also be conceived of as representing the *magnitude of sensory activation* resulting from such stimulation. The ordinate denotes the probability of an event occurring. Hence, the N distribution shows the

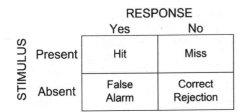

Figure 8.1 Stimulus–response matrix or table showing the four possible outcomes for any given test trial. Correct responses may be "hits" or "correct rejections," whereas errors may also be of two possible types, "misses" or "false alarms."

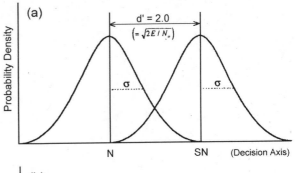

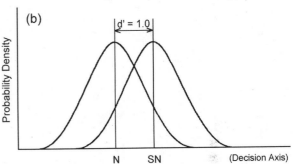

Figure 8.3 The separation between the distribution for the noise alone (N) and the distribution for the signal-plus-noise (SN) determines the value of d′.

probability of occurrence of a noise alone as a function of x, and the SN curve shows the chances of a signal-plus-noise as a function of x. The convention is to use the term "probability density" (as opposed to "probability") for the y-axis in order to reflect the fact that values of x change continuously rather than in discrete steps. The subject's response is a decision between "yes" ("I hear the signal as well as the noise") and "no" ("I hear the noise alone").

The N and SN distributions in Fig. 8.3 show the probability functions of noise alone (N) and signal-plus-noise (SN). We might think of these curves as showing the chances (or likelihood) of there being, respectively, a noise alone or a signal-plus-noise during a particular test trial. Obviously, there must always be more energy in SN than in N, due to the presence of the signal. The separation between the N and SN curves thus becomes a measure of sensitivity. This is an unbiased measure because the separation between the two curves is not affected by the subject's criteria for responding (biases). The separation is determined solely by the energy in the signals and the sensitivity of the auditory system. This separation is measured in terms of a parameter called **d prime (d′)**. The value of d′ is equal to the difference between the means ($\overline{x}$) of the N and SN distributions divided by their standard deviation (σ):

$$d' = \frac{\overline{x}_{SN} - \overline{x}_N}{\sigma}$$

Comparing Figs. 8.3 8.3a and 8.3b, we see that the greater the separation between N and SN distributions, the larger the value of d′. This value does not change even when different experimental methods are used (Swets, 1959).

	RESPONSE		
STIMULUS		Yes	No
Present		0.78	0.22	1.00
Absent		0.17	0.83	1.00

Figure 8.2 Hypothetical results in the form of proportions for 100 test trials actually containing stimuli and 100 test trials actually without stimuli ("catch trials").

Several points will be of interest to the quantitatively oriented reader. It is assumed that SN and N are normally distributed with equal variances. Since σ is the square root of the variance, and the variances of SN and N are assumed to be equal, then only one value of σ need be shown. The value of d′ is equal to the square root of twice the energy in the signal (2E) divided by the noise power (N_O) in a band that is one cycle wide (Swets, Tanner, and Birdsall, 1961), or

$$d' = \sqrt{\frac{2E}{N_O}}$$

Tables of d′ are available in the literature (Elliot, 1964); however, a corrected value of d′ may be a more valid measure because the standard deviation of SN is actually larger than that of N in some cases (Theodore, 1972).

How, then, does a subject decide whether to say "yes" or "no" for a given separation between the N and SN curves? Consider the N and SN distributions in Fig. 8.4. A vertical line has been drawn through the overlapping N and SN distribution in each frame of this figure. This line represents the subject's **criterion** for responding. Whenever the energy is greater than that corresponding to the criterion the subject will say "yes." This occurs to the right of the criterion along the x-axis. On the other hand, the subject will say "no" if the energy is less than (to the left of) the criterion value. The value (or placement) of this criterion depends on several factors, which we will examine next.

161

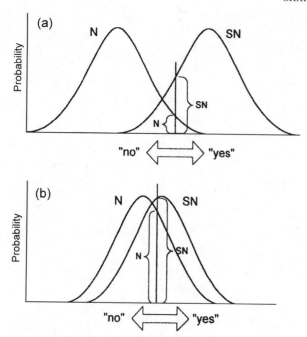

Figure 8.4 Criterion points (shown by vertical lines) for two degrees of overlapping of the noise alone (N) and signal-plus-noise (SN) distributions. The probabilities corresponding to the SN and N distributions at the criterion point are highlighted by brackets. Values of x below (to the left of) the criterion result in "no" decisions and those greater than (to the right of) the criterion yield "yes" decisions.

The first factor affecting the criterion may be expressed by the question "What is the probability that there is a noise alone compared to the probability that there is a signal-plus-noise for a given value of x?" For any point along the decision axis, this question is the same as comparing the height of the N curve with the height of the SN curve (Fig. 8.4). Otherwise stated, this value is the ratio of the likelihoods that the observation is from the N versus SN distributions for the two overlapping curves at any value of x. The ratio of these two probabilities is called **beta** (β). The value of the criterion is affected by the amount of overlap between the N and SN distributions, and by what the subject knows about the relative chances of a signal actually being presented.

Comparison of Figs. 8.4a and 8.4b shows how overlapping of the N and SN functions affects this ratio. At any point, the heights of the two curves becomes close as the separation between them decreases from that in Fig. 8.4a to that in Fig. 8.4b. An **ideal observer**, which is actually a mathematical concept rather than a real individual, would place the criterion point at the ratio which minimizes the chances of error, that is, at the point at which misses and false alarms are minimized. However, the placement of the criterion point will also be adjusted somewhat by what the subject knows about the chances of occurrence of a noise alone versus a signal-plus-noise. Let us now address ourselves to this factor.

Up to this point, it has been assumed that N and SN will be presented on a fifty-fifty basis. However, if the subject knows that a signal will actually be presented one-third of the time, then he will of course adjust his criterion β accordingly. In other words, he will adopt a stricter criterion. Alternatively, if the subject knows that a signal will occur more often than the noise alone, then he will relax his criterion for responding, adjusting for the greater chances of the signal actually being presented. The theoretical ideal observer always knows these probabilities; a real subject is often, but not always, told what they are.

The last factor that we will discuss which affects the final value of the criterion β has to do with how much a correct response is worth and how much a wrong response will cost. We are therefore concerned with the chance of an error associated with a particular criterion for responding. These chances are shown in Fig. 8.5. The subject will say "no" whenever the actual presentation falls to the left of the criterion, and will say "yes" when the presentation is to the right of the criterion. As a result of the fact that the N and SN distributions are overlapping, it turns out that there will be both "yes" and "no" decisions for a certain proportion of *both* signal and no-signal presentations. With the criterion placed as shown in the figure, most of the "yes" decisions will be in response to actual SN presentations; that is, the subject will say "yes" when there actually was a signal present. Recall that such a correct identification of the presence of the signal is called a *hit*. On the other hand, a certain percentage of the N trials will fall to the right of the criterion, so the subject will say "yes" even though there was actually no signal presented. This incorrect decision that a signal was present even though it really was not there is a *false alarm*. A stimulus–response table similar to the one in Fig. 8.1 is shown next to the N and SN distributions in Fig. 8.5 to illustrate how

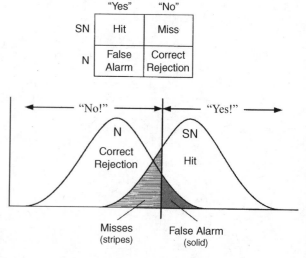

Figure 8.5 The four possible outcomes of a "yes" or "no" response based upon a given criterion value (*vertical line*). The corresponding stimulus–response table is shown to the right.

the two curves and the criterion relate to the possible outcomes of an experiment.

Now, suppose that a subject is told that it is imperative that he never miss a signal. He would thus move the criterion point toward the left to increase the hit rate; however, this shift would also have the effect of increasing the number of false alarms. This result would occur because moving the criterion toward the left increases the proportions of both the N and SN curves that fall inside of the "yes" region. On the other hand, suppose that the subject were advised that a false alarm is the worst possible error. Under such circumstances, the criterion point would be shifted toward the right, minimizing false alarms. Of course, this shift would also increase the number of misses, because a larger portion of the SN curve would now be in the "no" region.

Instead of telling the subject that one or another type of response is more (or less) important, the subject might be given a nickel for each correct response, lose three cents for a false alarm, etc. This, too, would cause the subject to adjust the criterion point so as to maximize the payoff associated with his responses. In effect, then, a set of values is attached to the responses so that each correct response has a **value** and each erroneous response has a **cost**.

An optimum criterion point (**optimum β**) is based upon the probabilities of the noise alone (p_N) and of the signal-plus-noise (p_{SN}) combined with the payoff resulting from the costs and values of each response. The *payoff* is the net result of the values of hits (V_H) and correct rejections (V_{CR}) and of the costs of misses (C_M) and false alarms (C_{FA}). In other words,

$$\text{optimum } \beta = \left(\frac{p_N}{p_{SN}} \right) \left(\frac{V_{CR} - C_{FA}}{V_H - C_M} \right)$$

The decision criterion is an attempt to maximize the payoff associated with the task. However, the subject in the real world is either not aware of all factors, or not able to use them as efficiently as the mathematically ideal observer. Therefore, the actual performance observed in an experiment generally falls short of what would have resulted had the subject been an ideal observer.

In summary, two types of information are obtained from the subject's responses in a TSD paradigm. One of these, d', is a measure of *sensitivity*, which is determined strictly by the separation between the noise and signal-plus-noise distributions and by the ability of the auditory system to make use of this separation. The other measure is the subject's *criterion* for responding, which does not affect the actual measure of sensitivity.

How can we show all of this information at the same time in a meaningful manner? Consider the effects of several different response criteria for the same value of d'. These criteria may be obtained by changing the directions given to the subject, or by changing the payoff scheme. Another way would be to have the subject rank the degree of certainty with which he makes each yes/no decision (see the discussion of TSD methods, below, for the rationale of this approach).

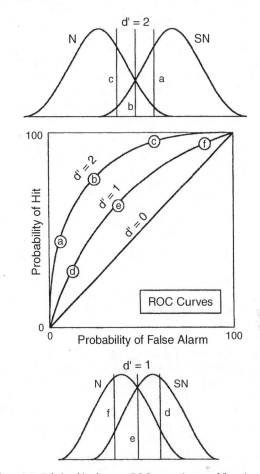

Figure 8.6 Relationships between ROC curves (center of figure) and the noise alone (N) and signal-plus-noise (SN) distributions for two values of d'. Sensitivity is depicted by the distance of the ROC curve from the diagonal. The upper set of distributions shows d' = 2, and the lower distributions show d' = 1. Various response criteria are indicated by the letters a–f.

For a given amount of sensitivity (i.e., a given value of d'), different criteria will result in different proportions of hits and false alarms. This result is shown for two arbitrarily selected values of d' in Fig. 8.6. We may plot the proportions of hits versus false alarms for each criterion point, as in the center of Fig. 8.6. Such a graph is called a **receiver-operating characteristic** or **ROC curve**. Notice that the ROC curve allows both the effects of sensitivity and response criterion to be illustrated at the same time. Sensitivity is shown by the distance of the ROC curve from the diagonal (at which d' = 0), or by the area under the ROC curve. On the other hand, the response criterion is indicated by the particular point along the ROC curve. Specifically, points a, b, and c in the figure (where d' = 2) differ in terms of sensitivity from points d, e, and f (for which d' = 1). However, even though points a, b, and c are the same in terms of sensitivity (d' = 2), they differ from each other in terms of response criteria. A similar relationship exists among points d, e, and f, where d' = 1.

PSYCHOPHYSICAL METHODS IN TSD

Yes/No Methods

This discussion of the theory of signal detection has dealt primarily with the yes/no method. To recapitulate: The subject is presented with a large number of trials for each stimulus level, and a large proportion of these are actually catch trials. For each trial, the subject says "yes" when a signal is detected and "no" when a signal is not detected. Fundamentally, then, the yes/no method in TSD is somewhat akin to the classical method of constant stimuli, although there are obvious differences in the number of trials, the large proportion of catch trials, and the manner of data analysis.

As in the classical methods, the TSD experiment is easily modified for use in a study of differential sensitivity. In this case, two signals are presented in a trial and the subject's task is to say "yes" ("they are different") or "no" ("they are not different").

The yes/no method is actually a subcategory of a larger class of experiments in which each trial contains one or two alternative signals. In this general case, the subject's task is to indicate which of two possible signals was present during the trial. For example, in the differential sensitivity experiment mentioned in the last paragraph, the decision is "same" versus "different", or else the subject might be asked to decide between two alternative speech sounds (e.g., /p/ and /b/) while some parameter is varied. In this light, the yes/no method might be thought of as a **single-interval forced-choice** experiment. In other words, the subject is presented with a stimulus interval during each trial and is required to choose between signal-plus-noise (one of the alternatives) and noise alone (the other alternative).

Two-Interval and N-Interval Forced-Choice Methods

Just as the subject may be asked to choose between two alternatives in a single-interval trial, he might also be asked to decide which of two successive intervals contained a signal. This approach is called the **two-interval forced-choice (2IFC)** or **two-alternative forced-choice (2AFC)** method. In this method, a test trial consists of two intervals, A and B, presented one after the other. One of the intervals (SN) contains the signal and the other one (N) does not. The subject must indicate whether the signal was presented in interval A or in interval B.

Experiments involving a choice between more than two choices are termed **multiple** or **N-interval** (or **alternative**) **forced-choice**, where N refers to the number of choices. For example, a 4IFC task would include four intervals (alternatives) in each test trial, among which the subject must choose the one that contained the signal.

Confidence Rating Methods

Recall that various points along the same ROC curve represent different response criteria with the same sensitivity d'. We might think of the response criterion as a reflection of how much confidence a subject has in his decision. In other words, a **strict** criterion means that the subject must have a great deal of confidence in his decision that the signal is present before he is willing to say "yes." In this case, the criterion value β is pushed toward the right along the decision axis. Alternatively, a **lax criterion** means that the subject does not require as much confidence in his "yes" decision, which moves the criterion point toward the left.

We might apply this relationship between the confidence in the decision and the criterion point by asking the subject to rate how much confidence he has in each of his responses. For example, the subject might be instructed to rate a "yes" response as "five" when he is absolutely positive that there was a signal, and "four" when he thinks there was a signal. A rating of "three" would mean "I'm not sure whether there was a signal or no signal." "Two" would indicate that there probably was no signal present, and a rating of "one" would suggest that the subject is positive that a signal was not presented. This procedure is the same as adopting a series of criterion points located successively from right to left along the decision axis. Thus, the use of **confidence ratings** enables the experimenter to obtain several points along the ROC curve simultaneously. This approach results in data comparable to those obtained by the previously discussed methods (Egan, Schulman, and Greenberg, 1959).

SOME IMPLICATIONS OF TSD

The theory of signal detection has importance in psychoacoustics because its application allows the experimenter to ferret out the effects of sensitivity and response criterion. Furthermore, TSD lends itself to experimental confirmation and can be used to test theories and their underlying assumptions. A key application of TSD has been the testing of the classical concept of threshold as an absolute boundary separating sensation from no sensation. It is implicit in this discussion that such a concept of a clear-cut threshold is not supported by TSD. However, the more general concept of threshold remains unresolved. Threshold theory is beyond the scope of this text. The interested student is therefore referred to the very informative discussions that may be found in the papers by Swets (1961) and by Krantz (1969).

REFERENCES

Egan, JP. 1975. Signal Detection Theory and ROC Analysis. New York, NY: Academic Press.

Egan, JP, Schulman, AI, Greenberg, GZ. 1959. Operating characteristics determined by binary decisions and by ratings. *J Acoust Soc Am* 31, 768–773.

Elliot, PB. 1964. Tables of d'. In: JA Swets (ed.), *Signal Detection and Recognition by Human Observers*. New York, NY: Wiley, 651—684.

Greene, DM, Swets, JA. 1974. *Signal Detection Theory and Psychophysics*. New York: Krieger.

Krantz, DH. 1969. Threshold theories of signal detection. *Psychol Rev* 76, 308–324.

Swets, JA. 1959. Indices of signal delectability obtained with various psychophysical procedures. *J Acoust Soc Am* 31, 511–513.

Swets, JA. 1961. Is there a sensory threshold? *Science* 134, 168–177.

Swets, JA (ed.). 1965. *Signal Detection and Recognition by Human Observers*. New York, NY: Wiley.

Swets, JA, Tanner, WP Jr, Birdsall, TG. 1961. Decision processes in perception. *Psychol Rev* 68, 301–340.

Theodore, LH. 1972. A neglected parameter: Some comments on "A table for calculation of d′ and β". *Psychol Bull* 78 260–261.

9 Auditory Sensitivity

The ear's extremely wide range of sensitivity is one of the most striking aspects of audition. The preceding chapters emphasized that hearing measurements are affected by psychophysical methods and other nonauditory factors; nevertheless, a reliable picture of auditory sensitivity has been provided by research over the years. Briefly, the ear is sensitive to a range of intensities from about 0 dB SPL (which is an amplitude of vibration of about the size of a hydrogen molecule) to roughly 140 dB (at which pain and damage to the auditory mechanism ensue). This **dynamic range** of the approximately 140 dB corresponds to a pressure ratio of 10 million to 1. In other words, the most intense sound pressure that is bearable is on the order of 10 million times as great as the softest one that is perceivable under optimum listening conditions. In terms of frequency, humans can hear tones as low as 2 Hz (although roughly 20 Hz is required for a perception of "tonality") and as high as about 20,000 Hz. Furthermore, the auditory system is capable of resolving remarkably small temporal differences.

The frequency and intensity sensitivities of the ear interact, affecting each other to a greater or lesser degree. In addition, when the duration of a sound is less than about half of a second, it affects both frequency and intensity sensitivity. Longer durations may be thought of as being infinitely long as far as auditory sensitivity is concerned.

Finally, the ear is able to discriminate small differences in a wide range of stimuli; that is, it has remarkable differential sensitivity—the ability to detect very small differences between similar sounds. This ability applies to all three parameters: intensity, frequency, and time.

So much for sweeping generalizations. Let us now look at some of the details.

ABSOLUTE SENSITIVITY

Minimum Audible Levels

The issue of **absolute sensitivity** is essentially one of describing how much sound intensity is necessary for a typical, normally hearing person to just detect the presence of a stimulus. We must realize at the outset that these values are actually measures of central tendencies (means, medians, and/or modes) that describe a group of ostensibly normal subjects. In addition, it is essential to know how and where the minimum audible sound intensity is measured.

Two fundamental methods have been used to measure the intensity of a minimum audible stimulus (Sivian and White, 1933). The first involves testing a subject's thresholds through earphones, and then actually monitoring the sound pressures in the ear canal (between the earphone and eardrum) that correspond to these thresholds. This procedure yields a measure of **minimum audible pressure (MAP)**. The alternative approach

is to seat the subject in a sound field and test his thresholds for sounds presented through a loudspeaker. The subject then leaves the sound field and the threshold intensity is measured with a microphone placed where his head had been. This method measures the **minimum audible field (MAF)**. It is important to dichotomize between the MAP and MAF methods because they result in different threshold values.

Ostensibly, MAP refers to the sound pressure at the eardrum. This quantity is monitored by placing a probe tube in the subject's ear canal. The probe tube passes through the earphone enclosure and leads to a microphone, which measures the sound pressure at the tip of the probe tube. Because it is difficult to place the probe right at the drum (as well as potentially painful and dangerous), the probe is generally located somewhere in the ear canal, as close to the drum as is practicable.

Minimum audible pressures are often stated in terms of the sound pressure generated by an earphone in a standardized 6-cc metal cavity (*6-cc coupler*), which approximates the volume under an earphone on the subject's ear. Such coupler pressures form the reference levels used in audiometric standards (see below). These **coupler-referred MAP** values are more appropriately called **MAPC** to distinguish them from the probe-tube MAP data obtained from actual ear canals (Killion, 1978).

Sivian and White reported the results of their classical MAP and MAF experiments in 1933. Their work was essentially confirmed by Dadson and King (1952) and by Robinson and Dadson (1956), whose data are shown in the lower portion of Fig. 9.1. These curves show monaural MAP and binaural MAF (from a loudspeaker located directly in front of the subject, i.e., at 0° azimuth) as a function of frequency. Monaural MAP values extending to very low frequencies are also shown. The MAP values for frequencies between 10,000 and 18,000 Hz are shown in the figure on an expanded frequency scale. As these MAP and MAF curves clearly show, human hearing is most sensitive between about 2000 and 5000 Hz, and reasonably good sensitivity is maintained in the 100 to 10,000 Hz range. Absolute sensitivity becomes poorer above and below these frequencies.

While the general relationship between auditory sensitivity and frequency is well established, one should be aware that subsequent experiments have provided detailed estimates of absolute sensitivity in the lower and upper frequency ranges. For example, one should refer to Berger (1981) for a detailed analysis of hearing sensitivity in the low-frequency range (50–1000 Hz), and to Schechter et al. (1986) for a detailed analysis of thresholds for the high frequencies (8000–20,000 Hz).

Notice in Fig. 9.1 that the MAF curve falls consistently below the MAP curve. In other words, a lower intensity is needed to reach threshold in a sound field (MAF) than under earphones (MAP). This fact was first demonstrated by Sivian and White (1933), and the discrepancy of 6 to 10 dB is called the "missing

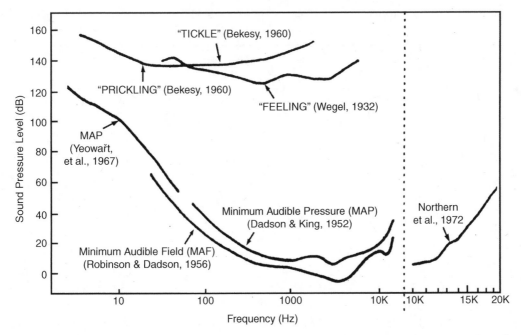

Figure 9.1 Minimal auditory field (MAF) after Robinson and Dadson (1956), and monaural minimal auditory pressure (MAP) after Dadson and King (1952) and Yeowart et al. (1967). The high-frequency MAP curve after Northern et al. (1972) is shown on the expanded scale to the right for clarity. Upper limits of "usable" hearing after Bekesy (1960) and Wegel (1932).

6 dB" (Munson and Wiener, 1952). Sivian and White proposed that the MAP/MAF discrepancy might be due to physiological noises picked up by the ear when it is covered by an earphone. These physiological noises would partially mask (see Chap. 10) the signal presented by the earphone, so that more sound pressure would be needed to achieve MAP than for the unmasked MAF. Although this explanation accounted for part of the missing 6 dB problem, it fell short of accounting for the whole difference.

Subsequent studies have formed the basis for resolving the MAP/MAF difference (Rudmose, 1963, 1982; Villchur, 1969, 1970, 1972; Morgan and Dirks, 1974; Stream and Dirks, 1974; Killion, 1978). This explanation was presented in a cohesive manner by Killion (1978). To begin with, recall from Chapter 3 that diffraction and ear canal resonance enhance the pressure of a free-field signal reaching the eardrum (Shaw, 1974). Thus, a corrected version of the international standard reference MAF curve (ISO-1961) may be converted to eardrum pressure by applying Shaw's (1974) head-related transfer function data. The correction accounts for an apparent error in the low-frequency MAF levels (Killion, 1978). Since binaural thresholds are somewhat better than monaural ones (see Chap. 13), a correction is also made to account for the advantage of binaural MAF over monaural MAP. By accounting for differences between real ear (MAP) and coupler (MAPC) values, the effects of impedance changes and ear canal distortion due to the placement of the earphone, and the effects of physiological noises, the MAP/MAF discrepancy is essentially resolved.

Threshold Microstructure

The MAP and MAF curves in Fig. 9.1 are drawn as smooth curves. It is commonly (and generally implicitly) assumed that an individual's threshold curve is similarly represented by a smooth line. The ubiquitous nature of this assumption is revealed by the fact that both clinicians and researchers make most of their threshold measurements at frequencies that are an octave apart, and very rarely sample at intervals that are less than a half-octave wide. However, this may not be the case (Elliot, 1958; van den Brink, 1970; Cohen, 1982; Long, 1984; Long and Tubis, 1988). Instead, a rippled or jagged configuration is often obtained when thresholds are sampled at numerous frequencies that are measured at very close intervals. Moreover, these patterns are highly repeatable. These irregularities in the threshold microstructure are associated with (particularly spontaneous) otoacoustic emissions, and it is believed that they reflect active processes in the cochlea (Wilson, 1980; Schloth, 1983; Zwicker and Schloth, 1983; Long, 1984; Long and Tubis, 1988; Talmadge et al., 1998, 1999). Discussions of active cochlear processes and otoacoustic emissions may be found in Chapter 4.

Upper Limits of Hearing

Just as we may conceive of the minimum audibility (MAP and MAF) curves as the lower limit of hearing sensitivity, the upper limits of hearing may be thought of as the sound pressure levels (SPLs) that are too loud or cause some kind of unpleasant sensation. These criteria are actually quite different. *Uncomfortable loudness* is usually what we mean by the upper limit of usable

Table 9.1 Reference Equivalent Threshold Sound Pressure Levels (RETSPLs) for Various Earphones in Decibels of Sound Pressure Level (dB SPL re: 20 μPa) in Appropriate Measurement Couplers

Frequency (Hz)	Supra-aural receivers in 6-cc [NBS-9A] coupler		Circumaural receivers in flat-plate coupler		Insert receivers (etymotic ER-3A & EARtone 3A) in:		
	Telephonics TDH-49 & 50	Telephonics TDH-39	Sennheiser HDA200	Koss HV/1A	HA-2 coupler	HA-1 coupler	Occluded ear simulator
125	47.5	45.0	30.5	–	26.0	26.5	28.0
250	26.5	25.5	18.0	–	14.0	14.5	17.5
500	13.5	11.5	11.0	–	5.5	6.0	9.5
750	8.5	8.0	6.0	–	2.0	2.0	6.0
1000	7.5	7.0	5.5	16.0	0.0	0.0	5.5
1500	7.5	6.5	5.5	–	2.0	0.0	9.5
2000	11.0	9.0	4.5	–	3.0	2.5	11.5
3000	9.5	10.0	2.5	–	3.5	2.5	13.0
4000	10.5	9.5	9.5	8.0	5.5	0.0	15.0
6000	13.5	15.5	17.0	–	2.0	−2.5	16.0
8000	13.0	13.0	17.5	16.5	0.0	−3.5	15.5
9000	–	–	18.5	21.0	–	–	–
10,000	–	–	22.0	25.5	–	–	–
11,200	–	–	23.0	24.5	–	–	–
12,500	–	–	28.0	26.0	–	–	–
14,000	–	–	36.0	33.0	–	–	–
16,000	–	–	56.0	51.0	–	–	–

Source: Based on ANSI S3.6-2004.

hearing. It refers to the level at which a sound is too loud to listen to for any appreciable period of time and is often referred to as the **uncomfortable loudness level (UCL)** or **loudness discomfort level (LDL)**. The LDL is associated with sound pressure levels approximating 100 dB (Hood and Poole, 1966, 1970; Hood, 1968; Morgan, Wilson, and Dirks, 1974), with higher mean LDLs of about 111 to 115 dB SPL reported by Sherlock and Formby (2005). On the other hand, the upper curves in Fig. 9.1 show that SPLs of about 120 dB or more produce sensations variously described as feeling, tickle, touch, tolerance, discomfort, or pain. Notice that these *unpleasant sensations* are actually *tactile* rather than auditory. High levels can produce temporary changes in hearing sensitivity and even permanent hearing loss and are discussed later in this chapter.

REFERENCE LEVELS

One might now ask what constitutes a reasonable conception of normal hearing sensitivity for the population as a whole. That is, how much SPL does the average person who is apparently free of pathology need to detect a particular sound? The answer permits standardization of audiometric instruments so that we may quantify hearing loss relative to "what normal people can hear."

Prior to 1964, several countries had their own standards for normal hearing and audiometer calibration based upon locally obtained data. For example, the 1954 British Standard (1954) was based upon one group of studies (Wheeler and Dickson,

1952; Dadson and King, 1952, whereas the 1951 American Standard (ASA-1951) reflected other findings (USPHS, 1935–1936; Steinberg et al., 1940). Unfortunately, these standards differed by about 10 dB, and the American Standard was too lax at 250 and 500 Hz, and too strict at 4000 Hz (Davis and Kranz, 1964). This situation was rectified in 1964 with the issuance of Recommendation R389 by the International Organization for Standardization (ISO-1964). This standard is generally referred to as ISO-1964. It was based upon a round-robin of loudness-balance and threshold experiments involving American, British, French, Russian, and German laboratories, and as a result equivalent reference SPLs were obtained for the earphones used by each country. These reference levels were subsequently incorporated into the S3.6 standard disseminated by the American National Standards Institute (ANSI S3.6-1969; now ANSI S3.6-2004).

The reference values for pure tone signals presented from various kinds of earphones are shown in Table 9.1.[1] These values are called **reference-equivalent threshold sound pressure levels (RETSPLs)** and are based on the current version of the *American National Standard Specification for Audiometers* (ANSI S3.6-2004), essentially corresponding to the ISO 389 standards

---

[1] The testing room must be very quiet in order to obtain auditory thresholds as low as those in Tables 9-1 to 9-3 (corresponding to 0 dB HL in Fig. 9.2). The maximum permissible noise levels for this purpose (ANSI S3.1−1999 [R2003]) are summarized in octave bands in Appendix 9-1 and in third-octave bands in Appendix 9-2.

Table 9.2 Sound Field Reference Equivalent Threshold Sound Pressure Levels (RETSPLs) in Decibels of Sound Pressure Level (dB SPL re: 20 μPa) at a Point Corresponding to the Listener's Head When Narrow Bands of Noise or Frequency Modulated Tones are Presented from Loudspeakers Located at Various Azimuths

| | Loudspeaker azimuth | | | |
| | 0° (front) | | 45° (side) | 90° (side) |
Center frequency[a] (Hz)	Monaural[b]	Binaural[c]	Monaural[b]	Monaural[b]
125	24.0	22.0	23.5	23.0
250	13.0	11.0	12.0	11.0
500	6.0	4.0	3.0	1.5
750	4.0	2.0	0.5	−1.0
1000	4.0	2.0	0.0	−1.5
1500	2.5	0.5	−1.0	−2.5
2000	0.5	−1.5	−2.5	−1.5
3000	−4.0	−6.0	−9.0	−6.5
4000	−4.5	−6.5	−8.5	−4.0
6000	4.5	2.5	−3.0	−5.0
8000	13.5	11.5	8.0	5.5

[a] Center frequencies of the narrow bands of noise or frequency-modulated tones used as test signals.
[b] Listening with one ear.
[c] Listening with both ears.
Source: Based on ANSI S3.6-2004.

(ISO-389-1-5,7, 1994a, 1994b, 1994c, 1998a, 1988b, 2005). Representative reference values for signals presented from loudspeakers are shown in Table 9.2 (ANSI S3.6-2004; ISO-389-7, 2005). Notice that these signals are narrow bands of noise or frequency modulated tones, which are employed because pure tones are subject to problems due to standing waves when used for sound field testing. In addition, separate values are provided for listening with one ear (monaurally) to sounds presented from different loudspeaker directions, and for listening with two ears (binaurally) when the speaker is located in front of the listener. Table 9.3 shows the reference values used when hearing is measured by bone conduction (ANSI S3.6-2004; ISO-389-3, 1994b). These values are called **reference-equivalent threshold force levels (RETFLs)** because they express the equivalent force (in dB re: 1 μN) on a measuring device known as a *mechanical coupler* or *artificial mastoid*, which corresponds to 0 dB HL when the bone-conduction vibrator is placed on a person's mastoid or forehead.

Hearing Level
Because each of the SPLs in Table 9.1 corresponds to minimum audibility, we may think of them as all representing the same **hearing level**. Thus, each RETSPL may also be referred to as 0 dB hearing level (0 dB HL) for its respective frequency. For example, the reference level for a 1000-Hz tone (for TDH-49 earphones) is 7.5 dB SPL so that 0 dB HL corresponds to 7.5 dB SPL at 1000 Hz. At 250 Hz, more sound pressure is required to reach the normal threshold so that 0 dB HL equals 26.5 dB SPL at this frequency. The relationship between SPL and HL is illustrated in Fig. 9.2. Figure 9.2a shows the minimally

audible (threshold) values in dB SPL as a function of frequency. As in Fig. 9.1, intensity increases upward on the y-axis. Figure 9.2b shows the same information in dB HL. Notice that the minimum audible values (0 dB HL) all lie along a straight line in terms of hearing level. In other words, the HL scale calls each zero reference SPL value "0 dB HL," so that thresholds can be measured in comparison to a straight line rather than a curved one.

The graph in Fig. 9.2b is the conventional **audiogram** used in audiology. Actually, the term "audiogram" may legitimately be used to describe any graph of auditory sensitivity as a function of frequency. By convention, increasing intensity (which indicates a hearing loss) is read downward on the y-axis when thresholds are plotted in dB HL.

Table 9.3 Reference Equivalent Threshold Force Levels (RETFLs) for Bone-Conduction Vibrators, Expressed in Decibels (dB) re: 1 μN Measured on a Mechanical Coupler (Artificial Mastoid)

Frequency (Hz)	Vibrator at mastoid	Vibrator at forehead
250	67.0	79.0
500	58.0	72.0
750	48.5	61.5
1000	42.5	51.0
1500	36.5	47.5
2000	31.0	42.5
3000	30.0	42.0
4000	35.5	43.5

Source: Based on ANSI S3.6-2004.

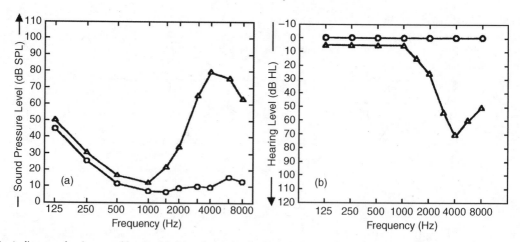

Figure 9.2 Audiograms showing normal hearing (*circles*) and a hearing loss in the high frequencies (*triangles*), expressed in (a) dB SPL and (b) dB HL. Note that intensity is shown downward on the clinical audiogram in dB HL.

Now, suppose that we measure the thresholds of a person whose cochlea has been partially damaged by excessive noise exposure. This kind of trauma often appears as a hearing loss in the higher frequencies. The triangles in Fig. 9.2 show the impaired thresholds in terms of both SPL and HL. The difference in dB between the impaired thresholds and the reference values (circles) is the amount of hearing loss at that frequency. For example, our hypothetical patient has a threshold of 5 dB HL at 1000 Hz. This means that he requires 5 dB HL to just detect the tone, as opposed to only 0 dB HL for a normal person. In SPL, this corresponds to a threshold of 12.5 dB (i.e., the 7.5 dB RETSPL) for 0 dB HL plus the 5 dB hearing loss. Had the threshold been 40 dB HL, the corresponding value would have been 47.5 dB SPL. Similarly, the 70 dB HL threshold at 4000 Hz is equivalent to 80.5 dB SPL (70 dB over the 10.5 dB RETSPL). As one might expect, audiometers are calibrated to dB HL values by measuring the output of the earphone in SPL at each frequency and then converting to HL by subtracting the appropriate RETSPL shown in Table 9.1.

Effects of Duration

Thus far we have been considering tones lasting for about 1 s or more. From the standpoint of audition, such durations may be viewed as infinite. Auditory sensitivity is altered, however, for durations much shorter than 1 s. Extremely short durations, on the order of 10 ms or less, result in transients that spread energy across the frequency range. These transients will confound the result of an experiment if they are audible (Wright, 1960, 1967), so that special care is needed in the design and interpretation of studies using short durations.

The perception of **tonality** appears to change in a somewhat orderly manner as the duration of a very short tone burst is increased (Burck et al., 1935; Doughty and Garner, 1947). A click is heard at the shortest durations, then a click with tonal qualities (*click pitch*) at slightly longer durations. For frequen-

cies below about 1000 Hz, a *tonal pitch* is perceived when the duration of the tone burst is long enough for the subject to hear several cycles (periods) of the tone. Thus, the duration threshold for tonality decreases from about 60 ms at 50 Hz to approximately 15 ms at 500 Hz. Above 1000 Hz, the threshold for tonality is essentially constant and is on the order of about 10 ms.

Absolute sensitivity decreases when the duration of a stimulus becomes much shorter than 1 s, and the nature of this phenomenon reveals an interesting property of the auditory system. Two observations are routinely encountered (Hughes, 1946; Zwislocki, 1960; Small et al., 1962; Campbell and Counter, 1969; Watson and Gengel, 1969). First, for durations up to roughly 200-300 ms, a 10-fold (decade) change in duration can offset an intensity change on the order of about 10 dB. In other words, reducing the duration of a tone burst at threshold from 200 to 20 ms (a decade reduction) reduces sensitivity to the degree that the intensity must be increased by 10 dB to re-attain threshold. Alternatively, the threshold intensity decreases by about 10 dB when the duration of a tone burst is increased from 20 to 200 ms. Second, durations longer than about 1/3 s are treated by the ear as though they are infinitely long. That is, increasing or decreasing durations that are longer than approximately 300 ms does not change the threshold level. These principles are shown in idealized form in Fig. 9.3.

The phenomenon under discussion is called **temporal integration** or **temporal summation**. It demonstrates that the ear operates as an energy detector that samples the amount of energy present within a certain time frame (or window). A certain amount of energy is needed within this time window for the threshold to be attached. This energy may be obtained by using a higher intensity for less time or a lower intensity for more time. The ear integrates energy over time *within* an integration time frame of roughly 200 ms. This interval might also be viewed as a period during which energy may be stored and can

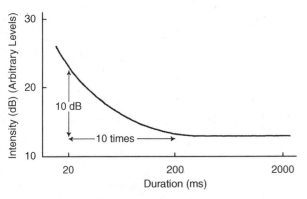

Figure 9.3 Idealized temporal integration function showing that a 10-times (decade) change in duration is offset by an intensity change of about 10 dB for stimulus durations up to about 200–300 ms.

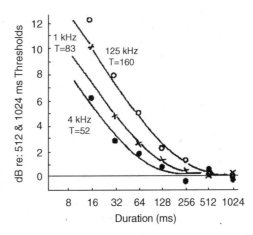

Figure 9.5 Effect of frequency on temporal integration. *Source*: Adapted from Watson and Gengel (1969), with Permission of *J. Acoust. Soc. Am.*

be measured as a time constant τ (Plomp and Bouman, 1959). Energy available for longer periods of time is not integrated with the energy inside the time window. This additional energy thus does not contribute to the detection of the sound, so that the threshold does not change for durations longer than 200 ms. Photographers might think of this situation as analogous to the interaction of a camera's f-stop (intensity) and shutter speed (duration) in summating the light energy for a certain film speed (integration time): The lens opening and shutter speed may be traded against one another as long as the same amount of light is concentrated upon the film. The trade-off between intensity and duration is illustrated conceptually in Fig. 9.4.

Figure 9.5 shows the effect of frequency upon temporal integration at threshold. Thresholds for shorter durations are shown relative to the threshold levels obtained for 512 ms, which are represented by the horizontal line. Notice that although temporal integration occurs for all frequencies shown, the functions become flatter (i.e., the time constant τ for integration becomes shorter) as frequency increases from 250 to 4000 Hz.

Temporal integration is observed at higher levels as well as at absolute threshold. Temporal summation of loudness is discussed in Chapter 11, and Chapter 3 covers this topic with respect to the acoustic reflex.

DIFFERENTIAL SENSITIVITY

Having examined the lower and upper bounds of hearing, we may now ask what is the smallest perceivable difference between two sounds. This quantity is called either the **difference limen (DL)** or the **just noticeable difference (jnd)**. These terms will be used interchangeably in this text. The DL is the smallest perceivable difference in dB between two intensities (ΔI) or the smallest perceivable change in hertz between two frequencies (Δf). We may think of the jnd in two ways. One is as the absolute difference between two sounds, and the other is as the relative difference between them. The latter is obtained by dividing the absolute DL by the value of the starting level. Thus, if the starting level I is 1000 units and the DL or ΔI is 50 units, then the relative DL, $\Delta I/I$, is 50/1000 = 0.05. This ratio, $\Delta I/I$, is called the **Weber fraction**.

A point about absolute versus relative DLs should be clarified before proceeding. The frequency DL or Δf is an absolute difference in hertz, as opposed to the relative frequency DL obtained by dividing Δf by the starting frequency f. Suppose it is necessary to change a 1000-Hz tone (f) by a 3.6 Hz Δf in order for a particular subject to just detect the frequency difference. His absolute frequency DL is thus 3.6 Hz, whereas his relative DL is 0.0036. However, the situation is different when the intensity DL is given in decibels, which is usually expressed as ΔI **in dB** or $10\log\frac{I+\Delta I}{I}$. Since decibels are actually ratios, ΔI in dB is really a relative value. (This is why ΔI and I were expressed as "units" in the above example.) Both $\Delta I/I$ and ΔI in dB are commonly encountered in the literature. Let's use two examples to illustrate the relationship between $\Delta I/I$ and ΔI in dB or $10\log\frac{I+\Delta I}{I}$.

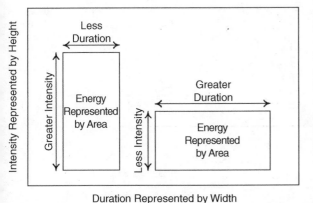

Figure 9.4 Artist's conceptualization of temporal integration depicting the trade-off between stimulus intensity and duration.

If $\Delta I/I = 1.0$, then ΔI in dB would be $10\log\frac{1+1}{1} = 10\log2$, or 3 dB. When $\Delta I/I$ is 0.5, then ΔI in dB $= 10\log\frac{1+0.5}{1} = 1.76$dB.

An important concept in psychophysics is known as **Weber's law**, which states that the value of $\Delta I/I$ (the Weber fraction) is a constant (k) regardless of stimulus level, or

$$\frac{\Delta I}{I} = k$$

Similarly, ΔI in dB or $10\log\frac{1+\Delta I}{I}$ would also be the same across stimulus levels. A classic conceptual illustration of Weber's law is the number of candles one must add to a number of candles that are already lit in order to perceive a difference in the amount of light (Hirsh, 1952). If 10 candles are lit, then only one more will produce a jnd of light (DL = 1). However, if there are originally 100 candles then 10 must be added to result in a perceptible difference, and to notice an increase in the light provided by 1000 candles, 100 must be added. Thus, the absolute value of the DL increases from 1 to 100, whereas the Weber fraction has remained constant, at k = 0.1 (since 1/10 = 10/100 = 100/1000 = 0.1), illustrating Weber's law.

Intensity Discrimination

Early differential sensitivity experiments (Knudsen, 1923) were plagued by audible transient noises due to the abrupt switching on and off of the stimuli, making it unclear whether subjects were responding to the stimulus or to the audible transient. In his classical study, Riesz (1928) overcame the switching noise problem by using **amplitude modulation (AM)** to produce intensity differences, as illustrated in Fig. 9.6a. Amplitude modulation was produced by simultaneously presenting two tones of slightly different frequencies, resulting in a tone that **beats** (fluctuates in intensity) at a rate equal to the difference in frequency between the two original tones. For example, combining a 1000-Hz tone with a 1003-Hz tone results in three beats per second, which Riesz found to be the optimal rate for

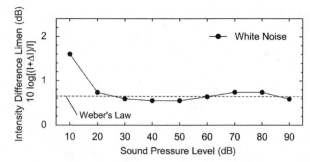

Figure 9.7 The intensity difference limen in decibels shown as a function of stimulus level for white noise based on the data of Houtsma, Durlach, and Braida (1980). The horizontal dashed line has been drawn through the data to represent Weber's law.

measuring intensity DLs in his study. To find the DL, Riesz's subjects adjusted the amplitude of one of the two beating tones until the beats became minimally audible. The intensity difference between the two tones was then taken as the measure of the DL. Technological advances made it possible for later studies to measure intensity DL by using pulsed pure tones, as illustrated in Fig. 9.6b.

The size of ΔI in dB is shown as a function of stimulus level for white noise in Fig. 9.7 and for pure tones in Fig. 9.8. Weber's law predicts that ΔI in dB should be the same at all stimulus levels, represented by the dashed horizontal lines in these figures. Weber's law appears to hold for broadband stimuli like white noise (e.g., Houtsma et al., 1980; Wojtczak and Viemeister, 2008). For example, Fig. 9.7 shows that the Weber fraction for white noise (expressed as $10\log\frac{1+\Delta I}{I}$) is constant at about 0.6 to 0.8 dB except for the faintest stimulus level.

The situation is different for narrow band signals like pure tones, for which the Weber fraction decreases somewhat as the stimulus level increases (Riesz, 1928; McGill and Goldberg, 1968a, 1968b; Viemeister, 1972; Moore and Raab, 1974;

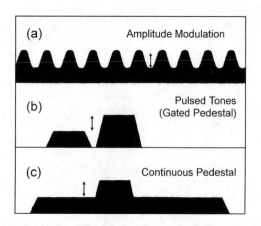

Figure 9.6 Artist's conceptualizations of various methods used to obtain the DL for intensity (see text): (a) amplitude modulation, (b) pulsed tones or gated pedestal, and (c) continuous pedestal.

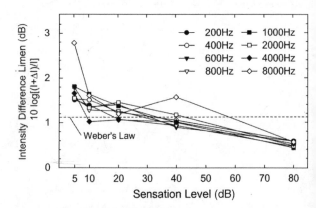

Figure 9.8 The intensity difference limen in decibels shown as a function of stimulus level for pure tones based on the data of Jesteadt, Wier, and Green (1977). The horizontal dashed line has been drawn through the data to represent Weber's law.

Jesteadt et al., 1977; Houtsma et al., 1980; Florentine et al., 1987; Viemeister and Bacon, 1988; Turner et al., 1989; Stellmack, Viemeister, and Byrne, 2004; Wojtczak and Viemeister, 2008). For example, Figure 9.8 shows that the Weber fraction decreases with increasing intensity from about 1.7 dB at a sensation level (SL) of 5 dB to about 0.5 dB at 80 dB SL. This slight deviation from Weber's law has come to be known as the **near miss to Weber's law** (McGill and Goldberg, 1968a, 1968b).[2]

Rabinowitz et al. (1976) combined and summarized the results for differential sensitivity at 1000 Hz. Their analysis suggested that Weber's law holds between 10 and 40 dB SL, although differential sensitivity changes with sensation level above and below this range. Viemeister and Bacon (1988) similarly suggested that the function relating the relative DL for intensity to sensation level can be approximated by a horizontal line segment between about 20 and 50 dB SL and a sloping one for higher levels. Informative discussions if Weber's law and the near miss are provided by, for example, Florentine et al. (1987), Viemeister and Bacon (1988), Green (1988), and Wojtczak and Viemeister (2008).

Riesz (1928), using the amplitude modulation method, reported that the Weber fraction is frequency dependent, becoming smaller as frequency increased from 35 Hz up to about 1000 Hz. The Weber fraction remained more or less constant for the frequencies above this, at least for SLs above 20 dB. However, this result has not been confirmed by subsequent studies (e.g., Harris, 1963; Schacknow and Raab, 1973; Penner et al., 1974; Jesteadt et al., 1977). For example, Jesteadt et al. (1977) found that $\Delta I/I$ does not change with frequency so that a single straight line could be used to show $\Delta I/I$ as a function of sensation level. The similarity of the functions relating ΔI in dB to sensation level at various frequencies can be seen Fig. 9.8. Florentine et al. (1987) investigated intensity DLs over a wide frequency range from 250 to 12,000 Hz. They did find a frequency dependency for the high frequencies, but not for the frequencies up to about 4000 Hz (similar to the findings by Jesteadt et al.).

Some of the variability existing in the intensity DL data may be due to the use of alternative methods of presenting the stimuli. Recall here that the DL experiment basically asks whether the subject can hear a difference (which is equal to ΔI) between a baseline signal presented at an intensity of I and a more intense signal presented at an intensity of $(I + \Delta I)$. We might call the baseline signal the pedestal. There are two general ways to present the increment.

One approach involves leaving the pedestal (I) on all the time and to add an intensity increment (ΔI) on top of it at various times. This is the **continuous pedestal** method and is shown schematically in lower frame (c) of Fig. 9.6. Alternatively, a pedestal alone (I), which may be presented for some period of time, and then be turned off, followed after a brief interval by the presentation of the pedestal together with the increment on top of it $(I + \Delta I)$. This strategy may be called the **gated pedestal** method and is shown in the middle frame (b) of Fig. 9.6. Turner, Zwislocki, and Filion (1989) pointed out that the continuous pedestal method is analogous to the types of listening conditions used in early DL studies (e.g., Riesz, 1928; Lüscher and Zwislocki, 1949; Jerger, 1952), while the pulsed-tone methods used by Jesteadt et al. (1977) and other more recent studies (e.g., Florentine and Buus, 1981; Florentine et al., 1987; Viemeister and Bacon, 1988; Turner et al., 1989) involve the gated pedestal technique.

Quite a few studies have directly or indirectly compared intensity DLs using the continuous and gated pedestal methods (e.g., Campbell and Lasky, 1967; Green, 1969; Green et al., 1979; Carlyon and Moore, 1986a; Viemeister and Bacon, 1988; Turner et al., 1989; Bacon and Viemeister, 1994). The general finding has been that smaller intensity DLs are produced by the continuous pedestal method than by the gated pedestal approach. Representative mean results from the study by Turner et al. are shown in Fig. 9.9 for stimuli presented at three frequencies. The reason(s) for the gated-continuous difference is not

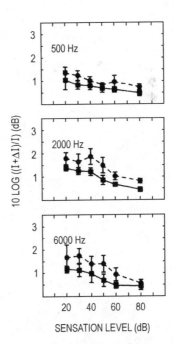

Figure 9.9 Intensity DLs in decibels (as $10\log\frac{I+\Delta I}{I}$) as a function of sensation level at three frequencies for the continuous (*squares/solid lines*) versus gated (*circles/dashed lines*) pedestal methods. *Source*: From Turner et al. (1989), with permission of *J. Acoust. Soc. Am.*

---

[2] A "severe departure" from Weber's law occurs under certain conditions (see Carlyon and Moore, 1984, 1986a, 1986b; Moore, 1984, 1986a,b). Here, a large increase in the Weber fraction is found at about 55–65 dB SPL for very brief high-frequency signals presented under the gated (versus continuous) pedestal condition, and for the detection of a signal in a band-reject masker, expressed as the signal-to-noise ratio.

clearly established. Turner et al. (1989) have suggested that it might involve a short-term memory effect, and that (citing data by Gescheider et al.) it is probably not a specifically auditory phenomenon because similar findings are also found for touch.

In summary, differential sensitivity for intensity follows Weber's law for wide-band noise and becomes slightly more acute with increasing sensation level in a manner that is a "near miss" to Weber's law for narrow-band stimuli like pure tones.

Frequency Discrimination

The early work (Knudsen, 1923) on differential sensitivity for frequency, like that on intensity discrimination was plagued by transient noise problems associated with the presentation of the stimuli. Shower and Biddulph (1931) circumvented this problem by using **frequency-modulated (FM)** tones as the stimuli. In other words, the test tone was varied continuously in frequency at a rate of twice per second. The subject's task was to detect the presence of a modulated tone as opposed to a steady tone. The DL was taken as the smallest difference in frequency that produced a perceptible modulation of the original tone. Since Shower and Biddulph's classic study included a very wide range of frequencies (62–11, 700 Hz) and sensation levels (5–80 dB), it has remained the most widely cited study of differential frequency sensitivity for many years. However, subsequent studies using pulsed tones have generally resulted in better (smaller) DLs at low frequencies and poorer (larger) DLs at higher frequencies than were found with the FM tones (Harris, 1952; Rosenblith and Stevens, 1953; Henning, 1967; Nordmark, 1968; Moore, 1973; Jesteadt and Wier, 1977; Wier et al., 1977; Nelson et al., 1983). We shall return to this point below. The most likely reason for the discrepancy is that frequency modulation results in a stimulus with a complex spectrum, so that we really cannot be sure what serves as the basis for the subject's responses.

Wier et al. (1977) reported the results of an extensive frequency-discrimination study using pulsed pure tones from 200 to 8000 Hz at sensation levels between 5 and 80 dB. They took the DL to be the smallest frequency difference Δf that the subject could detect 71% of the time. Fig. 9.10 shows some of their results at four sensation levels. The important observations are that Δf becomes larger as frequency increases, and that Δf becomes smaller as sensation level increases. Sensation level is relatively more important at low frequencies than at high ones, where the curves tend to converge. The best (smallest) values of Δf—on the order of 1 Hz—occur for low frequencies presented at about 40 dB SL or more. The DL increases substantially above about 1000 Hz so that Δf at 40 dB SL is roughly 16 Hz at 4000 Hz and 68 Hz by 8000 Hz. Figure 9.10 also shows that Δf is not simply a monotonic function of frequency; it does not always get larger as frequency increases. We see a departure from a monotonically rising function between 200 and 400 Hz. (There are also rather dramatic peaks in the vicinity of 800 Hz, although their origin is unclear.)

Other studies using pulsed tones at various frequencies and sensation levels are in essential agreement with the findings of

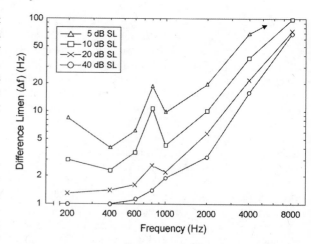

Figure 9.10 The frequency difference limen Δf is shown as a function of frequency at sensation levels of 5, 10, 20, and 40 dB, based the on data of Wier, Jesteadt, and Green (1977).

Wier et al. (Harris, 1952; Moore, 1973; Jesteadt and Wier, 1977; Nelson et al., 1983). Nordmark's data (1968) are in agreement with those of Wier et al. when the latter are corrected for differences in experimental methodology (Wier et al., 1976). Nelson et al. (1983) replicated the Wier et al. study using a somewhat different methodology. On the basis of their data, they developed a general equation to predict frequency discrimination given the frequency and level of the stimulus. This approach also predicted the data of Weir et al. extremely well and was also able to successfully estimate earlier frequency DL data of Harris (1952).

Relative differential sensitivity for frequency is shown as the Weber fraction $\Delta f/f$ for the data of Wier et al. (1977) in Fig. 9.11. Notice that $\Delta f/f$ improves (becomes smaller) as SL increases and

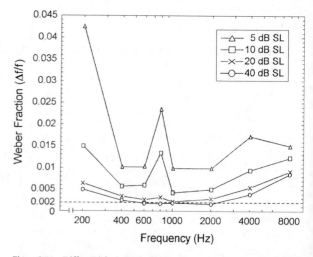

Figure 9.11 Differential sensitivity $\Delta f/f$ is shown as a function of frequency at sensation levels of 5, 10, 20, and 40 dB, based on the data of Wier, Jesteadt, and Green (1977).

is about 0.006 or less for frequencies as high as 4000 Hz when the tone level reaches 20 dB SL. The Weber fraction becomes as small as approximately 0.002 for frequencies between 400 and 2000 Hz at 40 dB SL, which corresponds to a frequency difference of just 0.2%. The value of $\Delta f/f$ is relatively constant for moderate sensation levels between about 400 and 2000 Hz, but becomes larger at higher and lower frequencies. In summary, then, $\Delta f/f$ is a somewhat complex function of both frequency and level, unlike ΔI in dB, which appears to depend principally upon stimulus level alone for a reasonably wide range of frequencies.

Profile Analysis

The discrimination of changes in spectral configuration is called **profile analysis** (Green, 1983, 1988). These differences in spectral shape are important factors contributing to the distinction between sound qualities or timbers (Chap. 12) and among speech sounds (Chap. 14).

Profile analysis experiments involve asking subjects to listen for a difference in the level of one component of a complex sound compared to the other components of the sound. This is a lot like an intensity DL, but instead of listening for a level difference between two sounds, the comparison is being made across frequencies within the same sound. The typical approach uses a two-alternative forced choice method, as illustrated in Fig. 9.12. Both intervals contain complex sounds made up of the same component frequencies. All of the components are equal in level in the comparison sound, illustrated by the left (interval 1) spectrum for trial a in the figure. In the target sound, all but one of the components are equal in level, but the remaining component is higher in level, as in the right (interval 2) spectrum for trial a. The larger component (highlighted with a thicker line) is the *signal* and the equal-level components are called the *background*. The subject's task is to choose the interval containing the target signal (interval 2 in this case). In this context, the threshold is the smallest level increment necessary to detect the signal above the background.

A special technique is needed to induce the subject to listen for a level difference across frequencies between the signal and the background instead of a difference between the overall levels of the two sounds. The approach is called **roving levels**, and it involves randomly varying the overall levels of both the comparison and target sounds over a large range (usually about 40 dB) from trial to trial. This concept is easily appreciated by seeing how the amplitudes of the spectra change across the six trials illustrated in Fig. 9.12. The ensuing jumble of levels prevents the subject from choosing the target sound by comparing its level to that of the comparison sound. In addition, the listener is given feedback (indicating which interval contained the target sound) after each response. As a result, the subject learns to pick the target sound based on the across-frequencies comparison between the signal and background (i.e., the spectral profile).

Figure 9.12 illustrates the typical profile analysis experiment, in which the components are equally spaced logarithmically in frequency, the signal (usually about 1000 Hz) is the center frequency, and the background frequencies all have the same level. Although our discussion focuses upon this basic arrangement, the student should be aware that others have also been used, such as multiple-component signals (e.g., Green and Kidd, 1983; Bernstein and Green, 1987; Green et al., 1987), jagged spectra (e.g., Kidd et al., 1991; Lenze and Richards, 1998), and signals involving decrements in level (e.g., Heinz and Formby, 1999).

Let us summarize several of the principal features of profile analysis. The interested student should refer to the papers cited and Green's (1988) classical book, *Profile Analysis*. Discriminations in profile analysis appear to be most sensitive (thresholds are lowest) when the signal frequency is in the midrange of the sound's spectrum, usually in the vicinity of about 500 to 2000 Hz (Green and Mason, 1985; Green et al., 1987). Thresholds become lower as the range of frequencies in the sound (bandwidth) widens and as the number of components within that range (spectral density) gets larger (Green et al., 1983, 1984; Bernstein and Green, 1987). However, the threshold becomes poorer due to masking (Chap. 10) when adding components that are close in frequency to the signal (Green et al., 1983; Bernstein and Green, 1987). Thresholds do not appear to be affected by the phase relationships among the components (Green et al., 1984; Green and Mason, 1985). In addition, Green and Mason (1985) found that the size of the increment (in dB) needed for a 1000-Hz signal to be discriminated from the background stayed the same for a range of background components from 30 to 70 dB SPL (although the increment became smaller at 80 dB). Thus, the intensity discrimination involved in profile analysis appears to follow Weber's law over a fairly wide range of levels. This is similar to what we saw for ΔI in dB for broadband noise earlier in the chapter.

Temporal Resolution

The importance of being able to make fine temporal discriminations should become obvious when one realizes that speech is made up of signals that change rapidly over time. We will briefly look at several general aspects of the temporal realm. The first deals with temporal resolution, the second with the nature of successiveness and temporal order, and the last is the difference limen for duration.

Temporal resolution refers to the shortest period of time over which the ear can discriminate two signals. One way to measure this period is by asking a subject to discriminate between signals that are exactly the same except for a phase difference. Green (1971, 1973a, 1973b) has referred to this quantity as **temporal auditory acuity** or **minimum integration time**. The latter phrase suggests that the ear's most sensitive temporal discriminations also provide an estimate of the shortest time period within which the ear can integrate energy. We could think of this time period as the "low end" of the scale for temporal integration, as discussed earlier in the chapter.

Temporal resolution has been studied using a variety of approaches, such as the temporal modulation transfer function and gap detection (e.g., Patterson and Green, 1970; Ronken,

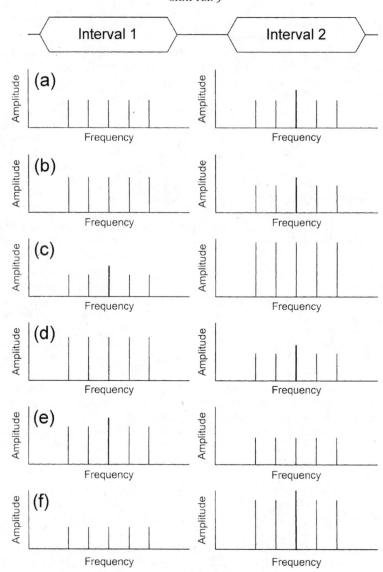

Figure 9.12 The typical profile-analysis experiment employs a two-interval forced choice procedure with roving levels. The time course of the two intervals is shown at the top of the figure, and the spectra of the sounds in intervals 1 and 2 are shown for six trials, labeled (a)–(f). The subject's task is to indicate which interval contains a level difference between the signal frequency (indicated by the thicker line) and the background frequencies. Notice that the overall levels of the comparison and target sounds are varied from trial to trial.

1970; Green, 1971, 1973a, 1973b, 1985; Viemeister, 1979; Forest and Green, 1987; Formby and Muir, 1988). The **temporal modulation transfer function** (TMTF) addresses the ability to detect the presence of amplitude modulation in a sound (e.g., Viemeister, 1979; Bacon and Viemeister, 1985; Formby and Muir, 1988). The basic method is illustrated in Fig. 13a, which shows the envelopes of two noises presented one after the other in a two-interval forced-choice paradigm. One of these signals is a noise that has been subjected to **sinusoidal amplitude modulation** (SAM), and the other signal is the same noise without modulation. The subject's task is to select the amplitude

modulated noise. This is a measure of temporal acuity because the amplitude fluctuations are occurring over time: the faster the **modulation rate** or **frequency** (the number of modulations per second), the closer together in time are the fluctuations (Fig. 9.13b). The listener's sensitivity for hearing the presence of amplitude modulation is measured in terms of **modulation depth**, or how deep the amplitude fluctuations must be in order for them to be detected (Fig. 9.13c).

Typical TMTFs are illustrated in Fig. 9.14 using data from two representative studies and show how much modulation depth is needed for modulation to be detected by the listener at

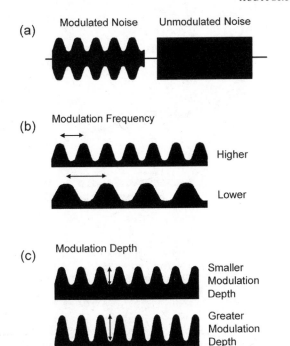

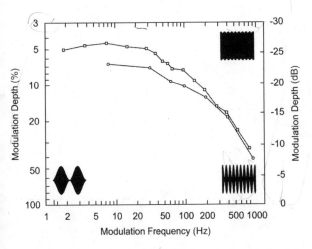

Figure 9.13 Artist's conceptualizations of (a) amplitude-modulated versus unmodulated noises, (b) different modulation rates, and (c) different modulation depths.

different modulation frequencies. Modulation depth is usually expressed in percent or decibels. When expressed in decibels, 0 dB corresponds to 100%, with smaller modulation depths given in decibels below 0 dB. For example, −6 dB would be 50%, −12 dB would be 25%, and −20 dB would be 10% modulation.

Figure 9.14 Examples of temporal modulation transfer functions based on the data of Bacon and Viemeister (1985; *squares*) and Formby and Muir (1988; *circles*). The inserts are artist's conceptualizations of stimulus waveforms to show that modulation frequency increases from left to right along the x-axis, and modulation depth decreases from bottom to top on the y-axis.

Moreover, TMTFs are plotted with maximum (100% or 0 dB) modulation depth and the bottom of the y-axis. The figure shows that the TMTF has a low-pass configuration. The ability to detect modulation is most sensitive for modulation frequencies up to about 50 Hz, and then decreases considerably above about 100 Hz.

A lucid appreciation of temporal resolution is provided by the **gap detection** technique, which has been employed by numerous investigators since it was introduced by Plomp in 1964 (e.g., Penner, 1977; Fitzgibbons, 1983; Shailer and Moore, 1983; Fitzgibbons and Gordon-Salant, 1987; Forest and Green, 1987; Formby and Muir, 1988; Moore et al., 1992; Schneider et al., 1994; Trehub et al., 1995; Phillips, Taylor, Hall, et al., 1997; Lister, Besing, and Koehnke, 2002; Phillips and Smith, 2004; Elangovan and Stuart, 2008). The basic strategy of the gap detection experiment is actually quite straightforward. Suppose we have a continuous burst of noise lasting 500 ms. We could "chop out" a short segment in the center of the noise lasting, say, 10 ms. We now have a (leading) noise burst lasting 245 ms, followed by a 10-ms silent period, followed by a (trailing) 245 ms noise burst. Hence, we have a *gap* lasting 10 ms surrounded in time by leading and trailing noise bursts. Three different gap durations are illustrated schematically in Fig. 9.15. The subject is asked whether he hears the gap, hence, the paradigm is called gap detection. The duration of the gap is varied according to some psychophysical method (see Chaps. 7 and 8) in order to find the shortest detectable gap between the two noise bursts, which is called the **gap detection threshold (GDT)**. Thus, the GDT reflects the shortest time interval we can resolve, and it is taken as a measure of temporal resolution.

The essential finding of GDT experiments is that auditory temporal resolution is on the order of 2 to 3 ms. Such GDTs are obtained when the noise signal contains the higher frequencies and when these are presented at levels that are adequately audible. That the ear can make temporal discriminations as small as about 2 ms is a consistent finding for the various approaches that have been used to study temporal auditory acuity, and is analogous to what Hirsh (1959) Hirsh and Sherrick (1961) described as auditory **successiveness** (versus simultaneity). Interested students will find detailed discussions of gap detection parameters in many sources (e.g., Fitzgibbons, 1983; Shailer and Moore, 1983; Buus and Florentine, 1985; Green, 1985; Forest and Green, 1987; Phillips, 1999; Elangovan and Stuart, 2008).

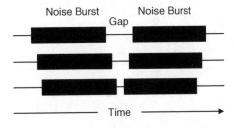

Figure 9.15 Artist's conceptualization of the gap detection paradigm with three different gap durations.

It is noteworthy, however, that 2 to 3 ms GDTs are found when the two sounds separated by the gap are the same, as in Fig. 9.16a. In contrast, GDTs are much longer (typically exceeding 20 ms) when the leading and following sounds differ in various ways, such as in terms of their spectra and/or durations (Phillips et al., 1997; Lister et al., 2002; Phillips and Smith, 2004; Elangovan and Stuart, 2008). Figure 9.16b shows an example, in which the two sounds differ in frequency. These examples reveal a distinction between with-channel and across-channel processing (e.g., Phillips, 1999; Elangovan and Stuart, 2008): Hearing the gap simply involves detecting a discontinuity between the two sounds when the two sounds are the same (i.e., within the same auditory filter channel), as in frame **a**, which can be accomplished by the peripheral auditory system. In contrast, the comparison is more complex when the two sounds are different (i.e., in different auditory channels), which requires central processing across auditory channels. Similarly longer temporal intervals are needed for **perceived temporal order**, which involves determining which of two different sounds came first (e.g., "high" and "low") as in Fig. 9.16b, and for detecting differences in the onset times of two otherwise simultaneous tones, as in Fig. 9.16c (e.g., Hirsh, 1959; Hirsh and Sherrick, 1961; Pisoni, 1977).

Temporal Discrimination

Earlier in this chapter, we saw that ΔI depends mainly upon intensity and that Δf is appreciably affected by both intensity and frequency. Differential sensitivity for the duration of a signal has also been investigated, although not as extensively as the other two parameters. The general finding is that the **difference limen for duration** (ΔT) becomes smaller as the overall duration decreases (Small and Campbell, 1962; Abel, 1972; Sinnott et al., 1987; Dooley and Moore, 1988). Abel (1972) studied ΔT

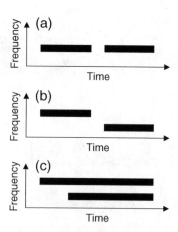

Figure 9.16 Examples of stimulus arrangements for tasks involving (a) gap detection when both signals are the same (within channel), (b) gap detection when the two sounds differ in frequency (between channels), and (c) detection of temporal onset time between two otherwise simultaneous signals differing in frequency. Arrangement (b) also shows the arrangement of a temporal order task, where the listener indicates whether the higher or lower signal came first.

for stimulus durations between 0.16 and 960 ms, using various bandwidths of noise from 200 to 300 Hz wide as well as 1000 Hz tone bursts. She presented subjects with two intervals, one containing a standard stimulus duration (T) and the other containing a slightly longer duration (T + ΔT). The subject listened to the two intervals (which were presented randomly) and indicated the one with the longer-duration signal. The smallest time difference correctly detected 75% of the time was taken as the DL for duration ΔT. As Figure 9.17 shows, ΔT decreases from about 50 ms at durations of 960 ms to on the order of

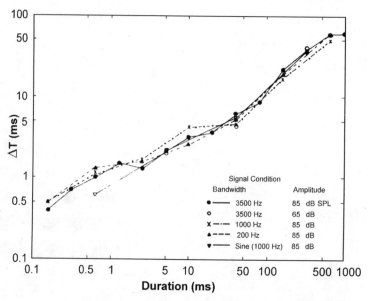

Figure 9.17 Values of ΔT as a function of duration from 0.16 to 960 ms. *Source*: From Abel (1972), with permission of *J. Acoust. Soc. Am.*

0.5 ms for durations of less than 0.5 ms. Differential sensitivity in terms of the Weber fraction $\Delta T/T$ is not a constant, but changes with duration so that $\Delta T/T$ is about 1.0 at 0.5 to 1 ms, roughly 0.3 at 10 ms, and approximately 0.1 from 50 to 500 ms. The results were essentially independent of bandwidth and intensity. Observations by Sinnott et al. (1987) and Dooley and Moore (1988) were in essential agreement with these findings.

Stimulus Uncertainty

Figure 9.18 illustrates a discrimination experiment in which the subjects are presented with pairs of tonal sequences (Watson et al., 1975, 1976; Watson and Kelly, 1981). Each sequence involves 10 brief tones arranged in a certain pattern of frequencies, one after the other. The sequences are the same in both intervals of each trial, except that the frequency of one of the tones may be changed in the second interval. The listener's task is to indicate whether the two sequences are the same or different. The smallest frequency difference that allows the subject to tell the two sequences apart constitutes a frequency DL, but the outcome is clearly being affected by the complexity of the task as well as by the frequency difference itself. (It is also possible to change more than one of the frequencies, or to vary the amplitude or duration.)

The nature of the task can be altered in various ways. The position of the tone being changed (shown by arrows in the figure) may be the same in every trial, such as always second (trial *a*) or always ninth (trial *b*), or it might occur in different positions from trial to trial. It is also possible for the overall pattern of the tones to be the same in every trial (e.g., *a* and *b*), or for the patterns to change from trial to trial (e.g., b and c). Stimulus arrangements that keep changing from trial to trial present the listener with considerably more uncertainty than trials that are always the same. In fact, the general observation has been that discrimination performance deteriorates when the listener must deal with greater amounts of stimulus uncertainty compared to lesser degrees of uncertainty about the stimuli (e.g., Watson et al., 1975, 1976; Watson and Kelly, 1981; Howard et al., 1984; Leek et al., 1991; Neff and Jesteadt, 1996; Kidd et al., 2002).

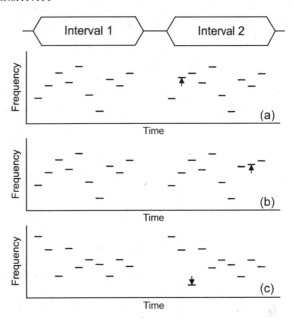

Figure 9.18 Schematic illustration of discrimination experiments in which subjects must determine whether pairs of 10-tone sequences are the same or different based on a frequency difference affecting one tone in the sequence. The frequency changes are highlighted by arrows and occur for the 2nd tone in trial a, the 9th tone in trial b, and the 3rd tone in trial c. Notice that the overall tonal patterns are similar in trials a and b, and is different in trial c.

Figure 9.19 illustrates the dramatic influence of stimulus uncertainty on the sizes of the DLs for frequency (Δf), intensity (ΔI), and time (ΔT), based on data reported by Watson and Kelly (1981). The term "informational masking" is used to describe the deterioration in perceptual performance due to uncertainty about the stimuli and will be revisited in Chapter 10.

TEMPORARY THRESHOLD SHIFT

It is not uncommon to experience a period of decreased hearing sensitivity, which lasts for some time, after being exposed to

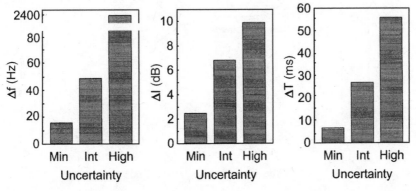

Figure 9.19 Increasing amounts of stimulus uncertainty [minimal (min), intermediate (int) and high] cause Δf, ΔI, and ΔT to increase considerably (informational masking). *Source*: Based on data by Watson and Kelly (1981).

high sound intensities, for example, after leaving a rock concert. This temporary shift in auditory threshold may last as long as roughly 16 h or more, improving gradually. The phenomenon is quite descriptively called **temporary threshold shift** (TTS) or **poststimulatory fatigue**.

Temporary threshold shift appears to be a manifestation of temporary changes in the hair cells as a result of exposure to the fatiguing stimulus. As one might expect, excessive and/or long-standing exposures may result in permanent threshold shifts, reflecting pathological changes or destruction of the hair cells and their associated structures. From the practical standpoint, the amount of TTS produced by exposure to a given fatiguing stimulus has been used as a predictor of individual susceptibility for noise-induced hearing loss. However, this approach is not unchallenged. Because space permits only brief coverage of TTS, the reader is referred to other sources for reviews of this topic and

related areas (e.g., Elliott and Fraser, 1970; Kryter, 1985; Ward, 1973, 1991; Miller, 1974; Henderson et al., 1976; Melnick, 1991; Schmiedt, 1984; Saunders et al., 1985; Clark, 1991; Hamernik et al., 1991; Gelfand, 2001).

It has long been known that TTS is related to the stimulus intensity (Hirsh and Bilger, 1955; Ward et al., 1958, 1959a, 1959b; Mills et al., 1970). Exposure levels below approximately 80 dB SPL are often described as **effective quiet** because they do not appear to produce any TTS. Above effective quiet, the amount of threshold shift increases as stimulus intensity is raised, as illustrated in the upper frame of Fig. 9.20 (Mills, JH, Gengle, RW, Watson, CS, Miller, JD, 1970). For a given intensity, the amount of TTS increases with the duration of the fatiguing stimulus in a manner that is proportional to the logarithm of exposure time. In addition, higher exposure levels produce greater amounts of threshold shift. However, the amount of

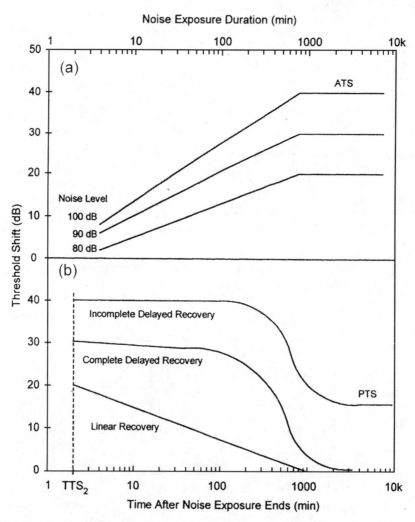

Figure 9.20   Upper frame: development of temporary threshold shift as a function of exposure duration (parameter is exposure level). *Lower frame*: patterns of recovery from temporary threshold shift with time after exposure ends. See text.

threshold shift eventually stops increasing after approximately 8 to 16 hours of exposure, when a maximum amount of TTS is achieved, called **asymptotic threshold shift (ATS)**.

It appears that higher frequency stimuli result in more TTS than do lower frequency fatiguers (Ward, 1963). The amount of TTS is smaller for intermittent sounds than for continuous stimulation (Ward et al., 1958, 1959a), and it appears to be related to the total or average time that the fatiguer is "on" during the course of stimulation (Ward, 1973). The frequency range over which TTS occurs becomes wider as the stimulus level is raised, and this affect is asymmetrical in that the higher frequencies (up to roughly 4000–6000 Hz) are the most severely affected. Temporary threshold shift reaches a maximum at a higher frequency than the fatiguer frequency, generally about one-half to one-octave above (Ward, 1962; Elliott and Fraser, 1970; Ward, 1973; Miller, 1974; Schmiedt, 1984; Saunders et al., 1985). Physiological work has also revealed that the greatest amount of TTS measured for single auditory neurons occurs when the animal is exposed to high-level sounds a half-octave below the neuron's characteristic frequency (Cody and Johnstone, 1981). The basis of this phenomenon appears to be that the location of the maximum basilar membrane vibration shifts in a basal (higher frequency) direction by an amount equivalent to about a half-octave at high levels of stimulation (Johnstone et al., 1986).

The course of recovery from TTS may be measured at various times after the fatiguing stimulus has been turned off. The recovery course is rather complicated within about 2 minutes following the offset of the fatiguer, during which time it is non-monotonic with a "bounce" occurring in the vicinity of the two-minute point (Hirsh and Ward, 1952; Hirsh and Bilger, 1955). This bounce is a reversal of the recovery after which the TTS begins to decrease again with time. For this reason, the amount of TTS produced by a given exposure is typically measured at the two-minute point and is therefore called **TTS$_2$**. The course of recovery of temporary threshold shift is then measured beginning from TTS$_2$. Three types of recovery are illustrated in the lower panel of Fig. 9.20. The normal course of recovery is seen as a straight line and progresses at a rate that is proportional to the logarithm of the time since exposure (Ward et al., 1959a, 1959b). Greater amounts of TTS begin their recovery after some delay. Both of these recovery patterns are complete, meaning that hearing sensitivity eventually returns to its pre-exposure level. In contrast, it is possible that large amounts of TTS may not resolve completely, leaving the person with a **permanent threshold shift (PTS)** or noise-induced hearing loss.

REFERENCES

Abel, SM. 1972. Duration discrimination of noise and tone bursts. *J Acoust Soc Am* 51, 1219–1223.

American National Standards Institute, ANSI–S3.6–1969. 1970. *Specifications for Audiometers.* New York, NY: ANSI.

American National Standards Institute, ANSI S3.1–1999 (R2003). 2003. *Maximum Permissible Ambient Noise Levels for Audiometric Test Rooms.* New York, NY: ANSI.

American National Standards Institute, ANSI–S3.6–2004. 2004. *American National Standard Specification for Audiometers.* New York, NY: ANSI.

American Standards Association, ASA–Z24.5–1951. 1951. *Specifications for Audiometers for General Diagnostic Purposes.* New York: ANA

Bacon, SP, Viemeister, NF. 1985. Temporal modulation transfer functions in normal-hearing and hearing-impaired listeners. *Audiology* 24, 117–134.

Bacon, SP, Viemeister, NF. 1994. Intensity discrimination and increment detection at 16 kHz. *J Acoust Soc Am* 95, 2616–2621.

Bekesy, G. 1960. *Experiments in Hearing.* New York, NY: McGraw-Hill.

Berger, H. 1981. Re-examination of the low-frequency 50-1000 Hz) normal threshold of hearing in free and diffuse sound fields. *J Acoust Soc Am* 70, 1635–1645.

Bernstein, LR, Green, DM. 1987. The profile-analysis bandwidth. *J Acoust Soc Am* 81, 1888–1895.

British Standards Institute, Standard 2497. 1954. *The Normal Threshold of Hearing for Pure Tones by Earphone Listening.*

Burck, W, Kotowski, P, Lichte, H. 1935. Die Lautstarke von Knacken. Gerauchen und Tonen. *Elek NachrTech* 12, 278–288.

Buus, S, Florentine, M. 1985. Gap detection in normal and impaired listeners: The effect of level and frequency. In: A Michelsen (ed.), *Time Resolution in Auditory Systems.* Berlin, Germany: Springer, 159–179.

Campbell, RS, Counter, SA. 1969. Temporal integration and periodicity pitch. *J Acoust Soc Am* 45, 691–693.

Campbell, RA, Lasky, EZ. 1967. Masker level and sinusoidal detection. *J Acoust Soc Am* 42, 972–976.

Carlyon, RR, Moore, BCJ. 1984. Intensity discrimination: A "severe departure" from Weber's law. *J Acoust Soc Am* 76, 1369–1376.

Carlyon, RR, Moore, BCJ. 1986a. Continuous versus gated pedestals and the "severe departure" from Weber's law. *J Acoust Soc Am* 79, 453–460.

Carlyon, RR, Moore, BCJ. 1986b. Detection of tones in noise and the "severe departure" from Weber's law. *J Acoust Soc Am* 79, 461–464.

Clark, WW. 1991. Recent studies of temporary threshold shift (TTS) and permanent threshold shift (PTS) in animals. *J Acoust Soc Am* 90, 175–181.

Cody, AR, Johnstone, BM. 1981. Acoustic trauma: Single neuron basis for the "half-octave shift". *J Acoust Soc Am* 70, 707.

Cohen, MF. 1982. Detection threshold microstructure and its effect on temporal integration data. *J Acoust Soc Am* 71, 405–409.

Dadson, RS, King, JH. 1952. A determination of the normal threshold of hearing and its relation to the standardization of audiometers. *J Laryngol Otol* 46, 366–378.

Davis, H, Krantz, FW. 1964. The international standard reference zero for pure-tone audiometers and its relation to the evaluation of impairment of hearing. *J Speech Hear Res* 7, 7–16.

Dooley, GJ, Moore, BCJ. 1988. Duration discrimination of steady and gliding tones: A new method for estimating sensitivity to rate of change. *J Acoust Soc Am* 84, 1332–1337.

Doughty, JM, Garner, WR. 1947. Pitch characteristics of short tones. 1. Two kinds of pitch threshold. *J Exp Psychol* 37, 351–365.

Elangovan, S, Stuart, A. 2008. Natural boundaries in gap detection are related to categorical perception of stop consonants. *Ear Hear* 29, 761–774.

Elliot, E. 1958. A ripple effect in the audiogram. *Nature* 181, 1076.

Elliott, DN, Fraser, W. 1970. Fatigue and adaptation. In: JV Tobias (ed.), *Foundations of Modern Auditory Theory, Vol. 1.* New York, NY: Academic Press, 115–155.

Fitzgibbons, PJ. 1983. Temporal gap detection in noise as a function of frequency, bandwidth and level. *J Acoust Soc Am* 74, 67–72.

Fitzgibbons, PJ, Gordon-Salant, S. 1987. Temporal gap resolution in listeners with high-frequency sensorineural hearing loss. *J Acoust Soc Am* 81, 133–137.

Florentine, M, Buus, S. 1981. An excitation-pattern model for intensity discrimination. *J Acoust Soc Am* 70, 1646–1654.

Florentine, M, Buus, S, Mason, CR. 1987. Level discrimination as a function of level for tones from 0.25 to 16 kHz. *J Acoust Soc Am* 81, 1528–1541.

Forest, TG, Green, DM. 1987. Detection of partially filled gaps in noise and the temporal modulation transfer function. *J Acoust Soc Am* 82, 1933–1943.

Formby, C, Muir, K. 1988. Modulation and gap detection for broadband and filtered noise signals. *J Acoust Soc Am* 84, 545–550.

Gelfand, SA. 2001. *Essentials of Audiology*, 2nd ed. New York, NY: Thieme.

Green, DM. 1969. Masking with continuous and pulsed tones. *J Acoust Soc Am* 46, 939–946.

Green, DM. 1971. Temporal auditory acuity. *Psychol Rev* 78, 540–551.

Green, DM. 1973a. Temporal acuity as a function of frequency. *J Acoust Soc Am* 54, 373–379.

Green, DM. 1973b. Temporal integration time. In: AR Møller (ed.), *Basic Mechanisms in Hearing.* New York, NY: Academic Press, 829–846.

Green, DM. 1983. Profile analysis: A different view of auditory intensity discrimination. *Am Psychol* 38, 133–142.

Green, DM. 1985. Temporal factors in psychoacoustics. In: A Michelsen (ed.), *Time Resolution in Auditory Systems.* New York, NY: Springer, 122–140.

Green, DM. 1988. *Profile Analysis: Auditory Intensity Discrimination.* New York, NY: Oxford University Press.

Green, DM, Kidd, G Jr, 1983. Further studies in auditory profile analysis. *J Acoust Soc Am* 73, 1260–1265.

Green, DM, Kidd, G Jr, Picardi, MC. 1983. Successive versus simultaneous comparison in auditory intensity discrimination. *J Acoust Soc Am* 73, 639–643.

Green, DM, Mason, CR. 1985. Auditory profile analysis: Frequency, phase, and Weber's law. *J Acoust Soc Am* 77, 1155–1161.

Green, DM, Mason, CR, Kidd, G Jr. 1984. Profile analysis: Critical bands and duration. *J Acoust Soc Am* 75, 1163–1167.

Green, DM, Nachmias, J, Kearny, JK, Jeffress, LA. 1979. Intensity discrimination with gated and continuous sinusoids. *J Acoust Soc Am* 66, 1051–1056.

Green, DM, Onsan, ZA, Forrest, TG. 1987. Frequency effects in profile analysis and detecting complex spectral changes. *J Acoust Soc Am* 81, 692–699.

Hamernik, RP, Ahroon, WA, Hsueh, KD. 1991. The energy spectrum of an impulse: Its relation to hearing loss. *J Acoust Soc Am* 90, 197–208.

Harris, JD. 1952. Pitch discrimination. *J Acoust Soc Am* 24, 750–755.

Harris, JD. 1963. Loudness Discrimination. *J Speech Hear Dis Monogr* Suppl 11, 1–63.

Heinz, MG, Formby, C. 1999. Detection of time- and bandlimited increments and decrements in a random-level noise. *J Acoust Soc Am* 106, 313–326.

Henderson, D, Hamernik, RP, Dosanjh, DS, Mills, JH. 1976. *Effects of Noise on Hearing.* New York, NY: Raven.

Henning, GB. 1967. Frequency discrimination in noise. *J Acoust Soc Am* 41, 774–777.

Hirsh, IJ. 1952. *The Measurement of Hearing.* New York, NY: McGraw-Hill.

Hirsh, IJ. 1959. Auditory perception of temporal order. *J Acoust Soc Am* 31, 759–767.

Hirsh, IJ, Bilger, RC. 1955. Auditory-threshold recovery after exposures to pure tones. *J Acoust Soc Am* 27, 1186–1194.

Hirsh, IJ, Sherrick, CE Jr. 1961. Perceived order in different sense modalities. *J Exp Psychol* 62, 423–432.

Hirsh, IJ, Ward, WD. 1952. Recovery of the auditory threshold after strong acoustic stimulation. *J Acoust Soc Am* 24, 131–141.

Hood, JD. 1968. Observations upon the relationship of loudness discomfort level and auditory fatigue to sound-pressure-level and sensation level. *J Acoust Soc Am* 44, 959–964.

Hood, JD, Poole, JD 1966. Tolerable limit of loudness: Its clinical and physiological significance. *J Acoust Soc Am* 40, 47–53.

Hood, JD, Poole, JP. 1970. Investigations on hearing upon the upper physiological limit of normal hearing. *Int Audiol* 9, 250–255.

Houtsma, AJM, Durlach, NI, Braida, LD. 1980. Intensity perception XI. Experimental results on the relation of intensity resolution to loudness matching. *J Acoust Soc Am* 68, 807–813.

Howard, JH, O'Toole, AJ, Parasuraman, R, Bennett, KB. 1984. Pattern-directed attention in uncertain-frequency detection. *Percept Psychophys* 35, 256–264.

Hughes, JW. 1946. The threshold of audition for short periods of stimulation. *Proc R Soc* B133, 486–490.

International Organization for Standardization, ISO 389-1. 1998a. *Acoustics—Reference Zero for Calibration of Audiometric Equipment—Part 1: Reference Equivalent Threshold Sound Pressure Levels for Pure Tone and Supraaural Earphones.* Geneva, Switzerland: ISO.

International Organization for Standardization, ISO 389-2. 1994a. *Acoustics—Reference Zero for Calibration of Audiometric Equipment—Part 2: Reference Equivalent Threshold Sound Pressure Levels for Pure Tone and Insert Earphones.* Geneva, Switzerland: ISO.

International Organization for Standardization, ISO 389-3. 1994b. *Acoustics—Reference Zero for Calibration of Audiometric Equipment–Part 3: Reference Equivalent Threshold Force Levels for Pure Tones and Bone Vibrators.* Geneva, Switzerland: ISO.

International Organization for Standardization, ISO 389-4. 1994c. *Acoustics—Reference Zero for Calibration of Audiometric Equipment—Part 4: Reference Levels for Narrow-Band Masking Noise.* Geneva, Switzerland: ISO.

International Organization for Standardization, ISO 389-5. 1998b. *Acoustics—Reference Zero for Calibration of Audiometric Equipment—Part 5: Reference Equivalent Threshold Sound Pressure Levels for Pure Tones in the Frequency Range 8 kHz to 16 kHz.* Geneva, Switzerland: ISO.

International Organization for Standardization, ISO 389-7. 2005. *Acoustics—Reference Zero for Calibration of Audiometric Equipment—Part 7: Reference Threshold of Hearing Under Free-Field and Diffuse-Field Listening Conditions.* Geneva, Switzerland: ISO.

Jerger, J. 1952. A difference limen recruitment test and its diagnostic significance. *Laryngoscope* 62, 1316–1332.

Jesteadt, W, Wier, CC. 1977. Comparison of monaural and binaural discrimination of intensity and frequency. *J Acoust Soc Am* 61, 1599–1603.

Jesteadt, W, Wier, CC, Green, DM. 1977. Intensity discrimination as a function of frequency and sensation level. *J Acoust Soc Am* 61, 169–177.

Johnstone, BM, Patuzzi, R, Yates, GK. 1986. Basilar membrane measurements and the traveling wave. *Hear Res* 22, 147–153.

Kidd, G Jr, Mason, CR, Arbogast, TL. 2002. Similarity, uncertainty, and masking in the identification of nonspeech auditory patterns. *J Acoust Soc Am* 111, 1367–1376.

Kidd, G Jr, Mason, CR, Uchanski, RM, Brantley, MA, Shah, P. 1991. The effects of amplitude perturbation and increasing numbers of components in profile analysis. *J Acoust Soc Am* 103, 535–541.

Killion, MC. 1978. Revised estimate of minimum audible pressure: Where is the "missing 6 dB?". *J Acoust Soc Am* 63, 1501–1508.

Knudsen, VO. 1923. The sensibility of the ear to small differences in intensity and frequency. *Physiol Rev* 21, 84–103.

Kryter, KD. 1985. *The Effects of Noise on Man,* 2nd ed. Orlando, FL: Academic Press.

Leek, MR, Brown, ME, Dorman, MF. 1991. Informational masking and auditory attention. *Percept Psychophys* 50, 205–214.

Lentz, JJ, Richards, VM. 1998. The effects of amplitude perturbation and increasing numbers of components in profile analysis. *J Acoust Soc Am* 103, 535–541.

Lister, J, Besing, J, Koehnke, J. 2002. Effects of age and frequency disparity on gap discrimination. *J Acoust Soc Am* 111, 2793–2800.

Long, GR. 1984. The microstructure of quiet and masked thresholds. *Hear Res* 15, 73–87.

Long, GR, Tubis, A. 1988. Modification of spontaneous and evoked otoacoustic emissions and associated psychoacoustic microstructure by aspirin consumption. *J Acoust Soc Am* 84, 1343–1353.

Luce, RD, Green, DW. 1974. Neural coding and physiological discrimination data. *J Acoust Soc Am* 56, 1554–1564.

Lüscher, E, Zwislocki, J. 1949. A simple method for indirect monaural determination of the recruitment phenomena (Difference limen in intensity in different types of deafness). *Acta Otol* Suppl 78, 156–168.

McGill, WJ, Goldberg, JP. 1968a. Pure-tone intensity discrimination as energy detection. *J Acoust Soc Am* 44, 576–581.

McGill, WJ, Goldberg, JP. 1968b. A study of the near-miss involving Weber's law and pure tone intensity discrimination. *Percept Psychophys* 4, 105–109.

Melnick, W. 1991. Human temporary threshold shift and damage risk. *J Acoust Soc Am* 90, 147—154.

Miller, JD. 1974. Effects of noise on people. *J Acoust Soc Am* 56, 729–764.

Mills, JH, Gengle, RW, Watson, CS, Miller, JD. 1970. Temporary changes in the auditory system due to exposure to noise for one or two days. *J Acoust Soc Am* 48, 524–530.

Moore, BCJ. 1973. Frequency difference limens for short duration tones. *J Acoust Soc Am* 54, 610–619.

Moore, BCJ, Peters, RW, Glassberg, BR. 1992. Detection of temporal gaps in sinusoids by elderly subjects with and without hearing loss. *J Acoust Soc Am* 92, 1923–1932.

Moore, BJC, Raab, DH. 1974. Pure-tone intensity discrimination: Some experiments relating to the "near-miss" to Weber's law. *J Acoust Soc Am* 55, 1049–1054.

Morgan, DW, Dirks, DD. 1974. Loudness discomfort level under earphone and in the free field: The effect of calibration. *J Acoust Soc Am* 56, 172–178.

Morgan, DW, Wilson, RH, Dirks, DD. 1974. Loudness discomfort level under earphone and in the free field: The effect of calibration. *J Acoust Soc Am* 56, 577–581.

Munson, WA, Wiener, FM. 1952. In search of the missing 6 dB. *J Acoust Soc Am* 24, 498–501.

Neff, DL, Jesteadt, W. 1996. Intensity discrimination in the presence of random-frequency, multicomponent maskers and broadband noise. *J Acoust Soc Am* 100, 2289–2298.

Nelson, DA, Stanton, ME, Freyman, RL. 1983. A general equation describing frequency discrimination as a function of frequency and sensation level. *J Acoust Soc Am* 73, 2117–2123.

Nordmark, JO. 1968. Mechanisms of frequency discrimination. *J Acoust Soc Am* 44, 1533–1540.

Northern, JL, Downs, MR, Rudmose, W, Glorig, A, Fletcher, J. 1972. Recommended high-frequency audiometric threshold levels 8000–18000 Hz. *J Acoust Soc Am* 52, 585–595.

Patterson, J, Green, DM. 1970. Discrimination of transient signals having identical energy spectra. *J Acoust Soc Am* 48, 894–905.

Penner, MJ. 1977. Detection of temporal gaps in noise as a measure of the decay of auditory sensation. *J Acoust Soc Am* 61, 552–557.

Penner, MJ, Leshowitz, B, Cudahy, E, Richard, G. 1974. Intensity discrimination for pulsed sinusoids of various frequencies. *Percept Psychophys* 15, 568–570.

Phillips, DP. 1999. Auditory gap detection, perceptual channels, and temporal resolution in speech perception. *J Am Acad Audiol* 10, 343–354.

Phillips, DP, Smith, JC. 2004. Correlations among within-channel and between-channel auditory gap-detection thresholds in normal listeners. *Perception* 33, 371–378.

Phillips, D, Taylor, T, Hall, S, Carr, M, Mossop, JE. 1997. Detection of silent intervals between noises activating different perceptual channels: Some properties of "central" auditory gap detection. *J Acoust Soc Am* 101, 3694–3705.

Pisoni, DB. 1977. Identification and discrimination of the relative onset time of two component tones: Implications for voicing perception in stops. *J Acoust Soc Am* 61, 1352–1361.

Plomp, R. 1964. Rate of decay auditory sensation. *J Acoust Soc Am* 36, 277–282.

Plomp, R, Bouman, MA. 1959. Relation between hearing threshold and duration for pure tones. *J Acoust Soc Am* 31, 749–758.

Rabinowitz, WM, Lim, LS, Braida, LD, Durlach, NI. 1976. Intensity perception: VI. Summary of recent data on deviations from Weber's law for 1000-Hz tone pulses. *J Acoust Soc Am* 59, 1506–1509.

Riesz, RR. 1928. Differential intensity sensitivity of the ear for pure tones. *Physiol Rev* 31, 867–875.

Robinson, DW, Dadson, RS. 1956. A re-determination of the equal loudness relations for pure tones. *Br J Appl Phys* 7, 166–181.

Ronken, DA. 1970. Monaural detection of a phase difference between clicks. *J Acoust Soc Am* 47, 1091–1099.

Rosenblith, WA, Stevens, KN. 1953. On the DL for frequency. *J Acoust Soc Am* 25, 980–985.

Rudmose, W. 1963. On the lack of agreement between earphone pressures and loudspeaker pressures for loudness balances at low frequencies. *J Acoust Soc Am* 35, S1906.

Rudmose, W. 1982. The case of the missing 6 dB. *J Acoust Soc Am* 71, 650–659.

Saunders, JC, Dear, SP, Schneider, ME. 1985. The anatomical consequences of hearing loss: A review and tutorial. *J Acoust Soc Am* 78, 833–860.

Schacknow, RN, Raab, DH. 1973. Intensity discrimination of tone bursts and the form of the Weber function. *Percept Psychophys* 14, 449–450.

Schechter, MA, Fausti, SA, Rappaport, BZ, Frey, RH. 1986. Age categorization of high-frequency auditory threshold data. *J Acoust Soc Am* 79, 767–771.

Schloth, E. 1983. Relation between spectral composition of spontaneous otoacoustic emissions and fine-structure of thresholds in quiet. *Acustica* 53, 250–256.

Schmiedt, RA. 1984. Acoustic injury and the physiology of hearing. *J Acoust Soc Am* 76, 1293–1317.

Schneider, BA, Pichora-Fuller, MK, Kowalchuk, D, Lamb, M. 1994. Gap detection and the precedence effect in young and old adults. *J Acoust Soc Am* 95, 980–991.

Shailer, MJ, Moore, BCJ. 1983. Gap detection as a function of frequency, bandwidth, and level. *J Acoust Soc Am* 74, 467–473.

Shaw, EAG. 1974. Transformation of sound pressure level from the free field to the eardrum in the horizontal plane. *J Acoust Soc Am* 56, 1848–1861.

Sherlock, P, Formby, C. 2005. Estimates of loudness, loudness discomfort, and the auditory dynamic range: Normative estimates, comparison of procedures, and test-retest reliability. *J Am Acad Audiol* 16, 85–100.

Shower, EG, Biddulph, R. 1931. Differential pitch sensitivity of the ear. *J Acoust Soc Am* 3, 275–287.

Sinnott, JM, Owren, MJ, Petersen, MR. 1987. Auditory duration discrimination in Old World monkeys (Macaca, Cercopithecus) and humans. *J Acoust Soc Am* 82, 465–470.

Sivian, LJ, White, SD. 1933. On minimum audible fields. *J Acoust Soc Am* 4, 288–321.

Small, AM, Brandt, JF, Cox, PG. 1962. Loudness as a function of signal duration. *J Acoust Soc Am* 34, 513–514.

Small, AM Jr, Campbell, RA. 1962. Temporal differential sensitivity for auditory stimuli. *Am J Psychol* 75, 401–410.

Steinberg, JC, Montgomery, HC, Gardner, MB. 1940. Results of the World's Fair hearing tests. *J Acoust Soc Am* 12, 291–301.

Stellmack, MA, Viemeister, NF, Byrne, AJ. 2004. Monaural and interaural intensity discrimination: Level effects and the "binaural advantage." *J Acoust Soc Am* 116, 1149–1159.

Stream, RW, Dirks, DD. 1974. Effects of loudspeaker on difference between earphone and free-field thresholds MAP and MAF. *J Speech Hear Res* 17, 549–568.

Talmadge, CL, Long, GR, Tubis, A, Dhar, S. 1999. Experimental confirmation of the two-source interference model for the fine structure of distortion product otoacoustic emissions. *J Acoust Soc Am* 105, 275–292.

Talmadge, CL, Tubis, A, Long, GR, Piskorski, P. 1998. Modeling otoacoustic and hearing threshold fine structure. *J Acoust Soc Am* 104, 1517–1543.

Trehub, SE, Schneider, BA, Henderson, JL. 1995. Gap detection in infants, children, and adults. *J Acoust Soc Am* 98, 2532–2541.

Turner, CW, Zwislocki, JJ, Filion, PR. 1989. Intensity discrimination determined with two paradigms in normal and hearing-impaired subjects. *J Acoust Soc Am* 86, 109–115.

U.S. Public Health Service. National Health Survey: Preliminary Reports, 1935–1936. Hearing Study Series Bulletins 1–7.

Van Den Brink, G. 1970. Experiments on binaural diplacusis and tone perception. In: R Plomp, GF Smoorenburg (eds.), *Frequency Analysis and Periodicity Detection in Hearing*. The Netherlands: Sitjhoff, 64–67.

Viemeister, NF. 1972. Intensity discrimination of pulsed sinusoids: The effects of filtered noise. *J Acoust Soc Am* 51, 1265–1269.

Viemeister, NF. 1979. Temporal modulation transfer functions based upon modulation thresholds. *J Acoust Soc Am* 66, 1364–1380.

Viemeister, NF, Bacon, SR. 1988. Intensity discrimination, and magnitude estimation for 1-kHz tones. *J Acoust Soc Am* 84, 172–178.

Villchur, E. 1969. Free-field calibration of earphones. *J Acoust Soc Am* 46, 1527–1534.

Villchur, E. 1970. Audiometer–earphone mounting to improve intersubject and cushion–fit reliability. *J Acoust Soc Am* 48, 1387–1396.

Villchur, E. 1972. Comparison between objective and threshold–shift methods of measuring real–ear attenuation of external sound by earphones. *J Acoust Soc Am* 51, 663–664.

Ward, WD. 1962. Damage–risk criteria for line spectra. *J Acoust Soc Am* 34, 1610–1619.

Ward, WD. 1963. Auditory fatigue and masking. In: J Jerger (ed.), *Modern Developments in Audiology*. New York, NY: Academic Press, 241–286.

Ward, WD. 1973. Adaptation and fatigue. In: J Jerger (ed.), *Modern Developments In Audiology*, 2nd ed. New York, NY: Academic Press, 301–344.

Ward, WD. 1991. The role of intermittence on PTS. *J Acoust Soc Am* 90, 164–169.

Ward, WD, Glorig, A, Sklar, DL. 1958. Dependence of temporary threshold shift at 4kc on intensity and time. *J Acoust Soc Am* 30, 944–954.

Ward, WD, Glorig, A, Sklar, DL. 1959a. Temporary threshold shift from octave-band noise: Applications to damage-risk criteria. *J Acoust Soc Am* 31, 522–528.

Ward, WD, Glorig, A, Sklar, DL. 1959b. Temporary threshold shift produced by intermittent exposure to noise. *J Acoust Soc Am* 31, 791–794.

Watson, CS, Gengel, RW. 1969. Signal duration and signal frequency in relation to auditory sensitivity. *J Acoust Soc Am* 46, 989–997.

Watson, CS, Kelly, WJ. 1981. The role of stimulus uncertainty in the discrimination of auditory patterns. In: DJ Getty, JH Howard Jr. (eds.), *Auditory and Visual Pattern Recognition*. Hillsdale, NJ: Erlbaum, 37–59.

Watson, CS, Kelly, WJ, Wroton, HW. 1976. Factors in the discrimination of tonal patterns. II. Selective attention and learning under various levels of uncertainty. *J Acoust Soc Am* 60, 1176–1186.

Watson, CS, Wroton, HW, Kelly, WJ, Benbasset, CA. 1975. Factors in the discrimination of tonal patterns. I. Component frequency, temporal position and silent intervals. *J Acoust Soc Am* 57, 1175–1185.

Wegel, RL. 1932. Physical data and physiology and excitation of the auditory nerve. *Ann Otol* 41, 740–779.

Wheeler, LJ, Dickson, EDD. 1952. The determination of the threshold of hearing. *J Laryngol Otol* 46, 379–395.

Wier, CC, Jesteadt, W, Green, DM. 1976. A comparison of method-of-adjustment and forced-choice procedures in frequency discrimination. *Percept Psychophys* 19, 75–79.

Wier, CC, Jesteadt, W, Green, DM. 1977. Frequency discrimination as a function of frequency and sensation level. *J Acoust Soc Am* 61, 178–184.

Wilson, JR. 1980. Evidence for a cochlear origin for acoustic re-emissions, threshold fine-structure and tonal tinnitus. *Hear Res* 2, 233–252.

Wojtczak, M, Viemeister, NF. 2008. Perception of suprathreshold amplitude modulation and intensity increments: Weber's law revisited. *J Acoust Soc Am* 123, 2220–2236.

Wright, HN. 1960. Audibility of switching transients. *J Acoust Soc Am* 32, 138.

Wright, HN. 1967. An artifact in the measurement of temporal summation at the threshold of hearing. *J Speech Hear Dis* 32, 354–359.

Yoewart, NS, Bryan, M, Tempest, W. 1967. The monaural MAP threshold of hearing at frequencies from 1.5 to 100 c/s. *J Sound Vib* 6, 335–342.

Zwicker, E, Schloth, E. 1983. Interrelation of different otoacoustic emissions. *J Acoust Soc Am* 75, 1148–1154.

Zwislocki, J. 1960. Theory of auditory summation. *J Acoust Soc Am* 32, 1046–1060.

APPENDIX 9.1

Maximum Permissible Room Noise Levels[a] (As Octave Band Levels in dB) Required for the Measurement of Thresholds As Low As the Reference Levels in Tables 9.1 to 9.3 and 0 dB HL in Fig. 9.2

Octave band center frequency (Hz)	Ears covered with		Ears not covered
	Supra-aural receivers	Insert receivers	
125	39[b] (35[c])	67[b] (59[c])	35[b] (29[c])
250	25	53	21
500	21	50	16
1000	26	47	13
2000	34	49	14
4000	37	50	11
8000	37	56	14

[a] Different room noise levels apply when the ears are covered versus uncovered because the amount of noise entering the ear is reduced by earphone muffs and insert receivers.
[b] Applies when 250 Hz is the lowest frequency tested.
[c] Applies when 125 Hz is the lowest frequency tested.
Source: Based on ANSI S3.1-1999 [R2003].

APPENDIX 9.2

Maximum Permissible Room Noise Levels[a] (As Third-Octave Band Levels in dB) Required for the Measurement of Thresholds As Low As the Reference Levels in Tables 9.1 to 9.3 and 0 dB HL in Fig. 9.2

Third-octave band center frequency (Hz)	Ears covered with		Ears not covered
	Supra-aural receivers	Insert receivers	
125	34[b] (30[c])	62[b] (54[c])	30[b] (24[c])
250	20	48	16
500	16	45	11
800	19	44	10
1000	21	42	8
1600	25	43	9
2000	29	44	9
3150	33	46	8
4000	32	45	6
6300	32	48	8
8000	32	51	9

[a] Different room noise levels apply when the ears are covered versus uncovered because the amount of noise entering the ear is reduced by earphone muffs and insert receivers.
[b] Applies when 250 Hz is the lowest frequency tested.
[c] Applies when 125 Hz is the lowest frequency tested.
Source: Based on ANSI S3.1-1999 [R2003].

10 Masking

The previous chapter dealt with auditory sensitivity. This one is concerned with masking, or how sensitivity for one sound is affected by the presence of another sound, and also with psychoacoustic phenomena that are for one reason or another typically associated with masking.

Suppose that the threshold for a sound A is found to be 10 dB SPL. A second sound B is then presented and the threshold of A is measured again, but this time in the presence of sound B. We now find that sound A must be presented at, say, 26 dB in order to be detected. In other words, sound A has a threshold of 10 dB when measured in quiet, but of 26 dB when determined in the presence of sound B. This increase in the threshold or *threshold shift* for one sound in the presence of another is called **masking**. Our definition of masking may be expanded to include the reduction in loudness that can occur when a second sound is presented, a process referred to as **partial masking** (Meyer, 1959; Scharf, 1964).

We may use the word "masking" to denote either the threshold shift, per se, or the amount (in dB) by which the threshold of a sound is raised due to the presence of another sound. Thus, sound A in our example has been *masked* by sound B, and the amount of *masking* due to the presence of B is equal to 26−10 dB, or 16 dB. In this case, 10 dB is the *unmasked threshold* of sound A, 26 dB is its *masked threshold*, and 16 dB is the *amount of masking*. These notions are illustrated in Fig. 10.1. We will adopt the convention of calling sound B the **masker**, and sound A the **signal**. (The signal is often referred to as the *test signal* or *probe signal*, and occasionally as the *maskee*.)

As will become obvious, masking not only tells us about how one sound affects another, but also provides insight into the frequency-resolving power of the ear. This is the case because the masking pattern to a large extent reflects the excitation pattern along the basilar membrane. In Chapter 13 we shall see how masking is modified under certain conditions of binaural hearing.

The basic masking experiment is really quite straightforward. First, the unmasked threshold of the test stimulus is determined and recorded. This unmasked threshold becomes the baseline. Next, the masker is presented to the subject at a fixed level. The test stimulus is then presented to the subject and its level is adjusted (by whatever psychoacoustic method is being used) until its threshold is determined in the presence of the masker. This level is the masked threshold. As just described, the amount of masking is simply the difference in decibels between this masked threshold and the previously determined unmasked (baseline) threshold. This procedure may then be repeated for all parameters of the test stimulus and masker. An alternative procedure is to present the test stimulus at a fixed level and then to vary the masker level until the stimulus is just audible (or just marked).

NATURE OF MASKING

The masking produced by a particular sound is largely dependent upon its intensity and spectrum. Let us begin with pure tones, which have the narrowest spectra. As early as 1894, Mayer had reported that, while low-frequency tones effectively mask higher frequencies, higher frequencies are not good maskers of lower frequencies. Masking, then, is not necessarily a symmetrical phenomenon. This spread of masking to frequencies higher than that of the masker has been repeatedly demonstrated for tonal maskers (Wegel and Lane, 1924; Ehmer, 1959a; Small, 1959; Finck, 1961). We must therefore focus our attention not only upon the amount of masking, but also upon the frequencies at which masking occurs.

Figure 10.2 shows a series of **masking patterns** (sometimes called **masking audiograms**) obtained by Ehmer (1959a). Each panel shows the amount of masking produced by a given pure tone masker presented at different intensities. In other words, each curve shows as a function of signal frequency how much the signal threshold was raised by a given masker presented at a given intensity. Masker frequency is indicated in each frame and masker level is shown near each curve. Several observations may be made from these masking patterns. First, the strongest masking occurs in the immediate vicinity of the masker frequency; the amount of masking tapers with distance from this "center" frequency. Second, masking increases as the intensity of the masker is raised.

The third observation deals with how the masking pattern depends upon the intensity and frequency of the masker. Concentrate for the moment upon the masking pattern produced by the 1000-Hz masker. Note that the masking is quite symmetric around the masker frequency for relatively low masker levels (20 and 40 dB). However, the masking patterns become asymmetrically wider with increasing masker intensity, with the greatest masking occurring for tones higher than the masker frequency, but with very little masking at lower frequencies. Thus, as masker intensity is raised, there is considerable spread of the masking effect upward in frequency but only a minimal effect downward in frequency. This phenomenon is aptly called **upward spread of masking**. Note too that there are peaks in some of the masking patterns corresponding roughly to the harmonics of the masker frequency. Actually, however, these peaks are probably not due to aural harmonics (see Chap. 12) because they do not correspond precisely to multiples of the masker (Ehmer, 1959a; Small, 1959). Small (1959) found that these peaks occurred when the masker frequency was about 0.85 times the test tone frequency.

Finally, notice that the masking patterns are very wide for low-frequency maskers and are considerably more restricted for high-frequency maskers. In other words, high-frequency

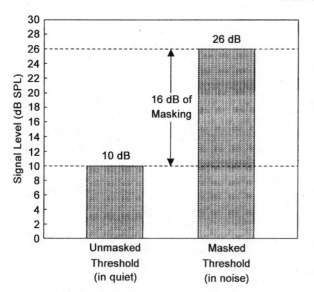

Figure 10.1 Hypothetical example in which a masker shifts the threshold of a test signal by 16 dB from 10 dB SPL to 26 dB SPL.

maskers only are effective over a relatively narrow frequency range in the vicinity of the masker frequency, but low frequencies tend to be effective maskers over a very wide range of frequencies.

These masking patterns reflect the activity along the basilar membrane, as illustrated in Fig. 10.3. Recall from Chapter 4 that the traveling wave envelope has a gradually increasing amplitude along its basal (high-frequency) slope, reaches a peak, and then decays rapidly with a steep apical (low-frequency)

slope. It is thus expected that higher (more basal) frequencies would be most affected by the displacement pattern caused by lower-frequency stimuli. In addition, the high-frequency traveling wave peaks and "decays away" fairly close to the basal turn, so that its masking effect would be more restricted. Lower frequencies, on the other hand, produce basilar membrane displacements along most of the partition. In addition, the excitation pattern becomes wider as the signal level increases.

Although a great deal of information about masking has been derived from studies using tonal maskers, difficulties become readily apparent when both the masker and test stimulus are tones. Two major problems are due to the effects of beats and combination tones.

Beats are audible fluctuations that occur when a subject is presented with two tones differing in frequency by only a few cycles per second (e.g., 1000 and 1003 Hz) at the same time. Consequently, when the masker and test tones are very close in frequency, one cannot be sure whether the subject has responded to the beats or to the test tone. These audible beats can result in notches at the peaks of the masking patterns when the masker and signal are close in frequency (Wegel and Lane, 1924). The situation is further complicated because combination tones are also produced when two tones are presented together. Combination tones are produced at frequencies equal to numerical combinations of the two original tones (f_1 and f_2), such as f_2-f_1 or $2f_1-f_2$. Beats and combination tones are covered in Chapter 12. Beats may be partially (though not totally) eliminated by replacing the tonal maskers with narrow bands of noise centered around given frequencies; however, the elimination of combination tones requires more sophisticated manipulations (Patterson and Moore, 1986). The results of narrow-band noise

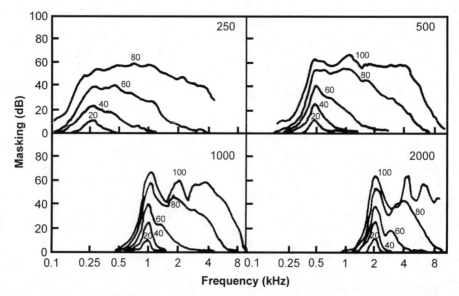

Figure 10.2 Masking patterns produced various pure tone maskers (masker frequency indicated in each frame). Numbers on curves indicate masker level. *Source*: Adapted from Ehmer (1959a, 1959b, with permission of *J. Acoust. Soc. Am.*

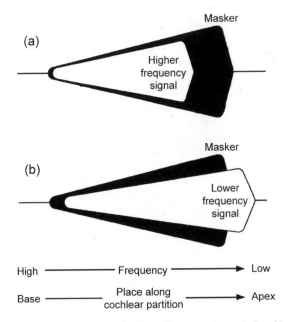

(a)

Masker

Higher frequency signal

(b)

Masker

Lower frequency signal

High ——————— Frequency ——————→ Low

Base ——————— Place along ——————→ Apex
cochlear partition

Figure 10.3 Artist's conceptualization of how upward spread of masking is related to traveling wave excitation patterns along the basilar membrane: The excitation pattern of a lower-frequency masker envelops that of a higher-frequency test signal (a), but a higher-frequency masker does not envelop the excitation pattern of a lower-frequency test signal (b).

masking experiments have essentially confirmed the masking patterns generated in the tonal masking studies (Egan and Hake, 1950; Ehmer, 1959b; Greenwood, 1961).

We have seen that upward spread of masking is the rule as masker level is increased. However, a very interesting phenomenon appears when the stimulus level is quite high, for example, at spectrum levels of about 60 to 80 dB. **Spectrum level** refers to the power in a one-cycle-wide band. In other words, spectrum level is level per cycle. It may be computed by subtracting 10 times the log of the bandwidth from the overall power in the band. Thus:

$$dB_{\text{spectrum level}} = dB_{\text{overall}} - 10 \log (\text{bandwidth})$$

If the bandwidth is 10,000 Hz and the overall power is 95 dB, then the spectrum level will be $95 - 10\log(10,000)$, or $95 - 40 = 55$ dB.

Higher-frequency maskers presented at intense levels can also produce masking at *low* frequencies (Bilger and Hirsh, 1956; Deatherage et al., 1957a, 1957b). This is called **remote masking** because the threshold shifts occur at frequencies below and remote from the masker. In general, the amount of remote masking increases when the bandwidth of the masking noise is widened or its spectrum level is raised (Bilger, 1958). Although the acoustic reflex can cause a threshold shift at low frequencies, it is unlikely that this is the cause of remote masking because remote masking has been shown to occur in the absence of

the acoustic reflex (Bilger, 1966). Instead, remote masking is most likely due primarily to envelope detection of distortion products generated within the cochlea at high masker intensities (Spieth, 1957; Deatherage et al., 1957a, 1957b). (See Chap. 4 for a discussion of cochlear distortion.)

It is apparent from Fig. 10.2 that masking increases as the level of the masker is raised. We may now ask how the amount of masking relates to the intensity of the masker. In other words, how much of a threshold shift results when the masker level is raised by a given amount? This question was addressed in the classical studies of Fletcher (1937) and Hawkins and Stevens (1950). Since the essential findings of the two studies agreed, let us concentrate upon the data reported by Hawkins and Stevens in 1950. They measured the threshold shifts for pure tones and for speech produced by various levels of a white noise masker. (It should be pointed out that although *white noise* connotes equal energy at all frequencies, the actual spectrum reaching the subject is shaped by the frequency response of the earphone or loudspeaker used to present the signal. Therefore, the exact masking patterns produced by a white noise depend upon the transducer employed, as well as on bandwidth effects that will be discussed in the next section.)

Figure 10.4 shows Hawkins and Stevens' data as masked threshold contours. These curves show the masked thresholds produced at each frequency by a white noise presented at various spectrum levels. The curves have been idealized in that the actual results were modified to reflect the masking produced by a true white noise. The actual data were a bit more irregular, with peaks in the curves at around 7000 Hz, reflecting the effects of the earphone used. The bottom contour is simply the unmasked threshold curve. The essential finding is that these curves are parallel and spaced at approximately 10-dB intervals, which is also the interval between the masker levels. This result suggests that a 10-dB increase in masker level produces a 10-dB

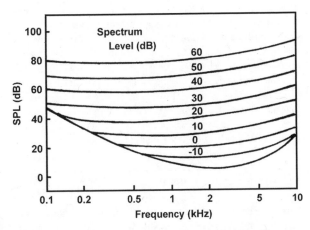

Figure 10.4 Masking contours showing masking as a function of frequency for various spectrum levels of an idealized white noise. Bottom curve is threshold in quiet. *Source*: Adapted from Hawkins and Stevens (1950), with permission of *J. Acoust. Soc. Am.*

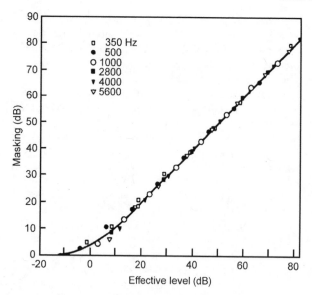

Figure 10.5 Masking produced at various frequencies as a function of the effective level of the masker. *Source*: Adapted from Hawkins and Stevens (1950), with permission of *J. Acoust. Soc. Am.*

increase in masked threshold; a point which will become clearer soon.

The actual amount of masking may be obtained by subtracting the unmasked threshold (in quiet) from the masked threshold. For example, the amount of masking produced at 1000 Hz by a white noise with a spectrum level of 40 dB is found by subtracting the 1000-Hz threshold in quiet (about 7 dB SPL) from that in the presence of the 40-dB noise spectrum level (roughly 58 dB). Thus, the amount of masking is $58-7 = 51$ dB in this example. Furthermore, because the masked thresholds are curved rather than flat, the white noise is not equally effective at all frequencies. We might therefore express the masking noise in terms of its effective level at each frequency. We may now show the amount of masking as a function of the effective level of the masking noise (Fig. 10.5). As Fig. 10.5 shows, once the masker attains an effective level, the amount of masking is a linear function of masker level. That is, a 10-dB increase in masker level results in a corresponding 10-dB increase in the masked threshold of the test signal. Hawkins and Stevens demonstrated that this linear relationship between masking and masker level is independent of frequency (as shown in the figure), and that it applies to speech stimuli as well as to pure tones.

FREQUENCY SELECTIVITY

Filters are used in our daily lives to select among various things that may be tangible or intangible. We have all seen change sorters. Even though mixed change is dropped into the same hole, dimes end up in one section, quarters in another, etc. The discrete and large size differences among coins make this

straightforward. However, a selection process must work within the limits of the filters. A clear albeit distasteful example of this point relates to the inevitable grading process in college courses. Grading represents a filtering process: The input to a bank of filters is a continuum from 70% to 100%, and the output is an "A" or a "B" or a "C." The "B" filter goes from 80% to 89%. Thus, it can select between 78% and 81%, or 89% and 90%, but it cannot differentiate between 83% and 85%. Otherwise stated, values that fall within the range of the same filter cannot be differentiated, whereas values that fall across the border of two filters can be isolated from one another. The same issue of selectivity applies to hearing. The ear's ability to analyze a sound so that we can separate one frequency from the other also implies a filtering capability, which we call frequency selectivity. Our ability to analyze the components of a sound depends on the width of our **auditory filters**.

What does all of this have to do with masking? As we shall see, masking and related experiments reveal the **frequency selectivity** of the ear and provide insight into the nature of the underlying auditory filter.

Because a tone may be masked by another tone or by a narrow band of noise as well as by white noise, it is reasonable to ask how much of the white noise actually contributes to the masking of a tone. Otherwise stated, does the entire bandwidth of the white noise contribute to the masking of a given tone, or is there a certain limited ("critical") bandwidth around the tone that alone results in masking? Fletcher (1940) attacked this problem by finding masked thresholds for tones produced by various bandwidths of noise centered around the test tones. He held the spectrum level constant and found that the masked threshold of a tone increased as the bandwidth of the masking noise was widened. However, once the noise band reached a certain critical bandwidth, further widening of the band did not result in any more masking of the tone. Thus, Fletcher demonstrated that only a certain critical bandwidth within the white noise actually contributes to the masking of a tone at the center of the band, a finding which has been repeatedly confirmed (Schaefer et al., 1950; Hamilton, 1957; Greenwood, 1961; Swets et al., 1962; Bos and deBoer, 1966).

This finding is easily understood if we think of the critical bandwidth as a filter. More and more of the energy in the white noise will be made available by the filter as the filter's bandwidth is widened. On the other hand, energy present in the white noise that lies above and below the upper and lower cutoff frequencies of the filter is "wasted" from the standpoint of the filter (Fig. 10.6). Now, if this filter defines the critical bandwidth that contributes to the masking of a tone at the center of the band, then it is easy to see how only that portion of the noise that is inside the filter will be useful in masking the tone. Adding to the noise band beyond the limits of this filter (the areas labeled "b" in Fig. 10.6) will not add any more masking, although it will cause the noise to sound louder (see Chap. 11).

Fletcher (1940) hypothesized that the signal power (S) would be equal to the noise power (No) located within the critical

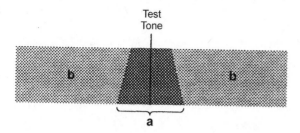

Figure 10.6 Energy within the critical band filter (a) contributes to the masking of the tone at the center, whereas energy outside of the filter (b) does not contribute to the masking (see text).

bandwidth (CB) when the tone was at its masked threshold: $S = CB \cdot No$. Thus, the **critical band** would be equal to the ratio of the signal power to the noise power, or $CB = S/No$. In decibels, this corresponds to $dB_S - dB_{No}$. Hawkins and Stevens (1950) found that the masked threshold of a 1000-Hz tone was approximately 58 dB in the presence of a white noise whose spectrum level was 40 dB. The resulting estimate of the critical band is therefore 58 dB − 40 dB = 18 dB, which corresponds to a bandwidth of 63.1 Hz. This estimate of the critical band is shown by the X in Fig. 10.7. Notice that this indirect estimate of the critical bandwidth based upon the power ratio of signal to noise is actually quite a bit narrower than the other more direct estimates of the critical band shown in the figure. For this reason, the indirect estimate based upon Fletcher's formula is

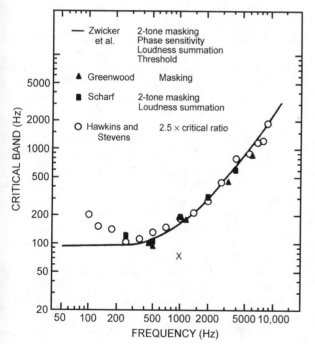

Figure 10.7 Critical bandwidth as a function of center frequency for various studies. The X is the critical ratio estimate of Hawkins and Stevens (1950) for a 1000-Hz tone. *Source*: Adapted from Scharf, Critical bands, in: *Foundations of Modern Auditory Theory* (J. V. Tobias, ed.), Vol. 1, ©1970, Academic Press.

referred to as **critical ratio**, as opposed to the **critical bands** obtained by other, direct means. Good correspondence to the critical band is obtained when the critical ratio is multiplied by a factor of 2.5 (Zwicker et al., 1957; Scharf, 1970). This correspondence is demonstrated by the open circles in Fig. 10.7, which are the values of the critical ratios multiplied by 2.5, based upon Hawkins and Stevens' (1950) data. Note that there is good agreement with Greenwood's (1961) masking data, as well as with the critical bands directly derived from loudness studies (see Chap. 11).

Bilger (1976) proposed that the listener performs an intensity discrimination between the noise power in the critical band and the combined power of the noise plus signal at the masked threshold; as a result the critical ratio is equated to the familiar Weber fraction (Chap. 9):

$$\frac{S}{CB \cdot N} = \frac{\Delta I}{I}$$

This equation is solved for critical bandwidth by multiplying S/N by the reciprocal of the Weber fraction

$$CB = \frac{S}{N} \cdot \frac{I}{\Delta I}$$

Since the critical ratio is multiplied by 2.5 to obtain the critical band, this leads to a Weber fraction of $1/2.5 = 0.4$, or a difference limen of 1.46 dB, a value that is in reasonable agreement with intensity DL data.

Figure 10.7 indicates that the critical band becomes wider as the center frequency increases. Scharf (1970) has provided a table of critical bandwidth estimates based upon the available data. Examples are a critical bandwidth of 100 Hz for a center frequency of 250 Hz, a 160-Hz band for 1000 Hz, and a 700-Hz band for 4000 Hz. Similar data and formulas for calculation of the critical bandwidth and critical band rate (the bark scale) have been provided by Zwicker and Terhardt (1980). Actually, one should be careful not to conceive of a series of discrete critical bands laid as it were end to end, but rather of a bandwidth around any particular frequency that defines the phenomenon we have discussed with respect to that frequency. [One should remember in this context Scharf's (1970, p. 159) elegant definition: "the critical band is that bandwidth at which subjective responses rather abruptly change."] We should thus think of critical bandwidths as overlapping filters rather than as discrete, contiguous filters.

It would appear that the original concept (Fletcher, 1940) of the critical bandwidth as defining an internal auditory filter is fundamentally correct. Its location is more than likely peripheral, with critical bandwidths probably corresponding to 1 to 2 mm distances along the human cochlear partition (Scharf, 1970). Thus, the critical band presents itself as a fundamental concept in the frequency-analysis capability of the cochlea, the physiological aspects of which are discussed in Chapter 4.

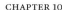

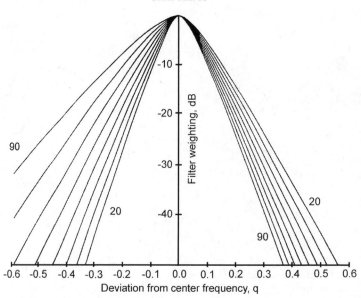

Figure 10.8 Shape and bandwidth (ERB) of the auditory filter expressed in terms of increasing level in 10 dB steps from 20 to 90 dB SPL/ERB. (Note the opposite directions in which the left- and right-hand slope change as level increases from 20 to 90 dB. The left-hand slope shown on these filters determines the high frequency aspect of the excitation pattern.) *Source*: From Moore and Glasberg (1987), with permission of *Hear Res.*

Detailed reviews of the critical band concept may be found in the work of Scharf (1970) and Bilger (1976).

The idea of the internal filter originally embodied in the critical band concept, particularly in its conceptualization as a rectangular filter around the center frequency (Fletcher, 1940), has been modified and updated by numerous investigators (Patterson, 1974, 1976; Houtgast, 1977; Weber, 1977; Moore and Glassberg, 1981, 1987; Patterson et al., 1982; Shailer and Moore, 1983; Fidell et al., 1983; Glasberg et al., 1984a, 1984b). Figure 10.8 shows the shapes of the auditory filter over a wide range of intensities, as derived in a paper by Moore and Glasberg (1987). The curves were based on raw data from young, normal hearing subjects from a variety of studies.[1] The figure reveals that the filter becomes increasingly more asymmetric with increasing level. The major aspect of this asymmetry is that the slope of the low-frequency (left-hand) branch of the filter decreases with increasing level. This widening of the left-hand branch of the filter that corresponds to the phenomenon of upward spread of masking has been discussed earlier in this chapter. We saw the reason is that the left-hand branch of this filter determines the high-frequency aspect of the excitation pattern.

With an idea of the shape of the auditory filter, we may ask how it is related to frequency and to the critical band (cf.

Fig. 10.7). To do this, we need to summarize the nature of the filters in some valid and convenient way. This can be done by using what is called the **equivalent rectangular bandwidth (ERB)** of the filter. An ERB is simply the rectangular filter that passes the same amount of power as would pass through the filter we are trying to specify. Thus, if a white noise is directed to the inputs of a filter of any given configuration and also through its ERB, then the power at their outputs (passed through them) would be the same. Using this approach, Moore and Glasberg (1983b) have shown how the auditory filter changes with frequency. Figure 10.9 shows the ERB of the auditory filter as a function of its center frequency. Here we see that the width of the auditory filter widens as frequency increases, and also that this relationship is quite consistent across several studies. Also shown in the figure is an equivalent line based upon the classical critical band. [The latter was derived using a formula by Zwicker and Terhardt (1980).] Observe that the more recent measurements of auditory filter width are slightly narrower but generally parallel with the older ones based upon classical critical band data. The parallel relationship breaks down below about 500 Hz, where unlike the earlier critical band data, the newer observations suggest that the auditory filter continues to be a function of frequency. One should refer to Patterson and Moore (1986), whose extensive discussion of this topic includes arguments addressing the discrepancy below 500 Hz in the light of differences in processing efficiency.

We have already seen that beats and combination tones can adversely affect tone-on-tone masking measurements. Now that we have an idea of the auditory filter, we may consider another factor that can confound masking (among other) experiments.

[1] The auditory filter tends to widen with age (Patterson and Moore, 1986). See Patterson et al. (1982) for other findings, and Gelfand (2001) for a general discussion of factors relating to aging and hearing impairment.

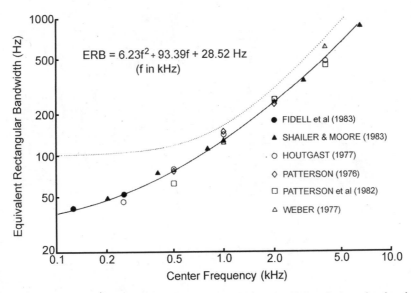

Figure 10.9   The solid line shows the width of the auditory filter (in terms of ERB) as a function of center frequency based on the data of various studies. The dotted line summarizes the same relationship for classical critical band data. *Source*: From Moore and Glasberg (1983b), with permission of *J. Acoust. Soc. Am.*

This phenomenon is **off-frequency listening** (Patterson, 1976; Patterson and Moore, 1986). Recall from the previous discussion the notion of a continuum of overlapping auditory filters. We typically presume that the subject is listening to some tone "through" the auditory filter which is centered at that test frequency. However, the subject might also "shift" to another auditory filter, which includes the test frequency but is not centered there. The example in Fig. 10.10 shows why this might happen. The vertical line depicts a tone of some frequency, and the bell curve portrays the auditory filter centered around this tone. The rectangle represents a low-pass noise masker. Look first at Fig. 10.10a. Notice that part of the masker falls within the auditory filter (shaded area). If the tone were presented *without* the noise, then the signal-to-noise (S/N) ratio coming out of this auditory filter would be very high. Hence, the subject would detect the tone. When the *noise is presented* along with the tone, then the portion of the noise falling inside of this auditory filter causes the S/N ratio to be diminished. This, in turn, reduces the chances that the subject will detect the tone.

All of this supposes that the only way to listen to the tone is through the auditory filter centered at that tone's frequency. However, the dashed curve in Fig. 10.10b shows that a sizable proportion of this test tone is also passed by a neighboring auditory filter, which itself is centered at a slightly higher frequency. Moreover, a much smaller part of the masking noise is passed by this neighboring filter. Hence, that the S/N ratio between the test tone and the masking noise is increased when the subject listens "through" this shifted auditory filter. Consequently, the likelihood that the tone will be detected is improved due to such off-frequency listening.

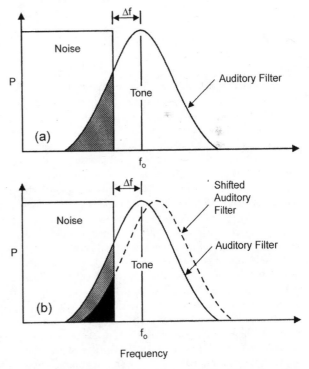

Figure 10.10   In both graphs, the solid curve represents the auditory filter centered at the test tone and the rectangle at the left portrays a lower frequency masking noise. Off-frequency listening occurs when the subject shifts to another auditory filter (indicated by the dashed curve in graph b) in order to detect the presence of a test signal. *Source*: Adapted from Patterson (1976), with permission of *J. Acoust. Soc. Am.*

193

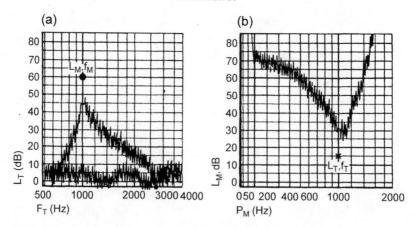

Figure 10.11 (a) Thresholds of sweeping-frequency *test* tones (LT, dB) as a function of frequency (of the test tones, FT, Hz) in quiet (*lower tracing*) and in the presence of a fixed masker (*upper tracing*). The filled circle shows the level and frequency of the fixed masker (60 dB, 1000 Hz; LM, FM). (b) These tracings show the levels of sweeping-frequency *masker* tones (LM, dB) needed to just mask the fixed test tone of 1000 Hz at 15 dB (LT, FT). *Source*: From Zwicker and Schorn (1978), with permission of *Audiology*.

An effective approach to minimize the confounding effects of off-frequency listening is to present the signals involved in an experiment (such as the test tone and masker tone) along with additional noise(s) which will mask out the frequencies above and below the range of interest (O'Loughlin and Moore, 1981).

PSYCHOACOUSTIC TUNING CURVES

So far, we have described masking in terms of the level of the tone (or other signal), which has been masked. Thus, the masking patterns in Fig. 10.2 expressed the amount of masking produced for various test tones as a function of frequency by a given masker (at some fixed level). That is, "30 dB of masking" on one of these graphs means that the masker caused the threshold of the test signal to be increased by 30 dB above its unmasked threshold. If this experiment were done using the Bekesy tracking method (Chap. 7), the "raw" results might look something like the left panel in Fig. 10.11. Here, the lower tracing shows the threshold of the test signal, which is a tone sweeping in frequency from 500 to 4000 Hz. The upper tracing shows the masked threshold tracing in the presence of a fixed masker (which is a 1000-Hz tone at 60 dB). Subtracting the lower (unmasked) tracing from the upper (masked) threshold tracing would result in a familiar masking pattern similar to those in Fig. 10.2.

Another way to look at masking was initiated by Chistovich (1957), Small (1959), and Zwicker (1974). This approach essentially asks the question, what levels of the masker are needed to mask the test signal? Now, the test tone (signal) is kept at a fixed level and frequency, and the level of the *masker* tone is adjusted until it just masks the test tone. This is done at many different frequencies of the masker, resulting in a curve very different from the familiar masking audiogram seen above.

This approach is easily understood by referring to the right panel of Fig. 10.11. (A careful look at this graph will reveal

differences from the left panel not only in the tracing but also in the captions for the x- and y-axes.) The tonal signal (i.e., the signal being masked) is a 1000-Hz tone at 15 dB (indicated by the *X*). Now it is the *masker* tone, which sweeps across the frequency range, and the subject uses the Bekesy tracking method to keep the masker at a level that will just mask the fixed test tone. The resulting diagram shows the level of the masker needed to keep the test tone just masked as a function of the masker frequency.

It should be apparent to the reader that this tracing bears a striking resemblance to the auditory neuron tuning curves seen in earlier chapters. It is thus called a **psychoacoustic** (or **psychophysical**) **tuning curve (PTC)**. Psychophysical tuning curves provide a very good representation of the ear's frequency selectivity. This occurs based on the notion that we are sampling the output of just one auditory filter when a very low-level signal is used. As the masker gets closer and closer to the frequency of the test signal, less and less level will be required to mask it, and hence the function of masker level needed to just mask the tone provides a picture of the filter.

However, one must avoid the temptation to think of the PTC as the psychoacoustic analogy of an individual neural tuning curve. It is clear that much more than a single neuron is being sampled, and that PTCs are wider than neural tuning curves. Moreover, the earlier discussions dealing with the implications of beats, combination tones, and off-frequency listening in masking are particularly applicable to PTCs. For example, PTCs become wider when off-frequency listening is minimized by the use of notched noise (Moore et al., 1984). A notched noise is simply a band-reject noise (see Chap. 1) in which the band being rejected is centered where we are making our measurement. Therefore, the notched noise masks the frequency regions above and below the one of interest, so that off-frequency listening is reduced.

Figure 10.12 shows two sets of individual PTCs at four test-tone frequencies (500–4000 Hz) from a more recent

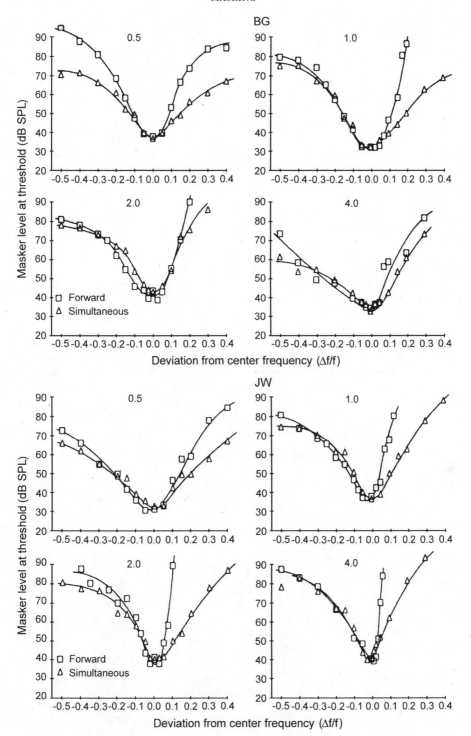

Figure 10.12 Individual psychoacoustic tuning curves at 500, 1000, 2000, and 4000 Hz for two listeners. Triangles are simultaneous masking data and squares are forward masking data. Notice that the forward masking PTCs show sharper tuning. *Source*: From Moore et al. (1984), with permission of *J. Acoust. Soc. Am.*

experiment. These PTCs were obtained by using simultaneous masking (triangles) versus forward masking (squares). As the figure shows, PTCs generated under forward masking conditions generally show sharper tuning than those described for simultaneous masking conditions (e.g., Houtgast, 1972; Duifhuis, 1976; Wightman et al., 1977; Weber, 1983; Lufti, 1984; Moore et al., 1984). These differences go beyond the current scope, but the interested reader will find several informative discussions on this topic (e.g., Weber, 1983; Jesteadt and Norton, 1985; Patterson and Moore, 1986; Lufti, 1988).

COMODULATION MASKING RELEASE

Recall that only a certain critical bandwidth of noise around a signal tone is involved in the masking of that tone: The masked threshold of the signal will not be changed by widening the noise bandwidth beyond the CB or adding one or more other bands outside of the CB. However, a different situation occurs when the masking noise is amplitude modulated, as illustrated by the following example.

It will be convenient for the noise band centered on the test tone to be called the *on-signal band*, and for any other bands of noise to be called *flanking* or *off-frequency bands*. We will begin by masking a pure tone signal by an on-signal band of noise that is being amplitude modulated, as illustrated by the waveform in the panel labeled "on-signal band alone" in upper portion of Fig. 10.13. The graph in the lower part of the figure shows that the masked threshold of the signal is 50 dB in presence of this amplitude modulated on-signal noise. We will now add another band of noise that is outside of the CB of the test tone. The off-signal band will be amplitude modulated in exactly the same way as the on-signal band, as illustrated in the panel labeled "comodulated bands" in Fig. 10.13. These two noise bands are said to be *comodulated bands* because the envelopes of their modulated waveforms follow the same pattern over time even though they contain different frequencies. We do not expect any change in masking with the comodulated bands because adding the off-frequency band is outside of the signal's critical band. However, we find that the masked threshold of the signal actually becomes better (lower) for the comodulated bands compared to what it was for just the on-signal band alone. This improvement is called **comodulation masking release (CMR)** (Hall, Haggard, and Fernandes, 1984). In the hypothetical example of Fig. 10.13, the masked threshold of the tone improved from 50 dB in the presence of just the on-signal band (left bar) to 39 dB for the comodulated bands (middle bar), amounting to a CMR of 11 dB. Notice that the masked threshold does not improve (right bar) if the on-signal and off-signal noise bands are *not* comodulated (panel labeled

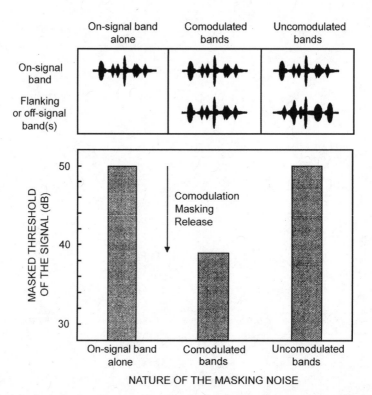

Figure 10.13 Hypothetical modulated noise band waveform envelopes (*above*) and masked threshold results (*below*) illustrating comodulation masking release. See text.

"uncomodulated bands"). Comodulation masking release also occurs for complex signals (made up of, e.g., 804, 1200, 1747, and 2503 Hz) even if there is some spectral overlap between the signal and the masker (Grose, Hall, Buss, and Hatch, 2005)

Comodulation masking release reveals that the auditory system is able to capitalize upon information provided across critical band filters, although a cohesive model explaining CMR is not yet apparent. One type of explanation suggests that the information provided by the off-signal band(s) helps the subject know when the troughs or "dips" occur in the modulating noise. Listening for the signal during these dips would result in a lower threshold (less masking) compared to times when the noise level is higher. Another type of model suggests that the auditory system compares the modulation patterns derived from the outputs of auditory filters in different frequency regions. This pattern would be similar for the filters that do not contain a signal but would be modified for the filter that contains a signal. Detecting a disparity between the outputs of the filters would thus indicate the presence of a signal. The interested student should see the informative review by Moore (1990) and the many contemporary discussions of CMR parameters, models, and related effects (e.g., Buus, 1985; Hatch et al., 1995; Hall and Grose, 1990; Moore et al., 1990; Hicks and Bacon, 1995; Bacon et al., 1997; Grose et al., 2005).

OVERSHOOT

The masked threshold of a brief signal can be affected by the temporal arrangement of the signal and a masking noise. The typical experiment involves a very brief signal and a longer duration masker, with various timing relationships between them. For example, the signal onset might be presented within a few milliseconds of the masker onset (as in Fig. 10.14a), in the middle of the masker (Fig. 10.14e), or the signal onset might trail the masker onset by various delays between these extremes (as in Fig. 10.14b to d). Compared to the amount of masking that takes place when the signal is in the middle of the masker, as much as 10 to 15 dB more masking takes place when the signal onset occurs at or within a few milliseconds of the masker onset. In other words, a brief signal is subjected to a much larger threshold shift at the leading edge of a masker compared to when it is placed in the temporal middle of the masker. This phenomenon was originally described by Elliott (1965) and Zwicker (1965a, 1965b) and is known as **overshoot**.

The amount of masking overshoot decreases as the signal delay gets longer, usually becoming nil by the time the delay reaches about 200 ms (e.g., Elliott, 1969; Zwicker, 1965a; Fastl, 1976). Masking overshoot is maximized for signals with high frequencies (above 2000 Hz) and short durations (under 30 ms) (e.g., Elliott, 1967, 1969; Zwicker, 1965a; Fastl, 1976; Bacon and Takahashi, 1992; Carlyon and White, 1992), and when the masker has a very wide bandwidth, much broader than the

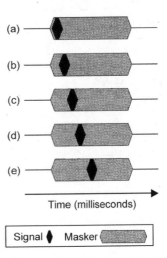

Figure 10.14 Timing relationships between a masker and brief signal. The signal onset is within a few milliseconds of the masker onset in the first frame and occurs at increasing delays in the subsequent frames. The signal is presented in the temporal middle of the masker in the last frame.

critical band (e.g., Zwicker, 1965b; Bacon and Smith, 1991). In addition, overshoot becomes greater as the masker increases from low to moderate levels, but it declines again as the masker continues to increase toward high levels (Bacon, 1990).

The different amounts of overshoot produced by narrow versus broad band maskers has been addressed by Scharf, Reeves, and Giovanetti (2008), who proposed that overshoot is caused (or at least affected) by the listener's ability to focus on the test frequency at the onset of the noise. This is disrupted by the wide range of frequencies in a broadband masker, but is focused by the narrow band masker because its spectrum is close to the signal frequency. Consistent with their explanation, they found that narrow band maskers caused little if any overshoot when the test tone always had the *same* frequency (stimulus *certainty*), as in the typical overshoot experiment. In contrast, narrow maskers produced more overshoot when the test frequency was *changed randomly* between trials (stimulus *uncertainty*). The opposite effect occurred with wide band maskers, in which case stimulus uncertainty produced less overshoot.

Although the precise origin of overshoot is not definitively known, the most common explanation is based on adaptation in auditory neurons (e.g., Green, 1969; Champlin and McFadden, 1989; Bacon, 1990; McFadden and Champlin, 1990; Bacon and Healy, 2000). Recall from Chapter 5 that the initial response of an auditory neuron involves a high discharge rate, which declines over a period of roughly about 10 to 20 ms. The neural response produced by the masker would thus be greatest at its leading edge and would weaken thereafter. As a result, more masking would be produced at the beginning of the masker than in the middle of it. Other hypotheses suggest that the basis for masking overshoot may be related to processes associated with the basilar membrane input–output function (von Klitzing and Kohlrausch, 1994; Strickland, 2001; Bacon and Savel, 2004), or a disruption in the listener's ability to attend to the signal frequency (Scharf et al., 2008).

Masking overshoot can also occur when the signal is very close to the offset of the masker, although it is considerably smaller than the onset effect (e.g., Elliott, 1969; Bacon and Viemeister, 1985; Bacon and Moore, 1986; Bacon et al., 1989; Formby et al., 2000). A peripheral origin for offset overshoot is unlikely because the increased spike rate seen at the onset of auditory neuron firing patterns does not also occur at offset. Hence, overshoot at masker offset has been attributed to central processes (e.g., Bacon and Viemeister, 1985; Bacon and Moore, 1986).

TEMPORAL MASKING

So far, we have been considering situations in which the masker and test signal occur simultaneously. Let us now examine masking that occurs when the test signal and masker do not overlap in time, referred to as **temporal** or **nonsimultaneous masking**. This phenomenon may be understood with reference to the diagrams in Fig. 10.15, which show the basic arrangements used in temporal masking experiments. In Fig. 10.15a, the signal is presented and terminated, and then the masker is presented after a brief time delay following signal offset. Masking occurs in spite of the fact that the signal and masker are not presented together. This arrangement is called **backward masking** or **pre-masking** because the masker is preceded by the signal, that is, the masking effect occurs backward in time (as shown by the arrow in the

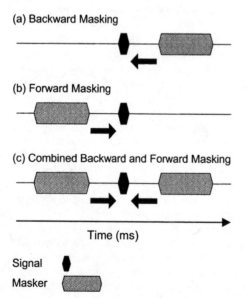

Figure 10.15 Temporal masking paradigms: (a) in backward masking the masker follows the signal, (b) in forward masking the masker precedes the signal, and (c) combined forward and backward masking. The heavy arrows show the direction of the masking effect.

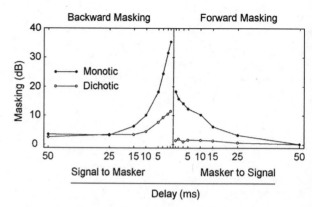

Figure 10.16 Temporal masking in decibels as a function of the interval between signal and masker. (Signal: 10 ms, 1000 Hz tone bursts; masker: 50 ms broadband noise bursts at 70 dB SPL.) *Source*: Adapted from Elliott (1962a), with permission of *J. Acoust. Soc. Am.*

figure). **Forward masking** or **post-masking** is just the opposite (Fig. 10.15b). Here, the masker is presented first, and then the signal is turned on after an interval following masker offset. As the arrow shows, the masking of the signal now occurs forward in time.

The amount of masking of the test signal produced under backward, forward, or combined forward/backward masking conditions is determined while various parameters of the probe and masker are manipulated. These parameters may be the time interval between signal and masker, masker level, masker duration, etc.

Figure 10.16 shows some examples of temporal masking data from Elliott's (1962a) classic paper. The ordinate is the amount of masking produced by 50-ms noise bursts presented at 70 dB SPL for a test signal of 1000 Hz lasting 10 ms. The abscissa is the time interval between masker and test signal for the backward and forward masking paradigms. Finally, the solid symbols show the amount of masking produced when the masker and signal are presented to the same ear (monotically), and the open symbols reveal the masking that results when the noise goes to one ear and the signal goes to the other (dichotic masking). Notice that considerably more masking occurs monotically than dichotically.

The amount of temporal masking is related to the time gap between the signal and the masker. More masking occurs when the signal and masker are closer in time, and less masking occurs as the time gap between them widens. However, the backward and forward masking functions are not mirror images of each other. As the figure shows, Elliott found greater threshold shifts for backward masking than for forward masking. Similar findings were reported by some investigators (Lynn and Small, 1977; Pastore et al., 1980), but others found the opposite to occur (Wilson and Carhart, 1971).

Backward masking decreases dramatically as the delay between the signal and masker increases beyond about 15 to 20 ms, and then continues to decrease very slightly as the interval

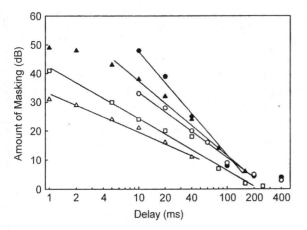

Figure 10.17 Examples of the more or less linear decrease of forward masking with the logarithm of the delay between the masker and the signal. *Source*: Based on data for various forward masking conditions from Wilson and Carhart (1971; *squares*), Smiarowski and Carhart (1975; *triangles*), and Weber and Moore (1981; *circles*).

is lengthened further. Forward masking also decreases with increasing delays, but more gradually. It declines linearly with the logarithm of the masker-signal delay (Fig. 10.17) and exists for intervals as long as about 200 ms depending on the study (e.g., Wilson and Carhart, 1971; Smiarowski and Carhart, 1975; Fastl, 1976, 1977, 1979; Widin and Viemeister, 1979; Weber and Moore, 1981; Jesteadt et al., 1982).

The amount of temporal masking increases as the level of the masker is increased, but not in the linear manner seen for simultaneous masking (Elliott, 1962a; Babkoff and Sutton, 1968; Jesteadt et al., 1981). Rather, with temporal masking, increasing the masker level by 10 dB may result in an additional threshold shift on the order of only about 3 dB.

The duration of the masker influences the amount of forward masking, but this does not appear to occur for backward masking (Elliott, 1967). The amount of forward masking increases as the masker duration gets longer up to about 200 ms (Zwicker, 1984; Kidd and Feth, 1982).

As we might expect, temporal masking is influenced by the frequency relationship between the signal and the masker (e.g., Wright, 1964; Elliott, 1967) just as we have seen for simultaneous masking. In other words, more masking occurs when the signal and masker are close together in frequency than when they are far apart. Formby et al. (2000) found that a 2500-Hz noise band produced temporal masking for a 500-Hz signal, demonstrating that remote masking can occur under temporal masking conditions.

The combined effects of forward and backward masking may be found by placing the signal between the two maskers, as shown in Fig. 10.15c. More masking occurs when backward and forward masking are combined than would result if the individual contributions of backward and forward masking were simply added together (Pollack, 1964; Elliott, 1969; Wilson and

Carhart, 1971; Robertson and Pollack, 1973; Penner, 1980; Pastore et al., 1980; Cokely and Humes, 1993; Oxenham and Moore, 1994, 1995). Such findings suggest that forward and backward masking depend upon different underlying mechanisms.

The underlying mechanisms of temporal masking are not fully resolved. Duifhuis (1973) suggested that the steep segments of the monotic temporal masking curves (Fig. 10.16) may be associated with cochlear processes, while the shallower segments at longer delays may be related to neural events. Several findings implicate some degree of central processing in temporal masking. For example, we have already seen that some degree of temporal masking occurs under dichotic conditions for forward and backward masking. In addition, masking level differences (a reduction in masking associated with binaural interactions; see Chap. 13), have been shown to occur for forward, backward, and combined forward-backing masking (e.g., Deatherage and Evans, 1969; Robertson and Pollack, 1973; Berg and Yost, 1976; Yost and Walton, 1977).

Although overlapping in time of the cochlear displacement patterns is a reasonable explanation at very short masker-signal delays, short-term neural adaptation caused by the masker is the predominant explanation of forward masking (Smith, 1977; Harris and Dallos, 1979; Kidd and Feth, 1982). However, even short-term adaptation cannot fully account for the extent of the forward masking measured in psychoacoustic experiments (Relkin and Turner, 1988; Turner et al., 1994). Moreover, forward masking also occurs in cochlear implant users even though the synapses between the hair cells and auditory neurons are bypassed in these patients (Chatterjee, 1999). Thus, the existing evidence seems to suggest that both peripheral and central processes are probably involved in forward masking.

Several lines of evidence in addition to the material describe above suggest that central processes are the principal factors in backward masking. Providing the listener with contralateral timing cues supplies information that affects the uncertainty of the task and has been shown to influence backward masking but not forward masking (Pastore and Freda, 1980; Puleo and Pastore, 1980). Moreover, performance decrements in backward masking (but not forward or simultaneous masking) have been found to be associated with disorders such as specific language impairment and dyslexia (Wright et al., 1997; Wright, 1998; Wright and Saberi, 1999; Rosen and Manganari, 2001).

CENTRAL MASKING

The typical arrangement of a masking experiment involves presenting both the masker and the test stimulus to the *same* ear. Up to now, we have been discussing this ipsilateral type of masking. Another approach is to present the masker to one ear and the test signal to the *opposite* ear. Raising the intensity of the masker will eventually cause the masker to become audible in the other ear, in which case it will mask the test stimulus (a process known as *cross-hearing* or *contralateralization* of the masker). This is actually a case of ipsilateral masking as well, because it is the amount of masker that crosses the head, so to speak, that causes the masking of the signal. However, it has been demonstrated that a masker presented to one ear can cause a threshold shift for a signal at the other ear even when the masker level is too low for it to cross over to the signal ear (Chocolle, 1957; Ingham, 1959; Sherrick and Mangabeira-Albarnaz, 1961; Dirks and Malmquist, 1964; Dirks and Norris, 1966; Zwislocki et al., 1967, 1968). This contralateral effect of the masker is most likely due to an interaction of the masker and test signal within the central nervous system, probably at the level of the superior olivary complex where bilateral representation is available (Zwislocki, 1972).

Central masking is in some ways similar to, yet in other ways quite different from, the monaural (direct, ipsilateral) masking discussed earlier. In general, the amount of threshold shift produced by central masking is far less than by monaural masking, and more central masking occurs for higher-frequency tones than for low. The amount of masking is greatest at masker onset and decays to a steady-state value within about 200 ms. Of particular interest is the frequency dependence of central masking. The greatest amount of central masking occurs when the masker and test tones are close together in frequency. This frequency dependence is shown rather clearly in Fig. 10.18, in which the masker is a 1000-Hz tone presented at a sensation level of 60 dB to the opposite ear. Note that the most masking occurs in a small range of frequencies around the masker frequency. This frequency range is quite close to the critical bandwidth. As the figure also shows, more central masking results when the masker and test tones are pulsed on and off together (curve a) rather than when the masker is continuously on and the signal is pulsed in the other ear (curve b). This is a finding common

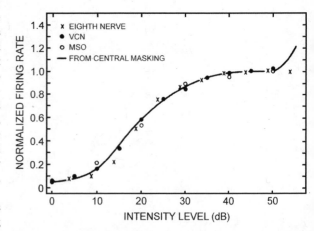

Figure 10.19 Relationship between actually obtained firing rates in the auditory (eighth cranial) nerve, ventral cochlear nucleus (VCN), and medial superior olive (MSO), and rates predicted from central masking data. *Source*: From Zwislocki, In search of physiological correlates of psychoacoustic characteristics, in: *Basic Mechanisms in Hearing* (A.R. Møller, ed.), © 1973 by Academic Press.

to most central masking experiments, although the amount of masking produced by a given masker level varies among studies and between subjects in the same study. Furthermore, central masking increases as the level of the masker is raised only for the pulsed masker/pulsed signal arrangement, whereas the amount of masking produced by the continuous masker/pulsed signal paradigm remains between about 1 and 2 dB regardless of masker level.

An excellent review of the relationships between the psychophysical and electrophysiological correlates of central masking may be found in two papers by Zwislocki (1972,1973). An example is shown in Fig. 10.19, which demonstrates the firing rates of neurons at various levels of the lower auditory nervous system (see Chaps. 5 and 6), and those predicted on the basis of central masking data. With few exceptions, the agreement shown in the figure for the intensity parameter also holds for frequency and time. Thus, central masking is shown to be related to activity in the lower auditory pathways.

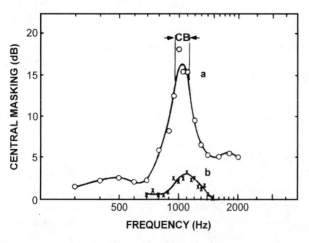

Figure 10.18 Central masking produced by a 1000-Hz tonal masker at 60 dB SL for an individual subject. Curve **a** is for a masker and a test signal pulsed on and off together; curve **b** is for a continuously on masker and a pulsed signal. *Source*: Adapted from Zwislocki et al. (1968), with permission of *J. Acoust. Soc. Am.*

INFORMATIONAL MASKING

The prior section dealt one type of central masking, in which the threshold for a signal presented to one ear is elevated by a masker in the opposite ear. This section addresses another kind of centrally mediated masking phenomenon, called informational masking. **Informational masking** refers to masking effects due to higher-level (central) processes rather than the interaction of the signal and masker in the cochlea. In this context, the term **energetic masking** is often used to describe peripheral masking effects. Informational masking effects in sound discrimination tasks are discussed in Chapter 9.

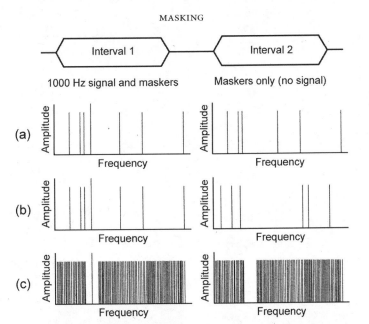

Figure 10.20 Informational masking experiments involve detecting a signal in the presence of a multiple-frequency masker. In each of these examples, the spectrum for interval 1 shows the signal and masker, and the spectrum for interval 2 shows the masker alone (no signal). The 1000-Hz signal is represented by a slightly taller line in each frame. No masker components occur within the critical band (protected range) around the signal frequency. (a) Spectra showing the same 6-component masker in both intervals. (b) Spectra showing the 6-masker components randomized between intervals. (c) Spectra showing the same 100-component masker in both intervals. (d) Spectra showing the 100 masker components randomized between intervals.

Informational masking has been studied in considerable detail (e.g., Neff and Green, 1987; Neff and Callaghan, 1988; Neff and Dethlefs, 1995; Kidd et al., 1994; Neff, 1995; Wright and Saberi, 1999; Richards et al., 2002; Arbogast, Mason, and Kidd, 2002; Gallum, Mason, and Kidd, 2005; Hall, Buss, and Grose, 2005). In the typical experiment, the listener must detect a pure tone signal in the presence of a multiple-frequency masker, although speech signals have also been used. The usual approach involves raising and lowering the signal to find its masked threshold using a two-interval forced-choice method, where one interval contains the signal and masker and the other interval contains just the masker (no signal). The subject's task is to indicate which interval contains the signal. Several examples are shown in Fig. 10.20, where the signal is a 1000-Hz pure tone. It is represented in the figure by the slightly taller line in interval 1 of each frame for illustrative purposes. The signal would actually be presented randomly in both intervals in a real experiment. The masker is a sound composed of two or more pure tone components within a certain frequency range (typically about 300–3000 Hz). The examples in the figure have maskers composed of 6 components (frames a and b) and 100 components (frames c and d). Masked thresholds are obtained separately for each masking condition (for 2-component maskers,

4-component maskers, 8-component maskers, etc.). All of the maskers have the same overall level regardless of how many components they contain or what the frequencies of the components happen to be. What is special about the informational masking situation is that the specific *frequencies of the masker components are randomized* from trial to trial. In other words, the frequencies making up the masker in one trial are different from what they are in another trial. In some conditions, the masker frequencies might also be randomized between the two intervals of the same trial.

In order to avoid or at least minimize the chances that the results might be confounded by effects due to peripheral (energetic) masking, informational masking experiments use a critical band-wide "protected region" around the signal frequency that does not contain any masker components. (Recall that in peripheral masking, a tone is masked by the part of the masker spectrum that is within a certain critical band around that tone.) All of the spectra in Fig. 10.20 have this protected range (most easily seen in frames c and d).

Figure 10.21 shows the amount of masking (for the 1000-Hz signal) produced by maskers with as few as 2 and as many as 150 components under two conditions: (1) when masker components *are* allowed to fall inside the critical band (as in the

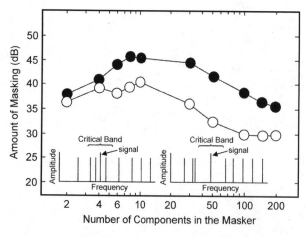

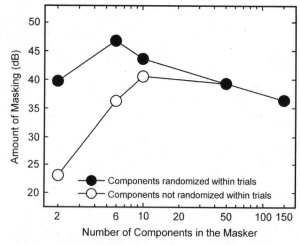

Figure 10.21 The graph shows amount of masking of a 1000-Hz signal produced by maskers with different numbers of components when masker components may fall within the critical band around the signal (*filled symbols*) compared to when none of the components are within the critical band (*open symbols*). *Source*: Adapted from Neff and Callaghan, 1988 with permission of *J. Acoust. Soc. Am. Insets*: The left spectrum shows some masker components falling *inside* the critical band around the signal. The right spectrum shows the same number of masker components, all falling *outside* the critical band.

Figure 10.22 The amount of masking of a 1000-Hz signal produced by maskers with different numbers of components. Open symbols show results when the masker frequencies are the same for both intervals (as in Fig. 10.20a and c). Closed symbols show results when the masker frequencies are randomized between intervals (as in Fig. 10.20b and d). *Source*: Adapted from Neff and Callaghan (1988) with permission of *J. Acoust. Soc. Am.*

left inset), and (2) when all of the components are outside of the critical band (as in the right inset). We see that more masking occurs when some of the masker components are within the critical band (filled symbols) than when they are all outside of the critical band (open symbols). However, there is still a considerable amount of masking even when all of the masker components are outside the critical band, that is, where they are too far from the signal to cause any appreciable energetic masking. This is informational masking. It is attributed to the *uncertainty* introduced into the listening task by randomizing the masker components, thereby interfering with the ability to detect the signal even though it has not be rendered inaudible at the periphery.

The influence of the degree of masker uncertainty is illustrated in Fig. 10.22. It shows the amount of masking (for the 1000-Hz signal) produced by multitone maskers composed of various numbers of components under two degrees of uncertainty. (1) The smaller degree of uncertainty occurs when the frequencies of the masker components are randomized between trials, but are the same for both intervals within a given trial (e.g., Fig. 10.20a for a 6-component masker and Fig. 10.20c for a 100-component masker). (2) Greater uncertainty occurs when the masker components are also randomized between the two intervals within each trial (e.g., Fig. 10.20b for 6 components and Fig. 10.20c for 100 components). The salient finding is that more informational masking occurs when there is a greater degree of uncertainty (components randomized within trials, filled symbols) than when there is less uncertainty (components not randomized within trials, open symbols). We also see that informational masking is greatest when the masker contains a

smaller number of components and smallest when there are a great many components.

It might seem odd that a smaller change in informational masking is produced by altering the degree of uncertainty when the masker contains a large number of components, but it makes sense with a simple visual analogy: Look at the spectra in Fig. 10.20, and notice that it is easier to see that the signal line is in interval 1 in frame a (where the few masker lines are the same for both intervals) than in frame b (where the few masker lines are different between the intervals). On the other hand, it is just as easy to see that the signal line is in interval 1 in frame d (where the many masker lines are different between the intervals) as it is in frame c (where they are the same for both intervals). It is as if a small number of masker components face the listener with a sparse and irregular background where knowing the details is very important; thus random changes in these details create a lot of uncertainty. On the other hand, a large number of components make the background more uniform so that knowing the details is relatively less important. Thus, random changes in its details do not cause as much uncertainty.

In summary, informational masking is the result of higher-level (central) processes related to uncertainty about the masker. The amount of informational masking is typically quite large, on the order of 40 to 50 dB or more, and the effect is greatest when the masker contains a relatively small number of components (generally about 20 or fewer). Before leaving this topic, it should be pointed out that informational masking is subject to a considerable amount of variability among subjects and is affected by a variety of factors (see, e.g., Neff and Callaghan, 1988; Neff and Dethlefs, 1995; Neff, 1995; Wright and Saberi, 1999; Richards et al., 2002).

REFERENCES

Arbogast, TL, Mason, CR, Kidd, G. 2002. The effect of spatial separation on informational and energetic masking of speech. *J Acoust Soc Am* 112, 2086–2098.

Babkoff, H, Sutton, S. 1968. Monaural temporal masking of transients. *J Acoust Soc Am* 44, 1373–1378.

Bacon, SP. 1990. Effect of masked level on overshoot. *J Acoust Soc Am* 88, 698–702.

Bacon, SP, Healy, EW. 2000. Effects of ipsilateral and contralateral precursors on the temporal effect in simultaneous masking with pure tones. *J Acoust Soc Am* 107, 589–1597.

Bacon, SP, Hendrick, MS, Grantham, DW. 1989. Temporal effects in simultaneous pure-tone masking in subjects with high-frequency sensorineural hearing loss. *Audiology* 27, 313–323.

Bacon, SP, Lee, J, Paterson, DN, Rainey, D.. 1997. Masking by modulated and unmodulated noise: Effects of bandwidth, modulation rate, signal frequency, and masker level. *J Acoust Soc Am* 76, 50–56.

Bacon, SP, Moore, BCJ. 1986. Temporal effects in masking and their influence on psychophysical tuning curves. *J Acoust Soc Am* 80, 1638–1645.

Bacon, SP, Savel, S. 2004. Temporal effects in simultaneous masking with on- and off-frequency noise maskers: Effects of signal frequency and masker level. *J Acoust Soc Am* 115, 1674–1683.

Bacon, SP, Smith, MA. 1991. Spectral, intensive, and temporal factors influencing overshoot. *Quart J Exp Psychol* 43A, 373–399.

Bacon, SP, Takahashi, GA. 1992. Overshoot in normal-hearing and hearing-impaired subjects. *J Acoust Soc Am* 91, 2865–2871.

Bacon, SP, Viemeister, NF. 1985. The temporal course of simultaneous pure-tone masking. *J Acoust Soc Am* 78, 1231–1235.

Berg, K, Yost, WA. 1976. Temporal masking of a click by noise in diotic and dichotic conditions. *J Acoust Soc Am* 60, 173–177.

Bilger, RC. 1958. Intensive determinants of remote masking. *J Acoust Soc Am* 30, 817–824.

Bilger, RC. 1966. Remote masking in the absence of intra-aural muscles. *J Acoust Soc Am* 39, 103–108.

Bilger, RC. 1976. A revised critical-band hypothesis. In: SK Hirsh, DH Eldredge (eds.), *Hearing and Davis: Essays Honoring Hallowell Davis*. St. Louis. MO: Washington University Press, 191–198.

Bilger, RC, Hirsh, IJ. 1956. Masking of tone by bands of noise. *J Acoust Soc Am* 28, 623–630.

Bos, CE, deBoer, E. 1966. Masking and discrimination. *J Acoust Soc Am* 39, 708–715.

Buus, S. 1985. Release from masking caused by envelope fluctuations. *J Acoust Soc Am* 78, 1958–1965.

Carlyon, RP, White, LJ. 1992. Effect of signal frequency and masker level on the frequency regions responsible for the overshoot effect. *J Acoust Soc Am* 91, 1034–1041.

Champlin, CA, McFadden, D. 1989. Reductions in overshoot following intense sound exposures. *J Acoust Soc Am* 85, 2005–2011.

Chatterjee, M. 1999. Temporal mechanisms underlying recovery from forward masking in multielectrode-implant listeners. *J Acoust Soc Am* 105, 1853–1863.

Chistovich, LA. 1957. Frequency characteristics of masking effect. Biophysics 2, 708–715.

Chocolle, R. 1957. La sensibility auditive differentielle dtintensite en presence d'un son contralateral de meme frequence. *Acustica* 7, 75–83.

Cokely, CG, Humes, LE. 1993. Two experiments on the temporal boundaries for nonlinear additivity of masking. *J Acoust Soc Am* 94, 2553–2559.

Deatherage, BH, Davis, H, Eldredge, DH. 1957a. Physiological evidence for the masking of low frequencies by high. *J Acoust Soc Am* 29, 132–137.

Deatherage, BH, Davis, H, Eldredge, DH. 1957b. Remote masking in selected frequency regions. *J Acoust Soc Am* 29, 512–514.

Deatherage, BH, Evans, TR. 1969. Binaural and masking: Backward, forward and simultaneous effects. *J Acoust Soc Am* 46, 362–371.

Dirks, DD, Malmquist, C. 1964. Changes in bone-conduction thresholds produced by masking of the non-test ear. *J Speech Hear Res* 7, 271–287.

Dirks, DD, Norris, JC. 1966. Shifts in auditory thresholds produced by pulsed and continuous contralateral masking. *J Acoust Soc Am* 37, 631–637.

Duifhuis, H. 1973. Consequences of peripheral frequency selectivity for nonsimultaneous masking. *J Acoust Soc Am* 54, 1471–1488.

Duifhuis, H. 1976. Cochlear nonlinearity and second filter. Possible mechanisms and implications. *J Acoust Soc Am* 59, 408–423.

Egan, JP, Hake, HW. 1950. On the masking pattern of a simple auditory stimulus. *J Acoust Soc Am* 22, 622–630.

Ehmer, RH. 1959a. Masking patterns of tones. *J Acoust Soc Am* 31, 1115–1120.

Ehmer, RH. 1959b. Masking by tones vs. noise bands. *J Acoust Soc Am* 31, 1253–1256.

Elliott, LL. 1962a. Backward masking: Monotic and dichotic conditions. *J Acoust Soc Am* 34, 1108–1115.

Elliott, LL. 1962b. Backward and forward masking of probe tones of different frequencies. *J Acoust Soc Am* 34, 1116–1117.

Elliott, LL. 1964. Backward masking: Different durations of the masker stimulus. *J Acoust Soc Am* 36, 393.

Elliott, LL. 1965.Changes in the simultaneous masked threshold of brief tones. *J Acoust Soc Am* 38, 738–756.

Elliott, LL. 1967. Development of auditory narrow-band frequency contours. *J Acoust Soc Am* 42, 143–153.

Elliott, LL. 1969. Masking of tones before, during, and after brief silent periods in noise. *J Acoust Soc Am* 45, 1277–1279.

Fastl, H. 1976. Temporal masking effects: I. Broad band noise masker. *Acustica* 35, 287–302.

Fastl, H. 1977. Temporal masking effects: II. Critical band noise masker. *Acustica* 36, 317–331.

Fastl, H. 1979. Temporal masking effects: III. Pure tone masker. *Acustica* 43, 283–294.

Fidell, S, Horonjeff, R, Teffeteller, S, Green, DM. 1983. Effective masking bandwidths at low frequencies. *J Acoust Soc Am* 73, 628–638.

Finck, A. 1961. Low-frequency pure tone masking. *J Acoust Soc Am* 33, 1140–1141.

Fletcher, H. 1937. Relation between loudness and masking. *J Acoust Soc Am* 9, 1–10.

Fletcher, H. 1940. Auditory patterns. *J Acoust Soc Am* 12, 47–65.

Formby, C, Sherlock, LP, Ferguson, SH. 2000. Enhancement of the edges of temporal masking functions by complex patterns of overshoot and undershoot. *J Acoust Soc Am* 107, 2169–2187.

Gallum, FJ, Mason, CR, Kidd, G. 2005. Binaural release from informational masking in a speech identification task. *J Acoust Soc Am* 118, 1605–1613.

Gelfand, SA. 2001. *Essentials of Audiology, 2nd edn.* New York, NY: Thieme Medical Publishers.

Glasberg, BR, Moore, BCJ, Nimmo-Smith, I. 1984a. Comparison of auditory filter shapes derived with three different maskers. *J Acoust Soc Am* 75, 536–544.

Glasberg, BR, Moore, BCJ, Patterson, RD, Nimmo-Smith, I. 1984b. Comparison of auditory filter. *J Acoust Soc Am* 76, 419–427.

Green, DM. 1969. Masking with continuous and pulsed sinusoids. *J Acoust Soc Am* 46, 939–946.

Greenwood, DD. 1961. Auditory masking and the critical band. *J Acoust Soc Am* 33, 484–502.

Grose, JH, Hall, JW, Buss, E, Hatch, DR. 2005. Detection of spectrally complex signals in comodulated maskers: Effects of temporal fringe. *J Acoust Soc Am* 118, 3774–3782.

Hall, JW, Buss, E, Grose, JH. 2005. Informational masking release in children and adults. *J Acoust Soc Am* 118, 1605–1613.

Hall, JW, Grose, JH. 1990. Effects of flanking band proximity, number, and modulation pattern on comodulation masking release. *J Acoust Soc Am* 87, 269–283.

Hall, JW, Haggard, MP, Fernandes, MA. 1984. Detection in noise by specto-temporal pattern analysis. *J Acoust Soc Am* 76, 50–56.

Hamilton, PM. 1957. Noise masked thresholds as a function of tonal duration and masking noise band width. *J Acoust Soc Am* 29, 506–511.

Harris, DM, Dallos, P. 1979. Forward masking of auditory nerve fiber responses. *J Neurophysiol* 42, 1083–1107.

Hatch, DR, Arne, BC, Hall, JW. 1995. Comodulation masking release (CMR): Effects of gating as a function of number of flanking bands and masker bandwidth. *J Acoust Soc Am* 97, 3768–3774.

Hawkins, JE, Stevens, SS. 1950. The masking of pure tones and of speech by white noise. *J Acoust Soc Am* 22, 6–13.

Hicks, ML, Bacon, SP. 1995. Some factors influencing comodulation masking release and across-channel masking. *J Acoust Soc Am* 98, 2504–2514.

Houtgast, T. 1972. Psychophysical evidence for lateral inhibition in hearing. *J Acoust Soc Am* 51, 1885–1894.

Houtgast, T. 1977. Auditory-filter characteristics derived from direct-masking data plus pulsation-threshold data with a rippled-noise masker. *J Acoust Soc Am* 62, 409–415.

Ingham, JG. 1959. Variations in cross-making with frequency. *J Exp Psychol* 58, 199–205.

Jesteadt, W, Bacon, SP, Lehman, JR. 1982. Forward masking as a function of frequency, masker level, and signal delay. *J Acoust Soc Am* 71, 950–962.

Jesteadt, W, Norton, SJ. 1985. The role of suppression in psychophysical measures of frequency selectivity. *J Acoust Soc Am* 78, 365–374.

Kidd, G, Feth, LL. 1982. Effect of masker duration on pure-tone forward masking. *J Acoust Soc Am* 72, 1384–1386.

Kidd, G Jr, Mason, CR, Deliwala, PS, Woods, WS, Colburn, HS. 1994. Reducing informational masking by sound segregation. *J Acoust Soc Am* 95, 3475–3480.

Kryter, KD. 1973. Impairment to hearing from exposure to noise. *J Acoust Soc Am* 53, 1211–1234. [Also: comments by A Cohen, H Davis, B Lempert, WD Ward, and reply by KD Kryter. *J Acoust Soc Am* 53, 1235–1252 (1973)]

Kryter, KD. 1985. *The Effects of Noise on Man, 2nd edn.* New York, NY: Academic Press.

Lufti, RA. 1984. Predicting frequency selectivity in forward masking from simultaneous masking. *J Acoust Soc Am* 76, 1045–1050.

Lufti, RA. 1988. Interpreting measures of frequency selectivity: Is forward masking special? *J Acoust Soc Am* 83, 163–177.

Lynn, G, Small, AM. 1977. Interactions of backward and forward masking. *J Acoust Soc Am* 61, 185–189.

Mayer, AM. 1894. Researches in acoustics. *Philos Mag* 37, 259–288.

McFadden, D, Champlin, CA. 1990. Reductions in overshoot during aspirin use. *J Acoust Soc Am* 87, 2634–2642.

Meyer, ME. 1959. Masking: Why restrict it to the threshold level? *J Acoust Soc Am* 31, 243.

Mills, JH, Gengel, RW, Watson, CS, Miller, JD. 1970. Temporary changes in the auditory system due to exposure to noise for one or two days. *J Acoust Soc Am* 48, 524–530.

Moore, BCJ. 1990. Co-modulation masking release: Spectro-temporal pattern analysis in hearing. *Brit J Audiol* 24, 131–137.

Moore, BCJ, Glasberg, BJ. 1983b. Suggested formulae for calculating auditory-filter bandwidths and excitation patterns. *J Acoust Soc Am* 74, 750–753.

Moore, BCJ, Glasberg, BR. 1981. Auditory filter shapes derived in simultaneous and forward masking. *J Acoust Soc Am* 70, 1003–1014.

Moore, BCJ, Glasberg, BR. 1987. Formulae describing frequency selectivity as a function of frequency and level, and their use in calculating excitation patterns. *Hear Res* 28, 209–225.

Moore, BCJ, Glasberg, R, Roberts, B. 1984. Refining the measurement of psychophysical tuning curves. *J Acoust Soc Am* 76, 1057–1066.

Moore, BCJ, Glasberg, BR, Schooneveldt, GP. 1990. Across-channel masking and across-channel masking. *J Acoust Soc Am* 87, 1683–1694.

Neff, DL. 1995. Signal properties that reduce masking by simultaneous random-frequency maskers. *J Acoust Soc Am* 98, 1909–1920.

Neff, DL, Callaghan, BP. 1988. Effective properties of multicomponent simultaneous maskers under conditions of uncertainty. *J Acoust Soc Am* 83, 1833–1838.

Neff, DL, Dethlefs, DL. 1995. Individual differences in simultaneous masking with random-frequency, multicomponent maskers. *J Acoust Soc Am* 98, 125–134.

Neff, DL, Green, DM. 1987. Masking produced by spectral uncertainty with multicomponent maskers. *Percept Psychophys* 41, 409–415.

O'Loughlin, BJ, Moore, BCJ. 1981. Improving psychoacoustic tuning curves. *Hear Res* 5, 343–346.

Oxenham, AJ, Moore, BCJ. 1994. Modeling the additivity of nonsimultaneous masking. *Hear Res* 80, 105–118.

Oxenham, AJ, Moore, BCJ. 1995. Additivity of masking in normally hearing and hearing-impaired subjects. *J Acoust Soc Am* 98, 1921–1934.

Pastore, RE, Freda, JS. 1980. Contralateral cueing effects in forward masking. *J Acoust Soc Am* 67, 2104–2105.

Pastore, RE, Harris, LB, Goldstein, L. 1980. Auditory forward and backward masking interaction. *Percept Psychophys* 28, 547–549.

Patterson, RD. 1974. Auditory filter shape. *J Acoust Soc Am* 55, 802–809.

Patterson, RD. 1976. Auditory filter shapes derived with noise stimuli. *J Acoust Soc Am* 59, 640–654.

Patterson, RD, Moore, BCJ. 1986. Auditory filters and excitation patterns as representations of frequency resolution. In: BCJ Moore (ed.), *Frequency Selectivity in Hearing*. London, UK: Academic Press, 123–177.

Patterson, RD, Nimmo-Smith, I, Webster, DL, Milroy, R. 1982. The deterioration of hearing with age: Frequency selectivity, the critical ratio, the audiogram, and speech threshold. *J Acoust Soc Am* 72, 1788–1803.

Penner, MJ. 1980. The coding of intensity and the interaction of forward and backward masking. *J Acoust Soc Am* 67, 608–616.

Pollack, I. 1964. Interaction of forward and backward masking. *J Aud Res* 4, 63–67.

Puleo, JS, Pastore, RE. 1980. Contralateral cueing effects in backward masking. *J Acoust Soc Am* 67, 947–951.

Relkin, EM, Turner, CW. 1988. A reexamination of forward masking in the auditory nerve. *J Acoust Soc Am* 84, 584–591.

Richards, VM, Tang, Z, Kidd G Jr. 2002. Informational masking with small set sizes. *J Acoust Soc Am* 111, 1359–1366.

Robertson, CE, Pollack, I. 1973. Interaction between forward and backward masking: A measure of the integrating period of the auditory system. *J Acoust Soc Am* 1313–1316.

Rosen, S, Manganari, E. 2001. Is there a relationship between speech and nonspeech auditory processing in children with dyslexia? *J Speech Lang Hear Res* 44, 720–736.

Schaefer, TH, Gales, RS, Shewaker, CA, Thompson, PO. 1950. The frequency selectivity of the ear as determined by masking experiments. *J Acoust Soc Am* 22, 490–497.

Scharf, B. 1964. Partial masking. *Acoustica* 14, 16–23.

Scharf, B. 1970. Critical bands. In: JV Tobias (ed.), *Foundations of Modern Auditory Theory, Vol. 1*. New York, NY: Academic Press, 157–202.

Scharf, B, Reeves, A, Giovanetti, H. 2008. Role of attention in overshoot: Frequency certainty versus uncertainty. *J Acoust Soc Am* 123, 1555–1561.

Shailer, MJ, Moore, BCJ. 1983. Gap detection as a function of frequency, bandwidth, and level. *J Acoust Soc Am* 74, 467–473.

Sherrick, CE, Mangabeira-Albarnaz, PL. 1961. Auditory threshold shifts produced by simultaneous pulsed contralateral stimuli. *J Acoust Soc Am* 33, 1381–1385.

Small, AM. 1959. Pure tone masking. *J Acoust Soc Am* 31, 1619–1625.

Smiarowski, RA, Carhart, R. 1975. Relations among temporal resolution, forward masking, and simultaneous masking. *J Acoust Soc Am* 57, 1169–1174.

Smith, RL. 1977. Short-term adaptation in single auditory nerve fibers: Some poststimulatory effects. *J Neurophysiol* 40, 1098–1112.

Spieth, W. 1957. Downward spread of masking. *J Acoust Soc Am* 29, 502–505.

Stelmachowicz, PG, Jesteadt, W. 1984. Psychophysical tuning curves in normal-hearing listeners: Test reliability and probe level effects. *J Speech Hear Res* 27, 396–402.

Strickland, EA. 2001. The relationship between frequency selectivity and overshoot. *J Acoust Soc Am* 109, 2062–2073.

Swets, JA, Green, DM, Tanner, WP. 1962. On the width of the critical bands. *J Acoust Soc Am* 34, 108–113.

Turner, CW, Relkin, EM, Doucet, J. 1994. Psychophysical and physiological forward masking studies: Probe duration and rise-time effects. *J Acoust Soc Am* 96, 795–800.

von Klitzing, R, Kohlrausch, A. 1994. Effect of masker level on overshoot in running- and frozen-noise maskers. *J Acoust Soc Am* 95, 2192–2201.

Weber, DL. 1977. Growth of masking and the auditory filter. *J Acoust Soc Am* 62, 424–429.

Weber, DL. 1983. Do off-frequency maskers suppress the signal? *J Acoust Soc Am* 73, 887–893.

Weber, DL, Moore, BCJ. 1981. Forward masking by sinusoidal and noise maskers. *J Acoust Soc Am* 69, 1402–1409.

Wegel, RL, Lane, CE. 1924. The auditory masking of one pure tone by another and its probable relation to the dynamics of the inner ear. *Physiol Rev* 23, 266–285.

Widin, GP, Viemeister, NF. 1979. Intensive and temporal effects in pure-tone forward masking. *J Acoust Soc Am* 66, 388–395.

Wightman, FL, McGee, T, Kramer, M. 1977. Factors influencing frequency selectivity in normal and hearing-impaired listeners. In: EF Evans, JP Wilson (eds.), *Psychophysics and Physiology of Hearing*. London. UK: Academic Press, 295–306.

Wilson, RH, Carhart, R. 1971. Forward and backward masking: Interactions and additivity. *J Acoust Soc Am* 49, 1254–1263.

Wright, HN. 1964. Backward masking for tones in narrow-band noise. *J Acoust Soc Am* 36, 2217–2221.

Wright, BA. 1998. Specific language impairment: Abnormal auditory masking and the potential for its remediation through training. In: AR Palmer, A Rees, AQ Summerfield, R Meddis (eds.), *Psychophysical and Physiological Advances in Hearing*. London, UK: Whurr, 604–610.

Wright, BA, Lombardino, LJ, King, WM, Puranik, CS, Leonard, CM, Merzenich, MM. 1997. Deficits in auditory temporal and spectral resolution in language-impaired children. *Nature* 387, 176–178.

Wright, BA, Saberi, K. 1999. Strategies used to detect auditory signals in small sets of random maskers. *J Acoust Soc Am* 105, 1765–1775.

Yost, WA, Walton, J. 1977. Hierarchy of masking-level differences for temporal masking. *J Acoust Soc Am* 61, 1376–1379.

Zwicker, E. 1965a. Temporal effects in simultaneous masking by white noise bursts. *J Acoust Soc Am* 37, 653–663.

Zwicker, E. 1965b. Temporal effects in simultaneous masking and loudness. *J Acoust Soc Am* 132–141.

Zwicker, E. 1974. On a psychoacoustical equivalent of tuning curves. In: E Zwicker, E Tehrhardt (eds.), *Facts and Models in Hearing*. Berlin, Germany: Springer, 95–99.

Zwicker, E. 1984. Dependence of post-masking on masker duration and its relation to temporal effects in loudness. *J Acoust Soc Am* 75, 219–223.

Zwicker, E, Flottrop, G, Stevens, SS. 1957. Critical bandwidth in loudness summation. *J Acoust Soc Am* 29, 548–557.

Zwicker, E, Schorn, K. 1978. Psychoacoustical tuning curves in audiology. *Audiology* 17, 120–140.

Zwicker, E, Terhardt, E. 1980. Analytical expressions of critical-band rate and critical bandwidth as a function of frequency. *J Acoust Soc Am* 68, 1523–1525.

Zwislocki, J. 1972. A theory of central masking and its partial validation. *J Acoust Soc Am* 52, 644–659.

Zwislocki, J. 1973. In search of physiological correlates of psychoacoustic characteristics. In: AR Møller (ed.), *Basic Mechanisms in Hearing*. New York, NY: Academic Press, 787–808.

Zwislocki, J, Buining, E, Glantz, J. 1968. Frequency distribution of central masking. *J Acoust Soc Am* 43, 1267–1271.

Zwislocki, J, Damianopoulus, EN, Buining, E, Glantz J. 1967. Central masking: Some steady-state and transient effects. *Percept Psychophys* 2, 59–64.

11   Loudness

The intensity of a sound refers to its physical magnitude, which may be expressed in such terms as its power or pressure. Turning up the "volume" control on a stereo amplifier thus increases the intensity of the music coming out of the loudspeakers. This intensity is easily measured by placing the microphone of a sound-level meter near the loudspeaker. The perception of intensity is called **loudness**; generally speaking, low intensities are perceived as "soft" and high intensities as "loud." In other words, intensity is the physical parameter of the stimulus and loudness is the percept associated with that parameter. However, intensity and loudness are not one and the same; although increasing intensity is associated with increasing loudness, there is not a simple one-to-one correspondence between the two. Furthermore, loudness is also affected by factors other than intensity. For example, it is a common experience to find that loudness changes when the "bass" and "treble" controls of a stereo amplifier are adjusted, even though the volume control itself is untouched. (*Bass* and *treble* are the relative contributions of the lower and higher frequency ranges, respectively. Thus, raising the bass emphasizes the low frequencies, and raising the treble emphasizes the high.)

LOUDNESS LEVEL

We may begin our discussion of loudness by asking whether the same amount of intensity results in the same amount of loudness for tones of different frequencies. For example, does a 100-Hz tone at 40 dB SPL have the same loudness as a 1000-Hz tone also presented at 40 dB? The answer is no. However, a more useful question is to ask how much intensity is needed in order for tones of different frequencies to sound equally loud. These values may be appropriately called **equal loudness levels**.

Although the exact procedures differ, the fundamental approach for determining equal loudness levels is quite simple. One tone is presented at a fixed intensity level, and serves as the reference tone for the experiment. The other tone is then varied in level until its loudness is judged equal to that of the reference tone. Subsequent studies have employed adaptive testing strategies (see Chap. 7) to accomplish loudness matching (e.g., Jesteadt, 1980; Schlauch and Wier, 1987; Florentine et al., 1996; Buus et al., 1997). The traditional reference tone has been 1000 Hz, but Stevens (1972) suggested the use of 3150 Hz, where threshold sensitivity is most acute. A third frequency tone may then be balanced with the reference tone; then a fourth, a fifth, and so on. The result is a list of sound pressure levels at various frequencies, all of which sound equal in loudness to the reference tone. We can then draw a curve showing these equally loud sound pressure levels as a function of frequency. If the experiment is repeated for different reference tone intensities, the result is a series of contours like the ones in Fig. 11.1.

The contour labeled "40 phons" shows the sound pressure levels needed at each frequency for a tone to sound equal in loudness to a 1000-Hz reference tone presented at 40 dB SPL. Thus, any sound that is equal in loudness to a 1000-Hz tone at 40 dB has a loudness level of 40 phons. A tone that is as loud as a 1000-Hz tone at 50 dB has a loudness level of 50 phons, one that is as loud as a 1000-Hz tone at 80 dB has a loudness level of 80 phons, etc. We may now define the **phon** as the unit of **loudness level**. All sounds that are equal in phons have the same loudness level even though their physical magnitudes may be different. Since we are expressing loudness level in phons relative to the level of a 1000-Hz tone, phons and decibels of sound pressure level are necessarily equal at this frequency.

The earliest equal loudness data were reported by Kingsbury in 1927. However, the first well-accepted **phon curves** were published in 1933 by Fletcher and Munson, and as a result, **equal-loudness contours** have also come to be known as **Fletcher–Munson curves**. Subsequently, extensive equal loudness contours were also published by Churcher and King (1937) and by Robinson and Dadson (1956). Equal loudness contours have also been reported for narrow bands of noise (Pollack, 1952). The curves shown in Fig. 11.1 reflect the values in the current international standard (ISO 226–2003).

At low loudness levels, the phon curves are quite similar in shape to the minimum audible field (MAF) curve. Thus, considerably more intensity is needed to achieve equal loudness for lower frequencies than for higher ones. However, notice that the phon curves tend to become flatter for higher loudness levels, indicating that the lower frequencies grow in loudness at a faster rate than the higher frequencies, overcoming, so to speak, their disadvantage at near-threshold levels. This effect can be experienced in a simple, at-home experiment. We begin by playing music from a CD at a moderate level, with the bass and treble controls set so that the music is as "natural sounding" as possible. If we decrease the volume to a much softer level, the music will also sound as though the bass was decreased, demonstrating the de-emphasis of the low (bass) frequencies at lower loudness levels. If we raise the volume to a quite loud level, then the music will sound as though the bass was turned up as well. This "boomy" sound reflects the faster rate of growth for the lower frequencies with increasing loudness levels.

Since the same sound pressure level will be associated with different loudness levels as a function of frequency, it would be convenient to have a frequency-weighting network that could be applied to the wide-band sounds encountered in the environment. Such a weighting function would facilitate calculating the loudness of such sounds as highway noise, sonic booms, etc. This has been done to some extent in the construction of electronic-weighting networks for sound level meters. These networks are rough approximations to various phon curves. For example, the **A-weighting** network approximates the general shape of the

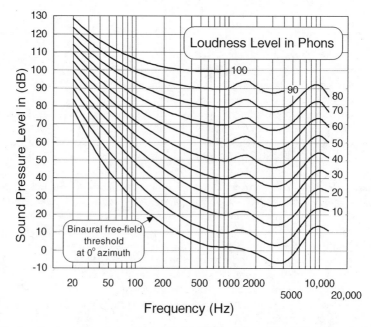

Figure 11.1 Equal loudness-level or phon curves (based on values in ISO 226–2003) and binaural free-field auditory threshold curve (based on values in ANSI S3.6–2004 and ISO 389–7-2005). Notice how the loudness level in phons corresponds to the number of decibels at 1000 Hz.

40-phon curve by de-emphasizing the low frequencies and more efficiently passing the high. The **B-weighting** network roughly corresponds to the 70-phon loudness level, and the **C-weighting** network is designed to mimic the essentially flat response of the ear at high loudness levels. These weightings are illustrated in Fig. 11.2. Sound levels that reflect the A-weighting network are expressed as **dB-A**, and **dB-C** refers to C-weighted sound levels (**dB-B** refers to B-weighted sound levels, but are rarely used).

The use of loudness levels represents a significant improvement over such vague concepts, as "more intense sounds are

louder." However, the phon itself does not provide a direct measure of loudness, per se. We must still seek an answer to the question of how the loudness percept is related to the level of the physical stimulus.

LOUDNESS SCALES

Loudness scales show how the loudness percept is related to the level of the sound stimulus. Since we are interested not only in the loudness of a particular sound, but also in how much louder one sound is than another, the relationship between loudness and sound level is best determined with direct ratio scaling techniques (see Chap. 7). This approach was pioneered and developed by Stevens (1955), 1956a, 1956b, 1957a, 1959, 1975), whose earliest attempts to define a ratio scale of loudness used the fractionalization method (Stevens, 1936). Stevens later adopted the use of magnitude estimation and magnitude production (Stevens, 1956a, 1956b), and the preponderance of subsequent work has employed these techniques alone or in combination (e.g., Hellman and Zwislocki, 1963, 1964, 1968; Stevens and Guirao, 1964; Stevens and Greenbaum, 1966; Rowley and Studebaker, 1969; Hellman, 1976).

The intensity difference limen (DLI), or just noticeable difference (jnd), has also been proposed as a basis for loudness scaling, as has been the partitioning of the audible intensity range into equal loudness categories. However, the consensus of data supports ratio scaling. See Robinson's (1957) review and study, and also Gardner (1958) and Stevens (1959) for summaries of

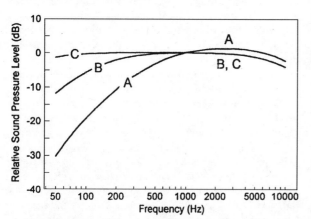

Figure 11.2 Frequency response curves for the A, B, and C weightings. Notice how the lower frequencies are de-emphasized significantly by the A weighting and less so by the B weighting, while the C-weighting network has a frequency response that is almost flat.

the controversy, as well see Marks (1974a) and Stevens (1975) for informative treatments within the more general context of psychophysics.

The unit of loudness is called the **sone** (Stevens, 1936), such that one sone is the **loudness** of a 1000-Hz tone presented at 40 dB SPL. Since sound pressure level in decibels and loudness level in phons are equivalent at 1000 Hz, we may also define one *sone* as the *loudness* corresponding to a *loudness level* of 40 *phons*. We may therefore express loudness in sones as a function of loudness level in phons (Robinson, 1957) as well as a function of stimulus level. Since loudness level does not vary with frequency (i.e., 40 phons represents the same loudness level at any frequency even though the SPLs are different), we can ignore frequency to at least some extent when assigning loudness in sones to a tone, as long as sones are expressed as a function of phons.

The **sone scale** is illustrated in Fig. 11.3 and is easily understood. Having assigned a value of one sone to the reference sound, we assign a loudness of two sones to the intensity that sounds twice as loud as the reference, 0.5 sones to the level that sounds half as loud, etc. For the most part, loudness in sones is a straight line when plotted as a function of sound level on log–log coordinates, revealing a **power function** relationship. In other words, the perception of loudness (L) may be expressed as a power (e) of the physical stimulus level (I), according to the formula

$$L = kI^e \qquad (11.1)$$

where k is a constant. (The value of the constant k depends upon the units used to express the magnitudes.) The manner in which loudness is related to the intensity of a sound is usually considered to be a case of **Stevens' power law** (1957b), which states that sensation grows as a power of stimulus level. Notice in the figure, however, that the straight-line function actually applies above about 40 dB. The exponent indicates the rate at which the sensation grows with stimulus magnitude. Thus, an exponent of 1.0 would mean that the magnitude of the sensation increases at the same rate as the stimulus level (as is the case for line length). Exponents less than 1.0 indicate that the sensation grows at a slower rate than physical stimulus level (examples are *loudness* and *brightness*), whereas exponents greater than 1.0 indicate that the perceived magnitude grows faster than the physical level (examples are *electric shock* and *heaviness*). Conveniently, the exponent also corresponds to the slope of the function.

Early studies resulted in a median exponent of 0.6 for loudness as a function of sound pressure level so that a 10-dB level increase would correspond to a doubling of loudness (Stevens, 1955); and Robinson (1957) reported that loudness increased twofold with a change in loudness level of 10 phons. This is essentially equivalent to saying that a doubling of loudness corresponds to a tripling of signal level. However, not all studies have reported this value. For example, Stevens and Guirao (1964) reported exponents averaging 0.77, and Stevens (1972) proposed an exponent of 0.67 (in which case a dou-

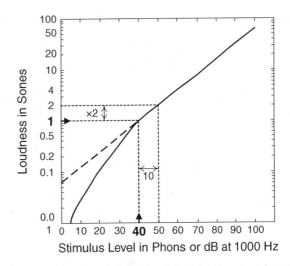

Figure 11.3 The sone scale depicts the relationship between loudness and stimulus level, where 1 sone is the loudness of a 40-dB tone at 1000 Hz (or 40 phons at other frequencies). Loudness doubles (halves) when the stimulus increases (decreases) by 10 dB (phons). Instead of continuing as a straight line for lower stimulus levels (represented by the dashed segment), the solid curve (based on values in ANSI S3.4–2007, Table 7) shows that the actual function curves downward below 40 phons, revealing faster growth of loudness at lower stimulus levels.

bling of loudness would correspond to a 9-dB increase). There is a fair amount of variability in loudness function exponents among subjects, although the individual exponents are very reliable (Logue, 1976; Walsh and Browman, 1978; Hellman, 1981; Hellman and Meiselman, 1988). Overall, the preponderance of the available data seems to point to an exponent of 0.6 as the most representative value (Marks, 1974b; Hellman, 1976, 1981; Scharf, 1978; Canevet et al., 1986; Hellman and Meiselman, 1988, 1993).

The straight-line relationship between loudness in sones and stimulus level in phons (or dB at 1000 Hz), as just described, actually does not occur at stimulus levels below about 40 dB (e.g., Hellman and Zwislocki, 1961, 1963; Scharf, 1978; Canevet et al., 1986; Buus, Muesch, and Florentine, 1998; ANSI S3.4–2007). Instead, the loudness function actually becomes steeper at lower stimulus levels, indicating faster loudness growth. Thus, the function actually curves downward below 40 phons as in Fig. 11.3. Moreover, instead of auditory threshold having a loudness level of 0 phons and a loudness of 0 sones, the ANSI S3.4–2007 incorporates the more correct actual values of 2.2 phons and 0.003 sones (see, e.g., Moore et al., 1997; Buus et al., 1998; Glasberg and Moore, 2006).

Various methods for calculating the loudness of a given actual sound have been developed over the years (e.g., Zwicker, 1958; Stevens, 1961, 1972; ISO 532–1975; ANSI S3.4–1980; Moore, Glasberg, and Baer, 1997; Zwicker and Fastl, 1999; Glasberg and Moore, 2006; ANSI S3.4–2007). The current approach is described in ANSI S3.4–2007 and is based on a model by Moore and colleagues (Moore et al., 1997; Glasberg and Moore, 2006).

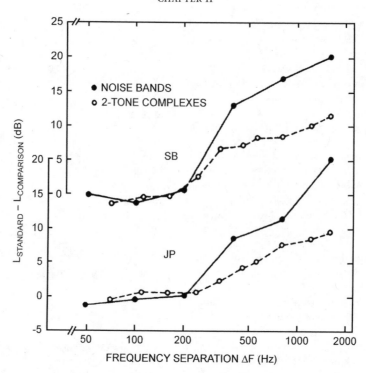

Figure 11.4   Effect of critical bandwidth upon loudness summation for a two-tone complex (open circles) and bands of noise (filled circles) for two subjects (SB and JP). Test level was 65 dB SPL and center frequency was 1000 Hz (see text). *Source*: From Florentine et al. (1978), with permission of *J. Acoust. Soc. Am.*

It can be used to calculate the loudness of any continuous sound containing noise and/or tonal components, presented either monaurally (to one ear) or binaurally (to both ears). The procedure itself should be performed by using computer software that is readily available (Glasberg and Moore, 2007; ANSI S3.4–2007) because it is quite laborious when done manually. We will not attempt to outline the details, but the general framework is as follows. The spectrum reaching the cochlea is determined by adjusting the stimulus spectrum to account for the transfer functions (a) from the sound field [1] or the earphones to the eardrum, and (b) through the middle ear (see Chap. 3). From this, the excitation level in the cochlea is determined for each auditory filter, expressed as the equivalent rectangular bandwidth (ERBs; see Chap. 10),[2] which is in turn converted into loudness values in sones per ERB. The overall loudness of the sound in sones is then calculated by summing the values for all of the ERBs. Consistent with existing data (Fletcher and Munson, 1933; Hellman and Zwislocki, 1963; Marks, 1978, 1987), binaural loudness is calculated to be twice that of monaural loudness when the same sound is presented to both ears.

[1] Different transfer functions are provided for free field and diffuse field measurements.
[2] The current approach employs ERBs instead of the critical bands used in earlier methods (e.g., ANSI S3.4–1980;), among other considerations.

LOUDNESS AND BANDWIDTH

The critical band concept was introduced with respect to masking in the last chapter. As we shall see, loudness also bears an intimate relationship to the critical bandwidth, and loudness experiments provide a direct estimate of the width of the critical band. As Scharf (1970) pointed out, it is convenient to think of the **critical band** as the bandwidth where abrupt changes occur. Consider the following experiment with this concept in mind.

Suppose pairs of simultaneous tones are presented to a subject, both tones always at the same fixed level. The first pair of tones presented is very close together in frequency, and the subject compares their loudness to the loudness of a standard tone. The frequency difference between the two tones is then increased, and the resulting loudness is again compared to the standard. We find that the loudness of the two tones stays about the same as long as the tones are separated by less than the critical bandwidth, but that there is a dramatic increase in loudness when the components are more than a critical bandwidth apart. The open circles in Fig. 11.4 show typical results for two subjects. In this figure, the amount of **loudness summation** is shown as the level difference between the standard and comparison stimuli (ordinate) as a function of bandwidth (abscissa). Notice that the loudness of the two-tone complex stays essentially the same for frequency separations smaller than the critical bandwidth (roughly 200 Hz in this example), whereas loudness increases

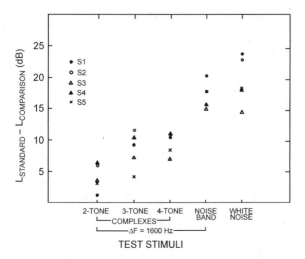

Figure 11.5 Loudness summation for tonal complexes and for noise (symbols show data for individual subjects). *Source*: From Florentine et al. (1978), with permission *J. Acoust. Soc. Am.*

when the frequency difference is greater than the width of the critical band.

That loudness remains essentially the same for bandwidths (or frequency separations) smaller than the critical band, but increases when the critical band is exceeded, has been demonstrated for two-tone and multitone complexes, and also for bands of noise (Zwicker and Feldtkeller, 1955; Zwicker and Feldtkeller, 1955; Feldtkeller and Zwicker, 1956; Zwicker et al., 1957; Scharf, 1959; Florentine et al., 1978). This loudness summation effect is minimal at near-threshold levels, and the greatest loudness increases occur for moderate signal levels (Zwicker and Feldtkeller, 1955; Zwicker et al., 1957; Scharf, 1959). As Figure 11.5 shows, loudness summation becomes greater as the number of components of a multitone complex is increased, with the most loudness summation occurring for bands of noise wider than the critical band (Florentine, Buus, and Bonding, 1978). This relation is shown in Fig. 11.4, in which the same loudness results from both two-tone complexes (open circles) and noise bands (filled circles) narrower than the critical band, but much greater loudness summation results for the noise when the critical bandwidth is exceeded.

TEMPORAL INTEGRATION OF LOUDNESS

Temporal integration (summation) at threshold was discussed in Chapter 9, where we found that sensitivity improves as signal duration increases up to about 200 to 300 ms, after which thresholds remain essentially constant. Temporal integration was also covered with respect to the acoustic reflex in Chapter 3. A similar phenomenon is also observed for loudness (e.g., Miller, 1948; Small et al., 1962; Creelman, 1963; Ekman et al., 1966; J.C. Stevens and Hall, 1966; Zwislocki, 1969; McFadden,

1975; Richards, 1977). Increasing the duration of a very brief signal at a given level above threshold will, within the same general time frame as in the cases previously discussed, cause it to sound louder.

There are two basic techniques that may be used to study the temporal integration of loudness. One method is similar to that used in establishing phon curves. The subject is presented with a reference sound at a given intensity and is asked to adjust the level of a second sound until it is equal in loudness with the first one (Miller, 1948; Small et al., 1962; Creelman, 1963; Richards, 1977). In such cases, one of the sounds is "infinitely" long (i.e., long enough so that we may be sure that temporal integration is maximal, say 1 s), and the other is a brief tone burst (of a duration such as 10 ms, 20 ms, 50 ms, etc.). Either stimulus may be used as the reference while the other is adjusted, and the result is an equal loudness contour as a function of signal duration. The alternate method involves direct magnitude scaling from which equal loudness curves can be derived (Ekman et al., 1966; J.C. Stevens and Hall, 1966; McFadden, 1975).

Figure 11.6 shows representative curves for the temporal integration of loudness. These curves are based upon the findings of Richards (1977). In his experiment, test tones of various durations were balanced in loudness to a 500-ms reference tone presented at either 20, 50, or 80 dB SPL. The ordinate shows the test tone levels (in dB SPL) needed to achieve equal loudness with the reference tone. This quantity is plotted as a function of test-tone duration on the abscissa. Notice that loudness increases (less intensity is needed to achieve a loudness balance with the reference tone) as test-tone duration increases. This

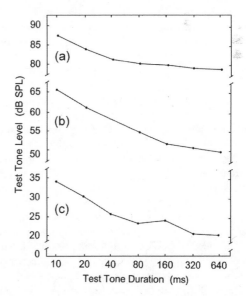

Figure 11.6 Temporal integration of loudness at 1000 Hz based upon loudness balances to a 500-ms tone presented at (a) 20 dB SPL, and (b) 50 dB SPL, and (c) 80 dB SPL. The steeper portions of the functions have slopes of (a) 10.5, (b) 12.5, and (c) 12.0 dB per decade duration change. *Source*: Based upon data by Richards (1977).

increase in loudness is greater for increases in duration up to about 80 ms, and then tends to slow down. In other words, increases in duration from 10 to about 80 ms have a steeper loudness summation slope than increases in duration above 80 ms. However, Richards did find that there was still some degree of additional loudness integration at longer durations.

These data are basically typical of most findings on temporal integration of loudness. That is, there is an increase of loudness as duration is increased up to some "critical duration," and loudness growth essentially stops (or slows down appreciably) with added duration. On the other hand, the critical duration is quite variable among studies and has generally been reported to decrease as a function of sensation level (e.g., Miller, 1948; Small et al., 1962), though not in every study (e.g., J.C. Stevens and Hall, 1966). In addition, the rate at which loudness has been found to increase with duration varies among studies. McFadden (1975) found large differences also among individual subjects. Richards (1977) fitted the steeper portions of the temporal integration functions with straight lines and found that their slopes were on the order of 10 to 12 dB per decade change in duration. The mean values are shown in Fig. 11.6 and agree well with other studies (Small et al., 1962; J.C. Stevens and Hall, 1966).

Temporal integration for loudness is also affected by the sensation level (SL) at which the loudness matches are made, with a greater amount of temporal integration occurring at moderate levels (between roughly 20–50 dB SL) compared to higher or lower sensation levels (Florentine et al., 1996; Buus et al., 1997). One might note at this point that the results of loudness integration experiments have been shown to be affected by the methodology used, and by the precise nature of the instructions given to the patients, and also by confusions on the part of subjects between loudness and duration of the signal (Stephens, 1974).

INDUCED LOUDNESS REDUCTION (LOUDNESS RECALIBRATION)

Induced loudness reduction (ILR) or **loudness recalibration** is a commonly encountered phenomenon in which the loudness of a test tone decreases when it follows the presentation of a stronger tone (e.g., Mapes-Riordan and Yost, 1999; Arieh and Marks, 2003a, 2003b; Nieder, Buus, Florentine, and Scharf, 2003; Arieh, Kelly, and Marks, 2005; Wagner and Scharf, 2006). For example, Wagner and Scharf (2006) asked listeners to make loudness magnitude estimates for a series of 70-dB test-tone bursts presented either alone or following 80-dB SPL inducer tone bursts at the same frequency. Figure 11.7 summarizes their results, which are averaged across frequencies because mean ILRs did not differ with frequency between 500 and 8000 Hz. The average loudness magnitude estimate for the test tone alone was 5.6, represented by the left-most filled symbol in the figure (labeled "without inducer"). In contrast, the loudness estimates were lower when the test tones are preceded by

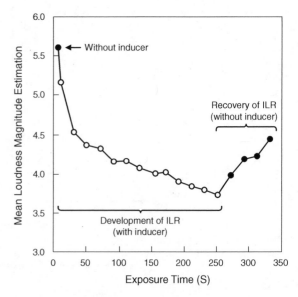

Figure 11.7 The development and recovery from induced loudness reduction (ILR) or loudness recalibration. Loudness magnitude estimates for 70-dB SPL test tone bursts presented alone (filled symbols) and following 80-dB SPL inducer tone bursts (open symbols). See text. *Source*: Reprinted with permission from Wagner and Scharf, 2006, *Journal of Acoustical Society of America, Vol 119*, p. 1017, © 2006, Acoustical Society of America.

the stronger inducer tones, shown by the open symbols. Notice that the amount of ILR increased with continued presentations of the inducer tones over time [labeled "development of ILR (with inducer)"] and began to decrease with time after the stronger inducer tones were discontinued [labeled "recovery of ILR (without inducer)"].

In general, induced loudness reduction occurs when the test tone and the stronger inducer tone are the same or relatively close in frequency, and the inducer ends at least several tenths of a second before the test tone starts. Moreover, as we observed in the example, the amount of ILR increases as the stronger inducer tone is repeated over time, and then decreases over time after the inducer is removed. The underlying mechanism of ILR is not known, but similarities between it and loudness adaptation (discussed next) suggest that these phenomena may involve a common mechanism (Nieder et al., 2003; Wagner and Scharf, 2006).

LOUDNESS ADAPTATION

Loudness adaptation refers to the apparent decrease in the loudness of a signal that is continuously presented at a fixed level for a reasonably long period of time. In other words, the signal appears to become softer as time goes on even though the sound pressure level is the same. Hood's (1950) classic experiment demonstrates this phenomenon rather clearly. A 1000-Hz tone is presented to the subject's right ear at 80 dB.

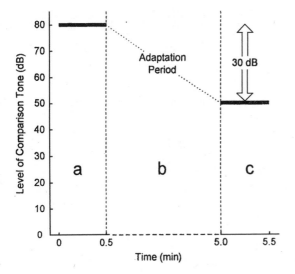

Figure 11.8 Loudness adaptation as shown by the level of the comparison stimulus. *Source*: Based on drawings by Hood (1950).

This adapting stimulus remains on continuously. At the start, a second 1000-Hz tone is presented to the left ear, and the subject adjusts the level of this second (comparison) tone to be equally loud as the adapting tone in the right ear (part a in Fig. 11.8). Thus, the level of the comparison tone is used as an indicator of the loudness of the adapting tone in the opposite ear. This first measurement represents the loudness prior to adaptation (the preadaptation balance).

The comparison tone is then turned off, while the adapting tone continues to be applied to the right ear (adaptation period b in Fig. 11.8). After several minutes of adaptation, the comparison signal is reapplied to the opposite ear, and the subject readjusts it to be equally loud with the 80-dB adapting tone. This time, however, the comparison tone is adjusted by the subject to only 50 dB in order to achieve a loudness balance with the adaptor (segment c in Fig. 11.8), indicating that the loudness of the adapting tone has decreased by an amount comparable to a 30-dB drop in signal level. Thus, there has been 30 dB of adaptation due to the continuous presentation of the tone to the right ear. Because the loudness decrease occurs during stimulation, the phenomenon is also called perstimulatory adaptation. This phenomenon contrasts, of course, with the temporary threshold shift (TTS) described in the previous chapter, which constitutes poststimulatory fatigue.

The method just described for the measurement of adaptation may be considered a simultaneous homophonic loudness balance. In other words, the subject must perform a loudness balance between two tones of the same frequency that are presented, one to each ear, at the same time. Other studies employing this approach have reported similar findings (Egan, 1955; Wright, 1960;; Small and Minifie, 1961).

A problem inherent in these early studies of loudness adaptation was their use of simultaneously presented adapting and comparison tones of the same frequency. Although the presumed task was a loudness balance between the ears, the experiments were confounded by the perception of a fused image due to the interaction of the identical stimuli at the two ears. As we shall see in Chapter 13, the relative levels at the two ears will determine whether the fused image is perceived centralized within the skull or lateralized toward one side or the other. It is therefore reasonable to question whether the loudness adaptation observed in such studies is confounded by interactions between the ears, such as lateralization.

One way around the problem is to use a comparison tone having a different frequency than the adapting tone. This procedure would reduce the lateralization phenomenon because the stimuli would be different at each ear. In 1955, Egan found no significant difference in the amount of loudness adaptation caused by this heterophonic method and the homophonic approach described above. Subsequently, however, Egan and Thwing (1955) reported that loudness balances involving lateralization cues did in fact result in greater adaptation than techniques that kept the effects of lateralization to a minimum.

Other studies have shown that loudness adaptation is reduced or absent when binaural interactions (lateralization cues) are minimized (Stokinger and Studebaker, 1968; Fraser et al., 1970; Petty et al., 1970; Stokinger et al., 1972a, 1972b; Morgan and Dirks, 1973). This may be accomplished by using adapting and comparison tones of different frequencies (heterophonic loudness balances), or by a variety of other means. For example, Stokinger and colleagues (Stokinger et al., 1972a, 1972b) reduced or obliterated loudness adaptation by shortening the duration of the comparison tone and by delaying the onset of the comparison tone after the adapting tone was removed. Both of these approaches had the effect of reducing or removing the interaction of the two tones between the ears. Moreover, the presentation of an intermittent tone to one ear induces adaptation of a continuous tone in the other ear (Botte et al., 1982; Scharf, 1983). Thus, it appears that lateralization methods foster misleading impressions about loudness adaptation effects, especially with regard to monaural adaptation (Scharf, 1983).

What, then, do we know about loudness adaptation based upon experimentation which directly assesses the phenomenon? Scharf (1983) has provided a cohesive report of a large number of loudness adaptation experiments using, for the most part, magnitude estimations of loudness that were obtained at various times during the stimulus. Several of his findings may be summarized for our purposes as follows. First, there appears to be a noticeable amount of variability among people in terms of how much adaptation they experience. Second, the loudness of a pure tone adapts when it is presented to a subject at levels up to approximately 30 dB sensation level (i.e., 30 dB above his threshold). This relationship is shown in Fig. 11.9, although one might note that adaptation was found to continue beyond the value of 70 s shown in the graph. The relationship between sensation level and loudness adaptation was subsequently qualified by Miskiewicz et al. (1993), who

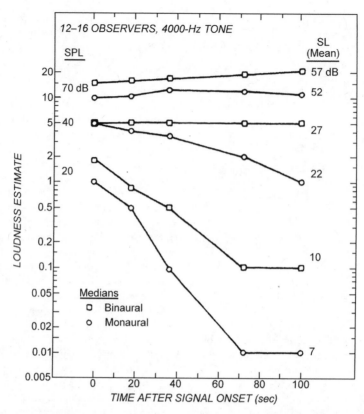

Figure 11.9 Adaptation (medians) for a 4000-Hz tone measured by successive magnitude estimations as a function of the duration of the tone. The parameter is sensation level, or the number of decibels above the subjects' thresholds. See text. *Source*: From Scharf, Loudness adaptation, in *Hearing Research and Theory, Vol. 2* (J.V. Tobias and E.D. Schubert, eds.), Vol. 2, ©1983 by Academic Press.

found that loudness adaptation also occurs above 30 dB SL for high-frequency sounds (12,000, 14,000, and 16,000 Hz). Third, there is more adaptation for higher-frequency tones than for lower-frequencies tones or for noises. Fourth, adaptation appears to be the same whether the tones are presented to one ear or to both ears. In the latter case, the amount of adaptation that is measured seems to be primarily determined by the ear with less adaptation. For example, if the right ear adapts in 90 s and the left ear in 105 s, then the binaurally presented tone would be expected to adapt in 105 s. Here, of course, we are assuming that both ears are receiving similar continuous tones. Clearly, these points represent only a brief sampling of Scharf's extensive findings and theoretical arguments. The student should consult his paper for greater elucidation as well as for an excellent coverage of the overall topic.

NOISINESS AND ANNOYANCE

It is interesting to at least briefly consider the "objectionability" of sounds before leaving the topic of loudness. After all, it is probably fair to say that louder sounds are often more objectionable than softer ones. Some common examples include the noises of airplane fly-overs, sirens, traffic, and construction equipment, as well as somebody else's loud music. On the other hand, some sounds are quite objectionable regardless of their intensities, such as the noise of squeaky floorboards and the screech of fingernails on a blackboard. Thus, sounds (generally noises) may be experienced as objectionable above and beyond their loudness, per se.

The term **perceived noisiness** (or just **noisiness**) is often used to describe the *objectionability* or *unwantedness* of a sound (Kryter, 1985). Specifically, noisiness is the unwantedness of a sound that does *not* produce fear or pain and is neither unexpected nor surprising. Moreover, noisiness is *not* related to the meaning or implications of the sound. In other words, noisiness has to do with the physical parameters of the noise. The amount of noisiness is given in **noys**, analogous to loudness in sones, and equally objectionable sounds share the same number of **perceived noise decibels** (**PNdB**) analogous to loudness level in phons (Kryter, 1959; Kryter and Pearsons, 1963, 1964). Thus, if sound A has twice the noisiness of sound B, then A will have double the number of noys and it will be 10 PNdB higher. As we would expect, the physical parameters that increase loudness also increase noisiness (e.g., noisiness increases as the sound level rises). Noisiness is also influenced by other parameters of the offending sound, such as its time course and spectrum: Lengthening the duration of a sound beyond 1 s increases the amount of noisiness. Sounds that rise in level over time are noisier than sounds that fall in level over the same amount of time, and noisiness increases as the build-up gets longer. A noise whose spectrum has a lot of energy concentrated inside of a narrow range of frequencies is noisier than a noise with a smoother spectrum.

In contrast to noisiness, the term **annoyance** describes the objectionability of a sound involving such things as its meaning or interpretation, implications for the listener, novelty, etc., as well as its physical parameters, per se (Kryter, 1985). Hence, it is not surprising that in addition to its obvious dependence on the level of the offending noise, annoyance is also related to a variety of other factors, such as the source of the noise and the individual's noise susceptibility. For example, residential noise annoyance appears to be affected by concerns about the dangers and other (including nonnoise) consequences of the noise source, attitudes about the importance of the noise source, the amount of isolation from noise at home, beliefs about noise prevention, and the person's general noise sensitivity (Fields, 1993). Transportation noise annoyance appears to be greatest for aircraft (followed by road traffic and then by railroad noises) and is substantially affected by fears about the noise source, concerns about how noise and pollution affect health, perceived disturbance from the noise, self-assessed noise sensitivity, coping capacity, and perceived ability to control the noise situation (Miedema and Vos, 1998, 1999; Kroesen, Molin, and van Wee, 2008). Several informative discussions of noise sensitivity and related matters are readily available for the interested reader (e.g., Job, 1988; Fields, 1993; Miedema and Vos, 2003).

REFERENCES

American National Standards Institute, ANSI S3.4–1980. 1980. *American National Standard Procedure for the Computation of Loudness of Noise.* New York, NY: ANSI.

American National Standards Institute, ANSI S3.4–2007. 2007. *American National Standard Procedure for the Computation of Loudness of Steady Sounds.* New York, NY: ANSI.

Arieh, Y, Kelly, K, Marks, LE. 2005. Tracking the time to recovery after induced loudness reduction. *J Acoust Soc Am* 117, 3381–3384.

Arieh, Y, Marks, LE. 2003a. Time course of loudness recalibration: Implications for loudness enhancement. *J Acoust Soc Am* 114, 1550–1556.

Arieh, Y, Marks, LE. 2003b. Recalibrating the auditory system: A speed-accuracy analysis of intensity perception. *J Exp Psychol Hum Percept Perform* 29, 523–536.

Botte, MC, Canevet, G, Scharf, B. 1982. Loudness adaptation induced by an intermittent tone. *J Acoust Soc Am* 72, 727–739.

Buus, S, Florentine, M, Poulsen, T. 1997. Temporal integration of loudness, loudness discrimination and the form of the loudness function. *J Acoust Soc Am* 101, 669–680.

Buus, S, Muesch, H, Florentine, M. 1998. On loudness at threshold. *J Acoust Soc Am* 104, 399–410.

Canevet, G, Hellman, RP, Scharf, B. 1986. Group estimation of loudness in sound fields. *Acustica* 277–282.

Churcher, BG, King, AJ. 1937. The performance of noise meters in terms of the primary standard. *J Inst Elec Eng* 81, 57–90.

Creelman, CD. 1963. Detection, discrimination, and the loudness of short tones. *J Acoust Soc Am* 35, 1201–1205.

Egan, JP. 1955. Perstimulatory fatigue as measured by heterophonic loudness balances. *J Acoust Soc Am* 27, 111–120.

Egan, JP, Thwing, EJ. 1955. Further studies on perstimulatory fatigue. *J Acoust Soc Am* 27, 1225–1226.

Ekman, E, Berglund, G, Berglund, V. 1966. Loudness as a function of duration of auditory stimulation. *Scand J Psychol* 7, 201–208.

Feldtkeller, J, Zwicker, E. 1956. *Das Ohr als Nachrichtenempfanger.* Stuttgart, Germany: Hirzel.

Fields, JM. 1993. Effect of personal and situational variables on noise annoyance in residential areas. *J Acoust Soc Am* 93, 2753–2763.

Fletcher, H, Munson, WA. 1933. Loudness, its definition, measurement, and calculation. *J Acoust Soc Am* 5, 82–105.

Florentine, M, Buus, S, Bonding, P. 1978. Loudness of complex sounds as a function of the standard stimulus and the number of components. *J Acoust Soc Am* 64, 1036–1040.

Florentine, M, Buus, S, Poulsen, T. 1996. Temporal integration of loudness as a function of level. *J Acoust Soc Am* 99, 1633–1644.

Fraser, WD, Petty, JW, Elliott, DN. 1970. Adaptation: Central or peripheral. *J Acoust Soc Am* 47, 1016–1021.

Gardner, WR. 1958. Advantages of the discriminability criteria for a loudness scale. *J Acoust Soc Am* 30, 1005–1012.

Glasberg, BR, Moore, BCJ. 2006. Prediction of absolute thresholds and equal-loudness contours using a modified loudness model. *J Acoust Soc Am* 120, 585–588.

Glasberg, BR, Moore, BCJ. 2007. Program for Calculation of Loudness According to a Modified Version of ANSI S3.4–2007 "*Procedure for the Computation of Loudness of Steady Sounds.*" Available at http://hearing.psychol.cam.ac.uk/Demos/demos.html.

Hellman, RP. 1976. Growth of loudness at 1000 and 3000 Hz. *J Acoust Soc Am* 60, 672–679.

Hellman, RP. 1981. Stability of individual loudness functions obtained by magnitude estimation and production. *Percept Psychophys* 29, 63–70.

Hellman, RP, Meiselman, CH. 1988. Prediction of individual loudness exponents from cross-modality matching. *J Speech Hear Res* 31, 605–615.

Hellman, RP, Meiselman, CH. 1993. Rate of loudness growth for pure tones in normal and impaired hearing. *J Acoust Soc Am* 93, 966–975.

Hellman, RP, Zwislocki, J. 1961. Some factors affecting the estimation of loudness. *J Acoust Soc Am* 33, 687–694.

Hellman, RP, Zwislocki, J. 1963. Monaural loudness function at 1000 cps and interaural summation. *J Acoust Soc Am* 35, 856–865.

Hellman, RP, Zwislocki, J. 1964. Loudness function of a 1000-cps tone in the presence of a masking noise. *J Acoust Soc Am* 36, 1618–1627.

Hellman, RP, Zwislocki, J. 1968. Loudness determination at low sound frequencies. *J Acoust Soc Am* 43, 60–64.

Hood, JD. 1950. Studies on auditory fatigue and adaptation. *Acta Otolaryngol* Suppl 92.

International Standards Organization, ISO 532–1975. 1975. *Method for Calculating Loudness Level.* Geneva, Switzerland: ISO.

International Standards Organization, ISO 226–2003. 2003. *Acoustics—Normal Equal-Loudness-Level Contours.* Geneva, Switzerland: ISO.

Jesteadt, W. 1980. An adaptive procedure for subjective judgments. *Percept Psychophys* 28, 85–88.

Job, RFS. 1988. Community response to noise: A review of factors influencing the relationship between noise exposure and reaction. *J Acoust Soc Am* 83, 991–1001.

Kingsbury, BA. 1927. A direct comparison of the loudness of pure tones. *Phys Rev* 29, 588–600.

Kroesen, M, Molin, EJE, van Wee, B. 2008. Testing a theory of aircraft noise annoyance: A structural equation analysis. *J Acoust Soc Am* 123, 4250–4260.

Kryter, KD. 1959. Scaling human reactions to sound from aircraft. *J Acoust Soc Am* 31, 1415–1429.

Kryter, KD. 1968. Concepts of perceived noisiness, their implementation and application. *J Acoust Soc Am* 43, 344–361.

Kryter, KD. 1985. *The Effects of Noise on Man,* 2nd Ed. Orlando, FL: Academic Press.

Kryter, KD, Pearsons, KS. 1963. Some effects of spectral content and duration on perceived noise level. *J Acoust Soc Am* 35, 866–883.

Kryter, KD, Pearsons, KS. 1964. Modification of noy tables. *J Acoust Soc Am* 36, 394–397.

Logue, AW. 1976. Individual differences in magnitude estimation of loudness. *Percept Psychophys* 19, 279–280.

Mapes-Riordan, D, Yost, WA. 1999. Loudness recalibration as a function of level. *J Acoust Soc Am* 106, 3506–3511.

Marks, LE. 1974a. *Sensory Processes: The New Psychophysics.* New York, NY: Academic Press.

Marks, LE. 1974b. On scales of sensation: Prolegomena to any future psychophysics that will be able to come forth as science. *Percept Psychophys* 16, 358–376.

Marks, LE. 1978. Binaural summation of loudness of pure tones. *J Acoust Soc Am* 64, 107–113.

Marks, LE. 1987. Binaural versus monaural loudness: Super-summation of tone partially masked by noise. *J Acoust Soc Am* 81, 122–128.

McFadden, D. 1975. Duration–intensity reciprocity for equal-loudness. *J Acoust Soc Am* 57, 701–704.

Miedema, HME, Vos, H. 1998. Exposure–response relationships for transportation noise. *J Acoust Soc Am* 104, 3432–3445.

Miedema, HME, Vos, H. 1999. Demographic and attitudinal factors that modify annoyance from transportation noise. *J Acoust Soc Am* 105, 3336–3344.

Miedema, HME, Vos, H. 2003. Noise sensitivity and reactions to noise and other environmental conditions. *J Acoust Soc Am* 113, 1492–1504.

Miller, GA. 1948. The perception of short bursts of noise. *J Acoust Soc Am* 20, 160–170.

Miskiewicz, A, Scharf, B, Hellman, R, Meiselman, C. 1993. Loudness adaptation at high frequencies. *J Acoust Soc Am* 94, 1281–1286.

Moore, BCJ, Glasberg, BR, Baer, T. 1997. A model for the prediction of thresholds, loudness and partial loudness. *J Audio Eng Soc* 45, 224–240.

Morgan, DE, Dirks, DD. 1973. Suprathreshold loudness adaptation. *J Acoust Soc Am* 53, 1560–1564.

Nieder, B, Buus, S, Florentine, M, Scharf, B. 2003. Interactions between test- and inducer-tone durations in induced loudness reduction. *J Acoust Soc Am* 114, 2846–2855.

Petty, JW, Fraser, WD, Elliott, DN. 1970. Adaptation and loudness decrement: A reconsideration. *J Acoust Soc Am* 47, 1074–1082.

Pollack, I. 1952. The loudness of bands of noise. *J Acoust Soc Am* 24, 533–538.

Richards, AM. 1977. Loudness perception for short-duration tones in masking noise. *J Speech Hear Res* 20, 684–693.

Robinson, DW. 1957. The subjective loudness scale. *Acustica* 7, 217–233.

Robinson, DW, Dadson, RS. 1956. A redetermination of the equal loudness relations for pure tones. *Brit J Appl Phys* 7, 166–181.

Rowley, RR, Studebaker, GA. 1969. Monaural loudness–intensity relationships for a 1000-Hz tone. *J Acoust Soc Am* 45, 1186–1192.

Scharf, B. 1959. Critical bands and the loudness of complex sounds near threshold. *J Acoust Soc Am* 31, 365–380.

Scharf, B. 1970. Critical bands. In: JV Tobias (ed.), *Foundations of Modern Auditory Theory. Vol. 1,* New York, NY: Academic Press, 157–202.

Scharf, B. 1978. Loudness. In: EC Carterette, MP Friedman (eds.), *Handbook of Perception, Vol. IV, Hearing.* New York, NY: Academic Press, 187–242.

Scharf, B. 1983. Loudness adaptation. In: JV Tobias, ED Schubert (eds.), Hearing Research and Theory, Vol. 2. New York, NY: Academic Press, 156.

Schlauch, RS, Wier, CC. 1987. A method for relating loudness-matching and intensity-discrimination data. *J Speech Hear Res* 30, 13–20.

Small, AM, Brandt, JF, Cox, PG. 1962. Loudness as a function of signal duration. *J Acoust Soc Am* 34, 513–514.

Small, AM, Minifie, FD. 1961. Effect of matching time on per-stimulatory adaptation. *J Acoust Soc Am* 33, 1028–1033.

Stephens, SDG. 1974. Methodological factors influencing loudness of short duration tones. *J Sound Vib* 37, 235–246.

Stevens, SS. 1936. A scale for the measurement of a psychological magnitude: Loudness. *Psychol Rev* 43, 405–416.

Stevens, SS. 1956a. Calculation of the loudness of complex noise. *J Acoust Soc Am* 28, 807–832.

Stevens, SS. 1956b. The direct estimation of sensory magnitudes—Loudness. *Am J Psychol* 69, 1–25.

Stevens, SS. 1955. The measurement of loudness. *J Acoust Soc Am* 27, 815–829.

Stevens, SS. 1957a. Concerning the form of the loudness function. *J Acoust Soc Am* 29, 603–606.

Stevens, SS. 1957b. On the psychophysical law. *Psychol Rev* 54, 153–181.

Stevens, SS. 1959. On the validity of the loudness scale. *J Acoust Soc Am* 31, 995–1003.

Stevens, SS. 1961. Procedure for calculating loudness: Mark VI. *J Acoust Soc Am* 33, 1577–1585.

Stevens, SS. 1972. Perceived level of noise by Mark VII and decibels (E). *J Acoust Soc Am* 51, 575–601.

Stevens, SS. 1975. In: G Stevens (ed.), *Psychophysics: Introduction to Its Perceptual, Neural and Social Prospects*. New York, NY: Wiley.

Stevens, SS, Greenbaum, H. 1966. Regression effect in psychophysical judgment. *Percept Psychophys* 1, 439–446.

Stevens, JC, Guirao, M. 1964. Individual loudness functions. *J Acoust Soc Am* 36, 2210–2213.

Stevens, JC, Hall, JW. 1966. Brightness and loudness as a function of stimulus duration. *Percept Psychophys* 1, 319–327.

Stokinger, TE, Cooper, WA, Meissner, WA, Jones, KO. 1972b. Intensity, frequency, and duration effects in the measurement of monaural perstimulatory loudness adaptation. *J Acoust Soc Am* 51, 608–616.

Stokinger, TE, Cooper, WA, Meissner, WA. 1972a. Influence of binaural interaction on the measurement of perstimulatory loudness adaptation. *J Acoust Soc Am* 51, 602–607.

Stokinger, TE, Studebaker, GA. 1968. Measurement of perstimulatory loudness adaptation. *J Acoust Soc Am* 44, 250–256.

Wagner, E, Scharf, B. 2006. Induced loudness reduction as a function of exposure time and signal frequency. *J Acoust Soc Am* 119, 1012–1020.

Walsh, JL, Browman, CP. 1978. Intraindividual consistency on a crossmodality matching task. *Percept Psychophys* 23, 210–214.

Wright, HN. 1960. Measurement of perstimulatory auditory adaptation. *J Acoust Soc Am* 32, 1558–1567.

Zwicker, E. 1958. Uber psychologische and methodische Grundlagen der Lautheit. *Acustica* 1, 237–258.

Zwislocki, J. 1969. Temporal summation of loudness: An analysis. *J Acoust Soc Am* 46, 431–441.

Zwicker, E, Fastl, H. 1999. *Psychoacoutics: Facts and Models*, 2nd ed. Berlin, Germany: Springer.

Zwicker, E, Feldtkeller, J. 1955. Uber die Lautstarke von gleichformigen Gerauschen. *Acustica* 5, 303–316.

Zwicker, E, Flottrop, G, Stevens, SS. 1957. Critical bandwidth in loudness summation. *J Acoust Soc Am* 29, 548–557.

12 Pitch

In this chapter, we will deal with several attributes of sounds grossly classified as **pitch**, along with several associated topics. Like "loudness," the word "pitch" denotes a perception with which we are all familiar. Pitch is generally described as the psychological correlate of frequency, such that high-frequency tones are heard as being "high" in pitch and low frequencies are associated with "low" pitches (ANSI, 2004). However, we saw in Chapter 9 that not all changes in frequency are perceptible. Instead, a certain amount of frequency change is needed before the difference limen (DL) is reached. In other words, the frequency difference between two tones must be at least equal to the DL before they are heard as being different in pitch. Moreover, we shall see that pitch does not follow frequency in a simple, one-to-one manner along a monotonic scale from low to high. Instead, the perception of pitch appears to be multifaceted, and it may be that there are various kinds of pitch. In addition, although we know that pitch involves both the place and temporal mechanisms of frequency coding discussed in earlier chapters, the precise interaction of frequency and temporal coding is not fully resolved.

Pitch can be expressed in a variety of ways. Perhaps the most common approach is to express pitch and pitch relationships in terms of musical notes and intervals. Another very useful method is to ask listeners to find the best match between the pitch of a certain sound and the pitches of various pure tones, and then to express the pitch of that sound in terms of the frequency of matched pure tone. For example, if a complex periodic sound is matched to a 500-Hz pure tone, then that sound has a pitch of 500 Hz. Similarly, if the pitch of a certain noise is matched to a 1700-Hz tone, then the noise is said to have a pitch of 1700 Hz. Another way to approach pitch is to construct a pitch scale analogous to the sone scale of loudness (Chap. 11), which will be our first topic.

MEL SCALES OF PITCH

Stevens, Volkmann, and Newman (1937) asked listeners to adjust the frequency of a tone until its pitch was one-half that of another (standard) tone. The result was a scale in which pitch is expressed as a function of frequency. This scale was revised by Stevens and Volkmann (1940), whose subjects had to adjust the frequencies of five tones within a certain frequency range until they were separated by equal pitch intervals. In other words, their task was to make the distance in pitch between tones A and B equal to that between tones B and C, C and D, and so on. Stevens and Volkmann also repeated the earlier fractionalization experiment except that a 40-Hz tone that was arbitrarily assigned a pitch of zero. Based on direct estimates of the pitch remaining below 40 Hz and extrapolations, 20 Hz was identified as being the lowest perceptible pitch. This

estimate agreed with Bekesy's (1960) observation that the lowest frequency yielding a sensation of pitch is approximately 20 Hz.

Stevens and Volkmann's (1940) revised **mel scale** is shown by the solid curve in Fig. 12.1a. On this graph, frequency in hertz is shown along the abscissa and pitch in units called **mels** is shown along the ordinate. The reference point on this scale is 1000 mels, which is defined as the pitch of a 1000-Hz tone presented at 40 phons. Doubling the pitch of a tone doubles the number of mels, and halving the pitch halves the number of mels. Thus, a tone that sounds twice as high as the 1000-mel reference tone would have a pitch of 2000 mels, while a tone that is half as high as the reference would have the pitch of 500 mels. The dotted curve shows what the relationship would look like *if* frequency and pitch were the same (if mels = hertz). Notice that frequency and pitch correspond only for low frequencies. However, the solid (mel scale) curve becomes considerably shallower than the dotted curve as frequency continues to rise. This reveals that pitch increases more slowly than frequency, so that the frequency range up to 16,000 Hz is focused down to a pitch range of only about 3300 mels. For example, notice that tripling the frequency from 1000 to 3000 Hz only doubles the pitch from 1000 to 2000 mels.

Other pitch scales have also been developed (e.g., Stevens et al., 1937; Beck and Shaw, 1962, 1963; Zwicker and Fastl, 1999), and it should not be surprising that the various scales are somewhat different from one another due to methodological and other variations. For example, the solid curve in Fig. 12.1b shows the mel scale formulated by Zwicker and Fastl (1999). This scale is based on ratio productions in which listeners adjusted the frequency of one tone to sound half as high as another tone. The reference point on the Zwicker and Fastl scale is 125 mels, which is the pitch of a 125-Hz tone. As in the upper frame, the dotted curve shows what the relationship would look like *if* pitch in mels was the same as frequency in hertz. Here, too, we see that pitch increases much slower than frequency, with the frequency range up to 16,000 Hz compressed into a pitch range of just 2400 mels. For example, a 2:1 change in pitch from 1050 to 2100 mels involves increasing the frequency by a factor of more than 6:1, from 1300 to 8000 Hz.

There is reasonably good correspondence between pitch in mels, critical band intervals in barks (see Chap. 10), and distance along the basilar membrane (e.g., Stevens and Volkmann, 1940; Scharf, 1970; Zwicker and Fastl, 1999; Goldstein, 2000). Zwicker and Fastl (1999) suggested that 100 mels corresponds to one bark and a distance of approximately 1.3 mm along the cochlear partition. These relationships are illustrated in Fig. 12.2. Goldstein (2000) reported that the Stevens–Volkmann (1940) mel scale is a power function of the frequency–place map for the human cochlea (Greenwood, 1990).

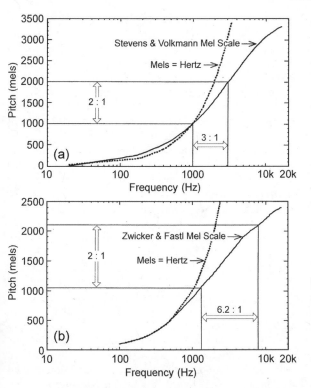

Figure 12.1 The relationship between frequency in hertz and pitch in mels based on the findings of (a) Stevens and Volkmann (1940) and (b) Zwicker and Fastl (1999). The dotted curves labeled Mels = Hertz illustrate what the relationship would look like if pitch in mels was the same as frequency in hertz.

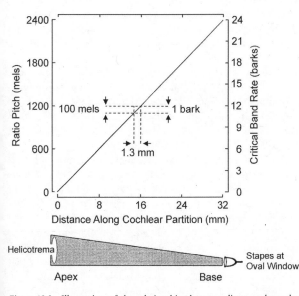

Figure 12.2 Illustration of the relationships between distance along the cochlear partition, pitch in mels, and critical band rate in barks. Notice the orientation of the basilar membrane. Based on scales by Zwicker and Fastl (1999).

BEATS, HARMONICS, AND COMBINATION TONES

The topics of audible beats, harmonics, and combination tones are often discussed in the context of how we perceive frequency. We will divert our attention to these phenomena early in this chapter not only because they are topics of interest in their own right, but also because they will be encountered as tools used to study various aspects of pitch perception in the discussion that follows.

We have seen in several contexts that a pure tone stimulus will result in a region of maximal displacement along the basilar membrane according to the place principle. Now, suppose that a second tone is added whose frequency (f_2) is slightly higher than that of the first sinusoid (f_1), a in Fig. 12.3. If the frequency difference between the two tones ($f_2 - f_1$) is small (say 3 Hz), then the two resulting excitation patterns along the cochlear partition will overlap considerably so that the two stimuli will be indistinguishable. However, the small frequency difference between the two tones will cause them to be in phase and out of phase cyclically in a manner that repeats itself at a rate equal to the frequency difference $f_2 - f_1$. Thus, a combination of a 1000-Hz tone and a 1003-Hz tone will be heard as a 1000-Hz tone that **beats**, or waxes and wanes in level, at a rate of three times per second. This perception of aural beats therefore reflects the limited frequency-resolving ability of the ear.

If the two tones are equal in level, then the resulting beats will alternate between maxima that are twice the level of the original tones and minima that are inaudible due to complete out-of-phase cancellation. Such beats are aptly called **best beats**. Tones that differ in level result in smaller maxima and incomplete cancellation. As one would expect, the closer the levels of the two tones, the louder the beats will sound.

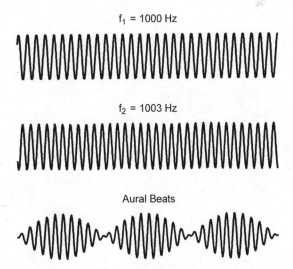

Figure 12.3 Tones of slightly different frequency, f_1 and f_2, result in beats that fluctuate (wax and wane) at a rate equal to the difference between them ($f_2 - f_1$).

As the frequency difference between the two tones widens, the beats become faster. These rapid amplitude fluctuations are perceived as **roughness** rather than as discernible beats, as discussed earlier in the chapter. Further widening of the frequency separation results in the perception of the two original tones, in addition to which a variety of combination tones may be heard. Combination tones, as well as aural harmonics, are the result of **nonlinear distortion** in the ear.

Distortion products are those components at the output of the system that were not present at the input. A simple example demonstrates how nonlinear distortions produce outputs that differ from the inputs. Consider two levers, one rigid and the other springy. The rigid lever represents a **linear system**. If one moves one arm of this lever up and down sinusoidally (the input), then the opposite arm will also move sinusoidally (the output). On the other hand, the springy lever illustrates the response of a **nonlinear system**. A sinusoidal input to one arm will cause the other arm to move up and down, but there will also be superimposed overshoots and undershoots in the motion, due to the "bounce" of the springy lever arms. Thus, the responding arm of the lever will move with a variety of superimposed frequencies (distortion products) even though the stimulus is being applied sinusoidally.

The simplest auditory distortion products are **aural harmonics**. As their name implies, these are distortion products which have frequencies that are multiples of the stimulus frequency. For example, a stimulus frequency f_1, when presented at a high enough level, will result in aural harmonics whose frequencies correspond to $2f_1$, $3f_1$, etc. Therefore, a 500-Hz primary tone (f_1) will result in aural harmonics that are multiples of 500 Hz ($2f_1 = 1000$ Hz, $3f_1 = 1500$ Hz, etc.). Two primary tones are illustrated in Fig. 12.4. The 800-Hz primary tone (f_1) is associated with an aural harmonic at 1600 Hz ($2f_1$) and the 1000-Hz primary (f_2) is associated with the aural harmonic at 2000 Hz ($2f_2$).

If two primary tones f_1 and f_2 are presented together, nonlinear distortion will result in the production of various **combination tones** due to the interactions among the primaries and the harmonics of these tones. For convenience, we will call the lower-frequency primary tone f_1 and the higher one f_2. There are several frequently encountered combination tones that we shall touch upon. [See Boring (1942) and Plomp (1965) for interesting historical perspectives, and Goldstein et al. (1978) for an classic review of the compatibility among physiological and psychoacoustic findings on combination tones.]

It is necessary to devise methods that enable us to quantify the aspects of combination tones. A rather classical method takes advantage of the phenomenon of aural beats discussed above. Recall that best beats occur when the beating tones are of equal amplitudes. Generally stated, this technique involves the presentation of a probe tone at a frequency close enough to the combination tone of interest so that beats will occur between the combination and probe tones. Characteristics of the combination tone are inferred by varying the amplitude of the probe until the subject reports hearing best beats (i.e., maximal amplitude variations). The **best beats method**, however, has been the subject of serious controversy (Lawrence and Yantis, 1956, 1957; Meyer, 1957; Chocolle and Legouix, 1957), and has been largely replaced by a cancellation technique (Zwicker, 1955; Goldstein, 1967; Hall, 1975). The **cancellation method** also employs a probe tone, but in this method, instead of asking the subject to detect best beats, the probe tone is presented at the frequency of the combination tone, and its phase and amplitude are adjusted until the combination tone is canceled. Cancellation occurs when the probe tone is equal in amplitude and opposite in phase to the combination tone. The characteristics of the combination tone may then be inferred from those of the probe tone that cancels it. A lucid description of and comparison among all of the major methods has been provided by Zwicker (1981).

Techniques such as these have resulted in various observations about the nature of combination tones. The simplest combination tones result from adding or subtracting the two primary tones. The former is the **summation tone** ($f_1 + f_2$). As illustrated in Fig. 12.4, primary tones of 800 Hz (f_1) and 1000 Hz (f_2) will result in the production of the summation tone $1000 + 800 = 1800$ Hz. We will say little about the summation tone except to point out that it is quite weak and not always audible. On the other hand, the **difference tone** ($f_2 - f_1$) is a significant combination tone that is frequently encountered. For the 800- and 1000-Hz primaries in the figure, the difference tone would be $1000 - 800 = 200$ Hz. The difference tone is heard only when the primary tones are presented well above threshold. Plomp (1965) found, despite wide differences among his subjects, that the primaries had to exceed approximately 50 dB sensation level in order for the difference tone to be detected.

The **cubic difference tone** ($2f_1 - f_2$) is another significant and frequently encountered combination tone. These distortion products appear to be generated by the active processes in the

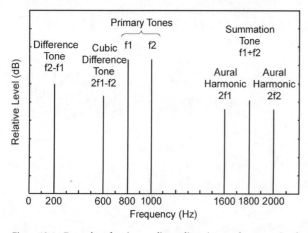

Figure 12.4 Examples of various auditory distortion products associated with stimulus (primary) tones of 800 Hz (f_1) and 1000 Hz (f_2).

cochlea and have already been encountered when distortion-product otoacoustic emissions were discussed in Chapter 4. For the 800- and 1000-Hz primary tones in Fig. 12.4, the resulting cubic difference tone is $2(800) - 1000 = 600$ Hz. A particularly interesting aspect of the cubic difference tone is that it is audible even when the primaries are presented at low sensation levels. For example, Smoorenburg (1972) demonstrated that $2f_1 - f_2$ is detectable when the primaries are only 15 to 20 dB above threshold, although he did find variations among subjects.

When the primary tones exceed 1000 Hz, the level of the difference tone $f_2 - f_1$ tends to be rather low (approximately 50 dB below the level of the primaries); in contrast, the difference tone may be as little as 10 dB below the primaries when they are presented below 1000 Hz (Zwicker, 1955; Goldstein, 1967; Hall, 1972a, 1972b). On the other hand, the cubic difference tone $2f_1 - f_2$ appears to be limited to frequencies below the lower primary f_1, and its level increases as the ratio f_2/f_1 becomes smaller (Goldstein, 1967; Hall, 1972a, 1972b, 1975; Smoorenburg, 1972). Furthermore, the cubic difference tone has been shown to be within approximately 20 dB of the primaries when the frequency ratio of f_2 and f_1 is on the order of 1.2:1 (Hall, 1972a; Smoorenburg, 1972). The student with an interest in this topic should also refer to the work of Zwicker (1981) and Humes (1985a, 1985b) for insightful reviews and analyses of the nature of combination tones.

An interesting attribute of combination tones is their stimulus-like nature. In other words, the combination tones themselves interact with primary (stimulus) tones as well as with other combination tones to generate beats and higher-order (secondary) combination tones, such as $3f_1-2f_2$ and $4f_1-2f_2$. Goldstein et al. (1978) have shown that such **secondary combination tones** have properties similar to those of combination tones generated by the primaries.

MUSICAL PITCH

As already mentioned, pitch is usually considered in musical terms. Here, tones are separated by perceptually relevant intervals. The intervals themselves are based on *ratios* between the frequencies of the tones (f_2/f_1) rather than on the differences between them ($f_2 - f_1$). For example, the principal interval is the **octave**, which is a 2:1 frequency ratio. It is helpful to discuss musical pitch scales with reference to Fig. 12.5, which depicts a standard piano keyboard with 88 keys.[1] The white keys are grouped in sets of 7, which are labeled in the order

C, D, E, F, G, A, B, next C.

The frequency of a particular C is exactly twice the frequency of the prior one so that each octave is divided into seven intervals. This order is called the *major scale* and is also associated

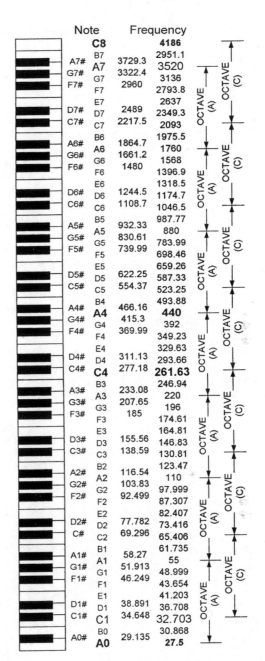

Figure 12.5 The musical scaling of pitch intervals (equal temperament) with reference to the keys on the piano keyboard.

with the familiar singing scale (*do, re, mi, fa, sol, la, ti, do*). Octaves can also be divided into 12 intervals, which are labeled in the order

C, C#[2], D, D#, E, F, F#, G, G#, A, A#, B, next C.

---

[1] For an online application that provides the musical note corresponding to a given frequency, see Botros (2001).

[2] The symbol # is read as "sharp"; hence, C# is C-sharp, D# is D-sharp, etc.

These 12-note groupings form the *chromatic scale* and correspond to the sets of 12 (7 white and 5 black) keys on the piano. Intervals within octaves are discussed below.

The musical scaling of pitch may be viewed in terms of two attributes, height and chroma (Révész, 1913; Bachem, 1948, 1950; Shepard, 1964). **Tone height** pertains to the monotonic increase from low to high pitch as frequency rises, and it is represented by the vertical arrow in Fig. 12.6. It has been suggested that mel scales of pitch are related to the dimension of tone height (Ward and Burns, 1982; Goldstein, 2000). In contrast, chroma is related to a perceptual similarity or sameness among tones that are separated by 2:1 frequency intervals, called **octave equivalence**. As a result, these tones have the same pitch class or chroma and share the same name. For example, every doubling of frequency beginning with 27.5 Hz in Fig. 12.5 produces a note called *A*, labeled *A0* at 27.5 Hz through *A7* at 3520 Hz. (The note called *A4*, which has a frequency of 440 Hz, is most commonly used as a standard or reference pitch for musical tuning.) Similarly, every doubling of frequency starting with 32.703 Hz in Fig. 12.5 is a note called *C*, from *C1* (at 32.703 Hz) to *C8* (4186 Hz). It should now be apparent that chroma changes from *C* through *B* within each octave, and that this patterns recycles at a higher frequency beginning at the next *C*. For example, *C1*, *D1#*, and *F1* differ in terms of chroma, whereas *A3*, *A5*, and *A6* have the same chroma but different tone heights. Thus, chroma is conceptualized in the form of the helix in Fig. 12.6.

It is interesting to note in this context that Demany and Armand (1984) found that 3-month-old infants were less sensitive to frequency shifts of exactly one octave than to smaller or larger shifts. These findings provide evidence of octave equivalence, supporting the existence of chroma perception in babies. Moreover, a topographically organized representation of musical keys in the rostromedial prefrontal cortex was identified by functional magnetic resonance imaging (fMRI) in musically experienced listeners performing musical perception tasks (Janata et al., 2002).

Just as there is a 2:1 frequency ratio between one *C* and the next one, the intervals within an octave also take the form of frequency ratios; however, a variety of different scaling schemes are available. For example, the **just (diatonic) scale** is based on three-note groupings (triads) having frequency ratios of 4:5:6, in order to maximize the consonance of thirds, fourths, and fifths. The **Pythagorean scale** concentrates on fourths and fifths. In contrast, the **equal temperament scale** employs logarithmically equal intervals. These scales are compared in Table 12.1. Each scale has advantages and limitations in music, although we will concentrate on the equal temperament scale. Several informative discussions of musical scales are readily available (e.g., Campbell and Greated, 1987; Rossing, 1989).

The equal temperament scale divides the octave into logarithmically equal **semitone** intervals corresponding to the groupings of 12 (7 white and 5 black) keys on the piano (Fig. 12.5). In order to split the 2:1 frequency ratio of a whole octave into 12 logarithmically equal intervals from *C* to the next *C*, each interval must be a frequency ratio of $2^{1/12}$:1 or 1.0595:1 (an increment of roughly 6%). For example, the semitone interval from *C* to *C#* constitutes a frequency ratio of $2^{1/12}$:1, which is the equivalent to 1.0595:1; two semitones from *C* to *D* is ($2^{1/12} \times 2^{1/12}$):1 = $2^{2/12}$:1 = 1.12246:1; and 12 semitones corresponding to one octave from one *C* to the next *C* is $2^{12/12}$:1 = 2:1.

Each equal temperament semitone is further divided into 100 logarithmically equal intervals called **cents**. The use of cents notation often facilitates pitch scaling. For example, cents notation makes it easier to compare the musical intervals involved in the equal temperament, just, and Pythagorean scales (Table 12.1). Since there are 100 cents per semitone and 12 semitones per octave, there are 1200 cents per octave. Thus, 1 cent corresponds to a frequency ratio[3] interval of $2^{1/1200}$:1 or 1.00058:1, which is an increment of less than 0.06%. This is considerably smaller than the relative difference limen for frequency ($\Delta f/f$) of about 0.002 encountered in Chapter 9, which corresponds to 0.2%. In this sense, it takes more than a few cents to achieve a perceptible pitch change. In fact, a study of perceptible tuning changes by Hill and Summers (2007) found that the difference

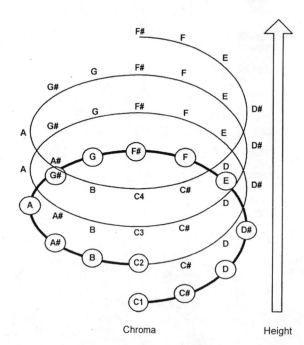

Figure 12.6 Chroma changes going around the helix, and this pattern of tone classes is repeated every octave. Tone height increases monotonically with frequency, as suggested by vertical arrow. Notice that tones with the same chroma and different tone heights appear above each other. Based on Shepard's (1964) conceptualization.

[3] A *frequency ratio* (f_2/f_1) can be converted into *cents* (c) with the formula c = $1200 \times \log_2(f_2/f_1)$; or c = $3986.31 \times \log_{10}(f_2/f_1)$ if one prefers to use common logarithms.

Table 12.1 Frequency Ratios and Cents for Musical Intervals with the Equal Temperament, Just, and Pythagorean Scales

From C to ...	Name	Equal temperament	Just	Pythagorean	Equal temperament	Just	Pythagorean
		Frequency ratio (f_2/f_1)			Cents		
C (itself)	Unison	$2^0 = 1.0595$	$1/1 = 1.0000$	$1/1 = 1.0000$	0	0	0
C#	Minor second	$2^{1/12} = 1.0595$	$16/15 = 1.0667$	$256/243 = 1.0535$	100	112	90
D	Major second	$2^{2/12} = 1.1225$	$10/9 = 1.1111$	$9/8 = 1.1250$	200	182	204
D#	Minor third	$2^{3/12} = 1.1892$	$6/5 = 1.2000$	$32/27 = 1.1852$	300	316	294
E	Major third	$2^{4/12} = 1.2599$	$5/4 = 1.2500$	$81/64 = 1.2656$	400	386	408
F	Fourth	$2^{5/12} = 1.3348$	$4/3 = 1.3333$	$4/3 = 1.3333$	500	498	498
F#	Tritone	$2^{6/12} = 1.4142$	$45/32 = 1.4063$	$1024/729 = 1.4047$	600	590	588
G	Fifth	$2^{7/12} = 1.4983$	$3/2 = 1.5000$	$3/2 = 1.5000$	700	702	702
G#	Minor sixth	$2^{8/12} = 1.5874$	$8/5 = 1.6000$	$128/81 = 1.5802$	800	814	792
A	Major sixth	$2^{9/12} = 1.6818$	$5/3 = 1.6667$	$27/16 = 1.6875$	900	884	906
A#	Minor seventh	$2^{10/12} = 1.7818$	$7/4 = 1.7500$	$16/9 = 1.7778$	1000	969	996
B	Major seventh	$2^{11/12} = 1.8877$	$15/8 = 1.8750$	$243/128 = 1.8984$	1100	1088	1110
(Next) C	Octave	$2^{12/12} = 2.0000$	$2/1 = 2.0000$	$2/1 = 2.0000$	1200	1200	1200

limen is about 10 cents and that category widths approximated 70 cents.

Recall that frequency is coded by both temporal and place mechanisms, with the former taking on a more important role for lower frequencies and the latter predominating for higher frequencies. Since auditory nerve firing patterns reflect phase locking for stimulus frequencies as high as roughly 5000 Hz (Chap. 5), it would appear that the temporal mechanism is operative up to about this frequency. With these points in mind, it is interesting to be aware of several lines of evidence indicating that the perception of pitch chroma is limited to the frequencies below roughly 5000 Hz, although pitch height continues to increase for higher frequencies.

The restriction of chroma perception to 5000 Hz and below has been shown in various ways. Bachem (1948) and Ohgushi and Hatoh (1989) found that listeners with absolute pitch could identify the chroma of pure tones was limited to the frequencies up to about 4000 to 5000 Hz. **Absolute (perfect) pitch** is the very rare ability to accurately identify or produce pitches in isolation, that is, without having to rely on a reference tone (Ward, 1963a, 1963b). Ward (1954) found that musicians could adjust the frequency of a (higher) tone to be an octave above another (lower) tone, providing both tones were less than 5500 Hz. In addition, Atteave and Olson (1971) found that the ability of musicians to transpose a familiar three-tone sequence (in effect, a simple melody) deteriorated above about 5000 Hz. Semal and Demany (1990) asked musicians to transpose a sequence of two pure tones until the higher tone in the pair was perceived to be "just above the upper limit of musical pitch." On average, this limit occurred at approximately 4700 Hz.

Consonance and Dissonance

In addition to their perceptual similarity, two simultaneously presented tones differing by octave intervals are also perceived

as being consonant. Such combinations of two or more simultaneous tones are often referred to as **chords**. **Consonance** simply means that when two sounds are presented together they result in a pleasant perception; in contrast, **dissonance** refers to sounds that appear unpleasant when presented together. Consonance versus dissonance for pairs of tones depends upon the difference between the two frequencies, and how well these frequencies can be resolved by the ear (Plomp and Levelt, 1965; Plomp and Steeneken, 1968; Kameoka and Kuriyagawa, 1969; Schellenberg and Trehub, 1994). Dissonance occurs when two tones are close enough in frequency to be less than a critical band apart. In this case, they are not completely resolved because their vibration patterns interact along the basilar membrane, leading to a sensation of **roughness** due to rapid beats between the two tones. This roughness is perceived as being unpleasant or dissonant. In contrast, the two tones will not interact if they are separated by more than a critical band, in which case there is no roughness, and if they are experienced as consonant.

Complex tones, such as musical notes, contain other frequencies in addition to their fundamentals. In music, the terms **partials** and **overtones** are used to refer these frequencies and are usually used as synonyms for harmonics. (However, one should be aware that many instruments, such as chimes and pianos, also produce "inharmonic" partials at frequencies that are not exact multiples of the fundamental). Thus, dissonance can be introduced by interactions among these partials, as well as between the fundamentals. With these points in mind, consonance is associated with notes composed of frequencies that are related by simple (small) integer ratios, such as 2:1 (octave, e.g., C4 and C5), 3:2 (perfect fifth, e.g., C4 and G4), and 4:3 (perfect fourth, C4 and F4). In contrast, dissonance occurs when their frequencies are related by complex (large) ratios such as 45:32 (tritone, e.g., F3 and B3). In terms of the musical intervals, two tones will be consonant when they are separated by 0 and

12 semitones (i.e., unison and octave), and dissonance occurs when the two notes are separated by intervals of 1–2, 6, and 10–11 semitones.

In contrast to two-tone combinations, the perception of chords becomes more involved when three or more tones are involved. A consonant three-tone chord (triad) is perceived as being **stable** when the spacing between the low and middle tones is different than the interval between the middle and high tones. However, **tension** is experienced when these two intervals are equal, in which case the chord is perceived as being unstable or ambiguous even though there is no dissonance (Meyer, 1956). Cook and colleagues have shown that the harmonious perception of triads depends on the effects of both dissonance and tension involving the fundamentals and partials of the notes that make up the chord (Cook, 2001; Cook and Fujisawa, 2006; Cook and Hayashi, 2008).

PITCH AND INTENSITY

In a classic study by Stevens (1935), subjects were asked to adjust the intensity of a tone until it had the same pitch as a standard tone of slightly different frequency. Results for one subject who was a "good responder" showed that increasing the intensity of the tone increased its pitch for frequencies 3000 Hz and above, and lowered its pitch for frequencies 1000 Hz and below. The pitch stayed essentially constant as intensity was varied for tones between 1000 and 3000 Hz.

Although Stevens' study has frequently been cited to illustrate how intensity affects pitch, subsequent studies did not find large pitch changes associated with intensity increases (Morgan et al., 1951; Ward, 1953; Cohen, 1961; Terhardt, 1979; Zwicker and Fastl, 1999). Figure 12.7 shows how the pitches of pure tones change as the sound pressure level is increased above a reference level of 40 dB (Terhardt, 1979; Zwicker and Fastl, 1999). Increasing level does cause pitch to fall for low-frequency tones and to rise for high-frequency tones. However, the sizes of these pitch shifts are quite small, amounting to less than 2% to 3% as the level increases from 40 to 80 dB.

PITCH OF COMPLEX SOUNDS

Pitch perception is not limited to pure tones. On the contrary, real-world sounds are complex, and common experience reveals that pitch perceptions are associated with them. When dealing with *aperiodic* sounds, the perceived pitch is related to the spectrum of the noise (Small and Daniloff, 1967; Fastl, 1971). In general, the pitches of low- and high-pass noises are related to their cut-off frequencies, and the pitches of band-pass noises are associated with their center frequencies. Moreover, the distinctiveness of the pitch sensation (**pitch strength**) elicited by narrow bands of noise can be quite strong, but it lessens as the bandwidth gets wider and becomes quite weak when the critical band is exceeded.

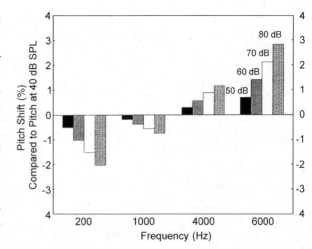

Figure 12.7 Change in pitch (pitch shift) compared to the pitch at 40 dB SPL for tones presented at sound pressure levels of 50, 60, 70, and 80 dB, at selected frequencies. Pitch shifts are upward for high frequencies and downward for low frequencies by about 2% to 3% or less. Based on data by Zwicker and Fastl (1999).

For complex *periodic* sounds, such as those produced by the human voice and many musical instruments, consider, for example, a woman's voice that is composed of many harmonics of 220 Hz (220, 440, 660, 880, 1100, 1320 Hz, etc.). Comparing the pitch of her voice to various pure tones, a match would be made with a 220-Hz tone. Here, the pitch is that of the fundamental frequency and is dominated by its lower harmonics. Classical experiments emphasized the importance of the first five harmonics in determining the pitch of complex tones (e.g., Plomp, 1964, 1967; Ritsma, 1967; Bilsen and Ritsma, 1967). However, the dominant range does not appear to be a fixed, and it is affected by factors such as the frequency of the fundamental, the levels of the harmonics, and duration (e.g., Patterson and Wightman, 1976; Moore et al., 1984, 1985; Gockel et al., 2005, 2007).

What is odd, however, is that the woman just described would still have a vocal pitch of 220 Hz even if the 220-Hz fundamental frequency is missing (in which case the lowest harmonic actually present would be 440 Hz). Demonstrating this phenomenon does not even require a trip to the laboratory—it is actually an every day occurrence because telephones do not provide any frequencies below about 300 Hz. This perception of the **missing fundamental** was first described by Seebeck in 1841, and was reintroduced a century later by Schouten (1940).

The missing fundamental is perhaps the best-known example of what has descriptively been called **periodicity pitch**, **virtual pitch**, **residue pitch**, **low pitch**, and **repetition pitch**. Another case is provided by signals that are periodically interrupted or amplitude modulated (Thurlow and Small, 1955; Burns and Viemeister, 1976, 1981). For example, Thurlow and Small (1955) found that if a high-frequency tone is interrupted periodically, then the subject will perceive a pitch corresponding to the frequency whose period is equal to the interruption rate. Thus, if the high-frequency tone is interrupted every 10 ms (the period of a 100-Hz tone), then subjects will match the pitch of the interrupted high-frequency tone to that of a 100-Hz tone.

Studies by Ritsma (1962, 1963) indicate that the existence region of virtual pitches extends up to about 800 Hz, but others have shown that periodicity pitches can be perceived as high as roughly 1400 Hz with a large enough number of harmonics (Plomp, 1967; Moore, 1973).

The classical *resonance-place theory* would suggest that the missing fundamental is due to energy present at the fundamental frequency as a result of distortions. In other words, the difference tone $f_2 - f_1$ would be the same as the missing fundamental since, for example, $1100 - 1000 = 100$ Hz. However, this supposition is not true because the missing fundamental differs from combination tones in several dramatic ways. For example, the missing fundamental is heard at sound pressure levels as low as about 20 dB (Thurlow and Small, 1955; Small and Campbell, 1961), whereas difference tones are not heard until the primary tones are presented at sound pressure levels of 60 dB or more (Bekesy, 1960; Plomp, 1965). Also, if a probe tone is presented to a subject at a frequency close to that of a difference tone (which is actually represented at a place along the basilar membrane), then aural beats are heard. However, beats do not occur when the probe is added to the missing fundamental (Schouten, 1940).

Further evidence against the supposition that the missing fundamental is the result of energy at the apex of the cochlea due to distortions (or other means) comes from masking studies (Licklider, 1954; Small and Campbell, 1961; Patterson, 1969). These experiments demonstrated that masking of the frequency range containing the missing fundamental does not obliterate its audibility. In other words, real low-frequency tones and difference tones can be masked, but the missing fundamental cannot be.

The concept that the missing fundamental results from distortions due to interactions among the harmonics within the cochlea is further weakened by studies which preclude this by using dichotic stimulation (Houtsma and Goldstein, 1972) or by presenting the harmonics sequentially rather than simultaneously (Hall and Peters, 1981). Dichotic stimulation refers to the presentation of different stimuli to the two ears (see Chap. 13). Houtsma and Goldstein (1972) presented one harmonic to each ear and asked their subjects to identify melodies based upon the perception of missing fundamentals. If the missing fundamental were really the result of interacting harmonics in the cochlea, then the subjects in this dichotic experiment would not hear it because only one tone was available to each cochlea. They found that the missing fundamental was perceived when the harmonics were presented separately to the two ears. This finding indicates that the phenomenon occurred within the central auditory nervous system, since this is the only region where the harmonics were simultaneously represented.

Hall and Peters (1981) showed that subjects could hear the missing fundamental when presented with three harmonics one

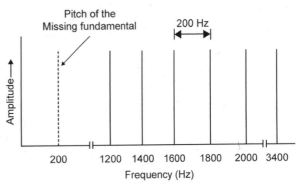

Figure 12.8 Spectrum illustrating the perception of the missing fundamental. Based on Patterson (1973), with permission of *J. Acoust. Soc. Am.*

after the other rather than simultaneously. Their stimuli were sequences of three harmonics (e.g., 600, 800, and 1000 Hz) each lasting 40 ms and separated by 10 ms pauses. An interaction among the harmonics was precluded because they were present at different times. These stimuli were presented alone (in quiet) and also in the presence of a noise. Pitch discrimination and matching tests revealed that their subjects heard the pitches of the harmonics in quiet, but that they heard the missing fundamental in noise.

Schouten's (1940, 1970) *residue theory* proposed that the perception of this missing fundamental is based upon the *temporal pattern* of the complex periodic sound's waveform. Consider a complex periodic tone containing energy only above 1200 Hz, spaced as shown in Fig. 12.8. This spectrum shows energy only for higher harmonics of 200 Hz (1200, 1400, 1600 Hz, etc.), but no energy at the 200-Hz fundamental frequency. Nevertheless, subjects presented with this complex tone will match its pitch to that of a 200-Hz tone. This would occur because the auditory system is responding to the period of the complex periodic tone (5 ms or 0.005 s), which corresponds to the period of 200 Hz (1/0.005 s = 200 Hz). If the components were separated by 100 Hz (e.g., 2000, 2100, 2200, 2300 Hz), then the waveform would have a period of 10 ms or 0.01 s, corresponding to 100 Hz. This can occur because all of the harmonics are separated by the same frequency difference (200 Hz in our example), but auditory filters (critical bandwidths) get wider as frequency increases. As a result, lower harmonics would fall into separate low-frequency auditory filters and would thus be perceived separately from one another. However, two or more higher harmonics will fall into the same (wider) high-frequency auditory filter. Interference between the harmonics within an auditory filter constitutes a complex periodic wave that repeats itself over time at the rate of the fundamental.

Raising each of the frequencies making up the complex by the same increment causes a slight increase in the pitch of the missing fundamental, as illustrated in Fig. 12.9. Here, the components of the complex sound have been increased by 60 Hz compared to the frequencies in the preceding figure so that

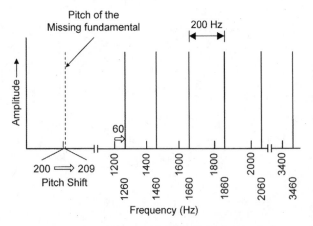

Figure 12.9 Spectrum illustrating the pitch shift of the missing fundamental. Based on Patterson (1973), with permission of *J. Acoust. Soc. Am.*

they are now 1260, 1460, 1660 Hz, etc. Notice that the missing fundamental is now matched to 209 Hz even though the components frequencies are still 200 Hz apart. This **pitch shift** of the missing fundamental was also originally described by (Schouten, 1940) and has been confirmed by many others (e.g., deBoer, 1956; Schouten et al., 1962; Smoorenburg, 1971; Patterson, 1973; Wightman, 1973a; Buunen et al., 1974). It has been suggested that the pitch shift may be based on the fine structure of the repeated waveform (e.g., Schouten 1940; Thurlow and Small, 1955; deBoer, 1956), as illustrated in Fig. 12.10. When the harmonics are exact multiples of 200 Hz (1200, 1400 Hz, etc.), there is exactly 5 ms between equivalent peaks in the repeated waveform. The upward shift of the harmonics by 60 Hz results in a slightly shorter interval between the equivalent peaks as the waveform is repeated, so that the pitch shifts upwards a bit. Ambiguities of pitch would result when the nearly but not exactly equivalent peaks are compared, as in Fig. 12.10.

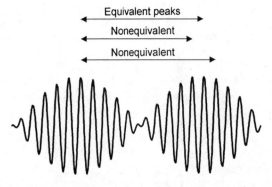

Figure 12.10 Comparison of the intervals between equivalent and nonequivalent peaks on repetitions of a waveform. Pitch ambiguity results when the pitch-extracting mechanism compares the peak of one repetition to peaks not equivalent to it on the next repetition of the waveform. Based on Schouten et al. (1962), with permission of *J. Acoust. Soc. Am.*

More recent explanations of virtual pitch involve *pattern perception models*. These explanations begin with a frequency analysis and go on to evaluate the pitch using some kind of higher-level processing. Pattern recognition may be thought of as the extraction of those similar attributes of a stimulus that allow it to be recognized as a member of a class in spite of variations in details. For example, the letter "A" is recognized whether it is printed upper- or lowercase, in italics, or even in this author's illegible penmanship.

Terhardt's (1974, 1979; Terhardt et al., 1982a, 1982b) *virtual pitch model* involves the perception of an auditory gestalt calling upon previously learned cues. These cues are subharmonics associated with various frequencies in complex sounds and are learned in the course of one's ongoing experience with the complex periodic sounds in speech. When we hear a sound, dominant resolved components are provided by the initial spectral analysis, and then the pitch processor compares the subharmonics of these components to those of the learned cues. The pitch is assigned based on the greatest degree of coincidence. The *optimum processor model* proposed by Goldstein (1973; Gerson and Goldstein, 1978) looks for the best match between a template of harmonics and the components of the complex periodic sound resolved by the initial frequency analysis. The virtual pitch is based on the fundamental frequency of the best-fitting template. In the *pattern transformation model* (Wightman, 1973b) the neural pattern resulting from a Fourier analysis at the peripheral level is examined by a pitch extractor that looks for important features shared by stimuli having the same pitch. Interested students will find detailed discussions of these and other models in several reviews (e.g., Plomp, 1976; Houtsma, 1995), in addition to the original sources.

Several studies provide physiological support for Shouten's explanation of virtual pitch (e.g., Brugge et al., 1969; Javel, 1980; Horst et al., 1986). For example, Javel (1980) found that both the envelopes and fine structures of amplitude-modulated tones were represented in auditory nerve firing patterns. However, perceptual evidence has revealed that his residue theory fails to provide a complete explanation for the perception of complex tones. The main problem is that it depends on interactions among the higher harmonics of a complex sound that are unresolved because they fall inside the same critical band filter(s). Yet, recall that the lower harmonics are dominant in determining the pitch of complex tones. The previously described results of Hall and Peters (1981) and Houtsma and Goldstein (1972) are also problematic for the Shouten's residue model. Recall that virtual pitches were heard even when the harmonics could not interact because they were presented sequentially or in different ears, implicating the involvement of more central mechanisms.

These issues are strengths for the pattern perception models, which rely upon the resolved lower harmonics and central pitch processors. However, these models also fall short of providing a complete explanation of virtual pitch. A key limitation here is that in spite of fact that the lower harmonics are the most important ones for hearing a virtual pitch, it is possible for a virtual pitch to be perceived (although generally not as well) based on just the higher frequency harmonics (e.g., Moore, 1973; Houtsma and Smurzynski, 1990). Thus, neither approach by itself provides a comprehensive account of virtual pitch perception, and it is not surprising that models involving aspects of both approaches have been suggested (e.g., Moore, 1977, 1997; van Noorden, 1982).

TIMBRE

Timbre, often referred to as **sound quality**, is typically defined as the sensory attribute of sound that enables one to judge differences between sounds having the same pitch, loudness, and duration (e.g., Plomp, 1970; ANSI, 2004). For example, it is timbre that distinguishes between the same musical note played on a violin, piano, guitar, or French horn; different vowels spoken by the same person; or a normal voice compared to one that is hoarse, harsh, or breathy. These examples show that timbre is multidimensional, being affected by both the ongoing or steady-state features of a sound as well as by its dynamic characteristics. The term **tone color** is sometimes used to refer to the timbre of steady-state sounds.

The interplay between the steady-state and dynamic attributes of timbre is illustrated in Fig. 12.11, which shows the results of a study in which listeners were asked to make similarity judgments among pairs of notes played on different instruments (Iverson and Krumhansl, 1993). An analysis of these judgments revealed that they involved two dimensions corresponding to (1) steady-state spectral features (a dull-bright continuum), shown vertically in the figure, and (2) dynamic characteristics (separating percussive from blown instruments), shown horizontally. Notice that the trumpet, saxophone, and tuba differed considerably vertically but were quite close in terms of the horizontal dimension. On the other hand, the piano and saxophone were similar along the vertical dimension but far apart horizon-

tally. The piano and tuba were perceptually far apart along both continua.

The steady-state and dynamic features of timbre have been studied in some detail (e.g., Berger, 1964; Strong and Clark, 1967; Wedin and Goude, 1972; von Bismark, 1974a, 1974b; Grey, 1977; Grey and Gordon, 1978; Wezel, 1979; Krumhansl, 1989; Iverson and Krumhansl, 1993; McAdams et al., 1999). Among the *steady-state* features of a sound that influence its timbre are the shape of the spectral envelope, its centroid, or center of gravity,[4] whether the spectral envelope is smooth or irregular, and whether there are noise-like (aperiodic) components present. (The vertical dimension in Fig. 12.11 is mainly associated with the centroid frequency of the spectrum.) For example, sounds with spectra emphasizing the higher frequencies have a bright character, whereas sounds emphasizing the lows are heard as dull. The locations of resonance peaks or formants distinguish between different vowels (see Chap. 14) and also between various musical instruments. Timbre is also affected when certain harmonics are absent. For example, a hollow quality is heard when complex tones are composed of just odd harmonics (i.e., even harmonics are missing).

The *dynamic* features affecting timbre include the amplitude envelope of the waveform (or how amplitude changes over time) and changes in the spectral envelope over time. (The horizontal dimension in Fig. 12.11 is associated with the amplitude envelope.) It is important to stress that these dynamic aspects include the onset (attack) and offset (release or decay) characteristics of a sound, as well as those occurring during its overall duration. For example, notes played on one musical instrument can sound like they are being played on another instrument when onsets are removed from the remainder of the sound, or when a recording of a piano section is played backward instead of forward.

REFERENCES

American National Standards Institute, ANSI S1–1994 (R2004). 2004. *American National Standard Acoustical Terminology.* New York, NY: ANSI.

Attneave, F, Olson, RK. 1971. Pitch as a medium: A new approach to psychophysical scaling. *Am J Psychol* 84, 147–166.

Bachem, A. 1948. Chroma fixation at the ends of the musical frequency scale. *J Acoust Soc Am* 20, 704–705.

Bachem, A. 1950. Tone height and chroma as two different pitch qualities. *Acta Psychol* 7, 80–88.

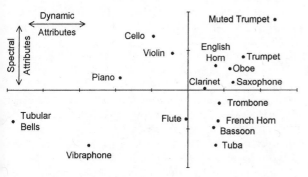

Figure 12.11 Two-dimensional similarity judgments among various musical instruments. Vertical dimension represents steady-state (spectral) characteristics. Horizontal dimension represents dynamic (amplitude envelope) characteristics. *Source*: Modified from Iverson and Krumhansl (1993), with permission of *J. Acoust. Soc. Am.*

[4] The centroid of the spectrum is its average frequency, weighted according to amplitude. The usual formula for it is

$$c = \frac{\sum f_i a_i}{\sum a_i}$$

where c is the centroid, f_i is the frequency of a component in the spectrum, and a_i is the amplitude of that component.

Beck, J, Shaw, WA. 1962. Magnitude estimations of pitch. *J Acoust Soc Am* 34, 92–98.

Beck, J, Shaw, WA. 1963. Single estimates of pitch magnitude. *J Acoust Soc Am* 35, 1722–1724.

Bekesy, G. 1960. *Experiments in Hearing*. New York, NY: McGraw-Hill.

Berger, KW. 1964. Some factors in the recognition of timbre. *J Acoust Soc Am* 36, 1888–1891.

Bilsen, FA, Ritsma, RJ. 1967. Repetition pitch mediated by temporal fine structure at dominant spectral regions. *Acustica* 19, 114–116.

Boring, EG. 1942. *Sensation and Perception in the History of Experimental Psychology*. New York, NY: Appleton-Century.

Botros, A. 2001. *Frequency to Musical Note Converter*. Available at http://www.phys.unsw.edu.au/music/note/.

Brugge, JF, Anderson, DJ, Hind, JE, Rose, JE. 1969. Time structure of discharges in singled auditory nerve fibers of the squirrel monkey in response to complex periodic sounds. *J Neurophysiol* 32, 386–401.

Burns, EM, Viemeister, NF. 1976. Nonspectral pitch. *J Acoust Soc Am* 60, 863–869.

Burns, EM, Viemeister, NF. 1981. Played-again SAM: Further observations on the pitch of amplitude-modulated noise. *J Acoust Soc Am* 70, 1655–1660.

Buunen, TJF, Festen, JM, Bilsen, FA, Van Den Brink, G. 1974. Phase effects in a three-component signal. *J Acoust Soc Am* 55, 297–303.

Campbell, M, Greated, C. 1987. *The Musician's Guide to Acoustics*. New York, NY: Schirmer.

Chocolle, R, Legouix, JP. 1957. On the inadequacy of the method of beats as a measure of aural harmonics. *J Acoust Soc Am* 29, 749–750.

Cohen, A. 1961. Further investigations of the effects of intensity upon the pitch of pure tones. *J Acoust Soc Am* 33, 1363–1376.

Cook, ND. 2001. Explaining harmony. The roles of interval dissonance and chordal tension. *Ann N Y Acad Sci* 930(1), 382–385.

Cook, ND, Fujisawa, TX. 2006. The psychophysics of harmony perception: Harmony is a three-tone phenomenon. *Emper Mus Rev* 1, 106–126.

Cook, ND, Hayashi, T. 2008. The psychoacoustics of harmony perception. *Am Sci* 96, 311–319.

deBoer, E. 1956. *On the residue in hearing*. Ph.D. Dissertation. Amsterdam, The Netherlands: University of Amsterdam.

Demany, L, Armand, F. 1984. The perceptual reality of tone chroma in early infancy. *J Acoust Soc Am* 76, 57–66.

Fastl, H. 1971. Über Tonhöhenempfindungen bei Rauschen. *Acustica* 25, 350–354.

Gerson, A, Goldstein, JL. 1978. Evidence for a general template in central optimal processing for pitch of complex tones. *J Acoust Soc Am* 63, 498–510.

Gockel, HE, Carlyon, RP, Plack, CJ. 2005. Dominance region for pitch: Effects of duration and dichotic presentation. *J Acoust Soc Am* 117, 1326–1336.

Gockel, HE, Moore, BCJ, Carlyon, RP, Plack, CJ. 2007. Effects of duration on the frequency discrimination of individual partials in a complex tone and on the discrimination of fundamental frequency. *J Acoust Soc Am* 121, 373–382.

Goldstein, JL. 1967. Auditory nonlinearity. *J Acoust Soc Am* 41, 676–689.

Goldstein, JL. 1973. An optimum processor theory for the central formation of the pitch of complex tones. *J Acoust Soc Am* 54, 1496–1516.

Goldstein, JL. 2000. Pitch perception. In: AE Kazdin (ed.), *Encyclopedia of Psychology*, Vol. 6. Oxford, UK: Oxford University Press, 201–210.

Goldstein, JL, Buchsbaum, G, Furst, M. 1978. Compatibility between psychophysical and physiological measurements of aural combination tones. *J Acoust Soc Am* 63, 474–485.

Greenwood, DD. 1990. A cochlear frequency-position function for several species—29 years later. *J Acoust Soc Am* 87, 2592–2605.

Grey, JM. 1977. Multidimensional perceptual scaling of musical timbres. *J Acoust Soc Am* 61, 1270–1277.

Grey, JM, Gordon, JW. 1978. Perceptual effects of spectral modifications of musical timbres. *J Acoust Soc Am* 63, 1493–1500.

Hall, JL. 1972a. Auditory distortion products f_2-f_1 and $2f_1-f_2$. *J Acoust Soc Am* 51, 1863–1871.

Hall, JL. 1972b. Monaural phase effect: Cancellation and reinforcement of distortion products f_2-f_1 and $2f_1-f_2$. *J Acoust Soc Am* 51, 1872–1881.

Hall, JL. 1975. Nonmonotonic behavior of distortion product $2f_1-f_2$; Psychophysical observations. *J Acoust Soc Am* 58, 1046–1050.

Hall, JW, Peters, RW. 1981. Pitch for nonsimultaneous successive harmonics in quiet and noise. *J Acoust Soc Am* 69, 509–513.

Hill, TJW, Summers, IR. 2007. Discrimination of interval size in short tone sequences. *J Acoust Soc Am* 121, 2376–2383.

Horst, JW, Javel, E, Farley, GR. 1986. Coding of fine structure in the auditory nerve. I. Fourier analysis of period and interspike histograms. *J Acoust Soc Am* 79, 398–416.

Houtsma, AJM. 1995. Pitch perception. In: BCJ Moore (ed.), *Hearing*. 2nd ed. San Diego, CA: Academic Press, 267–297.

Houtsma, AJM, Goldstein, JL. 1972. The central origin of the pitch of complex tones: Evidence from musical interval recognition. *J Acoust Soc Am* 51, 520–529.

Houtsma, AJM, Smurzynski, J. 1990. Pitch identification and discrimination for complex tones with many harmonics. *J Acoust Soc Am* 87, 304–310.

Humes, LR. 1985a. Cancellation level and phase of the (f_2-f_1) distortion product. *J Acoust Soc Am* 78, 1245–1251.

Humes, LR. 1985b. An excitation-pattern algorithm for the estimation of $(2f_1-f_2)$ and (f_2-f_1) cancellation level and phase. *J Acoust Soc Am* 78, 1252–1260.

Iverson, P, Krumhansl, C. 1993. Isolating the dynamic attributes of musical timbre. *J Acoust Soc Am* 94, 2595–2563.

Janata, P, Birk, JL, van Horn, JD, Leman, M, Tillmann, B, Bharucha, JJ. 2002. The cortical topography of tonal structures underlying western music. *Science* 298, 2167–2170.

Javel, E. 1980. Coding of AM tones in the chinchilla auditory nerve: Implications for the pitch of complex tones. *J Acoust Soc Am* 68, 133–146.

Kameoka, A, Kuriyagawa, M. 1969. Consonance theory. Part I: Consonance of dyads. *J Acoust Soc Am* 45, 1451–1459.

Krumhansl, CL. 1989. Why is musical timbre so hard to understand? In: J Nielzen, O Olsson (eds.), *Structure and Electroacoustic Sound and Music*. Amsterdam, The Netherlands: Elsevier (Excerpta Medica), 43–53.

Lawrence, M, Yantis, PJ. 1956. Onset and growth of aural harmonics in the overloaded ear. *J Acoust Soc Am* 28, 852–858.

Lawrence, M, Yantis, PJ. 1957. In support of an "inadequate" method for detecting "fictitious" aural harmonics. *J Acoust Soc Am* 29, 750–751.

Licklider, JCR. 1954. Periodicity pitch and place pitch. *J Acoust Soc Am* 26, 945.

McAdams, S, Beauchamp, JW, Meneguzzi, S. 1999. Discrimination of musical instrument sounds resynthesized with simplified spectrotemporal parameters. J Acoust Soc Am 105, 882–897.

Meyer, LB. 1956. *Emotion and Meaning in Music*. Chicago, IL: University of Chicago Press.

Meyer, MF. 1957. Aural harmonics are fictitious. *J Acoust Soc Am* 29, 749.

Moore, BCJ. 1973. Some experiments relating to the perception of complex tones. *Q J Exp Psychol* 25, 451–475.

Moore, BCJ. 1977. *An Introduction to the Psychology of Hearing*. London, UK: Academic.

Moore, BCJ. 1997. *An Introduction to the Psychology of Hearing*, 4th ed. London, UK: Academic Press.

Moore, BCJ, Glasberg, BR, Peters, RW. 1985. Relative dominance of individual partials in determining the pitch of complex tones. *J Acoust Soc Am* 77, 1853–1860.

Moore, BCJ, Glasberg, BR, Shailer, MJ. 1984. Frequency and intensity limens for harmonics within complex tones. *J Acoust Soc Am* 75, 550–561.

Morgan, CT, Garner, WR, Galambos, R. 1951. Pitch and intensity. *J Acoust Soc Am* 23, 658–663.

Ohgushi, K, Hatoh, T. 1989. On the perception of the musical pitch of high frequency tones. *Proceedings of the 13th International Congress on Acoustics* (Belgrade), 3, 27–30

Patterson, RD. 1969. Noise masking of a change in residue pitch. *J Acoust Soc Am* 45, 1520–1524.

Patterson, RD. 1973. The effects of relative phase and the number of components on residue pitch. *J Acoust Soc Am* 53, 1565–1572.

Patterson, RD, Wightman, FL. 1976. Residue pitch as a function of component spacing. *J Acoust Soc Am* 59, 1450–1459.

Plomp, R. 1964. The ear as a frequency analyzer. *J Acoust Soc Am* 36, 1628–1636.

Plomp, R. 1965. Detect ability threshold for combination tones. *J Acoust Soc Am* 37, 1110–1123.

Plomp, R. 1967. Pitch of complex tones. *J Acoust Soc Am* 41, 1526–1533.

Plomp, R. 1970. Timbre as a multidimensional attribute of complex tones. In: R Plomp, GF Smoorenburg (eds.), *Frequency Analysis and Periodicity Detection in Hearing*. Leiden, The Netherlands: Sijtthoff, 397–414.

Plomp, R. 1976. *Aspects of Tone Sensation*. London, UK: Academic.

Plomp, R, Levelt, WJM. 1965. Tonal consonance and critical bandwidth. *J Acoust Soc Am* 38, 548–560.

Plomp, R, Steeneken, HJM. 1968. Interference between two simple tones. *J Acoust Soc Am* 43, 883–884.

Révész, G. 1913. Zur Grundlegung der Tonspchologie. Leipzig: Veit. [English translation: de Courcy, G. 1954. *Introduction to the Psychology of Music*. Norman, France: University of Oklahoma Press.]

Ritsma, R. 1962. Existence region of the tonal residue. I. *J Acoust Soc Am* 34, 1224–1229.

Ritsma, R. 1963. Existence region of the tonal residue. II. *J Acoust Soc Am* 35, 1241–1245.

Ritsma, RJ. 1967. Frequencies dominant in the perception of the pitch of complex tones. *J Acoust Soc Am* 42, 191–198.

Rossing, TD. 1989. *The Science of Sound*. Reading, MA: Addison-Wesley.

Scharf, B. 1970. Critical bands. In: JV Tobias (ed.), *Foundations of Modern Auditory Theory*, Vol. I. New York, NY: Academic Press, 157–202.

Schellenberg, EG, Trehub, SE. 1994. Frequency ratios and the perception of tone patterns. *Psychon Bull Rev* 1, 191–201.

Schouten, JF. 1940. The residue, a new concept in subjective sound analysis. *Proc K Ned Akad* 43, 356–365.

Schouten, JF. 1970. The residue revisited. In: R Plomp, GF Smoorenburg (eds.), *Frequency Analysis and Periodicity Detection in Hearing*. Leiden, The Netherlands: Sijtthoff, 41–58

Schouten, JF, Ritsma, R, Cardozo, B. 1962. Pitch of the residue. *J Acoust Soc Am* 34, 1418–1424.

Seebeck, A. 1841. Beohachtungen uber einige Bedingungen der Entstehung von Tonen. *Ann Phys Chem* 53, 417–436.

Semal, C, Demany, L. 1990. The upper limit of "musical" pitch. *Music Perception* 8, 165–176.

Shepard, RN. 1964. Circularity of judgments of relative pitch. *J Acoust Soc Am* 36, 2346–2353.

Small, A, Campbell, RA. 1961. Masking of pulsed tones by bands of noise. *J Acoust Soc Am* 33, 1570–1576.

Small, A, Daniloff, TG. 1967. Pitch of noise bands. *J Acoust Soc Am* 41, 506–512.

Smoorenburg, G. 1971. Pitch perception of two-frequency stimuli. *J Acoust Soc Am* 48, 924–942.

Smoorenburg, GF. 1972. Audibility region of combination tones. *J Acoust Soc Am* 52, 603–614.

Stevens, SS. 1935. The relation of pitch to intensity. *J Acoust Soc Am* 6, 150–154.

Stevens, SS, Volkmann, J, Newman, EB. 1937. A scale for the measurement of the psychological magnitude pitch. *J Acoust Soc Am* 8, 185–190.

Stevens, SS, Volkmann, J. 1940. The relation of pitch to frequency: A revised scale. *Am J Psych* 53, 329–353.

Strong, W, Clark, M. 1967. Perturbations of synthetic orchestral wind-instrument tones. J Acoust Soc Am 41, 277–285.

Terhardt, E. 1974. Pitch, consonance, and harmony. *J Acoust Soc Am* 55, 1061–1069.

Terhardt, E. 1979. Calculating virtual pitch. *Hear Res* 1, 155–182.

Terhardt, E, Stoll, G, Seewann, M. 1982a. Pitch of complex signals according to virtual-pitch theory: Tests, examples, and predictions. *J Acoust Soc Am* 71, 671–678.

Terhardt, E, Stoll, G, Seewann, M. 1982b. Algorithm for extraction of pitch and pitch salience from complex tonal signals. *J Acoust Soc Am* 71, 679–688.

Thurlow, WR, Small, AM. 1955. Pitch perception of certain periodic auditory stimuli. *J Acoust Soc Am* 27, 132–137.

von Bismark, G. 1974a. Timbre of steady sounds: A factorial investigation of its verbal attributes. *Acustica* 30, 146–159.

von Bismark, G. 1974b. Sharpness as an attribute of timbre of steady sounds. *Acustica* 30, 159–172.

van Noorden, L. 1982. Two-channel pitch perception. In: M Clynes (ed.), *Music, Mind and Brain*. New York, NY: Plenum, 217–225.

Ward, WD. 1953. The subjective octave and the pitch of pure tones. Ph.D. Dissertation. Cambridge, MA: Harvard University.

Ward, WD. 1954. Subjective musical pitch. *J Acoust Soc Am* 26, 369–380.

Ward, WD. 1963a. Absolute pitch. Part I. *Sound* 2(3), 14–21.

Ward, WD. 1963b. Absolute pitch. Part II. *Sound* 2(4), 33–41.

Ward, WD, Burns, EM. 1982. Absolute pitch. In: D Deutch (ed.), *The Psychology of Music*. London, UK: Academic Press, 431–451.

Wedin, L, Goude, G. 1972. Dimensional analysis of the perception of instrumental timbre. *Scand J Psychol* 13, 228–240.

Wezel, DL. 1979. Timbre space as a musical control structure. *Comput Music J* 3, 45–52.

Wightman, FL. 1973a. Pitch and stimulus fine structure. *J Acoust Soc Am* 54, 397–406.

Wightman, FL. 1973b. The pattern-transformation model of pitch. *J Acoust Soc Am* 54, 407–416.

Zwicker, E. 1955. Der Ungewohnliche Amplitudengang der Nichtilinearen Vertzerrungen des Ohres. *Acustica* 5, 67–74.

Zwicker, E. 1981. Dependence of level and phase of the $(2f_1-f_2)$-cancellation tone on frequency range, frequency difference, and level of primaries, and subject. *J Acoust Soc Am* 70, 1277–1288.

Zwicker, E, Fastl, H. 1999. *Psychoacoustics: Facts and Models*, 2nd ed. Berlin, Germany: Springer-Verlag.

13   Binaural and Spatial Hearing

In this chapter, we explore several aspects of binaural hearing, that is, hearing with both ears instead of just one. We shall see that binaural hearing offers a number of advantages over monaural hearing, which have obvious implications for daily living. In particular, we will examine how we use hearing to determine the locations of sounds in space, which relies upon time and level differences between the ears and spectral variations caused by the pinna, head, and torso, all of which are affected by the direction of the sound source.

BINAURAL SUMMATION

Although Sivian and White (1933) did not find significant differences between the minimal audible field (MAF) for the better ear and binaural MAF, subsequent studies demonstrate that the intensity needed to reach threshold is lower when listening with two ears than with one. The essential finding is that, if one first corrects for any difference in monaural threshold between the two ears so that they are equal in terms of sensation level, then the binaural threshold will be approximately 3 dB better (lower) than the monaural thresholds (Causse and Chavasse, 1941, 1942a; Keys, 1947; Shaw et al., 1947). For example, to correct for the difference between monaural thresholds of 11 dB in the right ear and 16 dB in the left, the binaural stimulus would be presented 5 dB higher in the left ear. The resulting binaural threshold would be about 3 dB below these equated monaural thresholds. Hirsh (1948a) refers to this threshold advantage that occurs when listening with two ears as **binaural summation at threshold**. Similar binaural advantages have been demonstrated when the stimulus is white noise (Pollack, 1948) or speech (Keys, 1947; Shaw et al., 1947).

Loudness is also enhanced by binaural hearing. Based upon loudness level measurements, Fletcher and Munson (1933) concluded that a stimulus presented at a given SPL will sound twice as loud binaurally as monaurally. **Binaural summation of loudness** (Hirsh, 1948a) was shown as a function of sensation level by Causse and Chavasse (1942b), who performed loudness balances between binaurally and monaurally presented tones. At sensation levels close to threshold, they found that a binaural tone had to be about 3 dB lower in intensity than a monaural tone in order to produce the same sensation of loudness. This binaural advantage increased gradually with sensation level so that equal loudness was produced by a binaural tone 6 dB softer than the monaural stimulus at about 35 dB sensation level. This difference remained essentially constant at approximately 6 dB for higher sensation levels.

Perfect binaural summation means that a sound is twice as loud binaurally as it is monaurally. That loudness summation actually occurs at the two ears was questioned by Reynolds and Stevens (1960), who found that rate of binaural loudness growth had a slope of 0.6 compared to 0.54 for monaural loudness growth, and less than perfect binaural summation was found by Scharf and Fishken (1970). However, most findings suggest that a sound is twice as loud binaurally as it is monaurally (Fletcher and Munson, 1933; Hellman and Zwislocki, 1963; Marks, 1978, 1987). For example, Marks (1978) reported on the binaural summation of loudness for tones using magnitude estimation (and also loudness matches for corroboration). His findings are summarized in Fig. 13.1 The circles and squares show the loudness estimates for the left and right ears, respectively. The dotted lines show what the binaural estimates should be if summation is perfect. Notice that the actual binaural loudness estimates (shown by the triangles) fall almost exactly along the predicted functions. This indicates essentially perfect binaural summation at each frequency. Marks (1987) subsequently demonstrated complete binaural summation of loudness at 1000 Hz, as revealed by a 2:1 ratio of the loudness of a binaural tone to the monaural one. Recall from Chapter 11, in this context, that the calculated loudness of a binaural sound is taken to be twice that of a monaural sound (ANSI S3.4–2007).

DIFFERENTIAL SENSITIVITY

Various studies suggest that differential sensitivity for both intensity (Churcher et al., 1934; Harris, 1963; Rowland and Tobias, 1967; Jesteadt et al., 1977a, 1977b) and frequency (Shower and Biddulph, 1931; Pickler and Harris, 1955; Jesteadt et al., 1977a, 1977b) is better binaurally than when listening with only one ear. A problem, however, has been that the small differences detected between monaural and binaural difference limens (DLs) may have been the result of loudness summation. Pickler and Harris (1955) highlighted this problem. They found that the frequency DL was better binaurally than monaurally at low sensation levels. Recall from Chapter 9 that the effect of intensity upon differential sensitivity is greatest at low sensation levels, and that binaural hearing enhances sensitivity (or loudness) by roughly 3 to 6 dB. Thus, the smaller binaural DL may be due to summation rather than to some binaural mechanism for discrimination. To test this idea, Pickler and Harris adjusted the binaural signal level to account for the loudness advantage, and also tested DLs at a high level where differential sensitivity should not be affected by intensity. In both cases, the difference between monaural and binaural DLs disappeared. It was thus unclear whether the binaural DL is smaller than it is monaurally, or whether the difference just reflects a level difference.

This issue was essentially resolved in a study by Jesteadt et al. (1977a). They obtained intensity and frequency DLs at 70 dB SPL for 250-, 1000-, and 4000-Hz tones by using a two-interval forced-choice method. Their results are shown in Fig. 13.2 Note that binaural differential sensitivity is uniformly

DECIBELS SPL (400 Hz)

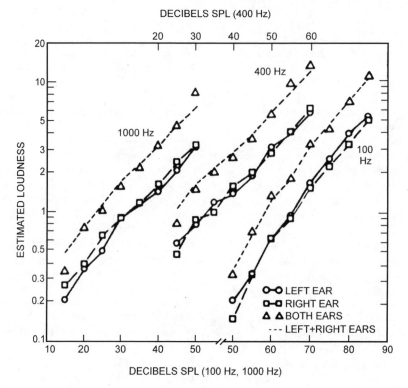

Figure 13.1 Loudness magnitude estimates for each ear and binaurally at 100, 400, and 1000 Hz. The dotted lines are predicted values for perfect summation. (See text.) *Source*: From Marks (1978), with permission of *J. Acoust. Soc. Am.*

better (the DL is smaller) than monaural, and that the difference is largely the same regardless of frequency. The ratio of the monaural to the binaural DL is on the order of 1.65 for intensity and 1.44 for frequency. The binaural–monaural differences obtained by Jesteadt et al. are not attributable to a loudness advantage for binaural hearing, because a difference of about 30 dB would have been needed to produce the observed binaural DL advantages (Shower and Biddulph, 1931; Jesteadt et al., 1977a, 1977b); and binaural summation is equivalent to only about 3 to 6 dB. Stellmack, Viemeister, and Byrne (2004) found that average intensity DLs were about 2 dB better binaurally (interaural intensity differences) than monaurally, which was significant for broadband noise but not for 4000-Hz tones.

BINAURAL FUSION AND BEATS

Even though the sounds of daily life reach the two ears somewhat differently in terms of time, intensity, and spectrum, we still perceive a single image. As Cherry (1961) pointed out, we perceive one world with two ears. More precisely, the similar but nonidentical signals reaching the two ears are fused into a single, coherent image (gestalt). This process is called **binaural fusion**.

Binaural fusion experiments require earphone listening because this allows us to precisely control the stimuli presented to the two ears, as well as how these signals are related. Gener-

ally, the experimenter is looking for a combination of stimuli that results in a *fused image lateralized to the center (midline) of the head*. The essential finding is that, although completely dissimilar signals are not fused, the auditory system does achieve binaural fusion as long as the signals presented to the two ears are similar in some way (Cherry, 1953; Cherry and Sayers, 1956; Sayers and Cherry, 1957; Broadbent, 1955; Leakey et al., 1958). The low frequencies, below roughly 1500 Hz, appear to be the most important. Thus, if each ear is presented with a 300-Hz tone at the same time, the subject will perceive a fused image in the center of his head.

A second example will demonstrate an important property of binaural fusion. If two different high-frequency tones are presented one to each ear, they will be heard as two separate signals. However, if a single low-frequency tone is superimposed upon both high frequencies so that they are caused to modulate at the frequency of the low tone, the listener will report a fused image (Leakey et al., 1958). This result shows that the auditory system uses the low-frequency envelopes of the complex signals (their macrostructures) for fusion even though the details of the signals (their microstructures) are different. Fusion of speech can be shown to occur, for example, when only the high-frequency components of the speech waveform are directed to one ear and only the lows are presented to the other (Broadbent, 1955). Even

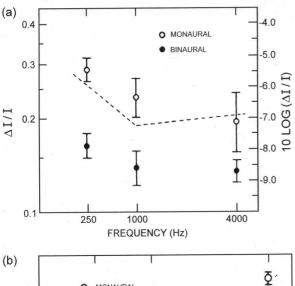

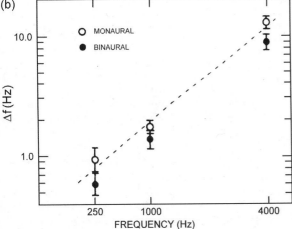

Figure 13.2 (a) Mean values of binaural and monaural ΔI//I. Dotted line shows predicted monaural values from Jesteadt et al. (1977a). (b) Mean binaural and monaural values of Δf. Dotted line shows predicted monaural DLs from Wier et al. (1977). *Source:* From Jesteadt et al. (1977b), with permission of *J. Acoust. Soc. Am.*

though neither ear alone receives enough of the speech signal for identification, the resulting fused image is readily identified.

The binaural fusion mechanism has been described in terms of a model by Cherry and Sayers (Cherry and Sayers, 1956; Sayers and Cherry, 1957) in which the central auditory nervous system carries out a running cross-correlation between the inputs to the two ears. In other words, the signals entering the ears are viewed as statistical events, and the fusion mechanism operates by looking for commonalities between the inputs coming from the two ears on an ongoing basis.

A very interesting phenomenon occurs when one tone is presented to the right ear and a second tone of slightly different frequency is presented to the left. The result is the perception of beats (see Chap. 12) in the fused image. Recall that beats occur when one combines two tones slightly different

in frequency because phase differences between the tones result in alternating increases and decreases in amplitude. The intriguing aspect of **binaural beats** is that they occur even though the two signals are acoustically completely isolated from one another. Obviously, binaural beats must result from some interaction between the neural codings of the signals from the two ears taking place within the central nervous system. [Cells have been identified in the superior olive that are responsive to the envelope of binaural beats (e.g., Wernick and Starr, 1966). They are probably at least partially involved in subserving the perception of binaural beats.]

Binaural beats differ from monaural beats in several ways (Licklider et al., 1950; Tobias, 1963; Groen, 1964). Whereas monaural beats can be heard for interacting tones across the audible frequency range, binaural beats are associated with the lower frequencies, and the best responses are for tones between about 300 and 600 Hz. Binaural beats can still be heard even if the frequency difference between the ears is relatively wide, although the perception of the image changes with frequency separation (see below). In addition, binaural beats can be perceived even if there is a substantial difference in sound level between the ears. (Recall from Chap. 5 that phase locking to stimulus cycle occurs at the very lowest levels at which an auditory neuron responds.) There have also been reports that binaural beats can be detected if one of the tones is presented at a level below the behavioral threshold for that ear (Lehnhardt, 1961; Groen, 1964); however, subsequent experiments have failed to confirm these findings (Tobias, 1963; Gu et al., 1995).

Licklider et al. (1950) reported that perceptual differences occur as the frequency separation widens between the ears. When identical frequencies are presented to two ears, the listener hears a fused image. When the frequencies are 2–10 Hz apart, the subject reports loudness fluctuations, which give way to a perception of "roughness" when the frequency difference reaches about 20 Hz. As the frequency separation becomes wider and wider, the fused image appears first to split into two smooth tones, and these tones then migrate in perceived location to the respective ears.

AUDITORY SCENE ANALYSIS

Before proceeding to the question of directional hearing, let us consider the different but related issue of how we differentiate among the many sounds that surround us at any particular time. One very familiar experience of this kind is the aptly named **cocktail party effect**, which refers to our ability to follow what one person is saying when one or more other people are talking at the same time (Cherry, 1953). Of course, this is certainly not the only situation in which we separate one sound from the other. For example, we regularly separate the words of a song from the accompanying music, and are able to differentiate among the many sound sources in a busy work or home environment. This phenomenon has been described as **auditory scene analysis** (Bregman, 1990) or **sound source determination** (Yost, 1993, 1997; Yost and Sheft, 1993).

A variety of acoustical parameters have been considered as contributors to this process, including spectral profile, spectral separation, harmonicity, spatial separation, temporal onsets and offsets, temporal modulation, and temporal separation (Yost, 1993, 1997; Yost and Sheft, 1993). For example, the spatial separation of a signal (target) and a masker has been shown to reduce both energetic and informational masking (see Chap. 10; see, e.g., Arbogast et al., 2002; Hawley, Litovsky, and Culling, 2004; Gallum, Mason, and Kidd, 2005; Kidd, Mason, Brughera, and Hartmann, 2005; Wu, Wang, Chen, et al., 2005). This **spatial release from masking** (or **spatial unmasking**) occurs because (1) separating the target and the masker provides an acoustical advantage by increasing the target-to-masker ratio at one of the ears, and (2) the advantages provided by binaural processing, which are discussed in this chapter.

Auditory scene analysis may also be addressed in the context of gestalt psychology principles for the grouping of objects in the visual field [1] (Bregman, 1990; Bregman and Ahad, 1996). We will briefly consider a few basic aspects of this approach as a foundation for further study.

Fundamentally, auditory scene analysis involves grouping the sounds impinging on the listener's ears into *perceptual units* called **streams** based on certain criteria or *grouping principles*. For example, the grouping factors of **proximity** and **similarity** pertain to how close or far apart sounds are in terms of their physical parameters. In other words, sounds tend to be grouped together when they are close and/or similar with respect to parameters such as frequency, spectral shape, timing, harmonicity (harmonics of a common fundamental frequency), intensity, and direction or spatial origin. On the other hand, sounds that are far apart or dissimilar in terms of these parameters tend not to be grouped together, but are perceived as separate streams. This is illustrated in Fig. 13.3 which represents the perception of alternating higher- and lower-frequency tones. In the upper frame, the two tones are relatively close in frequency, and they are perceptually grouped into a *single stream* of alternating pitches (*ABABABAB*) that is heard to be coming from the same sound source. However, when the two tones are far apart in frequency, they are heard as *two separate streams* of interrupted tones (*A...A...A...A* and *B...B...B...B*) coming from different sound sources, as in the lower frame. The former case illustrates **stream fusion** (or **stream integration**), and the latter case is **stream segregation**.

Other gestalt grouping principles are also involved in auditory streaming including, among others, common fate and good continuation. **Common fate** is the tendency for stimuli that change together over time to be grouped perceptually, implying a common origin. This would apply to sounds that have similar onsets, offsets, and variations in frequency, harmonicity, or level

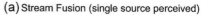
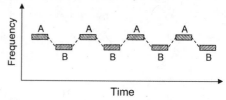

(a) Stream Fusion (single source perceived)

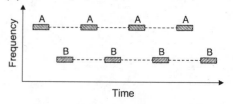

(b) Stream Segregation (different sources perceived)

Figure 13.3 Both panels show a sequence of alternating higher-(*A*) and lower-(*B*) frequency tones. (a) When the two frequencies are close enough, they are heard as a single stream of alternating pitches (*ABABABAB*), which is coming from one sound source. (b) When the two frequencies are sufficiently different, they are heard as two separate streams of interrupted tones (*A...A...A...A* and *B...B...B...B*), each coming from a different sound source.

over time. **Good continuation** applies to smooth changes in the physical parameters of a sound so that abrupt changes or discontinuities imply a change in the source.

Auditory streaming involves both primitive and schema-based processes (Bregman, 1990). **Primitive processes** are innate, automatic, and unconscious, and may be viewed as operating on the acoustical aspects of the signal in a bottom-up fashion. Thus, the streaming of alternating high- and low-frequency tones illustrated in Fig. 13.3 is an example of a primitive process. On the other hand, **schema-based processes** operate in a top-down fashion, involving learned information and cognitive effort to "hear out" a signal (e.g., listening for a familiar tune being played within the din of sounds in a university cafeteria). Increasing the speed of a schema-based streaming task results in poorer performance, but this is not the case for tasks that involve primitive processes. Primitive processes are symmetrical; for example, there is no difference between listening for just the higher tones or just the lower tones when presented with a sequence containing both, as in Fig. 13.3 However, schema-based processes are *asymmetrical*. Thus, it is easier to extract familiar names than the other sounds with which they are intermixed in the cacophony of a busy cafeteria.

DIRECTIONAL HEARING

Localization

How do we determine the direction of a sound source? Intuitively, we expect that some sort of comparison between the two ears must be involved. We are usually concerned with binaural

---

[1] See Palmer (1999) for an extensive review of visual perception.

listening in a sound field (stereophony), but we sometimes use earphones for personal entertainment or to precisely control experimental conditions, as described above. Interestingly, stereophonic and headphone listening can result in different perceptions of space. Sounds presented from loudspeakers are perceived to be coming from *outside* the head (*externalized*) from a source that can be **localized** in the environment. On the other hand, sounds presented from earphones are generally perceived to be *inside* the head (*internalized*), coming from an apparent source that is **lateralized** along a plane between the two ears. This difference between *extracranial* **localization** and *intracranial* **lateralization** is easily experienced by comparing the way music from the same compact disc album sounds through loudspeakers versus earphones. In general, identical sounds impinging at the same time upon the two ears are localized directly in front of (or behind) the listener or, through earphones, from an apparent source lateralized in the center of the head. However, one should be aware that externalization can be a matter of degree, as opposed to being an all-or-none experience (see Blauert, 1997; Hartmann and Wittenberg, 1996). For a review of this topic, see Durlach et al. (1992).

Horizontal directions are expressed as angles of **azimuth** around the head, illustrated in Fig. 13.4a Sounds coming from straight ahead have an azimuth 0° and those coming from directly behind have an azimuth of 180°. Other azimuths are usually given as the number of degrees right (+) or left (−) of center. For example, a loudspeaker that is off center toward the right by 45° has an azimuth of 45° right or +45°, and a loudspeaker located 45° off center toward the left has an azimuth of 45° left or −45°. Azimuths are sometimes expressed in terms of the total number of degrees going around the head toward the right, in which case 45° right would be 45°, and 45° left would be 315°. Vertical directions are expressed as angles of **elevation** (usually along the medial plane from front to back), as illustrated in Fig. 13.4b. In this case, 0° elevation means straight ahead, an elevation of 90° is directly above the head, and 180° is directly behind the head.

The traditional **duplex theory** explains localization on the basis of *time* differences between the ears at lower frequencies and *level* differences between the ears at higher frequencies (Lord Rayleigh, 1907).[2] Consider the arrangement in Fig. 13.5a. The signal from the speaker, which is off to the right, must follow a longer path to the far (left) ear than to the near (right) ear. As Fig. 13.5b. shows, low frequencies have wavelengths that are longer than the path around the head so that they "bend around" the head to the far ear (diffraction). Thus, **interaural time differences (ITDs)** are expected to provide localization cues for the lower frequencies, where the wavelength of the tone is larger than the distance the signal must travel from the near (right) ear to the far (left) ear. In contrast, higher frequencies have wavelengths smaller than the head so that they are

[2] Lord Rayleigh was John William Strutt (1842–1919).

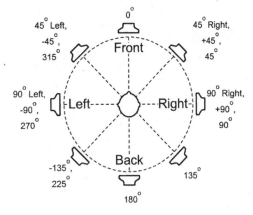

(a) Azimuth (Horizontal Plane)

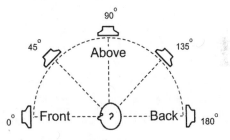

(b) Elevation (Medial Plane)

Figure 13.4 (a) Angles of azimuth horizontally around the head. Various ways of expressing azimuth angles are illustrated. (b) Angles of elevation vertically around the head in the medial plane.

"blocked" in the path to the far (left) ear (Fig. 13.5c). This **head shadow** causes a reduction in the intensity of the signal at the far ear, producing sound level differences between the ears. Thus, **interaural level differences (ILDs)** or **interaural intensity differences (IIDs)** are expected to provide localization cues for the higher frequencies. Our thresholds for interear differences are as small as approximately 10 μs for ITDs (Klumpp and Eady, 1956) and about 1 dB for ILDs (Mills, 1960; Blauert, 1997).

The traditional approach to interaural differences involves modeling the head as a solid sphere around which the ear-to-ear distance approximates 22 to 23 cm (Woodworth, 1938). This results in a time delay of roughly 660 μs for the sound to get from the near ear to the far ear, which in turn corresponds to a frequency of 1500 Hz. Thus, the greatest time delay occurs when a sound source is directly to one side or the other (90° azimuth), for which the ITD would be 660 μs, denoted by the peak of the curve in Fig. 13.6. Below 1500 Hz, the wavelength is greater than the distance around the head, and the phase difference at the two ears provides an unambiguous localization cue. However, the phase discrepancy becomes ambiguous (except for the first wavelength) as the frequency increases to 1500 Hz, where its wavelength approximates the distance around the head, resulting in localization errors. At higher frequencies, the wavelength

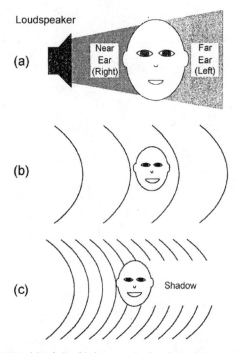

Loudspeaker

(a)

Near Ear (Right)   Far Ear (Left)

(b)

(c)   Shadow

Figure 13.5 (a) Relationship between a loudspeaker and the two ears. (b) Low frequencies bend around the head due to their large wavelengths. (c) High frequencies have wavelengths smaller than head diameter so that an acoustic shadow results at the far ear.

is shorter than the size of the head so that the resulting head shadow produces ILDs. The ILDs thus provide localization cues for the higher frequencies.

Feddersen et al. (1957) measured the interaural time and level differences for human heads as functions of angle around the head (azimuth) and frequency. Figure 13.6 shows that their ITD measurements were in good agreement with the Woodworth model. Notice that there was no difference between the ears when the signals (clicks) come from directly in front or behind (0° and 180°), because the ears are equidistant from the sound source in both cases. Interaural time differences developed as the loudspeaker moved around the head, bringing it closer to one ear than the other. The ITD increased to a maximum of about 660 μs when the loudspeaker was directly in front of one ear (90° azimuth), where the distance (and therefore the time delay) between the ears is greatest. Feddersen et al. also found that ILDs depend on both frequency and azimuth. As expected, ILDs were negligible at 200 Hz and increased with frequency to as much as about 20 dB at 6000 Hz. The ILDs were 0 dB directly in front and behind (at 0° and 180° azimuth), where the sound source is equidistant between ears and increased to as much as about 20 dB (depending on frequency), as the loudspeaker moved closer to side or the other, reaching a maximum where the loudspeaker directly in front of one ear (at 90°).

Woodworth's sphere model actually falls short of providing an accurate description of the interaural cues associated with the human head. This is not surprising because the configuration

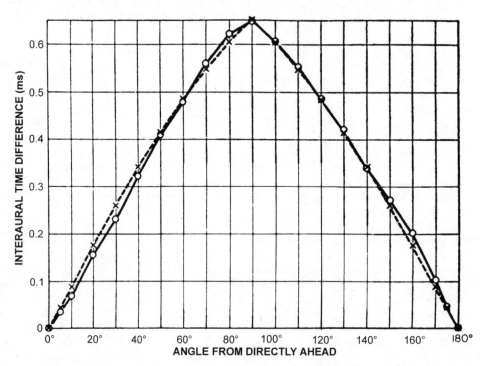

Figure 13.6 Interaural time differences for different loudspeaker azimuths. Crosses are calculated differences based on Woodworth's (1938) solid sphere model. Circles are measurements by Feddersen et al. (1957). *Source*: From Feddersen et al. (1957), permission of *J. Acoust. Soc. Am.*

of the head differs considerably from that of a sphere. Kuhn (1977) found that the ITDs for the higher frequencies came close to the 660 μs value predicted by the sphere model, but they do not change with frequency below 500 Hz or above 3000 Hz. He also found that the ITDs below about 500 Hz were about 800 to 820 μs instead of 660 μs. Middlebrooks (1999a) found that maximum interaural time delays among adults ranged from 657 to 792 μs. Taken together with other findings (e.g., Nordlund, 1962; Abbagnaro et al., 1975; Roth et al., 1980; Bronkhorst and Plomp, 1988), the implication is that the sphere model does not explain the nature of low-frequency ITDs, but applies principally to the higher frequencies and to the leading edges of clicks and click-like signals, for which the major directional cues are not the phase-derived ITDs. Even directional hearing for high-frequency complex sounds, which is principally associated with ILDs, is also affected by interaural time differences. Moreover, the duplex model alone falls short of completely explaining directional hearing because it does not adequately explain front-back distinctions, directionality above and below the horizontal plane, and monaural localization.

In addition to the effects of the ear canal resonance (Chap. 3), the spectrum of the sound arriving at the eardrum is affected by the pinna, head, and torso. In particular, **spectral cues** (also known as **pinna cues** and **monaural spectral cues**) at high frequencies introduced by the pinnae are important for the perception of elevation, front-back distinctions, and monaural localization (Blauert, 1969/70, 1997; Hebrank and Wright, 1974; Weinrich, 1982; Musicant and Butler, 1984; Middlebrooks and Green, 1991; Middlebrooks, 1992, 1997; Shaw, 1997; Wightman and Kistler, 1997). These pinna cues also contribute to the extracranialization of sound sources (Plenge, 1974; Blauert, 1997). Low-frequency cues (below about 3000 Hz) associated with head diffraction and torso reflections appear to be involved in vertical localization (e.g., Gardner, 1973; Algazi et al., 2001).

The manner in which the amplitude spectrum of a sound is modified going from a source in the environment to the eardrum is shown by the **head-related transfer function (HRTF)**. Families of HRTFs are shown for sources located *horizontally* at many azimuths around the head in Fig. 13.7 (Shaw, 1974),[3] and *vertically* at many elevations around the medial plane of the head in Fig. 13.8

The curves in these figures make it clear that the spectrum of the sound that finally arrives at the eardrum depends on the direction from which it came (see, e.g., Shaw, 1997). This is most easily seen for horizontal directions in Fig. 13.7 by comparing the shapes of HRTFs for sounds coming from the front (top panel), side (middle panel), and back (bottom panel) of the head. Also notice that the sound level reaching the eardrum gets weaker as the source moves from the same side of the

head around to the opposite side of the head. Consider a sound source located 45° to the right. In this case, the sound reaching the right (*near*) eardrum is affected by the HRTF labeled 45°, and the sound arriving at the left (*far*) eardrum is modified by the HRTF labeled −45°. (The 45° and −45° HRTFs are found in the upper panel in Fig. 13.7, or refer back to Fig. 3.2 for an uncluttered view.) It is easy to realize how these differences translate into ILDs. The same 0° curve applies to both ears if the source is directly ahead, and the same 180° curve applies to both ears if the sound is coming from directly behind (180°), in which case the ILDs are 0 dB.

Changes in elevation cause changes in the high-frequency aspects of the HRTF due to directionally dependent filtering by the pinna (Hebrank and Wright, 1974; Shaw, 1997). This is seen in Fig. 13.8 as a "pinna notch" that shifts between about 5000 and 11,000 Hz as the sound source moves up around the head. Scanning upward from the bottom of the figure, notice that there is a notch at about 6000 Hz when the sound source is *below* the head. The notch gets *higher* in frequency as the sound source moves *upward* toward the *front* and then continues up toward the top of the head (*above*), where the notch is essentially absent. Continuing around, the notch then gets *lower* in frequency as the source moves *downward* toward the *back* of the head and then *below* again.

Classical studies of localization were conducted by Stevens and Newman (1936) and Sandel, Teas, Feddersen, and Jeffress (1955). Stevens and Newman (1936) sat their subjects in a chair elevated about 12 f above the roof of the Harvard Biological Laboratories building to minimize the possible confounding effects of echoes and reverberation. The sound source was a loudspeaker mounted on a boom arm that extended 12 f from the listener. The loudspeaker was rotated around the subject in 15° steps from 0° to 180°, and the task was to listen for the signal and report its apparent direction. It is important to point out that their subjects regularly made *front-back confusions*. For example, sounds presented from 30° right of center *in front* of the subject (30° off center from 0° azimuth) were confused with sounds presented from 30° right of center *behind* (30° off center from 180° azimuth). These front-back reversals were treated as equivalent, correct responses, and the location of the sound source was judged relative to 0° or 180°, whichever was closer. With this in mind, Stevens and Newman's findings are shown as a function of frequency in Fig. 13.9 Localizations were most accurate below 1000 Hz and above 4000 Hz, with the greatest errors between about 2000 and 4000 Hz.

Sandel et al. (1955) asked subjects to localize sounds in an anechoic (echo-free) room. Loudspeakers placed at 0° and at 40° right and left were used to generate "phantom" sound sources at various azimuths, depending upon the phases of the signals. The subject indicated the perceived location of the tone source with an "acoustic pointer," which was a speaker that rotated on a boom around his or her head. A noise from this speaker alternated with the test tones, and the subject's task was to place the noise loudspeaker (pointer) at the apparent location

---

[3] This data may be found in tabular form in Shaw and Vaillancourt (1985).

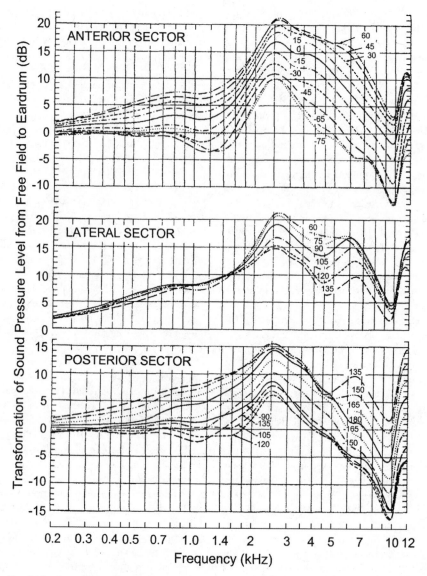

Figure 13.7 Horizontal head-related transfer functions for sound sources located at many angles of azimuth (θ) around the head based on data from 12 studies. *Source*: From Shaw (1974) with permission of *J. Acoust. Soc. Am.*

of the test tone source. They found that ITDs accounted for the localization of tones below about 1500 Hz, and that these were used to localize the high frequencies. Many random errors at 1500 Hz suggested that interaural cues are ambiguous around this frequency. These results were essentially consistent with those of Stevens and Newman.

The sizable localization errors and front/back confusions observed in these early studies imply that the directional cues provided by tonal signals are limited and ambiguous. It is interesting to note in this context that Stevens and Newman found better localization results for noises than for tones, which they attributed to quality (spectral) differences and ILDs for the

high-frequency energy in these noises. In contrast, accuracy is substantially improved and front/back errors are reduced when localizing *broad-band* signals (e.g., Butler and Planert, 1976; Oldfield and Parker, 1984; Butler, 1986; Makous and Middlebrooks, 1990). Broad-brand stimuli provide the listener with multiple cues across frequencies, including both interaural differences and spectral shape information (Wightman and Kistler, 1993, 1997). Recall, here, that the spectral shape cues due to pinna effects are found in the higher frequencies. It is interesting to note, for example, that Musicant and Butler (1984) found that front/back distinctions were best when their stimuli included high frequencies (above 4000 Hz), and that

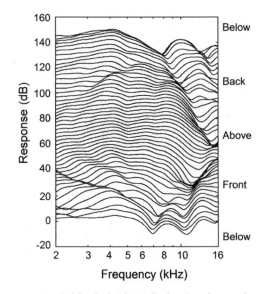

Figure 13.8 Vertical head-related transfer functions for sound sources located at many angles of elevation along the medial plane around the head of a representative subject. *Source*: Figure provided courtesy of Dr. Richard O. Duda, used with permission.

performance dropped considerably when the various depressions of the pinnae were occluded.

We learn more about the contributions of the higher frequencies from a study by Middlebrooks (1992). In this study, subjects were asked to localize high-frequency narrow-band noises presented from loudspeaker locations corresponding to 360 combinations of azimuth and elevation. The subject's task was to point the subject's nose at the perceived sound source location, and this response was in turn monitored by using special instrumentation to determine head orientation. The results demonstrated that *azimuth* was accurately localized and related to ILDs, while *front/back* and *elevation* localizations were related to spectral cues.

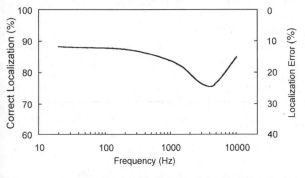

Figure 13.9 Accuracy of localization in percent (left axis) and localization error in percent (right axis) as a function of frequency, based on data reported by Stevens and Newman (1936).

Head Movements

There has been some controversy about whether the dynamic cues provided by head movements can improve localization accuracy (see, e.g., Middlebrooks and Green, 1991; Wightman and Kistler, 1993). Classical papers by Wallach (1939, 1940) presented findings and convincing arguments supporting the relevance of head movements as a means of reducing localization ambiguities, but some studies found that any benefits provided by head movements were either small or not significant (Pollack and Rose, 1967; Thurlow and Runge, 1967; Fisher and Freedman, 1968). However, questions about the impact of head movements on localization appear to have been resolved by contemporary experiments using real and virtual sound methods (e.g., Bronkhorst, 1995; Perrett and Noble, 1997a, 1997b; Wightman and Kistler, 1999; Macpherson and Middlebrooks, 2002). Although there is considerable intersubject variability, localization is improved by head movements, especially in terms of reducing front/back and vertical confusions.

Lateralization

Lateralization experiments have helped clarify and expand upon what we know about directional cues, because the use of earphones allows us to precisely control and manipulate the signals presented to the ears. Many studies have examined the effects of ITD and ILD cues upon lateralization (e.g., Klumpp and Eady, 1956; Zwislocki and Feldman, 1956; Mills, 1960; Yost et al., 1971; Yost, 1974; Grantham, 1984; Yost and Dye, 1988). While exact procedures vary, the general approach is to present two stimuli to the subject that differ with respect to interaural time (phase) or level, and to determine whether this interaural disparity results in a perceptible change in lateralization. The overall findings essentially agree with the localization data. That is, ITDs are most important up to about 1500 Hz, and ILDs take over as the primary lateralization cue for higher frequencies.

Yost (1974) performed a particularly interesting lateralization experiment addressing the discrimination of interaural time (actually phase) differences. He presented subjects with two stimuli. The first included a particular interaural time (actually phase) difference, θ. This difference, of course, resulted in a lateralization toward one side of the head analogous to the azimuth position. The second stimulus was the same except that the phase difference between the ears was larger by a slight amount $\Delta\theta$. Thus, it was $\theta + \Delta\theta$. The subjects had to detect the value of $\Delta\theta$ by discriminating between the two stimuli (θ vs. $\theta + \Delta\theta$). For any value of θ, the smaller the value of $\Delta\theta$ needed for a change in apparent lateralization, the better the discrimination of interaural phase. We might think of $\Delta\theta$ as analogous to the smallest perceptible change in azimuth (similar to the minimal audible angle discussed later in this chapter). The results are summarized in Fig. 13.10 Note that $\Delta\theta$ is smallest (best) when θ is 0° or 360°. These values of θ are midline lateralizations because 0° and 360° correspond to a zero phase disparity between the ears. Thus, the most acute interaural phase discriminations are made at the midline. On the other hand,

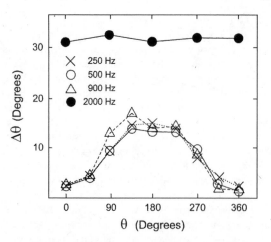

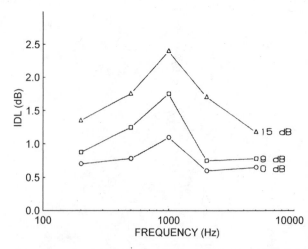

Figure 13.10 Changes in interaural phase ($\Delta\theta$) required in order to detect a difference in lateralization from a standard (reference) phase difference (θ). *Source*: Adapted from Yost (1974), with permission of *J. Acoust. Soc. Am.*

Figure 13.11 Thresholds for interaural differences in level (IDL) in decibels as a function of frequency from 200 to 5000 Hz. (Note that the scale of the ordinate is from 0 to 2.5 dB.) These findings were obtained when the standard stimulus itself was lateralized at midline (circles, marked 0 dB), halfway between midline and the left ear (squares, marked 9 dB), and at the left ear (triangles, marked 15 dB). The 0-, 9-, and 15-dB values are the interaural level differences needed to place the standard image at these locations. *Source*: From Yost and Dye (1988), with permission of *J. Acoust. Soc. Am.*

interaural phase discrimination was poorest ($\Delta\theta$ as largest) when θ was 180°; that is, when the signals were lateralized directly to one side.

Figure 13.10 also shows that $\Delta\theta$ was essentially the same for the frequencies up to 900 Hz. In contrast, interaural phase discrimination was substantially poorer at 2000 Hz, where it was constant at about 30°. Interaural phase had no effect at all for 4000 Hz (not shown on the graph). Thus, interaural phase was shown to be an important cue at low frequencies but unimportant for highs, in a manner consistent with the localization data.

Lateralization experiments have revealed that discrimination for ILDs is constant as a function of frequency within a range of about 2 dB, but with a curious increase in the size of the ILD at 1000 Hz (Mills, 1960; Grantham, 1984; Yost and Dye, 1988). These findings are illustrated in Fig. 13.11 The excellent interaural level discrimination at the high frequencies is, of course, expected from the previous discussion. Three sets of findings are shown in Fig. 13.11 depending upon whether the standard stimulus against which the discrimination was made was itself perceived to be (lateralized) at the midline, halfway between midline and the left ear, or at the left ear. These three lateralizations of the standards signal were achieved by using ILDs of 0, 9, and 15 dB, respectively (Yost, 1981). A comparison of these three curves makes it clear that ILD discrimination is most acute at midline, is least sensitive when the standard is lateralized off to one side, and is at some intermediate value when the discrimination is made between the midline and at the left ear.

Interaural time differences come into play whenever the signal contains low frequencies. For example, Yost et al. (1971) found that the lateralization of clicks is impaired by removing their low-frequency components, but not by eliminating the highs; others found that ITDs could result in lateralization differences

for high-frequency noise bursts and clicks (Klumpp and Eady, 1956; Hafter and DeMaio, 1975).

Lateralization has been used to study the relative salience of ILDs and ITDs by establishing the trade-off between the time and intensity cues. This was done by asking the subject to adjust the ILD (or ITD) until a midline image was perceived. Harris (1960) found trading ratios of 25 µs/dB for clicks with energy below 1500 Hz and 60 µs/dB for clicks with energy above 1500 Hz. These trading ratios imply that ITDs have greater salience for low frequencies (because a smaller ITD is needed to center the image) and ILDs are more salient for the highs (because a larger ITD is needed). However, these studies were marked by inconsistent results between subjects. For example, Moushegian and Jeffress (1959) found that the trading ratio for a 500-Hz tone was about 20 to 25 µs/dB for two subjects but only about 2.5 µs/dB for another subject.

Subjects in time-intensity trading studies often heard two lateralized images instead of one (Whitworth and Jeffress, 1961; Hafter and Jeffress, 1968; Jeffress and McFadden, 1971; Hafter and Carrier, 1972). One image was called the *time image* because it depended on ITDs (especially <1500 Hz) but was essentially unaffected by ILDs. The other was an *intensity image* and was responsive to both ILDs and ITDs at all frequencies. Typical trading ratios (for clicks) were on the order of 2 to 35 µs/dB for the time image and 85 to 150 µs/dB for the intensity image (Hafter and Jeffress, 1968). It may be that the intersubject differences reported by Harris (1960) and by Moushegian and Jeffress (1959) were due to responses to the time image by some subjects and to the intensity image by others.

Although high-frequency lateralization is typically associated with ILDs, it can be influenced by ITDs, such as when the high-frequency signal is amplitude-modulated at a low rate (e.g., Henning, 1974; Neutzel and Hafter, 1976, 1981). Let us borrow some examples from Henning (1974) to illustrate this. Consider three kinds of signals (each lasting 250 ms) presented binaurally to subjects with interaural time differences: (1) a low frequency (300 Hz), (2) a high frequency (3600 Hz), and (3) a high frequency (3900 Hz) that was sinusoidally amplitude-modulated (SAM) at 300 Hz. Listeners could lateralize the 300-Hz tone based on ITDs but could not do this for the 3600-Hz tone, but the 3900-Hz SAM signal also could be lateralized on the basis of ITDs (as well, in fact, as for the 300-Hz tone).

An interesting effect called **binaural interference** [4] occurs when a listener's experience of binaural phenomena for high frequencies is affected by the simultaneous presence of low frequencies (e.g., McFadden and Pasanen, 1976; Trahiotis and Bernstein, 1990; Buell and Hafter, 1991; Stellmack and Dye, 1993; Bernstein and Trahiotis, 1995; Heller and Trahiotis, 1995; Hill and Darwin, 1996; Best, Gallun, Carlile, and Shinn-Cunningham, 2007). This disruption is usually reported as poorer sensitivity for ITDs or lateralization changes at a high frequencies (signal) when the low frequency (interferer) are also present compared to when the high frequency signal is presented alone. Binaural interference appears to occur when the signal and interferer are grouped into a single perceptual unit, such as when they turn on and off simultaneously; however, it is reduced or eliminated when cues are provided that allow them to be segregated, such as when the signal and interferer frequencies turn on and off at different times.

Virtual Auditory Space Localization
The ability to take advantage of earphone testing to study directional hearing has been dramatically enhanced with the use of **virtual auditory space (VAS)** techniques. This approach uses an individual's own HRTFs for both ears (based on many sound source directions) to produce test signals that simulate naturally occurring free-field cues when they are presented to the subject through earphones (Wightman and Kistler, 1989a). These virtual stimuli have been found to accurately represent acoustical cues for localization (Wightman and Kistler, 1989a), and result in spatial position judgments similar to those found with real free-field signals, although front/back and vertical errors are more common (e.g., Wightman and Kistler, 1989b; Bronkhorst, 1995).

Unlike the *intracranially lateralized* images produced by the earlier earphone methods, VAS techniques appear to produce perceptions that are actually *localized extracranially* (e.g., Macpherson and Middlebrooks, 2002). Subjects in these virtual localization studies perceived a single apparent source as opposed to the split images often reported in the earlier lateralization studies (Wightman and Kistler, 1992; Macpherson and Middlebrooks, 2002). Wightman and Kistler (1992) compared the relative strengths of ITDs, ILDs, and spectral cues in establishing the perceived location of a sound. This was done by presenting broad-band noise signals containing conflicting localization cues. For example, the ITD would indicate that the sound source was at one location but the ILD and spectral cues would indicate that it was at a different location. In spite of the conflicting cues, their subjects perceived a single sound source at a location determined by the ITD. However, the dominance of the ITD cue was lost when the low frequencies were removed from the noise (by filtering), in which case the perceived location was determined by the ILD and spectral cues. More recently, Macpherson and Middlebrooks (2002) found that ITDs had greater salience than ILDs when localizing low-pass sounds, and that ILDs had greater salience than ITDs for high-pass sounds.

Considerable individual differences exist in the dimensions of the skull, pinna, etc., which are related to differences in HRTFs (Middlebrooks, 1999a). Testing with VAS techniques has made it possible to determine whether these individual differences affect directional hearing. To do this involves comparing an individual's localization performance for virtual sources based on his or her *own* ears versus virtual sources based on *another person's* ears (Wenzel et al., 1993; Møller et al., 1996; Middlebrooks, 1999b). Overall, it has been found that localization becomes less accurate when "listening through somebody else's ears" compared to "listening through your own ears," principally involving front/back confusions and elevation errors. It is interesting to note that this kind of manipulation of VAS sound sources has been found to produces changes in the spatial responses of the primary auditory cortex in the ferret (Mrsic-Flogel et al., 2001).

Minimum Audible Angle
Another aspect of directional hearing involves determining the smallest difference in location between two sound sources that results in a different perceived location. Since the two sound sources are viewed relative to the head, this is the same as asking what is the smallest angle (or difference in azimuth) that a listener can discriminate. Mills (1958, 1963, 1972) studied this phenomenon in depth and called it the **minimal audible angle (MAA)**. Specifically, he tested the MAA as a function of frequency when the sound sources were located in front of the subject (0°), and when they were 30°, 45°, 60°, and 75° off to the side. The logistics of the basic task are illustrated in Fig. 13.12 where we see that the listener must distinguish the difference between two points in space. Notice that the figure actually shows two different conditions, one in which the MAA is being determined when both sound sources are directly in front of the listener (at 0° azimuth) and another one in which the two sound sources are off to one side (at 45° azimuth).

---

[4] This term should not be confused with *clinical* binaural interference, in which some hearing-impaired patients have the atypical experience of poorer performance binaurally than monaurally.

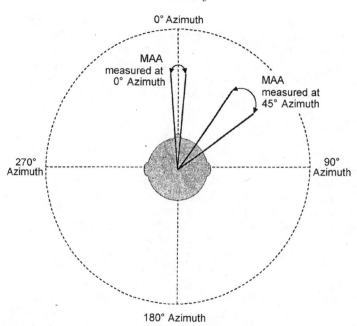

0° Azimuth

MAA
measured at
0° Azimuth

MAA
measured at
45° Azimuth

270°
Azimuth

90°
Azimuth

180° Azimuth

Figure 13.12 The minimal audible angle (MAA) is the smallest angular difference that can be perceived between two sound sources. This illustration shows the arrangement when the MAA is being measured under two different conditions. In one case, the MAA is being measured for loudspeakers directly in front of the listener (at 0° azimuth); in the other case, the loudspeakers are located at 45° azimuth.

In his classical studies, Mills found that the MAA was smallest (best) for the frequencies below about 1500 Hz and above approximately 2000 Hz, and was largest (poorest) between these frequencies. This result reflects the ambiguity of localization cues in the vicinity of 1500 Hz, thus confirming the previously mentioned findings. Mills also found that MAAs were most acute (approximately 1–2°) when the sound sources were directly in front of the head, and that they increased dramatically to very high values when the sources were at the side of the head. This result occurs because small changes in location in front of the head result in large interaural differences (especially ITDs). However, when the sources are off to one side of the head (facing one ear), the interaural differences remain largely the same in spite of relatively large changes in angle between the loudspeakers. We might thus conceive of a **cone of confusion** (Fig. 13.13) to one side of the head, within which the interaural differences do not vary when the sound sources change location (Mills, 1972). This image demonstrates the importance of head movements in localization, since these movements keep changing the position of the cone of confusion—the zone of ambiguity—thereby minimizing its detrimental effect.

The MAA described by Mills involved the discrimination of two stimuli presented sequentially. Perrott (1984) expanded upon the concept of the MAA using stimuli that were presented at the same time, describing the **concurrent minimum audible angle (CMAA)**. As for the MAA, the CMAA is also most acute for sounds presented directly in front of the subject and least sensitive when the stimuli are presented off to one side. However,

the CMAA is also affected by spectral differences between the two sounds whose locations are to be discriminated. Subjects were unable to distinguish a difference in the angular locations of the stimuli when their frequencies differed by only 15 Hz. When the signals differed in frequency by 43 Hz, the size of the CMAA increased from 4.5° when the two signals were presented from 0° azimuth to an angle of about 45° when they were

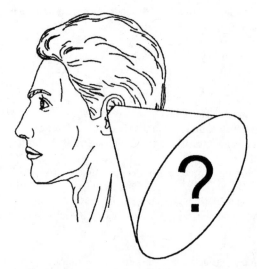

Figure 13.13 The cone of confusion (see text). *Source*: Modified after Mills (1972).

presented from 67° off to the left. On the other hand, signals 101 Hz apart had CMAAs of about 10° when the two sources were anywhere from straight ahead (0° azimuth) up to 55° off center. The CMAA then increased dramatically to about 30° when these signals were presented from 67° to the left. (An intermediate relationship between CMAA and azimuth was obtained for signals differing in frequency by 72 Hz.) As Perrott has pointed out, the CMAA involves the issue of sound source identification ("what") as well as that of localization ("where").

Minimum Audible Movement Angle

The MAA and CMAA describe the smallest perceptible difference in location between two *stationary* sound sources, A and B. We may also ask a similar question with regard to the *motion* of a sound source. How far (in degrees) must B travel away from A in order for us to know that B is moving? This smallest change in location that is needed for us to detect motion is called the **minimum audible movement angle (MAMA)** and has been the topic of considerable study (Harris and Sergeant, 1971; Perrott and Musicant, 1977; Grantham, 1986; Perrott and Tucker, 1988; Perrott et al., 1989; Saberi and Perrott, 1990a; Chandler and Grantham, 1992). Taken together, the evidence suggests that minimum audible movement angles depend on the same parameters that apply for stationary sources, plus the effect of how fast the moving sound source is moving. Using broad-band noise sources presented from directly in front of the head (0° azimuth), Chandler and Grantham (1992) found that the mean MAMA was 5.2° when the moving loudspeaker had a velocity of 10° per second (°/s), and 5.7° at 20°/s. However, the mean MAMA increased to 8.2° at 45°/s, 12° at 90°/s, and 17.3° at 180°/s. For noises presented from speakers at 60° azimuth, mean MAMAs increased from 8.3° at 10°/s to 28.4° at 180°/s. Notice that binaural sensitivity for motion becomes less sensitive for faster velocities. Saberi and Perrott (1990a) found that the minimum audible movement angle was most acute for velocities between 1.8°/s and 11°/s, and that it increased for slower velocities as well as for faster ones. Within this range, they were able to measure mean MAMAs as small as about 2° (approaching the size of the stationary MAA).

Distance

How do we judge distance with hearing? The answer to this question is not clear, although there has been renewed interest in this area. This section will outline several of the factors that have been considered as potential cues for perceiving the distance from a sound source. The interested student will find informative reviews in Coleman (1963), Blauert (1997), and Zahorik (1996). We will begin with sound level and the ratio of direct-to-reverberant energy. It appears that both can be salient distance cues, and that there is flexibility in their relative prominence in making distance judgments, depending on the nature of the sound (Zahorik, 2002a).

Sound level in a free field drops by 6 dB for each doubling of distance from the source (Chap. 1). Thus, sound level pro-

vides the listener with a distance cue. However, more than the expected decrease of 6 dB is required to perceive a doubling of distance so that apparent distance underestimates actual distance (Bekesy, 1938; Cochran, Throop, and Simpson, 1968; Gardner, 1969; Blauert, 1997; Petersen, 1990; Begault, 1991). For example, Blauert (1997) demonstrated that a doubling of perceived distance requires sound level reduction of about 20 dB instead of the expected value of 6 dB. Perceptual underestimates of actual distances appear to be ubiquitous findings in distance perception studies (Zahorik, 2002a).

Sounds reaching a listener in a real room involve both the *direct sound* from the source and *reverberation*, composed of multiple *reflections* from the walls, ceiling, floors, and various objects within the room. Under these conditions, the direct energy decreases with distance from the source (due to the inverse square law), but the reverberant energy remains pretty much uniform. As a result, the *ratio of direct-to-reverberant energy* changes with distance, enabling it to provide a distance perception cue for the listener (Blauert, 1997). The salience of the direct-to-reverberant energy ratio is fairly well established, and it is commonly found that distance performance is better in reverberant settings than in anechoic (echo-free) situations (Mershon and King, 1975; Mershon and Bowers 1979; Mershon et al., 1989; Wagenaars, 1990; Nielsen, 1993; Bronkhorst and Houtgast, 1999; Zahorik, 2002a, 2002b). Moreover, Zahorik (2002a) found that the direct-to-reverberant ratio had greater perceptual weight as a distance cue than sound level for noise signals. However, it appears to provide a coarsely grained distance cue because the threshold for discriminating direct-to-reverberant ratios is about 5 to 6 dB, roughly corresponding to a 2.5-fold change in distance (Zahorik, 2002b).

Spectral shape is another potential acoustical cue for distance perception when dealing with relatively long distances (Coleman, 1968; Butler et al., 1980; Little, Mershon, Cox, 1992; Blauert, 1997). The spectrum of a sound changes with distance from the sound source due to absorption as sound travels through the air, which causes the high frequencies to be attenuated with distance a great deal more than the lows.

Brungart (1999) showed that *binaural cues*, specifically *ILDs* for relatively *low* frequencies (<3000 Hz), contribute to distance perception when the sound source is less than 1 m from the head. This might seem odd because ILDs are generally associated with the high frequencies. However, low-frequency ILDs become significant when the source is close to the head and increase with proximity (Brungart and Rabinowitz, 1999; Duda and Martens, 1998).

There is at least some evidence which suggests that *familiarity* or *experience* with the sound source has some influence on distance perception. For example, experience with speech may provide the listener with a frame of reference that would be helpful in making distance judgments based on sound level, and it has been found that sound level is a salient cue for judging distance for speech (Gardner, 1969; Brungart and Scott, 2001). In addition, the accuracy of distance judgments is better for speech played forward compared to backward (McGregor et al., 1985). Also suggesting that familiarity improves auditory distance perception, Coleman (1962) found that the accuracy of distance judgments for unfamiliar sounds (1-s noise bursts) improved as experience with the stimulus accumulated over the course of repeated test trials. (The accuracy of azimuth localizations did not change with repeated trials.) Interestingly, Zahorik (2002a) found that sound level has a greater perceptual weight than the direct-to-reverberant ratio when making distance judgments for speech signals (a familiar sound), whereas the opposite is true for noise bursts (an unfamiliar sound). On the other hand, Nielsen (1991) did not find differences in judged distances for speech, noise, and two kinds of musical signals.

PRECEDENCE EFFECT

Consider two apparently unrelated situations. The first involves listening to a radio news broadcast through both speakers of a home sound system. (We are not using a stereo music CD because we want identical signals from both speakers.) Sitting equidistant from the speakers causes us to perceive a phantom sound source between them. However, sitting close to one speaker (so that the signal reaches our ears sooner from that direction than from the other speaker) gives us the impression that all of the sound is coming from the closer speaker. This occurs even though the other speaker is still on.

The second situation involves listening to someone talking in a hard-walled room. In this case, the sounds reaching our ears include the direct sound from the talker's lips plus reflections of these sounds from the walls. Because the reflected sounds take an indirect route (via the walls), they reach our ears later than the direct sound and also from different directions. Yet, we hear a single sound coming from the direction of the earlier-arriving direct sound (although the reflections will "color" the quality of what we hear).

These situations illustrate a phenomenon known as the **precedence effect**, **Haas effect**, or the **first wavefront principle** (Gardner, 1968; Blauert, 1997). In general terms, when a sound coming from one direction is very quickly followed by a second sound (the echo) from another direction, then the perceived sound will be dominated by the earlier-arriving signal. In other words, we could say that **echo suppression** has occurred.

The precedence effect may be described in terms of how listeners perceive a sequence of four clicks presented through earphones, as in the classic experiment by Wallach, Newman, and Rosenzweig (1949). Figure 13.14 shows that the first click (A) went to the left ear followed by click B to the right ear after a very short delay ($\tau 1$). If presented alone, this pair of clicks was heard as a *fused image coming from the left*. Click C went to the right ear followed after another very short delay ($\tau 2$) by click D to the left ear, and by itself this pair was heard as a *fused image from the right*. The composite four-click sequence was heard as a *fused image from the left*; that is, its perception

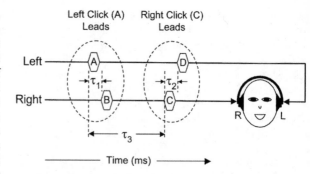

Figure 13.14 Arrangement of clicks presented through earphones to demonstrate the precedence effect, as used by Wallach, Newman, and Rosenzweig (1949).

was dominated by the left-leading onset rather than the right leading at its offset. Thus, the first-arriving signal determined the perceived location of the fused sound. Wallach et al. found that this precedence effect occurred for intervals between the two click pairs ($\tau 3$) up to 40 ms. However, longer durations of $\tau 3$ caused the listener to hear two separate signals, one at each ear.

Haas' (1949, 1951) classic demonstration of the precedence effect involved presenting speech from two loudspeakers, with a delay in the onset of the signal from one speaker compared to the other. These delays are analogous to interval $\tau 3$ in the Wallach et al. study. A *fused image* coming from the *leading* loudspeaker was heard for delays up to 35 ms. Longer delays caused listeners to detect the presence of the second (delayed) sound, although the signal was still localized toward the leading side. Delays longer than about 50 ms caused listeners to hear one sound from the leading speaker and a distinct echo coming from the delayed speaker. It is interesting to note that the precedence effect is robust with regard to some modifications of the temporal, spectral, and interaural characteristics of the stimuli (Dixon and Colburn, 2006).

Various studies have expanded on the classical descriptions of the precedence effect, revealing that the general phenomenon encompasses several identifiable aspects (for reviews, see Blauert, 1997; Litovsky et al., 1999). **Fusion** is the perception of the leading and trailing signals as a single, unified image, and occurs for delays up to about 5 to 10 ms for clicks (e.g., Ebata et al., 1968; Freyman et al., 1991; Yang and Grantham, 1997; Litovsky and Shinn-Cunningham, 2001) and roughly 40 to 50 ms for speech (e.g., Haas, 1951; Lochner and Burger, 1958). Longer delays cause two separate images to be heard. The delay at which the perception splits into two images is called the **echo threshold**.

The perceived location of the fused image is affected by the size of the delay between the two signals. **Summing localization** occurs for delays shorter than 1 ms, in which case the perceived location of the fused image is affected by both the leading and lagging clicks (Blauert, 1997), as illustrated in Fig. 13.15a. **Localization dominance** occurs when the location of the fused image

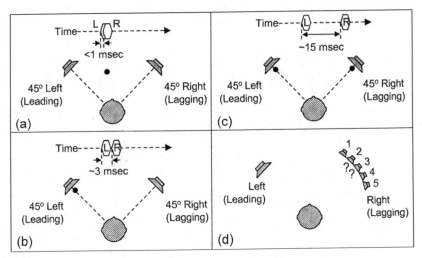

Figure 13.15   Aspects of the precedence effect shown in terms of signals presented from two loudspeakers, located 45° right and left of the listener. The left signal leads and the right signal(s) lags. In frames a to c, the filled circles indicate the locations of the perceived images, and the delay between the onsets of the two signals is shown along the top of each frame. In frame d, the task is to discriminate between the signals from the array of speakers on the (lagging) right side.

is determined by the leading signal (Fig. 13.15b). This occurs when the delay between the first and second clicks is between about 1 and 5 ms. Localization dominance breaks down as the delay lengthens, with the image splitting in two at the echo threshold, beyond which two images are heard, each coming from its own side (Fig. 13.15c).

Another aspect of the precedence effect is illustrated in Fig. 13.15d. Here, the listener is asked to discriminate between the azimuth locations of clicks on the lagging side (i.e., between speakers 1, 2, 3, etc.). Discrimination is poorer when the leading signal is present compared to what it is without the leading signal (e.g., Perrott et al., 1989; Freyman et al., 1991; Litovsky and Macmillan, 1994). An analogous effect occurs with earphones, where the presence of the leading signal affects the difference limens for ITDs or ILDs for the delayed signal (e.g., Zurek, 1980; Saberi and Perrott, 1990b; Shinn-Cunningham et al., 1993; Tollin and Henning, 1998). This effect occurs for delays up to about 5 ms and is aptly called **discrimination suppression**.

As suggested by the examples at the beginning of this section, the precedence effect suppresses the effects of reflections which would otherwise interfere with our perception of the direct sound, including speech. For example, Lochner and Burger (1964) found that speech discrimination was unaffected by reflections arriving up to 30 ms after the direct sound, although later-arriving reflections resulted in reduced intelligibility. Reflections that arrive beyond the time when the precedence effect is operative result in distortions and masking of the speech signal (e.g., Bolt and MacDonald, 1949; Kurtovic, 1975; Nabelek, 1976; Nabelek and Robinette, 1978; Gelfand and Silman, 1979; Nabelek and Dagenais, 1986; see Chap. 14).

Several interesting phenomena are encountered when the precedence effect is viewed in the context of the listener's immediate experience with the listening situation. Suppose we measure a listener's echo threshold several times: immediately after hearing leading/lagging click trains of various lengths (e.g., 3, 6, 9, 12, and 15 click pairs), and also without any preceding click pairs. [The upper left part of Fig. 13.16 (labeled a) shows an example of a train of 12 leading/lagging click pairs presented from right and left loudspeakers.] We would find that the echo threshold increases as the preceding click train gets longer (reaching a maximum at 12 pairs). Thus, there is a *build up of echo suppression* that is dependent upon the listener's immediate experience with the listening task (Clifton and Freyman, 1989; Freyman et al., 1991; Clifton et al., 1994). What's more, this build up of echo suppression appears to be *asymmetrical*, being greater when the right click leads than when the left click is leads (Clifton and Freyman, 1989; Grantham, 1996).

A *breakdown of echo suppression* called the **Clifton effect** occurs when the leading and lagging clicks switch directions (Clifton, 1987; Clifton and Freyman, 1989). The basic demonstration of the Clifton effect involves presenting the listener with a train of click pairs coming from right and left loudspeakers (Fig. 13.16). The leading click in each pair is from the left and the lagging click is from the right, so that each click pair is heard as a fused image coming from the left side (labeled a in the figure). After 12 pairs, the order of the clicks is *switched* so that now the right click leads and the left one lags. At this point, we would expect to hear a fused image from the now-leading right side, but this does not happen. Instead, the *precedence effect breaks down* and the listener hears *both* clicks, each coming from its own side (b in the figure). Then, after several right/left click pairs are presented, the listener again hears a fused image from

245

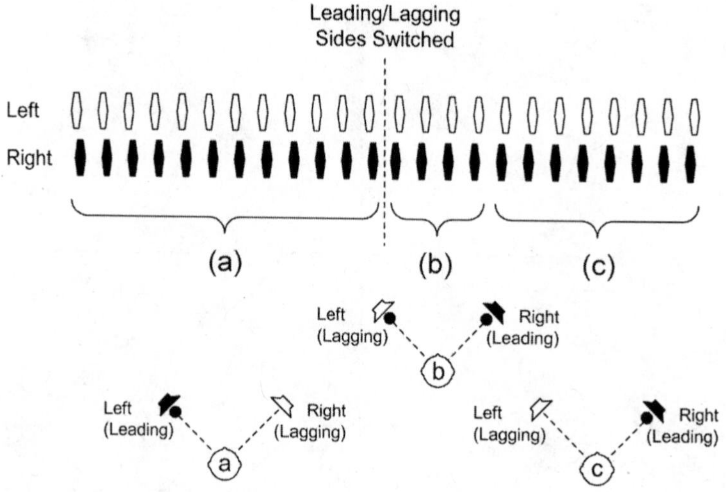

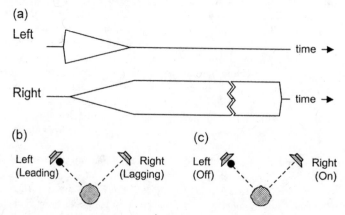

Leading/Lagging
Sides Switched

Left

Right

(a)   (b)   (c)

Left 🏠 Right
(Lagging) - (Leading)
ⓑ

Left 🏠   Right ◁   Left ◁   Right 🏠
(Leading)   (Lagging)   (Lagging)   (Leading)
ⓐ   ⓒ

Figure 13.16 The Clifton effect. (a) Left-leading click pairs are heard as a fused image coming from the left (represented by the filled circle in the lower drawing). (b) Switching to right-leading click pairs causes the precedence effect to break down, and both clicks are heard coming from their respective sides (represented by the two filled circles). (c) The precedence effect is then re-established, with a fused signal heard from the now-leading right side (represented by the filled circle).

the now-leading right side, which indicates that the precedence effect has been re-established (c in the figure).

A fascinating illusion called the **Franssen effect** (Franssen, 1960, 1962) is illustrated in Fig. 13.17 Here, a low-frequency tone (e.g., 500 Hz) is presented from two loudspeakers. The tone from the left speaker has an abrupt onset and then fades away over the course of, say, 100 ms. The tone from the right speaker builds up, while the left tone is fading away and may stay on for a few seconds. The amplitude envelopes of the two tones over time are represented in Fig. 13.17a. As expected, the listener initially localizes a fused image coming from the left speaker, attributable to the abrupt onset (Fig. 13.17b). What is odd, however, is that the listener continues localizing the tone to the *left* even after the *left* signal is *off* and the *only* signal is coming from the *right* speaker (Fig. 13.17c). This illusion can actually

persist for quite some time (Berkley, 1983, 1987). Interestingly, Hartmann and Rakerd (1989) showed that the Franssen effect fails to occur when the environment is anechoic (echo-free), and explained the illusion based on the **plausibility hypothesis**: The Franssen effect occurs in typical rooms, where reflections cause the ITDs for the steady-state tone from the right speaker (as in Fig. 13.17) to become so atypical that they are implausible as localization cues. The listener discounts these implausible cues and attributes the tone's direction to the unambiguous cue provided by the abrupt onset of the tone burst from the left speaker. The illusion does not occur in anechoic rooms because the ITDs are not distorted by reflections, and therefore provide the listener with plausible localization cues.

The build-up effect (including its right-left asymmetry), Clifton effect, and Franssen illusion reveal that the precedence

(a)
Left
⟶ time →

Right
⟶ time →

(b)   (c)
Left 🏠   Right ◁   Left 🏠   Right ◁
(Leading)   (Lagging)   (Off)   (On)

Figure 13.17 The Franssen effect (illusion). (a) Amplitude envelopes over time of the tones coming from the left and right loudspeakers. (b) Fused (filled circle) image initially localized to the leading left side. (c) Image (filled circle) continues being localized to the left side even after the left signal is off.

effect is influenced by, for example, experiences with and expectations about the listening task and environment, and the plausibility of the cues. Thus, higher-level central processes are involved in the precedence effect (e.g., Hafter et al., 1988; Hartmann and Rakerd, 1989; Freyman et al., 1991; Clifton et al., 1994; Grantham, 1996; Clifton and Freyman, 1997; Hartmann, 1997; Litovsky et al., 1999). There is also considerable physiological evidence of central involvement in the precedence effect (e.g., Litovsky, 1998; Litovsky et al., 1999; Litovsky and Delgutte, 2002). For example, in their comprehensive review, Litovsky et al. (1999) used physiological data from several studies in the literature to compare the time frames over which evidence of echo suppression occurred at various levels in the nervous system of cats. Suppression increased going from lower to higher levels of the auditory pathway from the auditory nerve to the auditory cortex.

MASKING LEVEL DIFFERENCES

The term **masking level difference (MLD)** may be a bit confusing at first glance. Obviously it refers to some sort of difference in masking. Consider a typical masking experiment (Chap. 10) in which a signal **S** is barely masked by a noise **N**. This can be done in one ear (**monotically**), as in Fig. 13.18a, or by presenting an *identical* signal and noise to both ears (**diotically**), as in Fig. 13.18b. (Identical stimuli are obtained by simply directing the output of the same signal and noise sources to both earphones in phase.) For brevity and clarity, we will adopt a shorthand to show the relationships among the stimuli and ears. The letter **m** will denote a monotic stimulus and **o** will refer to a diotic stimulus. Thus, **SmNm** indicates that the signal and noise are presented to one ear, and **SoNo** means that the same signal and the same noise are simultaneously presented to both ears. Either of these conditions can be used as our starting point.

Suppose that we add an identical noise to the unstimulated ear of Fig. 13.18a, so that the signal is still monotic but the noise is now diotic (**SmNo**), as in Fig. 13.18c. Oddly enough, the previously masked signal now becomes audible again! Starting this time from the masked situation in Fig. 13.18b (SoNo), we can make the signal audible again by reversing the phase of (inverting) the noise between the ears (Fig. 13.18d) or by reversing the phase of the signal between the ears (Fig. 13.18e). The phase reversal is indicated by the Greek letter π, since the stimuli are now 180° (or one radian, π) out of phase between the ears. (The phase reversal is accomplished by simply reversing the positive and negative poles at one of the earphones.) These new conditions are thus called **SoNπ** and **SπNo,** respectively. Note that the binaural advantage occurs only when the stimuli are in some way *different* at the two ears (dichotic). These fascinating observations were first reported in 1948 by Hirsh (1948b) for tonal signals and by Licklider (1948) for speech.

We may now define the MLD as the difference (advantage) in masked threshold between dichotically presented stimuli and

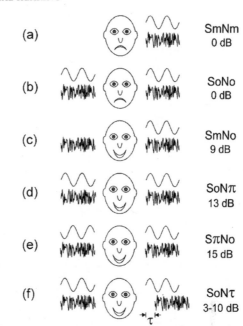

Figure 13.18 Masking level differences (MLDs) for various conditions (see text).

signals that are presented monotically (or diotically). It is not surprising to find that the MLD is also referred to as **binaural unmasking**, **binaural release from masking**, or the **binaural masking level difference (BMLD)**. We shall express the magnitude of the MLD as the difference in decibels between a particular dichotic arrangement and either the SmNm or SoNo conditions. Other MLD conditions are discussed below.

The size of the MLD varies from as large as about 15 dB for the SπNo condition (Green and Henning, 1969) to as little as 0 dB, depending upon a variety of parameters. Typical MLD magnitudes associated with various dichotic arrangements are shown in Fig. 13.18 The MLD becomes larger as the spectrum level of the masking noise is increased, especially when the noise is presented to both ears (No) at the same level (Hirsh, 1948a, 1948b; Blodgett et al., 1962; Dolan and Robinson, 1967; Dolan, 1968; McFadden, 1968).

The largest MLDs are obtained when either the signal (SπNo) or the noise (SoNπ) is opposite in phase at the two ears. The large MLDs obtained from these antiphasic conditions have been known since it was first described (Hirsh, 1948b) and have been repeatedly confirmed (e.g., Jeffress et al., 1952; Colburn and Durlach, 1965). Recall from Chapter 5 that the firing patterns of auditory nerve fibers are phase-locked to the stimulus, particularly at low frequencies. Thus, the large MLDs associated with antiphasic conditions may be related to this phase-locking in the neural coding of the stimuli (Green and Henning, 1969). Furthermore, since the degree of phase-locking is greatest at low frequencies, and decreases as frequency becomes higher,

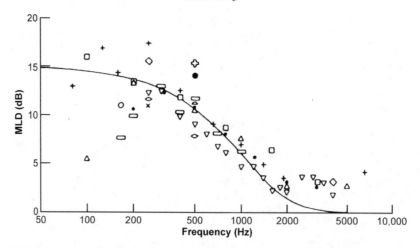

Figure 13.19 Magnitude of the MLD (SπNo–SoNo) as a function of frequency for many studies. *Source*: Adapted from Durlach, Binaural signal detection: equalization and cancellation theory, in *Foundations of Modern Auditory Theory 2* (J.V. Tobias, ed.), © 1972 by Academic Press.

we would expect the size of the MLD to be related to stimulus frequency as well.

Figure 13.19 shows the relationship between MLD size and stimulus frequency from several studies, as summarized by Durlach (1972). As expected, the MLD is largest for low frequencies—about 15 dB for 250 Hz—and decreases for higher frequencies until a constant of about 3 dB is maintained by about 1500 to 2000 Hz. (Look at the individual data points in Fig. 13.19 rather than at the smooth line, which is a statistical approximation of the actual results.) Note that the MLD (at least for SπNo) does not fall to zero above 1500 Hz, and recall in this context that statistically significant phase-locking is maintained as high as 5000 Hz (Chap. 5).

There is very good agreement about the size of the MLD for the frequencies above 250 Hz. At lower frequencies, there is a great deal of variation in the MLD sizes reported by different studies (e.g., Hirsh, 1948b; Webster, 1951; Durlach, 1963; Rabiner et al., 1966; Dolan, 1968). This is shown in Fig. 13.19 by the substantial spread among the data points for the lower frequencies. Much of this variation in the lower frequencies may be explained on the basis of differences in noise level. In particular, Dolan (1968) showed that the MLDs at 150 and 300 Hz increase with the spectrum level of the masker, attaining a value of approximately 15 dB when the noise spectrum level is 50 dB or more. Thus, the MLD becomes rather stable once moderate levels of presentation are reached.

We have been assuming that the noises at the two ears (SoNo) are derived from the same noise source, insuring that the waveforms are exactly the same at both ears. Another way to indicate identical waveforms is to say that the noises are perfectly correlated. Had we used two separate noise generators, then the noises would no longer be perfectly correlated. We would then say that the noises are uncorrelated (**Nu**). Robinson and Jeffress (1963) added noises from the same (correlated) and different (uncorrelated) generators to study how noise correlation affects

the size of the MLD. They found that the MLD resulting from uncorrelated noises is on the order of 3 to 4 dB, and that the MLD becomes larger as the degree of correlation decreases. The MLD resulting from uncorrelated noise may contribute to our ability to overcome the effects of reverberation. This relation was demonstrated by Koenig et al. (1977), who found that room reverberation decorrelates the noise reaching the two ears, resulting in an MLD of about 3 dB.

As only a certain critical bandwidth contributes to the masking of a tone (Chap. 10), it is not surprising that the MLD also depends upon the critical band (Sondhi and Guttman, 1966; Mulligan et al., 1967) around a tone. In fact, the MLD actually increases as the noise band narrows (Metz et al., 1967; Wightman, 1971). As it turns out, a very narrow band of noise looks much like a sinusoid that is being slowly modulated in frequency and amplitude. If we present such a narrow band noise to both ears and delay the wavefront at one ear relative to the other, then the degree to which the noises are correlated will change periodically as a function of the interaural time delay.

With this in mind, consider the arrangement in Fig. 13.18f. The noises presented to the two ears are from the same generator, but the noise is delayed at one ear relative to the other (Nτ). The interaural time delay decorrelates the noises in a manner dependent upon the time delay. This situation (SoNτ) results in MLDs, which are maximal when the time delay corresponds to half-periods of the signal and minimal when the time delays correspond to the period of the signal (Rabiner et al., 1966; Langford and Jeffress, 1964). Figure 13.20 shows examples at several frequencies. The effect is clearest at 500 Hz. The period of 500 Hz is 2 ms, and the half-period is thus 1 ms. As the figure shows, the MLDs are largest at multiples of the half-period (in the vicinity of 1 ms and 3 ms for 500 Hz) and are smallest at multiples of the full period (about 2 ms and 4 ms for 500 Hz). Also notice that successive peaks tend to become smaller and smaller.

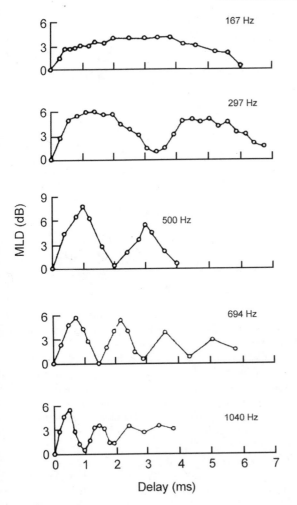

Figure 13.20 The MLD as a function of interaural time delay. *Source:* Adapted from Rabiner et al. (1966), with permission of *J. Acoust. Soc. Am.*

Licklider (1948) reported MLDs for speech about the same time that the phenomenon was described for tones (Hirsh, 1948a, 1948b). Interestingly enough, the unmasking of speech is associated with the MLDs for pure tones within the spectral range critical for speech perception (Carhart et al., 1967, 1968; Levitt and Rabiner, 1967a). This was shown quite clearly in a study by Levitt and Rabiner (1967a) that used monosyllabic words as the signal and white noise as the masker. The subjects were asked to indicate whether the test words were detectable in the presence of the noise while different parts of the speech spectrum were reversed in phase between the ears. They found MLDs (SπNo) on the order of 13 dB when the frequencies below 500 Hz were reversed in phase, indicating that the MLD for speech detection is primarily determined by the lower frequencies in the speech spectrum.

The MLD for speech detection obviously occurs at a minimal level of intelligibility. That is, a signal whose intelligibility

is zero (see Chap. 14) may still be barely detectable. Increasing the presentation level of the words would result in higher intelligibility, that is, a larger proportion of the words would be correctly repeated. The level at which half of the words are correctly repeated may be called the 50% intelligibility level; the 100% intelligibility level is the test level at which all of the words are repeated correctly. The speech MLD is quite large at near-detection levels. However, MLDs for speech are smallest at higher presentation levels where overall intelligibility is good (Schubert and Schultz, 1962; Green and Yost, 1975; Carhart et al., 1967, 1968; Levitt and Rabiner, 1967a).

Levitt and Rabiner (1967a, 1967b) suggested the term **binaural intelligibility level difference** (**BILD** or **ILD**)[5] to indicate the amount of unmasking for speech intelligibility. The BILD is the difference between the levels at which a particular percentage of the test words are correctly repeated for a dichotic condition and for SoNo. Levitt and Rabiner (1967a) found that the BILD was on the order of only 3 to 6 dB for an intelligibility level of 50%. Thus, the release from masking increases from about 3 to 13 dB as the intelligibility level goes down toward bare detection. At the lowest intelligibility level, where one can detect but not repeat the words, the BILD and MLD for speech are synonymous. In this light, we may consider the MLD as the limiting case of the BILD (Levitt and Rabiner, 1967b).

Although the speech MLD depends on frequencies below 500 Hz, Levitt and Rabiner (1967a) found that the entire speech spectrum makes a significant contribution to the BILD. In a later paper they presented a numerical method for predicting the BILD (Levitt and Rabiner, 1967b). The procedure assumes that the SπNo condition reduces the noise level in a manner that depends upon frequency and signal-to-noise ratio. That is, the lower frequencies are given greater relative importance at low signal-to-noise ratios where overall intelligibility is poor. This technique makes predictions that are in close agreement with the empirical data (Licklider, 1948; Schubert and Schultz, 1962; Levitt and Rabiner, 1967a).

Some work has also been done on MLDs for differential sensitivity and loudness (Townsend and Goldstein, 1972; Henning, 1973). We shall not go into detail in these areas, except to point out that MLDs for loudness and discrimination of intensity occur mainly at near-detection levels and become insignificant well above threshold. This situation, of course, is analogous to what we have seen for BILDs as opposed to MLDs for speech signals. However, Marks (1987) reported that binaural loudness summation for a 1000 Hz tone under MLD-like masking conditions was substantially greater than a doubling of loudness over the monaural condition.

Although a variety of models has been proposed to explain the mechanism of MLDs, we will take a brief look at two of the

---

[5] We will use BILD to avoid confusion because ILD also means interaural level difference.

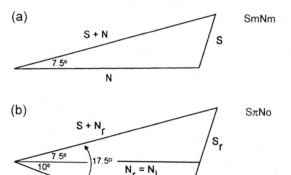

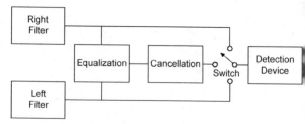

Figure 13.22 A simplified block diagram of Durlach's equalization–cancellation (EC) model.

Figure 13.21 Vector diagrams for the (a) SmNm and (b) SπNo conditions (see text). *Source*: Adapted from Jeffress, Binaural signal detection: Vector theory, in *Foundations of Modern Auditory Theory, vol. 2* (J.V. Tobias, ed.), © 1972 by Academic Press.

best-known approaches, the Webster–Jeffress lateralization theory (Webster, 1951; Jeffress, 1972) and Durlach's equalization–cancellation model (Durlach, 1963, 1972; Culling and Summerfield, 1995; Breebaart, van de Par, and Kohlrausch, 2001).

The Webster–Jeffress **lateralization theory** attributes MLDs to interaural phase and level differences. Recall that only a certain critical band contributes to the masking of a tone, and that this limited-bandwidth concept also applies to MLDs. Basically, the lateralization model compares the test tone to the narrow band of frequencies in the noise that contributes to its masking. Changing phase between the ears (SπNo) results in a time-of-arrival difference at a central mechanism, which provides the detection cue. The vector diagrams in Fig. 13.21 show how this system might operate for SπNo versus SmNm. Figure 13.21a shows the interaction between the noise (N) and signal (S) amplitudes as vectors 7.5° apart. The resulting S + N amplitude is too small for detection. Figure 13.21b shows the situation when the signal is reversed in phase at the two ears (SπNo). Now, the right and left noise amplitudes (N_r and N_l) are equal ($N_r = N_l$), but the signal vectors for the two ears (S_r and S_l) point in opposite directions due to the reversed phase. Thus, the signal in the right ear leads the noise in phase by 7.5°, while in the left ear it lags in phase by 10° so that the phase difference between the resulting S = N at the two ears is 17.5°. In other words, S + N at the right ear is now 17.5° ahead of that in the left. If the signal is a 500-Hz tone, this lag corresponds to a time-of-arrival advantage for the right S + N of 97 μs. In addition, the lengths of the S + N vectors indicate an amplitude advantage that is also available as a detection cue, since the right S + N is now substantially longer (more intense) than the left. That is, the SπNo condition causes the combined S + N from the right ear to reach a central detection mechanism sooner and with greater amplitude. This causes a lateralization of the result

(to the right in this example), which the model uses as the basis for detection of the signal.

Durlach's **equalization–cancellation (EC) model** is shown schematically in Fig. 13.22. The stimuli pass through critical-band filters at the two ears, and then follow both monaural and binaural routes to a detection device, which decides whether the signal is present. The detection device switches among the three possible channels (two monaural and one binaural), and will use the channel with the best signal-to-noise ratio as the basis for a response. The monaural channels go straight to the detection mechanism. The binaural channel, however, includes two special stages.

In the first stage, the inputs from the two ears are adjusted to be equal in amplitude (the equalization step). Then the inputs from the two ears are subtracted one from the other in the cancellation step.[6] Of course, if the signal and noise were identical in both ears (SoNo), then the entire binaural signal would be canceled. In this case, the detection device would choose among the monaural inputs so that no MLD resulted. However, for the SπNo condition, the subtraction cancels the in-phase noise and actually enhances the out-of-phase signal. Thus, if the EC model works perfectly, the signal-to-noise ratio will be improved infinitely. In reality, the mechanism operates less than perfectly so that cancellation is not complete. This imperfection is due to atypical stimuli that necessitate unusual types of equalization, or to random jitter in the process, which causes the cancellation mechanism to receive inputs that are imperfectly equalized.

REFERENCES

Abbagnaro, LA, Bauer, BB, Torick, EL. 1975. Measurements of diffraction and interaural delay of a progressive sound wave caused by the human head-II. *J Acoust Soc Am* 58, 693–700.

Algazi, VR, Avendano, C, Duda, RO. 2001. Elevation localization and head-related transfer function analysis at low frequencies. *J Acoust Soc Am* 109, 1110–1122.

American National Standards Institute, ANSI S3.4–2007. 2007. American National Standard Procedure for the Computation of Loudness of Steady Sounds. New York, NY: ANSI.

[6] Recall the rules for algebraic subtraction $(+1) - (+1) = 0$, as for the in-phase noise; $(+1) - (-1) = +2$, as for the out-of-phase signal.

Arbogast, TL, Mason, CR, Kidd, G. 2002. The effect of spatial separation on informational and energetic masking of speech. *J Acoust Soc Am* 112, 2086–2098.

Begault, DR. 1991. Preferred sound intensity increase for sensation of half distance. *Percept Motor Skill* 72, 1019–1029.

Bekesy, G. 1938. Über die Entstehung der Entfernungsempfindung beim Hören. Akustische Zeitschrif 3, 21–31.

Berkley, DA. 1983. Room acoustics and listening. *J Acoust Soc Am* 44, S17.

Berkley, DA. 1987. Hearing in rooms. In: WA Yost, G Gourevitch (eds.), *Directional Hearing*. New York, NY: Springer, 249–260.

Bernstein, LR, Trahiotis, C. 1995. Binaural interference effects measured with masking-level difference and with ITD- and IID-discrimination paradigms. *J Acoust Soc Am* 98, 155–163.

Best, V, Gallun, FJ, Carlile, S, Shinn-Cunningham, BG. 2007. Binaural interference and auditory grouping. *J Acoust Soc Am* 121, 1070–1076.

Blauert, J. 1969/70. Sound localization in the median plane. *Acustica* 22, 205–213.

Blauert, J. 1997. *Special Hearing: The Psychophysics of Human Sound Localization*. Revised Edition. Cambridge, MA: MIT Press.

Blodgett, HC, Jeffress, LA, Whitworth, RH. 1962. Effect of noise at one ear on the masking threshold for tones at the other. *J Acoust Soc Am* 34, 979–981.

Bolt, RH, MacDonald, AD. 1949. Theory of speech masking by reverberation. *J Acoust Soc Am* 21, 577–580.

Breebaart, J, van de Par, S, Kohlrausch, A. 2001. Binaural processing model based on contralateral inhibition. I. Model structure. *J Acoust Soc Am* 110, 1074–1088.

Bregman, AS. 1990. *Auditory Scene Analysis: The Perceptual Organization of Sound*. Cambridge, MA: Bradford Books, MIT Press.

Bregman, AS, Ahad, PA. 1996. *Demonstrations of Auditory Scene Analysis: The Perceptual Organization of Sound [Compact Disc]*. Cambridge, MA: MIT Press.

Broadbent, DE. 1955. A note on binaural fusion. *Q J Exp Psychol* 7, 46–47.

Bronkhorst, AW. 1995. Localization of real and virtual sources. *J Acoust Soc Am* 98, 2542–2553.

Bronkhorst, AW, Houtgast, T. 1999. Auditory distance perception in rooms. *Nature* 397, 517–520.

Bronkhorst, AW, Plomp, R. 1988. The effect of head-induced interaural time and level differences on speech intelligibility in noise. *J Acoust Soc Am* 83, 1508–1516.

Brungart, DS. 1999. Auditory localization of nearby sources. III. Stimulus effects. *J Acoust Soc Am* 106, 3589–3602.

Brungart, DS, Rabinowitz, WM. 1999. Auditory localization of nearby sources. Head-related transfer functions. *J Acoust Soc Am* 106, 1465–1479.

Brungart, DS, Scott, KR. 2001. The effects of production and presentation level on the auditory distance perception of speech. *J Acoust Soc Am* 106, 1465–1479.

Buell, TN, Hafter, ER. 1991. Combination of binaural information across frequency bands. *J Acoust Soc Am* 90, 1894–1900.

Butler, RA. 1986. The bandwidth effect on monaural and binaural localization. *Hear Res* 21, 67–73.

Butler, RA, Levy, ET, Neff, WD. 1980. Apparent distance of sounds recorded in echoic and anechoic chambers. *J Exp Psychol Human Percept Perf* 6, 745–750.

Butler, RA, Planert, N. 1976. The influence of stimulus bandwidth on localization of sound in space. *Percept Psychophys* 19, 103–108.

Carhart, R, Tillman, T, Dallos, P. 1968. Unmasking for pure tones and spondees: Interaural phase and time disparities. *J Speech Hear Res* 11, 722–734.

Carhart, R, Tillman, T, Johnson, K. 1967. Release of masking for speech through interaural time delay. *J Acoust Soc Am* 42, 124–138.

Causse, R, Chavasse, P. 1941. Recherches sur les seuil de l'audition binauriculaire compare au seuil monauriculaire en fonction de la frequence. *Comp R Soc Biol* 135, 1272–1275.

Causse, R, Chavasse, P. 1942a. Difference entre le seuil de l'audition binauriculaire et le seuil monauriculaire de la frequence. *Comp R Soc Biol* 136, 301.

Causse, R, Chavasse, P. 1942b. Difference entre l'ecoute binauriculaire et monauriculaire par la perception des intensites supraliminaires. *Comp R Soc Biol* 139, 405.

Chandler, DW, Grantham, DW. 1992. Minimum audible movement angle in the horizontal plane as a function of frequency and bandwidth, source azimuth, and velocity. *J Acoust Soc Am* 91, 1625–1636.

Cherry, C. 1961. Two ears-but one world. In: WA Rosenblith (ed.), *Sensory Communication*. Cambridge, MA: MIT Press, 99–117.

Cherry, EC. 1953. Some experiments on the recognition of speech, with one and with two ears. J Acoust Soc Am 25, 975–979.

Cherry, EC, Sayers, BMcA. 1956. "Human cross-correlator"—A technique for measuring certain parameters of speech perception. *J Acoust Soc Am* 28, 889–896.

Churcher, BG, King, AJ, Davies, H. 1934. The minimal perceptible change of intensity of a pure tone. *Phil Mag* 18, 927–939.

Clifton, RK. 1987. Breakdown of echo suppression in the precedence effect. *J Acoust Soc Am* 82, 1834–1835.

Clifton, RK, Freyman, RL. 1989. Effect of click rate and delay on breakdown of the precedence effect. *Percept Psychophys* 462, 139–145.

Clifton, RK, Freyman, RL. 1997. The precedence effect: Beyond echo suppression. In: R Gilkey, T Anderson (eds.), *Binaural and Spatial Hearing in Real and Virtual Environments*. Hillsdale, NJ: Erlbaum, 233–255.

Clifton, RK, Freyman, RL, Litovsky, RY, McCall, D. 1994. Listeners' expectations about echoes can raise or lower echo threshold. *J Acoust Soc Am* 95, 1525–1533.

Cochran, P, Throop, J, Simpson, WE. 1968. Estimation of distance of a source of sound. *Am J Psychol* 81, 198–206.

Colburn, HS, Durlach, NI. 1965. Time-intensity relations in binaural unmasking. *J Acoust Soc Am* 38, 93–103.

Coleman, PD. 1962. Failure to localize the source distance of an unfamiliar sound. *J Acoust Soc Am* 34, 345–346.

Coleman, PD. 1963. Analysis of cues to auditory depth perception in free space. *Psychol Bull* 60, 302–315.

Coleman, PD. 1968. Dual role of frequency spectrum in determination of auditory distance. *J Acoust Soc Am* 44, 631–632.

Culling, JF, Summerfield, Q. 1995. Perceptual separation of concurrent speech sounds: Absence of across-frequency grouping by common interaural delay. *J Acoust Soc Am* 98, 785–797.

Dixon, RM, Colburn, HS. 2006. The influence of spectral, temporal and interaural stimulus variations on the precedence effect. *J Acoust Soc Am* 119, 2947–2964.

Dolan, TR. 1968. Effects of masker spectrum level on masking-level differences at low signal frequencies. *J Acoust Soc Am* 44, 1507–1512.

Dolan, TR, Robinson, DE. 1967. An explanation of masking-level differences that result from interaural intensive disparities of noise. *J Acoust Soc Am* 42, 977–981.

Duda, RO, Martens, WL. 1998. Range dependence of the response of a spherical head model. *J Acoust Soc Am* 104, 3048–3058.

Durlach, NI. 1963. Equalization and cancellation theory of binaural masking level differences. *J Acoust Soc Am* 35, 1206–1218.

Durlach, NI. 1972. Binaural signal detection: Equalization and cancellation theory. In: JV Tobias (ed.), *Foundations of Modern Auditory Theory*, Vol. 2. New York, NY: Academic Press, 369–462.

Durlach, NI, Colburn, HS. 1978. Binaural phenomena. In: EC Carterette, MP Friedman (eds.), *Handbook of Perception, Vol. I -Hearing*. New York, NY: Academic Press, 365–466.

Durlach, NI, Rigopulos, A, Pang, XD, Woods, WS, Kulkarni, A, Colburn, HS, Wenzel, EM. 1992. On the externalization of auditory images. *Presence* 1, 251–257.

Ebata, M, Sone, T, Nimura, T. 1968. On the perception of direction of echo. *J Acoust Soc Am* 44, 542–547.

Feddersen, WE, Sandel, TT, Teas, DC, Jeffress, LA. 1957. Localization of high-frequency tones. *J Acoust Soc Am* 29, 988–991.

Fisher, HG, Freedman, SJ. 1968. The role of the pinna in auditory localization. *J Aud Res* 8, 15–26.

Fletcher, H, Munson, W. 1933. Loudness: Its definition, measurement and calculation. *J Acoust Soc Am* 5, 82–108.

Franssen, NV. 1960. Some considerations on the mechanism of directional hearing. Ph.D. Dissertation. Delft, The Netherlands: Technische Hogeschool.

Franssen, NV. 1962. *Stereophony*. Eindhoven, The Netherlands: Phillips Technical Library. [English translation, 1964.]

Freyman, RL, Clifton, RK, Litovsky, RY. 1991. Dynamic processes in the precedence effect. *J Acoust Soc Am* 90, 874–884.

Gallum, FJ, Mason, CR, Kidd, G. 2005. Binaural release from informational masking in a speech identification task. *J Acoust Soc Am* 118, 1605–1613.

Gardner, MB. 1968. Historical background of the Haas and/or precedence effect. *J Acoust Soc Am* 43, 1243–1248.

Gardner, MB. 1969. Distance estimation of 0 degrees or apparent 0 degree-oriented speech signals in anechoic space. *J Acoust Soc Am* 45, 47–53.

Gardner, MB. 1973. Some monaural and binaural facets of median plane localization. *J Acoust Soc Am* 54, 1489–1495.

Gelfand, SA, Silman, S. 1979. Effects of small room reverberation upon the recognition of some consonant features. *J Acoust Soc Am* 66, 22–29.

Grantham, DW. 1984. Interaural intensity discrimination: Insensitivity at 1000 Hz. *J Acoust Soc Am* 75, 1190–1194.

Grantham, DW. 1986. Detection and discrimination of simulated motion of auditory targets in the horizontal plane. *J Acoust Soc Am* 79, 1939–1949.

Grantham, DW. 1996. Left-right asymmetry in the buildup of echo suppression in normal-hearing adults. *J Acoust Soc Am* 99, 1118–1123.

Green, DM. 1966. Interaural phase effects in the masking of signals of different durations. *J Acoust Soc Am* 39, 720–724.

Green, DM, Henning, GR. 1969. Audition. *Ann Rev Psychol* 20, 105–128.

Green, DM, Yost, WA. 1975. Binaural analysis. In: WD Keidel, WD Neff (eds.), *Handbook of Sensory Physiology, Vol. V/2: Auditory System*. New York, NY: Springer-Verlag, 461–480.

Groen, JJ. 1964. Super- and subliminate binaural beats. *Acta Otol* 57, 224–230.

Gu, X, Wright, BA, Green, DM. 1995. Failure to hear binaural beats below threshold. *J Acoust Soc Am* 97, 701–703.

Haas, H. 1949. The influence of a single echo on the audibility of speech. *Library Com* 363. Garston, Watford, UK: Dept. Sci. Indust. Rest.

Haas, H. 1951. Über den Einfluss eines Einfachechos aud die Hörsamkeit von Sprache. *Acustica* 1, 49–58. [English translation: *J Audiol Eng Soc* 20, 146–159 (1972).]

Hafter, ER, DeMaio, J. 1975. Difference thresholds for interaural delay. *J Acoust Soc Am* 57, 181–187.

Hafter, ER, Bourbon, WT, Blocker, AS, Tucker, A. 1969. Direct comparison between lateralization and detection under antiphasic masking. *J Acoust Soc Am* 46, 1452–1457.

Hafter, ER, Buell, TN, Richards, V. 1988. Onset-coding in lateralization: Its form, site, and function. In: GM Edelman, WE Gall, WM Cowan (eds.), *Auditory Function: Neurobiological Bases of Hearing*. New York, NY: Wiley, 647–676.

Hafter, ER, Carrier, SC. 1970. Masking-level differences obtained with a pulsed tonal masker. *J Acoust Soc Am* 47, 1041–1048.

Hafter, ER, Carrier, SC. 1972. Binaural interaction in low-frequency stimuli: The inability to trade time and intensity completely. *J Acoust Soc Am* 51, 1852–1862.

Hafter, ER, Jeffress, LA. 1968. Two-image lateralization of tones and clicks. *J Acoust Soc Am* 44, 563–569.

Harris, GG. 1960. Binaural interactions of impulsive stimuli and pure tones. *J Acoust Soc Am* 32, 685–692.

Harris, JD. 1963. Loudness discrimination. *J Speech Hear Dis Monogr Suppl* 11.

Harris, JD, Sergeant, RL. 1971. Monaural/binaural minimum audible angle for a moving sound source. *J Speech Hear Res* 14, 618–629.

Hartmann, WM. 1997. Listening in a room and the precedence effect. In: R Gilkey, T Anderson (eds.), *Binaural and Spatial Hearing in Real and Virtual Environments*. Hillsdale, NJ: Erlbaum, 191–210.

Hartmann, WM, Rakerd, B. 1989. Localization of sound in rooms. IV: The Franssen effect. *J Acoust Soc Am* 86, 1366–1373.

Hartmann, WM, Wittenberg, A. 1996. On the externalization of sound images. *J Acoust Soc Am* 99, 3678–3688.

Hawley, ML, Litovsky, RY, Culling, JF. 2004. The benefits of binaural hearing in a cocktail party: Effect of location and type of interferer. *J Acoust Soc Am* 115, 833–843.

Hebrank, J, Wright, D. 1974. Spectral cues used in the localization of sound sources on the median plane. *J Acoust Soc Am* 56, 1829–1834.

Heller, LM, Trahiotis, C. 1995. Extents of laterality and binaural interference effects. *J Acoust Soc Am* 99, 3632–3637.

Hellman, RP, Zwislocki, J. 1963. Monaural loudness function at 1000 cps, and interaural summation. *J Acoust Soc Am* 35, 856–865.

Henning, GB. 1973. Effect of interaural phase on frequency and amplitude discrimination. *J Acoust Soc Am* 54, 1160–1178.

Henning, GB. 1974. Delectability of interaural delay in high-frequency complex waveforms. *J Acoust Soc Am* 55, 84–90.

Hill, NI, Darwin, CJ. 1996. Lateralization of a perturbed harmonic: Effects of onset asynchrony and mistuning. *J Acoust Soc Am* 100, 2352–2364.

Hirsh, IJ. 1948a. Binaural summation: A century of investigation. *Psychol Bull* 45, 193–206.

Hirsh, IJ. 1948b. The influence of interaural phase on interaural summation and inhibition. *J Acoust Soc Am* 20, 536–544.

Hirsh, IJ, Burgeat, M. 1958. Binaural effects in remote masking. *J Acoust Soc Am* 30, 827–832.

Jeffress, LA. 1972. Binaural signal detection: Vector theory. In: JV Tobias (ed.), *Foundations of Modern Auditory Theory*, Vol. 2. New York, NY: Academic Press, 349–368.

Jeffress, LA, Blodgett, HC, Deatheredge, BH. 1952. The masking of tones by white noise as a function of interaural phases of both components. *J Acoust Soc Am* 24, 523–527.

Jeffress, LA, McFadden, D. 1971. Differences of interaural phase and level in detection and lateralization. *J Acoust Soc Am* 49, 1169–1179.

Jesteadt, W, Wier, CC, Green, DM. 1977a. Comparison of monaural and binaural discrimination of intensity and frequency. *J Acoust Soc Am* 61, 1599–1603.

Jesteadt, W, Wier, CC, Green, DM. 1977b. Intensity discrimination as a function of frequency and sensation level. *J Acoust Soc Am* 61, 169–177.

Keys, J. 1947. Binaural versus monaural hearing. *J Acoust Soc Am* 19, 629–631.

Kidd, GK, Mason, CR, Brughera, A, Hartmann, WM. 2005. The role of reverberation in the release from masking due to spatial separation for speech intelligibility. *Acta Acustica with Acustica* 91, 526–536.

Klumpp, RG, Eady, HR. 1956. Some measurements of interaural time difference thresholds. *J Acoust Soc Am* 28, 859–860.

Koenig, AH, Allen, JB, Berkley, DA, Curtis, TH. 1977. Determination of masking-level differences in a reverberant environment. *J Acoust Soc Am* 61, 1374–1376.

Kuhn, GF. 1977. Model for the interaural time differences in azimuthal plane. *J Acoust Soc Am* 62, 157–167.

Kurtovic, H. 1975. The influence of reflected sound upon speech intelligibility. *Acustica* 33, 32–39.

Langford, TL, Jeffress, LA. 1964. Effect of noise cross-correlation on binaural signal detection. *J Acoust Soc Am* 36, 1455–1458.

Leakey, DM, Sayers, BMcA, Cherry, EC. 1958. Binaural fusion of low and high frequency sounds. *J Acoust Soc Am* 30, 222–223.

Lehnhardt, E. 1961. Die akustische Korrelation. *Arch Ohren Nasen Kehlkopfheilk* 178, 493–497.

Levitt, H, Rabiner, LR. 1967a. Binaural release from masking for speech and grain in intelligibility. *J Acoust Soc Am* 42, 601–608.

Levitt, H, Rabiner, LR. 1967b. Predicting binaural gain in intelligibility and release from masking for speech. *J Acoust Soc Am* 42, 820–829.

Licklider, JCR. 1948. The influence of interaural phase relations upon the masking of speech by white noise. *J Acoust Soc Am* 20, 150–159.

Licklider, JCR, Webster, JC, Hedlun, JM. 1950. On the frequency limits of binaural beats. *J Acoust Soc Am* 22, 468–473.

Litovsky, RY. 1998. Physiological studies on the precedence effect in the inferior colliculus of the kitten. *J Acoust Soc Am* 103, 3139–3152.

Litovsky, RY, Colburn, HS, Yost, WA, Guzman, SJ. 1999. The precedence effect. *J Acoust Soc Am* 106, 1633–1654.

Litovsky, RY, Delgutte, B. 2002. Neural correlates of the precedence effect in the inferior colliculus: Effect of localization cues. *J Neurophysiol* 87, 976–994.

Litovsky, RY, Macmillan, NA. 1994. Sound localization precision under conditions of the precedence effect: Effects of azimuth and standard stimuli. *J Acoust Soc Am* 96, 752–758.

Litovsky, RY, Shinn-Cunningham, BG. 2001. Investigation of the relationship among three common measures of precedence: Fusion, localization dominance, and discrimination suppression. *J Acoust Soc Am* 109, 346–358.

Little, AD, Mershon, DH, Cox, PH. 1992. Spectral content as a cue to perceived auditory distance. *Perception* 21, 405–416.

Lochner, JPA, Burger, JF. 1958. The subjective masking of short time delayed echoes, their primary sounds, and their contribution to the intelligibility of speech. *Acustica* 8, 1–10.

Lochner, JPA, Burger, JF. 1964. The influence of reflections on auditorium acoustics. *J Sound Vib* 1, 426–454.

Lord Rayleigh (Strutt, JW). 1907. Our perception of sound duration. *Phil Mag* 13, 214–232.

Macpherson, EA, Middlebrooks, JC. 2002. Listener weighting of cues for lateral angle: The duplex theory of sound localization revisited. *J Acoust Soc Am* 111, 2219–2236.

Makous, JC, Middlebrooks, JC. 1990. Two-dimensional sound localization by human listeners. *J Acoust Soc Am* 87, 2188–2200.

Marks, LE. 1978. Binaural summation of loudness of pure tones. *J Acoust Soc Am* 64, 107–113.

Marks, LE. 1987. Binaural versus monaural loudness: Super-summation of tone partially masked by noise. *J Acoust Soc Am* 81, 122–128.

McFadden, D. 1968. Masking-level differences determined with and without interaural disparities in masking intensity. *J Acoust Soc Am* 44, 212–223.

McFadden, D, Pasanen, EG. 1976. Lateralization at high frequencies based on interaural time differences. *J Acoust Soc Am* 59, 634–639.

McGregor, P, Horn, AG, Todd, MA. 1985. Are familiar sounds ranged more accurately? *Percept Motor Skills* 61, 1082.

Mershon, DH, Ballenger, WL, Little, AD, McMurtry, PL, Buchanan, JL. 1989. Effects of room reflectance and background noise on perceived auditory distance. *Perception* 18, 403–416.

Mershon, DH, Bowers, JN. 1979. Absolute and relative cues for the auditory perception of egocentric distance. *Perception* 8, 311–322.

Mershon, DH, King, LE. 1975. Intensity and reverberation as factors in the auditory perception of echocentric distance. *Percept Psychophys* 18, 409–415.

Metz, PJ, von Bismark, G, Durlach, NI. 1967. I. Further results on binaural unmasking and the EC model. II. Noise bandwidth and interaural phase. *J Acoust Soc Am* 43, 1085–1091.

Middlebrooks, JC. 1992. Narrow-band sound localization related to external ear acoustics. *J Acoust Soc Am* 92, 2607–2624.

Middlebrooks, JC. 1997. Spectral shape cues for sound localization. In: R Gilkey, T Anderson (eds.), *Binaural and Spatial Hearing in Real and Virtual Environments*. Hillsdale, NJ: Erlbaum, 77–97.

Middlebrooks, JC. 1999a. Individual differences in external ear transfer functions reduced by scaling in frequency. *J Acoust Soc Am* 106, 1480–1492.

Middlebrooks, JC. 1999b. Virtual localization improved by scaling nonindividualized external-ear transfer functions in frequency. *J Acoust Soc Am* 106, 1493–1510.

Middlebrooks, JC, Green, DM. 1991. Sound localization by human listeners. *Ann Rev Psychol* 42, 135–159.

Mills, AW. 1958. On the minimal audible angle. *J Acoust Soc Am* 30, 237–246.

Mills, AW. 1960. Lateralization of high-frequency tones. *J Acoust Soc Am* 32, 132–134.

Mills, AW. 1963. Auditory perception of spatial relations. *Proc Int Cong Tech Blind*, Vol. 2. New York, NY: American Foundation for the Blind.

Mills, AW. 1972. Auditory localization. In: JV Tobias (ed.), *Foundations of Modern Auditory Theory*, Vol. 2. New York, NY: Academic Press, 301–348.

Møller, H, Sorensen, MF, Jensen, CB, Hammershoi, D. 1996. Binaural technique: Do we need individual recordings? *J Audio Eng Soc* 44, 451–469.

Moushegian, G, Jeffress, LA. 1959. Role of interaural time and intensity differences in the lateralization of low-frequency tones. *J Acoust Soc Am* 31, 1441–1445.

Mrsic-Flogel, TD, King, AJ, Jenison, RL, Schnupp JWH. 2001. Listening through different ears alters special response fields in ferret primary auditory cortex. *J Neurophysiol* 86, 1043–1046.

Mulligan, BE, Mulligan, MJ, Stonecypher, JF. 1967. Critical band in binaural detection. *J Acoust Soc Am* 41, 7–12.

Musicant, A, Butler, R. 1984. The influence of pinnae-based spectral cues on sound localization. *J Acoust Soc Am* 75, 1195–1200.

Nabelek, AK. 1976. Reverberation effects for normal and hearing-impaired listeners. In: SK Hirsh, DH Eldridge, IJ Hirsh, SR Silverman (eds.), *Hearing and Davis: Essays Honoring Hallowell Davis*. St. Louis, MO: Washington University Press, 333–341.

Nabelek, AK, Dagenais, PA. 1986. Vowel errors in noise and in reverberation by hearing impaired listeners. *J Acoust Soc Am* 80, 741–748.

Nabelek, AK, Robinette, L. 1978. Influence of the precedence effect on word identification by normal hearing and hearing-impaired subjects. *J Acoust Soc Am* 63, 187–194.

Neutzel, JM, Hafter, ER. 1976. Lateralization of complex waveforms: Effects of fine structure, amplitude, and duration. *J Acoust Soc Am* 60, 1339–1346.

Neutzel, JM, Hafter, ER. 1981. Discrimination of interaural delays in complex waveforms: Spectral effects. *J Acoust Soc Am* 69, 1112–1118.

Nielsen, SH. 1991. Distance perception in hearing. Unpublished Ph.D. Dissertation. Aalborg, Denmark: Aalborg University.

Nielsen, SH. 1993. Auditory distance perception in different rooms. *J Audio Eng Soc* 41, 755–770.

Nordlund, B. 1962. Physical factors in angular localization. *J Acoust Soc Am* 54, 75–93.

Oldfield, SR, Parker, PA. 1984. Acuity of sound localisation: A topography of auditory space. I. Normal hearing conditions. *Perception* 13, 581–600.

Palmer, SE. 1999. *Vision Science: Photon to Phenomenology*. Cambridge, MA: MIT Press.

Perrett, S, Noble, W. 1997a. The contribution of head motion cues to localization of low-pass noise. *Percept Psychophys* 59, 1018–1026.

Perrett, S, Noble, W. 1997b. The effect of head rotations on vertical plane sound localization. *J Acoust Soc Am* 102, 2325–2332.

Perrot, DR, Marlborough, K. 1989. Minimum audible movement angle: Marking the end points of a path traveled by a moving sound source. *J Acoust Soc Am* 85, 1773–1775.

Perrott, DR. 1984. Concurrent minimum audible angle: A re-examination of the concept of auditory special acuity. *J Acoust Soc Am* 75, 1201–1206.

Perrott, DR, Marlborough, K, Merrill, P, Strybel, TZ. 1989. Minimum audible angle thresholds obtained under conditions in which the precedence effect is assumed to operate. *J Acoust Soc Am* 85, 282–288.

Perrott, DR, Musicant, A. 1977. Minimum audible movement angle: Binaural localization of moving sources. *J Acoust Soc Am* 62, 1463–1466.

Perrott, DR, Tucker, J. 1988. Minimum audible movement angle as a function of signal frequency and the velocity of the source. *J Acoust Soc Am* 83, 1522–1527.

Petersen, J. 1990. Estimation of loudness and apparent distance of pure tones in a free field. *Acustica* 70, 61–65.

Pickler, AG, Harris, JD. 1955. Channels of reception in pitch discrimination. *J Acoust Soc Am* 27, 124–131.

Plenge, G. 1974. On the difference between localization and lateralization. *J Acoust Soc Am* 56, 944–951.

Pollack, I. 1948. Monaural and binaural threshold sensitivity for tones and white noise. *J Acoust Soc Am* 20, 52–58.

Pollack, I, Rose, M. 1967. Effects of head movements on the localization of sounds in the equatorial plane. *Percept Psychophys* 2, 591–596.

Rabiner, LR, Lawrence, CL, Durlach, NI. 1966. Further results on binaural unmasking and the EC model. *J Acoust Soc Am* 40, 62–70.

Reynolds, GS, Stevens, SS. 1960. Binaural summation of loudness. *J Acoust Soc Am* 32, 1337–1344.

Robinson, DE, Jeffress, LA. 1963. Effect of varying the interaural noise correlation on the delectability of tonal signals. *J Acoust Soc Am* 35, 1947–1952.

Roth, RL, Kochhar, RK, Hind, JE. 1980. Interaural time differences: Implications regarding the neurophysiology of sound localization. *J Acoust Soc Am* 68, 1643–1651.

Rowland, RC, Tobias, JV. 1967. Interaural intensity difference limens. *J Speech Hear Res* 10, 745–756.

Saberi, K, Perrott, DR. 1990a. Minimum audible movement angles as a function of sound source trajectory. *J Acoust Soc Am* 88, 2639–2644.

Saberi, K, Perrott, DR. 1990b. Lateralization thresholds obtained under conditions in which the precedence effect is assumed to operate. *J Acoust Soc Am* 87, 1732–1737.

Sandel, TT, Teas, DC, Feddersen, WE, Jeffress, LA. 1955. Localization of sound from single and paired sources. *J Acoust Soc Am* 27, 842–852.

Sayers, BMcA, Cherry, EC. 1957. Mechanism of binaural fusion in the hearing of speech. *J Acoust Soc Am* 29, 973–987.

Scharf, B, Fishken, D. 1970. Binaural summation of loudness: Reconsidered. *J Exp Psychol* 86, 374–379.

Schenkel, KD. 1964. Über die Abhängigkeit der Mithörschwellen von der interauralen Phasenlage des Testchalls. *Acustica* 14, 337–346.

Schubert, ED, Schultz, MC. 1962. Some aspects of binaural signal selection. *J Acoust Soc Am* 34, 844–849.

Shaw, EAG. 1974. Transformation of sound pressure level from the free field to the eardrum in the horizontal plane. *J Acoust Soc Am* 56, 1848–1861.

Shaw, EAG. 1997. Acoustical features of the external ear. In: R Gilkey, T Anderson (eds.), *Binaural and Spatial Hearing in Real and Virtual Environments*. Hillsdale, NJ: Erlbaum, 25–47.

Shaw, EAG, Vaillancourt, MM. 1985. Transformation of sound–pressure level from the free field to the eardrum presented in numerical form. *J Acoust Soc Am* 78, 1120–1123.

Shaw, WA, Newman, EB, Hirsh, IJ. 1947. The difference between monaural and binaural thresholds. *J Exp Psycho* 37, 229–242.

Shinn-Cunningham, BG, Zurek, PM, Durlach, NI. 1993. Adjustment and discrimination measurements of the precedence effect. *J Acoust Soc Am* 93, 2923–2932.

Shower, EG, Biddulph, R. 1931. Differential pitch sensitivity of the ear. *J Acoust Soc Am* 3, 275–287.

Sivian, LJ, White, SD. 1933. On minimal audible fields. *J Acoust Soc Am* 4, 288–321.

Sondhi, MM, Guttman, N. 1966. Width of the spectrum effective in the binaural release of masking. *J Acoust Soc Am* 40, 600–606.

Stellmack, MA, Dye, RH. 1993. The combination of interaural information across frequencies: The effects of number and spacing of components, onset asynchrony, and harmonicity. *J Acoust Soc Am* 93, 2933–2947.

Stellmack, MA, Viemeister, NF, Byrne, AJ. 2004. Monaural and interaural intensity discrimination: Level effects and the "binaural advantage." *J Acoust Soc Am* 116, 1149–1159.

Stevens, SS, Newman, EB. 1936. The localization of actual sources of sound. *Am J Psychol* 48, 297–306.

Thurlow, WR, Runge, PS. 1967. Effect of induced head movements on localization of direction of sounds. *J Acoust Soc Am* 42, 480–488.

Tobias, JV. 1963. Application of a "relative" procedure to the binaural-beat problem. *J Acoust Soc Am* 35, 1442–1447.

Tollin, DJ, Henning, GB. 1998. Some aspects of the lateralization of echoed sound in man. I: Classical interaural delay-based precedence. *J Acoust Soc Am* 104, 3030–3038.

Townsend, TH, Goldstein, DP. 1972. Suprathreshold binaural unmasking. *J Acoust Soc Am* 51, 621–624.

Trahiotis, C, Bernstein, LR. 1990. Detectability of interaural delays over select spectral regions: Effects of flanking noise. *J Acoust Soc Am* 87, 810–813.

Wagenaars, WM. 1990. Localization of sound in a room with reflecting walls. *J Audio Eng Soc* 38, 99–110.

Wallach, H. 1939. On sound localization. *J Acoust Soc Am* 10, 270–274.

Wallach, H. 1940. The role of head movements and vestibular and visual cues in sound localization. *J Exp Psychol* 27, 339–368.

Wallach, H, Newman, EB, Rosenzweig, MR. 1949. The precedence effect in sound localization. *Am J Psychol* 62, 315–336.

Webster, FA. 1951. The influence of interaural phase on masked thresholds. I. The role of interaural time-duration. *J Acoust Soc Am* 23, 452–462.

Weinrich, S. 1982. The problem of front-back localization in binaural hearing. *Scand Audiol Suppl* 15, 135–145.

Wenzel, EM, Arruda, M, Kistler, DJ, Wightman, FL. 1993. Localization using nonindividualized head-related transfer functions. *J Acoust Soc Am* 94, 111–123.

Wernick, JS, Starr, A. 1966. Electrophysiological correlates of binaural beats in superior-olivary complex of cat. *J Acoust Soc Am* 40, 1276.

Whitworth, RH, Jeffress, LA. 1961. Time vs. intensity on the localization of tones. *J Acoust Soc Am* 33, 925–929.

Wier, CC, Jesteadt, W, Green, DM. 1977. Frequency discrimination as a function of frequency and sensation level. *J Acoust Soc Am* 61, 178–184.

Wightman, FL. 1971. Detection of binaural tones as a function of masker bandwidth. *J Acoust Soc Am* 50, 623–636.

Wightman, FL, Kistler, DJ. 1989a. Headphone simulation of free-field listening. I: Stimulus synthesis. *J Acoust Soc Am* 85, 858–867.

Wightman, FL, Kistler, DJ. 1989b. Headphone simulation of free-field listening. II: Psychophysical validation. *J Acoust Soc Am* 85, 868–878.

Wightman, FL, Kistler, DJ. 1992. The dominant role of low-frequency interaural time differences in sound localization. *J Acoust Soc Am* 91, 1648–1661.

Wightman, FL, Kistler, DJ. 1993. Sound localization. In: WA Yost, AN Popper, RR Fay (eds.), *Human Psychoacoustics.* New York, NY: Springer-Verlag, 155–192.

Wightman, FL, Kistler, DJ. 1997. Factors affecting the relative salience of sound localization cues. In: R Gilkey, T Anderson (eds.), *Binaural and Spatial Hearing in Real and Virtual Environments.* Hillsdale, NJ: Erlbaum, 1–23.

Wightman, FL, Kistler, DJ. 1999. Resolution of front-back ambiguity in spatial hearing by listener and source movement. *J Acoust Soc Am* 105, 2841–2853.

Woodworth, RS. 1938. *Experimental Psychology.* New York, NY: Holt, Rhinehart, and Winston.

Wu, X, Wang, C, Chen, J, Qu, H, Li, W, Wu, Y, Schneider, BA., Li, L. 2005. The effect of perceived spatial separation on informational masking of Chinese speech. *Hear Res* 199, 1–10.

Yang, X, Grantham, DW. 1997. Echo suppression and discrimination suppression aspects of the precedence effect. *Percept Psychophys* 59, 1108–1117.

Yost, WA. 1974. Discriminations of interaural phase differences. *J Acoust Soc Am* 55, 1299–1303.

Yost, WA. 1981. Lateral position of sinusoids presented with interaural intensive and temporal differences. *J Acoust Soc Am* 70, 397–409.

Yost, WA. 1993 Overview: Psychoacoustics. In: WA Yost, AN Popper, RR Fay (eds.), *Human Psychophysics.* New York, NY: Springer-Verlag, 1–12.

Yost, WA. 1997. The cocktail party problem: Forty years later. In: R Gilkey, T Anderson (eds.), *Binaural and Spatial Hearing in Real and Virtual Environments.* Hillsdale, NJ: Erlbaum, 329–347.

Yost, WA, Dye, RH Jr. 1988. Discrimination of interaural differences of level as a function of frequency. *J Acoust Soc Am* 83, 1846–1851.

Yost, WA, Sheft, S. 1993. Auditory perception. In: WA Yost, AN Popper, RR Fay (eds.), *Human Psychophysics.* New York, NY: Springer-Verlag, 193–236.

Yost, WA, Wightman, FL, Green, DM. 1971. Lateralization of filtered clicks. *J Acoust Soc Am* 50, 1526–1531.

Zahorik, P. 1996. Auditory distance perception: A literature review. Wisconsin: University of Wisconsin-Madison. http://www.waisman.wisc.edu/~zahorik/papers/dist.html.

Zahorik, P. 2002a. Assessing auditory distance perception using virtual acoustics. *J Acoust Soc Am* 111, 1832–1846.

Zahorik, P. 2002b. Direct-to-reverberant energy ratio sensitivity. *J Acoust Soc Am* 112, 2110–2117.

Zurek, PM. 1980. The precedence effect and its possible role in the avoidance of interaural ambiguities. *J Acoust Soc Am* 67, 952–964.

Zwislocki, J, Feldman, RS. 1956. Just noticeable differences in dichotic phase. *J Acoust Soc Am* 28, 860–864.

14 Speech and Its Perception

Pure tones, clicks, and the like enable us to study specific aspects of audition in a precise and controllable manner. On the other hand, we communicate with each other by speech, which is composed of particularly complex and variable waveforms. A knowledge of how we perceive simpler sounds is the foundation upon which an understanding of speech perception must be built. As one might suppose, speech perception and intimately related areas constitute a voluminous subject encompassing far more than hearing science, per se, and the interested student will find numerous sources addressing the topic at various levels (e.g., Miller, 1951; Fletcher, 1953; Fant, 1970; Flanagan, 1972; Massaro, 1987, 1998; Pickett, 1999; Miller et al., 1991; Kent and Read, 2002; Liberman, 1996; Ryalls, 1996; Jusczyk and Luce, 2002; Diehl et al., 2004; Galantucci et al., 2006; Ferrand, 2007; Raphael et al., 2007; Massaro and Chen, 2008).

Speech perception and speech production are inherently interrelated. We must be able to speak what we can perceive, and we must have the ability to perceive the sounds that our speech mechanisms produce. Traditionally, the sounds of speech have been described in terms of the vocal and articulatory manipulations that produce them. We too shall begin with production. For the most part, our discussion will focus upon phonemes.

By a **phoneme** we mean a group of sounds that are classified as being the same by native speakers of a given language. Let us see what the "sameness" refers to. Consider the phoneme /p/ as it appears at the beginning and end of the word "pipe." There are actually several differences between the two productions of /p/ in this word. For example, the initial /p/ is accompanied by a release of a puff of air (aspiration), whereas the final /p/ is not. In other words, the actual sounds are different, or distinct **phonetic elements**. (By convention, phonemes are enclosed between slashes and phonetic elements between brackets.) In spite of this, native speakers of English will classify both as belonging to the family designated as the /p/ phoneme. Such phonetically dissimilar members of the same phonemic class are called allophones of that phoneme. Consider a second example. The words "beet" and "bit" (/bit/ and /bIt/, respectively) sound different to speakers of English but the same to speakers of French. This happens because the phonetic elements [i] and [I] are different phonemes in English, but are allophones of the same phoneme in French. Since the French person classifies [i] and [I] as members of the same phonemic family, he hears them as being the same, just as English speakers hear the aspirated and unaspirated productions of /p/ to be the same.

This last example also demonstrates the second important characteristic of phonemes. Changing a phoneme changes the meaning of a word. Thus, /i/ and /I/ are different phonemes in English, because replacing one for the other changes the meaning of at least some words. However, [i] and [I] are not different phonemes in French; that is, they are **allophones**, because replacing one for the other does not change the meaning of words. Implicit in the distinction of phonetic and phonemic elements is that even elementary speech sound classes are to some extent learned. All babies the world over produce the same wide range of sounds phonetically; it is through a process of learning that these phonetic elements become classified and grouped into families of phonemes that are used in the language of the community.

SPEECH SOUNDS: PRODUCTION AND PERCEPTION

Our discussion of speech sounds will be facilitated by reference to the simplified schematic diagram of the vocal tract in Fig. 14.1 The power source is the air in the lungs, which is directed up and out under the control of the respiratory musculature. Voiced sounds are produced when the vocal folds (vocal cords) are vibrated. The result of this vibration is a periodic complex waveform made up of a fundamental frequency on the order of 100 Hz in males and 200 Hz in females, with as many as 40 harmonics of the fundamental represented in the spectrum (Flanagan, 1958) (Fig. 14.2a). Voiceless (unvoiced) sounds are produced by opening the airway between the vocal folds so that they do not vibrate. Voiceless sounds are aperiodic and noise-like, being produced by turbulences due to partial or complete obstruction of the vocal tract. Regardless of the source, the sound is then modified by the resonance characteristics of the vocal tract. In other words, the vocal tract constitutes a group of filters that are added together, and whose effect is to shape the spectrum of the waveform from the larynx. The resonance characteristics of the vocal tract (Fig. 14.2b) are thus reflected in the speech spectrum (Fig. 14.2c). The vocal tract resonances are called **formants** and are generally labeled starting from the lowest as the first formant (F1), second formant (F2), third formant (F3), etc. This is the essence of the **source-filter theory**, or the **acoustic theory of speech production** (Fant, 1970).

Vowels

Speech sounds are generally classified broadly as vowels and consonants. Vowels are voiced sounds whose spectral characteristics are determined by the size and shape of the vocal tract. (Certain exceptions are notable. For example, whispered speech is all voiceless, and vowels may also be voiceless in some contexts of voiceless consonants in connected discourse. Also, the nasal cavity is generally excluded by action of the velum unless the vowel is in the environment of a nasal sound.) Changing the shape of the vocal tract changes its filtering characteristics, which in turn change the formant structure, that is, the frequencies at which the speech signal is enhanced or de-emphasized (Fig. 14.2). Diphthongs such as /aI/ in "buy" and /oU/ in "toe" are heard when one vowel glides into another.

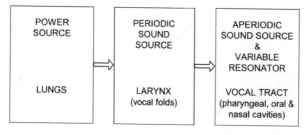

Figure 14.1 Schematic representation of speech production.

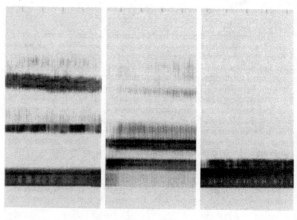

Figure 14.3 Spectrograms showing sustained production of the vowels /i/, /æ/, and /u/ (left to right). Timing marks along the top are 100 ms apart.

In general, the formant frequencies depend upon where and to what extent the vocal tract is constricted (Peterson and Barney, 1952; Stevens and House, 1955, 1961; Flanagan, 1972). The locations and degrees of these constrictions control the sizes and locations of the volumes in the vocal tract. For example, elevation of the back of the tongue results in a larger volume between this point of constriction and the lips than does elevation of the tongue tip. We may thus describe a vowel from front to back in terms of the amount of tongue elevation. Lip rounding is another important factor. In English, front vowels (/i, I, e, ɛ, æ/) are produced with retraction of the lips, while the lips are rounded when the back vowels (/u, U, o, ɔ, a/) are formed. Rounding the front vowel /i/ as in "tea" while keeping the high-front tongue placement results in the French vowel /y/, as in "*tu*." The degree of tenseness associated with the muscle contractions is also a factor in vowel production and perception, as in the differentiation of the tense /i/ ("peat") from the lax /I/ ("pit"). Tense vowels are generally more intense and longer in duration than their lax counterparts.

The middle vowels (/ʌ,ə,ɜ,ɝ,ɚ/) are produced when tongue elevation is in the vicinity of the hard palate. These include the *neutral vowel* or *schwa*, /ə/, associated mainly with unstressed syllables (e.g., "*about*" and "*support*").

Without going into great detail, the frequency of the **first format (F1)** is largely dependent upon the size of the volume behind the tongue elevation, that is, upon the larger of the vocal tract volumes. This volume must, of course, increase as the elevated part of the tongue moves forward. Thus, front tongue elevation produces a larger volume behind the point of constriction, which in turn is associated with lower F1 frequencies,

whereas back tongue elevations decrease the size of this volume, thereby raising the frequency of F1. The frequency of the **second formant (F2)** depends largely upon the size of the volume in front of the point of tongue elevation, becoming higher when the cavity is made smaller (when the tongue is elevated closer to the front of the mouth). Lip rounding lowers the first two formants by reducing the size of the mouth opening.

Figure 14.3 shows sustained productions of several vowels in the form of sound **spectrograms** (Koenig et al., 1946; Potter et al., 1947). Frequency is shown up the ordinate, time along the abscissa, and intensity as relative blackness or gray-scale. Thus, blacker areas represent frequencies with higher energy concentrations and lighter areas indicate frequency regions with less energy. The formants are indicated by frequency bands much darker than the rest of the spectrogram. These horizontal bands represent frequency regions containing concentrations of energy and thus reflect the resonance characteristics of the vocal tract. The vertical striations correspond to the period of the speaker's fundamental frequency.

The relationship between tongue position and the frequencies of F1 and F2 are shown for several vowels in Fig. 14.4. However, it should be noted that these formant frequencies are approximations based on average male values from just one study. Formant center frequencies and bandwidths tend to become higher going from men to women to children, which reflects the effect of decreasing vocal tract length (Fig. 14.5). Formant parameters vary appreciably among talkers and even between studies (e.g., Peterson and Barney, 1952; Hillenbrand et al., 1995); they are affected by such factors as neighboring phonemes, by whether the syllable is stressed or unstressed, etc.

The lower formants (especially F1 and F2, as well as F3) are primarily responsible for vowel recognition (Peterson, 1952; Peterson and Barney, 1952; Delattre et al., 1952; Hillenbrand et al., 1995). However, given the wide variations alluded to above, it is doubtful that vowels are identified on the basis of their formant frequencies, per se. The relationships among the

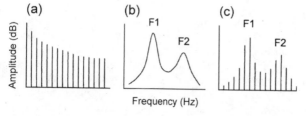

Figure 14.2 The source-filter theory (acoustic theory) of speech production: Idealized spectra showing that when the glottal source spectrum (a) is passed through the vocal tract filters (b) the resulting (output) spectrum (c) represents characteristics of the vocal tract. F1 and F2 indicate the first two formants.

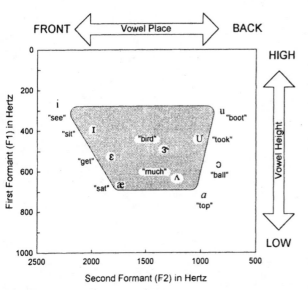

FRONT ← Vowel Place → BACK

HIGH

LOW

First Formant (F1) in Hertz

Second Formant (F2) in Hertz

Vowel Height

Figure 14.4 Vowel quadrilateral showing the approximate values of the first (F1) and second (F2) formants of several vowels as they relate to tongue height and place based on data for male talkers by Peterson and Barney (1952).

formants, as well as the environment of the vowel and its duration, provide important cues (Tiffany, 1953; Stevens and House, 1963; Lindblom and Studdert-Kennedy, 1967). It has been suggested that, for each individual speaker, the listener adjusts the "target" values of the formants according to the utterances of that speaker (e.g., Ladefoged and Broadbent, 1957; Lieberman, 1973); however, this is certainly not the only explanation for vowel perception. A lucid review of vowel perception issues and theories may be found in Kent and Read (2002), and more advanced students will find informative discussions in a series

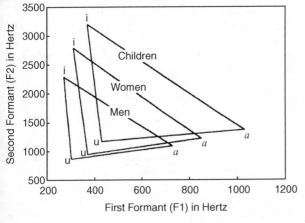

Figure 14.5 Average formant frequencies increase going from men to women to children, as illustrated here by the shifts in the average values of F1 and F2 for the vowels /i/, /a/, and /u/. *Source*: Based on data by Peterson and Barney (1952).

of papers by Miller (1989), Nearey (1989), and Strange (1989a, 1989b).

Consonants

The consonants are produced by either a partial or complete obstruction somewhere along the vocal tract. The ensuing turbulence causes the sound to be aperiodic and noise-like. The consonants are differentiated on the basis of manner of articulation, place of articulation, and voicing; that is, on how and where the obstruction of the vocal tract occurs, and on whether there is vocal cord vibration. Table 14.1 shows the English consonants, arranged horizontally according to place of articulation and vertically by manner of articulation and voicing. Examples are given where the phonetic and orthographic symbols differ.

The stops, fricatives, and affricates may be either voiced or voiceless, whereas the nasals and semivowels are virtually always voiced. The nasal cavities are excluded from the production of all consonants except the nasals by elevation of the velum. We shall briefly discuss the consonants in order of the manner of their articulation.

The **stops** are produced by a transition (see below) from the preceding vowel, a silent period on the order of roughly 30 ms during which air pressure is impounded behind a complete obstruction somewhere along the vocal tract, a release (burst) of the built-up pressure, and finally a transition into the following vowel (Cooper et al., 1952; Fischer-Jorgensen, 1954; Liberman et al., 1956; Halle et al., 1957). Of course, whether there is a transition from the preceding vowel and/or into the following vowel depends upon the environment of the stop consonant. Voiceless stops in the initial position are generally aspirated, or released with a puff of air. Initial voiced stops and all final stops tend not to be aspirated, although this does not apply always or to all speakers. The voiceless stops (/p,t,k/) and their voiced cognates (/b,d,g/) are articulated in the same way except for the presence or absence of voicing and/or aspiration. As a rule, the voiceless stops tend to have longer and stronger pressure buildups than do their voiced counterparts (Sharf, 1962; Arkebauer et al., 1967).

The six stops are produced at three locations. The **bilabials** (/p,b/) are produced by an obstruction at the lips, the **alveolars** (/t,d/) by the tongue tip against the upper gum ridge, and the **velars** (/k,g/) by the tongue dorsum against the soft palate. Whether the sound is heard as voiced or voiceless is, of course, ultimately due to whether there is vocal cord vibration. However, cues differ according to the location of the stop in an utterance. The essential voicing cue for initial stops is **voice onset time** (**VOT**), which is simply the time delay between the onset of the stop burst and commencement of vocal cord vibration (Lisker and Abramson, 1964, 1967). In general, voicing onset precedes or accompanies stop burst onset for voiced stops but lags behind the stop burst for voiceless stops. For final stops and those that occur medially within an utterance, the essential voicing cue appears to be the duration of the preceding

Table 14.1 Consonants of English.

	Bilabial	Labiodental	Linguadental	Alveolar	Palatal	Velar	Glottal
Stops							
Voiceless	p			t		k	
Voiced	b			d		g	
Fricatives							
Voiceless	ʍ(**wh**ich)	f	θ (**th**ing)	s	ʃ(**sh**oe)		
Voiced		v	ð (**th**is)	z	ʒ(beige)		
Affricates							
Voiceless					tʃ(ca**tch**)		h
Voiced					ʤ (do**dge**)		
Nasals[a]	m			n		ŋ (si**ng**)	
Liquids[a]					r, l		
Glides[a]	w					j (**y**es)	

[a]The nasals, liquids, and glides are voiced.

vowel (Raphael, 1972). Longer vowel durations are associated with the perception that the following stop is voiced. Voiceless stops are also associated with longer closure durations (Lisker, 1957a, 1957b), faster formant transitions (Slis, 1970), greater burst intensities (Halle et al., 1957), and somewhat higher fundamental frequencies (Haggard et al., 1970) than voiced stops.

Place of articulation (bilabial vs. alveolar vs. velar) for the stops has been related to the **second formant (F2) transition** of the associated vowel (Liberman et al., 1954; Delattre et al., 1955), along with some contribution from the F3 transitions (Harris et al., 1958). By a formant transition we simply mean a change with time of the formant frequency in going from the steady-state frequency of the vowel into the consonant (or vice versa). Formant transitions may be seen for several initial voiced stops in Fig. 14.6. The F2 transitions point in the direction of approximately 700 Hz for bilabial stops, 1800 Hz for the alveolars, and 3000 Hz for the velars (Liberman et al., 1954). The second formation transition **locus principle** is illustrated in Fig. 14.7 These directions relate to the location of vocal tract obstruction. That is, a larger volume is enclosed behind an obstruction at the lips (/p,b/) than at the alveolus (/t,d/) or the

velum (/k,g/) so that the resonant frequency associated with that volume is lower for more frontal obstructions. Moving the point of obstruction backward reduces the cavity volume and thus increases the resonant frequency. Additional place information is provided by the frequency spectrum of the stop burst. **Stop bursts** tend to have concentrations of energy at relatively low frequencies (500–1500 Hz) for the bilabials, at high frequencies (about 4000 Hz and higher) for the alveolars, and at intermediate frequencies (between around 1500 and 4000 Hz) for the velars (Liberman et al., 1956).

There tends to be a considerable amount of *variability* (often described as a *lack of invariance*) in the formant cues because the configurations of the formant transitions change according to the associated vowels. This variability is readily observed in Fig. 14.7 and is especially apparent for the alveolars. For example, the second formant transition from /d/ into the following vowel is different for /di/ and /du/. An invariant place of articulation cue has been proposed on the basis of several acoustical and perceptual studies (e.g., Stevens and Blumstein, 1978; Blumstein and Stevens, 1979, 1980; Blumstein, Isaacs, and Mertus, 1982; Kewley-Port, 1983; Kewley-Port and Luce, 1984; Furui, 1986). For example, Stevens, Blumstein, and colleagues demonstrated invariant patterns in the gross configurations of the spectra integrated over a period of roughly 20 ms in the vicinity of the consonant release. Figure 14.8 shows the general configurations of these **onset spectra**, which are (a) *diffuse and falling* for bilabials, /p,b/; (b) *diffuse and rising* for the alveolars, /t,d/; and (c) *compact* for the velars, /k,g/.

In addition to the perceptual findings, further support for this concept comes from experiments using computer models (Searle, Jacobson, and Rayment, 1979) and auditory nerve discharge patterns (Miller and Sachs, 1983). There is theoretical and experimental support for the notion that children use onset spectra as the primary cues for place of articulation for stops before they learn to use formant transitions as secondary perceptual cues (e.g., Blumstein and Stevens, 1979, 1980; Ohde et al., 1995), although there are contrary models and results,

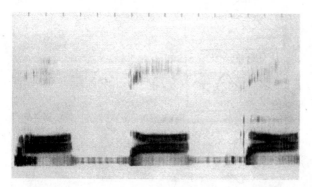

Figure 14.6 Spectrograms of /ba/, /da/, and / ga/ (left to right). Note second formant transitions.

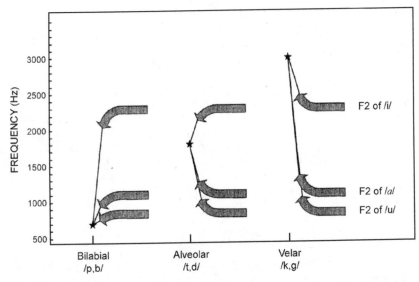

Figure 14.7 Artist's conceptualization of the second formant transition locus principle for stop consonant place of articulation. Stars indicate the locus (target frequency) toward which the second formant transitions point for bilabials, alveolars, and velars.

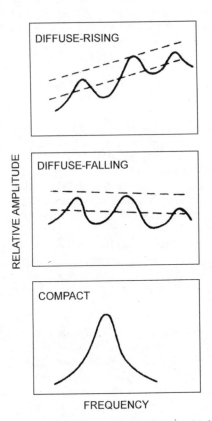

Figure 14.8 Invariant onset spectrum configurations associated with stop-consonant place of articulation: alveolars, diffuse, and rising; labials, diffuse, and falling; velars, compact. *Source*: Adapted from Blumstein and Stevens (1979), with permission of *J. Acoust. Soc. Am.*

as well (e.g., Walley and Carrell, 1983; Nittrouer and Studdert-Kennedy, 1987; Nittrouer, 1992). Repp and Lin (1989) have suggested that the onset spectrum may provide the listener with a very brief "acoustic snapshot of the vocal tract" that might be supplemented by the dynamic cues of formant transitions if more information is needed to accurately identify the sound.

The **fricatives** are produced by a partial obstruction of the vocal tract so that the air coming through becomes turbulent. The nature of the fricatives has been well described (House and Fairbanks, 1953; Huges and Halle, 1956; Harris, 1958; Strevens, 1960; Heinz and Stevens, 1961; Jassem, 1965; Guerlekian, 1981; Jongman, 1985; Behrens and Blumstein, 1988). Several examples of the fricatives are shown in the spectrograms in Fig. 14.9 Fricatives are distinguished from other manners of articulation by the continuing nature of their turbulent energy (generally lasting 100 ms or more). Vowels preceding fricatives

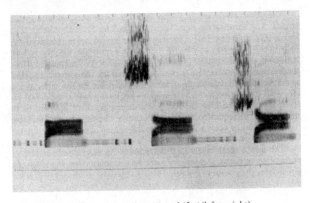

Figure 14.9 Spectrograms of /fa/, /sa/, and /ʃ,a/ (left to right).

261

tend to have greater power and duration, and somewhat longer fundamental frequencies, than vowels preceding stops. As is true for the stops, fricatives may be either voiced or voiceless. However, unlike the stops, the duration of the fricatives makes it possible for voicing to be cued by the presence versus absence of periodic energy during frication. In addition, fricative voicing is also cued by VOT and by the nature of the preceding vowel. Moreover, voiceless fricatives tend to have longer durations than their voiced counterparts.

Spectral differences largely account for place distinctions between the alveolar (/s,z/) and the palatal (/ʃ,ʒ/) sibilant fricatives. The palatals have energy concentrations extending to lower frequencies (about 1500–7000 Hz) than do the alveolars (roughly 4000–7000 Hz), most likely because of the larger volume in front of the point of vocal tract obstruction for /ʃ,ʒ/ than for /s,z/. On the other hand, /θ,ð/, and /f, v/ are differentiated largely on the basis of formant transitions. Because of resonation of the entire vocal tract above the glottis, /h/ possesses more low frequencies than the more anterior fricatives. The amplitudes of /s/ and /ʃ/ are considerably greater than those of /f/ and /θ/. However, perceptual experiments by Behrens and Blumstein (1988) have demonstrated that these amplitudes are less important than spectral properties in differentiating between these two groups of fricatives. The **affricates** are produced by the rapid release of their stop components into their fricative components.

The **nasals** are produced by opening the port to the nasal cavities at the velum. They are semivowels in that they are voiced and have some of the formant characteristics of vowels. However, they differ from other sounds by the coupling of the nasal and oral cavities. The characteristics of nasals have been described by Fujimura (1962) and others (Cooper et al., 1952; Malécot, 1956; House, 1957; Kurowski and Blumstein, 1987a, 1987b). The coupling of the nasal cavities to the volume of oral cavity behind the point of obstruction (the velum for /ŋ/, alveolus for /n/, and lips for /m/) constitutes a side-branch resonator. This results in antiresonances at frequencies that become lower as the volume of the side branch (oral cavity) becomes larger. Thus, we find that antiresonances appear in the frequency regions of roughly 1000 Hz for /m/ (where the side branch is the largest), 1700 Hz for /n/, and 3000 Hz for /ŋ/ (where the side branch is the shortest). Furthermore, overall intensity is reduced, and for the first formant is lower than for the vowels, constituting a characteristic low-frequency nasal murmur. Place of articulation is cued by differences in the spectrum of the nasal murmur (e.g., Kurowski and Blumstein, 1993), and spectral and amplitude changes at the juncture between the nasal and the adjoining vowel (e.g., Kurowski and Blumstein, 1987a, 1987b; Ohde, Haley, and Barnes, 2006).

The **semivowels** are /w,j/ and /r,l/. The former two are known as the **glides** and the latter ones are **liquids**. The semivowels have been described by O'Connor et al. (1957), Lisker (1957a, 1957b), and Fant (1970). The bilabial glide /w/ is produced

initially in the same way as the vowel /u/, with a transition into the following vowel over the course of about 100 ms. For the glide /j/, the transition into the following vowel is from /i/ and takes about the same amount of time as for /w/. The first formants of both /w/ and /j/ are on the order of 240 Hz, with the second formant transitions beginning below about 600 Hz for /w/ and above 2300 Hz for /j/. Furthermore, there appears to be relatively low-frequency frication-like noise associated with /w/ and higher-frequency noise with /j/, due to the degree of vocal tract constriction in their production.

The liquids (/r,l/) have short-duration steady-state portions of up to about 50 ms, followed by transitions into the following vowel over the course of roughly 75 ms. The /r/ is produced with some degree of lip rounding, and /l/ is produced with the tongue tip at the upper gum ridge so that air is deflected laterally. The first formants of the liquids are on the order of 500 Hz for /r/ and 350 Hz for /l/, which are relatively high, and the first and second formant transitions are roughly similar for both liquids. The major difference appears to be associated with the presence of lip rounding for /r/ but not for /l/. Since lip rounding causes the third formant to be lower in frequency, /r/ is associated with a rather dramatic third formant transition upward in frequency, which is not seen for /l/, at least not for transitions into unrounded vowels. The opposite would occur for /r/ and /l/ before a rounded vowel.

DICHOTIC LISTENING AND CEREBRAL LATERALIZATION

Dichotic listening studies involve asking listeners to respond to two different signals presented at the same time, one to the right ear and another to the left ear (see, e.g., Berlin and McNeil (1976). This approach was introduced to the study of speech perception by Broadbent (1954, 1956) as a vehicle for the study of memory, and was extended to the study of hemispheric lateralization for speech by Kimura (1961, 1967). Kimura asked her subjects to respond to different digits presented to the two ears. The result was a small but significant advantage in the perception of the digits at the right ear—the **right ear advantage (REA)**. On the other hand, there was a left ear advantage when musical material was presented dichotically (Kimura, 1964).

The study of dichotic listening was enhanced with the use of CV syllables by Shankweiler and Studdert-Kennedy (1967) and others (e.g., Studdert-Kennedy and Shankweiler, 1970; Studdert-Kennedy et al., 1970; Berlin et al., 1973; Cullen et al., 1974). The basic experiment is similar to Kimura's, except that the dichotic digits are replaced by a pair of dichotic CV syllables. Most often, the syllables /pa, ka, ta, ba, da, ga/ are used. The CV studies confirmed and expanded the earlier digit observations. For example, Studdert-Kennedy and Shankweiler (1970) found a significant REA for the CVs but not for vowels.

They further found that the REA was larger when the conso-nants differed in both place of articulation and voicing (e.g., /pa/ vs. /ga/) than when the contrast was one of place (e.g., /pa/ vs. /ta/) or voicing (e.g., /ta/ vs. /da/) alone. Similarly, Studdert-Kennedy and Shankweiler (1970) found that errors were less common when the dichotic pair had one feature (place or voicing) in common than when both place and voicing were different.

Since the primary and most efficient pathways are from the right ear to the left cerebral hemisphere and from the left ear to the right hemisphere, these have been interpreted as reveal-ing right-eared (left hemisphere) dominance for speech and left-eared (right hemisphere) dominance for melodic mate-rial. That the left hemisphere is principally responsible for the processing of speech material is also supported by physi-ological findings using a variety of approaches (Wood et al., 1971; Wood, 1975; Mäkelä et al., 2003, 2005; Josse et al., 2003; Tervaniemi and Hugdahl, 2003; Price et al., 2005; Shtyrov et al., 2005).

The robustness of the REA was demonstrated by Cullen et al. (1974), who showed that the REA is maintained until the signal to the right ear is at quite a disadvantage relative to the one presented to the left. Specifically, the REA was maintained until (1) the stimuli presented to the left ear were 20 dB stronger than those to the right, (2) the signal-to-noise ratio (SNR) in the right ear was 12 dB poorer than in the left, and (3) the CVs presented to the right ear were filtered above 3000 Hz while the left ear received an unfiltered signal. Interestingly, Cullen et al. also demonstrated that when the right-ear score decreased, the left ear score actually became proportionally better so that the total percent correct (right plus left) was essentially constant. This suggests that there is a finite amount of information that can be handled at one time by the speech-handling mechanism in the left hemisphere.

When the CV delivered to one ear is delayed relative to the presentation of the CV to the other ear, then there is an advan-tage for the ear receiving the *lagging* stimulus, particularly for delays on the order of 30 to 60 ms (Studdert-Kennedy et al., 1970; Berlin et al., 1973). This phenomenon is the **dichotic lag effect**. Since it also occurs for nonspeech (though speech-like) sounds, there is controversy over whether the lag effect is a speech-specific event or a more general phenomenon such as backward masking (Darwin, 1971; Pisoni and McNabb, 1974; Mirabile and Porter, 1975; Porter, 1975).

CATEGORICAL PERCEPTION

Liberman et al. (1961) prepared synthetic consonant–vowel (CV) monosyllables composed of two formants each. They asked their subjects to discriminate between these pairs of syn-thetic CVs as the second formant transition was varied, and obtained a finding that has had a profound effect upon the study of speech perception. Subjects' ability to *discriminate* between the two CVs in a pair was excellent when the consonants were *identifiable* as different phonemes, whereas discrimination was poor when the consonants were identified as belonging to the same *phonemic category*.

This phenomenon of **categorical perception** is illustrated in Fig. 14.10 which shows idealized results from a hypothetical study of how VOT affects the perception of initial alveolar stops. Recall that VOT is the voicing cue for initial stops, so we are dealing with the perception of /t/ versus /d/. The stimuli are CV syllables differing in VOT. For simplicity, we will identify VOTs by letters instead of actual durations in milliseconds. Two types of perceptual tasks are involved. In the first test, the amount of VOT is varied in 10 equal increments from A (the shortest) to J (the longest), and the subjects must identify the CVs as /ta/ or /da/. The upper frame of the figure shows that just about all of the shorter VOTs (A to E) were heard as /d/, whereas virtu-ally all of the longer VOTs (F to J) were heard as /t/. In other words, there was an abrupt change in the categorization of the stimuli as either voiced or voiceless between VOT increments E and F, constituting a *category boundary*. The second task is to

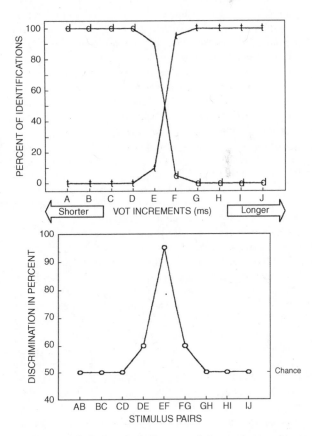

Figure 14.10 Idealized results for in a categorical perception experiment (see text).

discriminate between pairs of these stimuli; for example, between A–B, B–C, C–D, etc. Notice that the VOT difference (in milliseconds) is the same between the members of each pair. These results are shown in the lower frame of the figure, where 50% is random guessing (chance). Notice that the subjects can easily discriminate between E and F, where one member of the pair (E) is identified as /da/ and the other member of the pair (F) is identified as /ta/. On the other hand, they cannot discriminate between any of the other pairs, where both members were identified as /da/ (e.g., C vs. D) or as /ta/ (e.g., G vs. H). Thus, the CVs identified as belonging to the *same* category are poorly discriminated, whereas those identified as belonging to *different* categories are easily discriminated.

Categorical perception has been explored in many studies using a variety of speech and nonspeech stimuli (e.g., Fry et al., 1962; Lisker and Abramson, 1964, 1970; Liberman et al., 1961, 1967; Abramson and Lisker, 1970; Miller et al., 1976; Pisoni, 1977; Cutting and Rosner, 1974; Mitler et al., 1976; Stevens and Klatt, 1974; Repp, 1984; Schouten and vanHessen, 1992; for reviews, see Repp, 1984; Diehl, Lotto, and Holt, 2004). Categorical perception was originally observed for speech sounds (especially for consonants, and to a lesser extend for vowels), but not for nonspeech stimuli. Categorical perception has also been shown to occur in infants (Eimas et al., 1971; Eimas, 1974; Bertoncini et al., 1988). In addition, categorical perception is subject to **selective adaptation**, seen as changes in the boundary between categories (voiced–voiceless or different places of articulation) after hearing many repeated presentations of a prototype of just one of two opposing stimuli (e.g., Eimas and Corbit, 1973; Cooper and Blumstein, 1974). For example, hearing many repetitions of a /ba/ prototype (i.e., from the voiced end of the VOT continuum) will cause the listener's voiced–voiceless boundary between /pa/ and /ba/ to shift toward /ba/, thus favoring the perception of /pa/.

Findings like the ones just described were originally interpreted as suggesting that categorical perception reflects an innate **speech or phonetic module**, that is, an underlying process that is phonetic or speech-specific in nature rather than involving more general auditory mechanisms (e.g., Liberman et al., 1967; see below). However, the accumulated evidence has shown that categorical perception actually involves more general auditory mechanisms rather than phonetic or speech-specific processes. In particular, categorical perception and selective adaptation have been shown to occur for a variety of nonspeech materials, and there is an association of categorical perception with psychoacoustic phenomena such as perceived temporal order and across-channel gap detection (Miller et al., 1976; Pisoni, 1977; Cutting and Rosner, 1974; Tartter and Eimas, 1975; Mitler et al., 1976; Sawusch and Jusczyk, 1981; Formby et al., 1993; Nelson et al., 1995; Phillips et al., 1997; Phillips, 1999; Elangovan and Stuart, 2008). Experiments revealing categorical perception in a variety of animals provide even more impressive evidence for an underlying auditory rather than phonetic mechanism (Kuhl and Miller, 1975, 1978; Kuhl and

Padden, 1982, 1983; Nelson and Marler, 1989; Dooling et al., 1995).

THE SPEECH MODULE

Whether speech perception actually involves a specialized phonetic module as opposed to general auditory capabilities is an unresolved issue. We just considered this controversy while addressing categorical perception, which was originally considered to be evidence of a specialized speech mode, but is now understood to reflect underlying auditory capabilities. Other phenomena have also been implicated in the fundamental issue of whether speech perception involves a specialized speech module or general auditory processes, such as duplex perception, the perception of sine wave speech, and the McGurk effect.

Duplex perception (e.g., Whalen and Liberman, 1987) refers to hearing *separate speech and nonspeech sounds* when the listener is presented with certain kinds of stimuli. It can be demonstrated by splitting the acoustical characteristics of a synthetic consonant–vowel syllable like /da/, and presenting them separately to the two ears as shown in the lower part of Fig. 14.11. In this version of the duplex perception experiment, one ear receives only the syllable base, composed of F1 with its transition and F2 *without* its transition. The other ear receives only the second formant transition. Neither of these sounds is heard as speech when presented alone. However, when they are presented simultaneously, the listener hears *both* a *speech* sound (/da/) in one ear and a *nonspeech* sound (a chirp) in the other ear, as illustrated in the upper part of the figure. The ability of the same stimuli to evoke separate speech and nonspeech perceptions implies the existence of separate auditory and phonetic perceptual mechanisms. One should note, however, that Fowler and Rosenblum (1991) reported that they found duplex perception for a door slamming sound, a non-speech stimulus that would not involve a specialized speech module.

The perception of **sine wave speech** has often been associated with a specialized speech mode because it reveals how the same signal can be experienced as either speech or nonspeech (e.g., Remez, Rubin, Pisoni, and Carrel, 1981; Remez, Rubin, Berns, et al., 1994).[1] Sine wave speech is a synthetic signal composed of three or more pure tones that increase and decrease in frequency over time to mimic the changing formants of naturally spoken speech, but with all other aspects of the speech signal omitted. Naïve listeners experience these signals as peculiar complex tonal patterns, but subjects will perceive them as speech when told that they are listening to intelligible computer-generated speech.

---

[1] On-line demonstrations of sine wave speech by Robert Remez may be found at http://www.columbia.edu/~remez/Site/Musical%20Sinewave%20Speech.html, and by Christopher Darwin at http://www.lifesci.sussex.ac.uk/home/Chris_Darwin/SWS/.

Perceptions

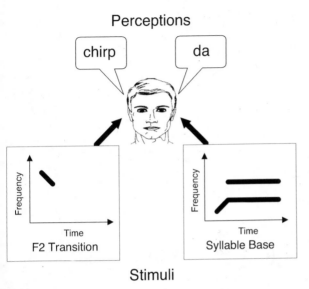

Figure 14.11 Idealized illustration of duplex perception. Presenting a syllable base without the second formant transition to one ear and just the second formant transition to other ear, causes the perception of both a speech sound (syllable /da/) in one ear and a nonspeech chirp-like sound in the other ear.

The **McGurk (McGurk–MacDonald) effect** illustrates the interaction of auditory and visual information in speech perception (McGurk and MacDonald, 1976; MacDonald and McGurk, 1978). To understand this effect, remember that real face-to-face conversations involve auditory and visual signals that agree: the listener *sees* lip and facial manipulations on the talker's face that correspond with what he *hears* the talker saying. For example, when a talker says /ba/, the listener hears /ba/ and also sees /ba/ on the talker's face, and, as expected, perceives /ba/. In contrast, the McGurk effect occurs when the listener is presented with *competing* auditory and visual representations of the speech. For example, the listener might be presented with an audio recording of /ba/ from earphones along with a video recording of a /ga/ on a screen. In this case, the listener perceives another syllable (e.g., /da/) or just one of the two originals, constituting the McGurk effect. This illusion is so strong that the listener even experiences it if he knows that two different stimuli were presented. The McGurk effect has been taken as evidence for a specialized speech module and/or the perception of speech gestures for some time (e.g., Liberman and Mattingly, 1985), but other interpretations also have been offered (e.g., Massaro, 1987, 1998). The accumulating physiological findings suggest that the McGurk effect involves mechanisms dealing with phonetic information, which are located in cortical auditory areas and have left hemispheric dominance (Sams et al., 1991; Näätänen, 2001; Colin et al., 2002, 2004; Möttönen et al., 2002; Saint-Amour et al., 2007).

Additional physiological evidence for a speech module has been provided by functional MRI (fMRI) studies (Benson, Whalen, Richardson, et al., 2001; Whalen, Benson, Richardson, et al., 2006), which found that changes in the complexity of speech versus nonspeech signals during passive listening resulted in different patterns of activation in the primary auditory and auditory association cortices.

POWER OF SPEECH SOUNDS

Several points about the power of speech sounds are noteworthy prior to a discussion of speech intelligibility. From the foregoing, we would expect to find most of the power of speech in the vowels, and since the vowels have a preponderance of low-frequency energy, we would expect the long-term average spectrum of speech to reflect this as well. This expectation is borne out by the literature (Fletcher, 1953). The weakest sound in English is the voiceless fricative /θ/ and the strongest is the vowel /ɔ/ (Sacia and Beck, 1926; Fletcher, 1953). If /θ/ is assigned a power of one, then the relative power of /ɔ/ becomes 680 (Fletcher, 1953). The relative power of the consonants range up to 80 for /ʃ/, are between 36 (/n/) and 73 (/ŋ/) for the nasals, are on the order of 100 for the semivowels, and range upward from 220 (/i/) for the vowels (Fletcher, 1953). As one would expect, the more powerful sounds are detected and are more intelligible at lower intensities than are the weaker ones.

The spectrograms shown earlier in this chapter show how the speech spectrum changes from moment to moment. In contrast, the spectrum of the speech signal over the long run is shown by the **long-term average speech spectrum (LTASS)**. Two sets of LTASS values are illustrated in Fig. 14.12 Here, we see the sound pressure levels at each frequency (actually in third-octave bands) when the overall speech level is 70 dB SPL. (If the overall speech level is higher or lower, then the

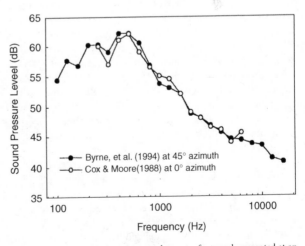

Figure 14.12 Long-term average speech spectra for speech presented at an overall level of 70 dB SPL. *Filled symbols*: composite of male and female speech samples from 12 languages at 45° azimuth (based on Byrne et al. (1994)). *Open symbols*: composite of male and female speech in English at 0° azimuth (based on Cox and Moore, 1988).

values shown on the y-axis would simply be scaled up or down proportionately.) The LTASS developed by Byrne et al. (1994) is identified by the closed symbols. This is an overall composite for male and female speech across 12 languages and was measured at an azimuth of 45°. Notice that these values are very similar to the LTASS described by Cox and Moore (1988) for combined male and female speech by using English materials presented from straight ahead of the listener (at 0° azimuth), which are identified by the open symbols.

The essential and expected implication of the material in Fig. 14.12 is that most of the energy in speech is found in the lower frequencies, particularly below about 1000 Hz, whereas intensity falls off as frequency increases above this range. It should be kept in mind that these curves show the relative speech spectrum averaged over time for male and female speakers combined. Although the LTASS tends to be similar for male and female speech in the 250 to 5000 Hz range, male levels are considerably higher at frequencies ≤160 Hz and female levels are slightly higher ≥6300 Hz (Byrne et al., 1994). The average overall sound pressure level of male speech tends to be on the order of 3 dB higher than that for females (e.g., Pearsons et al., 1977).

SPEECH INTELLIGIBILITY

In general, **speech intelligibility** refers to how well the listener receives and comprehends the speech signal. The basic approach to studying speech intelligibility is quite simple and direct. The subject is presented with a series of stimuli (syllables, words, phrases, etc.) and is asked to identify what he has heard. The results are typically reported as the percent correct, which is called the **speech recognition**, **discrimination**, or **articulation score** (Campbell, 1910; Fletcher and Steinberg, 1929; Egan, 1948). The approach may be further broken down into **open set** methods requiring the subject to repeat (or write) what was heard without prior knowledge of the corpus of test items (Egan, 1948; Hirsh et al., 1952; Peterson and Lehiste, 1962), and **closed set** methods that provide a choice of response alternatives from which the subject must choose (Fairbanks, 1958; House et al., 1965). These tests were originally devised in the development of telephone communication systems. The factors that contribute to speech intelligibility (or interfere with it) may be examined by obtaining articulation scores under various stimulus conditions and in the face of different kinds of distortions.

Audibility: Speech Level and Signal-to-Noise Ratio

It is well established that speech intelligibility improves as the speech signal becomes progressively more audible (Fletcher and Steinberg, 1929; French and Steinberg, 1947; Fletcher, 1953). The dependence of speech intelligibility on the audibility is seen as an increase in speech recognition performance with increasing speech level (Fig. 14.13a) or signal-to-noise ratio (Fig. 14.13b). In other words, there are **psychometric functions** for speech intelligibility as well as for the other psychoacoustic

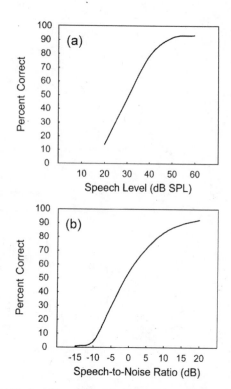

Figure 14.13 Speech recognition performance for single-syllable words improves with increasing (a) speech level and (b) speech-to-noise ratio. *Source*: Based on Gelfand (1998), used with permission.

phenomena we have discussed. As a rule, recognition performance generally becomes asymptotic when maximum intelligibility is reached for a given type of speech material; however, speech intelligibility may actually decrease if the level is raised to excessive levels.

Frequency

How much information about the speech signal is contained in various frequency ranges? The answer to this question is not only important in describing the frequencies necessary to carry the speech signal (an important concept if communication channels are to be used with maximal efficiency), but also may enable us to predict intelligibility. Egan and Wiener (1946) studied the effects upon syllable intelligibility of varying the bandwidth around 1500 Hz. They found that widening the bandwidth improved intelligibility, which reached 85% when a 3000-Hz bandwidth was available to the listener. Narrowing the passband resulted in progressively lower intelligibility; conversely, discrimination was improved by raising the level of the stimuli. That is, the narrower the band of frequencies, the higher the speech level must be in order to maintain the same degree of intelligibility.

French and Steinberg (1947) determined the intelligibility of male and female speakers under varying conditions of low- and high-pass filtering. Discrimination was measured while filtering out the high frequencies above certain cutoff points

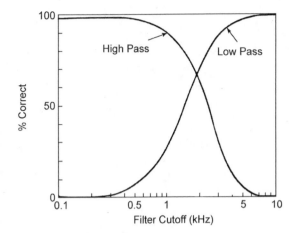

Figure 14.14 Syllable recognition as a function of high-pass and low-pass filtering. *Source*: Adapted from French and Steinberg (1947), with permission of *J. Acoust. Soc. Am.*

(low-pass), and while filtering out the lows below various cutoffs (high-pass). Increasing amounts of either high- or low-pass filtering reduced intelligibility, and performance fell to nil when the available frequencies (the passband) were limited to those below about 200 Hz or above roughly 6000 Hz. As illustrated in Fig. 14.14 the high- and low-pass curves intersected at approximately 1900 Hz, where discrimination was about 68%. In other words, roughly equivalent contributions accounting for 68% intelligibility each were found for the frequencies above and below 1900 Hz. (That the frequency ranges above and below 1900 Hz each accounted for 68% intelligibility is but one of many demonstrations of the redundancy of the speech signal.) One must be careful, however, not to attach any magical significance to this frequency or percentage. For example,

the crossover point dropped to about 1660 Hz only for male talkers. Furthermore, Miller and Nicely (1955) showed that the crossover point depends upon what aspect of speech (feature) is examined. Their high- and low-pass curves intersected at 450 Hz for the identification of nasality, 500 Hz for voicing, 750 Hz for frication, and 1900 Hz for place of articulation.

Amplitude Distortion

If the dynamic range of a system is exceeded, then there will be **peak-clipping** of the waveform. In other words, the peaks of the wave will be "cut off," as shown in Fig. 14.15 The resulting waveform approaches the appearance of a square wave, as the figure clearly demonstrates. The effects of clipping were studied by Licklider and colleagues (Licklider, 1946; Licklider et al., 1948; Licklider and Pollack, 1948), and the essential though surprising finding is that peak-clipping does not result in any appreciable decrease in speech intelligibility even though the waveform is quite distorted. On the other hand, if the peaks are maintained but the center portion of the wave is removed (*center-clipping*), then speech intelligibility quickly drops to nil.

Interruptions and Temporal Distortion

The effect of rapid interruptions upon word intelligibility was examined in a classical study by Miller and Licklider (1950). They electronically interrupted the speech waveform at rates from 0.1 to 10,000 times per second, and with speech–time fractions between 6.25 and 75%. The **speech–time fraction** is simply the proportion of the time that the speech signal is actually on. Thus, a 50% speech–time fraction means that the speech signal was on and off for equal amounts of time, while 12.5% indicates that the speech signal was actually presented 12.5% of the time.

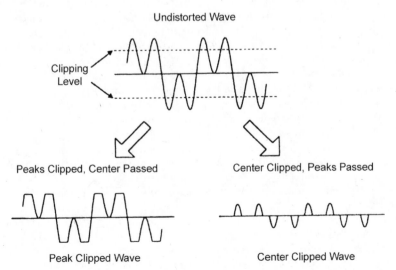

Figure 14.15 Effects of peak-clipping and center-clipping on the waveform. "Clipping level" indicates the amplitude above (or below) which clipping occurs.

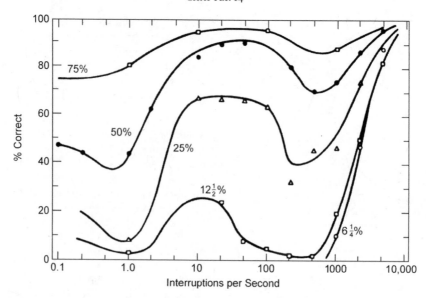

Figure 14.16 Discrimination as a function of interruption rate with speech–time fraction as the parameter. *Source*: Adapted from Miller and Licklider (1950), with permission of *J. Acoust. Soc. Am.*

For the lowest **interruption rate**, the signal was alternately on and off for several seconds at a time. Thus, the discrimination score was roughly equal to the percent of the time that the signal was actually presented. The results for faster interruption rates are also shown in Fig. 14.16 When the speech–time fraction was 50%, performance was poorest when the signal was interrupted about one time per second. This is an expected finding, because we would expect intelligibility to be minimal when the interruption is long enough to overlap roughly the whole test word. At much faster interruption rates, the subjects get many "glimpses" of the test word. That is, assuming a word duration of 0.6 s and five interruptions per second, there would be about three glimpses of each word, and so forth for higher interruption rates. (The dip in the function between 200 and 2000 interruptions per second may be due to an interaction between the speech signal and the square wave that was used to modulate the speech signal to produce the interruptions.) Looking now at the remaining curves in Fig. 14.16 we find that the more the speech signal was actually on, the better the discrimination performance; whereas when the speech–time fraction fell well below 50%, intelligibility dropped substantially at all interruption rates. Essentially similar findings were reported by Powers and Speaks (1973). We see from such observations the remarkable facility with which we can "piece together" the speech signal, as well as the considerable redundancy contained within the speech waveform.

Other forms of temporal distortion also substantially decrease speech intelligibility, and this is particularly so for speeding or time compression of the speech signal (e.g., Calearo and Lazzaroni, 1957; Fairbanks and Kodman, 1957; Beasley et al., 1972). Space and scope preclude any detailed discussion except

to note that intelligibility decreases progressively with speeding (or time compression) of the speech signal. An excellent review may be found in Beasley and Maki (1976).

Masking and Reverberation
The presentation of a noise has the effect of **masking** all or part of a speech signal. The general relationship between the effective level of the masker and the amount of masking for tones (Chap. 10) also holds true for the masking of speech by a broad-band noise (Hawkins and Stevens, 1950). That is, once the noise reaches an effective level, a given increment in noise level will result in an equivalent increase in speech threshold. Furthermore, this linear relationship between masker level and speech masking holds true for both the detection of the speech signal and intelligibility.

Recall from Chapter 10 that masking spreads upward in frequency, so that we would expect an intense low-frequency masker to be more effective in masking the speech signal than one whose energy is concentrated in the higher frequencies. This was confirmed by Stevens et al. (1946) and by Miller (1947). Miller also found that when noise bands were presented at lower intensities, the higher-frequency noise bands also reduced speech discrimination. This effect reflects the masking of consonant information concentrated in the higher frequencies.

Miller and Nicely (1955) demonstrated that the effect of a wide-band noise upon speech intelligibility is similar to that of low-pass filtering. This is expected, since a large proportion of the energy in the noise is concentrated in the higher frequencies. Both the noise and low-pass filtering resulted in rather systematic confusions among consonants, primarily affecting the correct identification of place of articulation. On the other hand, voicing and nasality, which rely heavily upon the lower frequencies, were minimally affected.

Reverberation is the persistence of acoustic energy in an enclosed space after the sound source has stopped; it is due to multiple reflections from the walls, ceiling, and floor of the enclosure (normally a room). The amount of reverberation is expressed in terms of **reverberation time**, which is simply how long it takes for the reflections to decrease by 60 dB after the sound source has been turned off.

It is a common experience that intelligibility decreases in a reverberant room, and this has been demonstrated in numerous studies, as well (e.g., Knudsen, 1929; Bolt and MacDonald, 1949; Nabelek and Pickett, 1974; Gelfand and Hochberg, 1976; Nabelek, 1976; Nabelek and Robinette, 1978; Gelfand and Silman, 1979; Helfer, 1994). The amount of discrimination impairment becomes greater as the reverberation time increases, particularly in small rooms where the reflections are "tightly packed" in time.

In one sense, reverberation appears to act as a masking noise in reducing speech intelligibility; however, this is an oversimplification. The reflected energy of reverberation overlaps the direct (original) speech signal, so that perceptual cues are masked, but there are at least two distinguishable masking effects: In **overlap masking**, a subsequent phoneme is masked by energy derived from a preceding speech sound, whereas **self-masking** occurs when cues are masked within the same phoneme. In addition, reverberation distorts phoneme cues by causing a smearing of the speech signal over time, thereby also causing confusions that are not typical of masking. As a result, we are not surprised to find that, for example, stops are especially susceptible to the effects of reverberation, and final consonants are affected to a greater extent than are initial ones (e.g., Knudsen, 1929; Gelfand and Silman, 1979).

Different speech intelligibility outcomes have been associated with reverberation, masking, and the two combined: Lower percent-correct scores are obtained with noise-plus-reverberation than what would have been predicted from the scores obtained with masking alone and reverberation alone (e.g., Nabelek and Mason, 1981; Harris and Reitz, 1985; Helfer, 1992); and differences have also been found between the patterns of the perceptual errors obtained with reverberation, masking, and the two combined (e.g., Nabelek et al., 1989; Tanaka and Nabelek, 1990; Helfer, 1994). In addition, reverberation and noise have been found to produce different errors for vowels, which were often associated with the time course of the signal (Nabelek and Letowski, 1985; Nabelek and Dagenais, 1986). The student will find several informative reviews of reverberation effects in the literature (e.g., Nabelek, 1976; Helfer, 1994; Nabelek and Nabelek, 1994). With these and the preceding points in mind, one should be aware that contemporary standards for classroom acoustics call for unoccupied noise levels of 35 dBA and reverberation times of 0.4 s (40 dBA

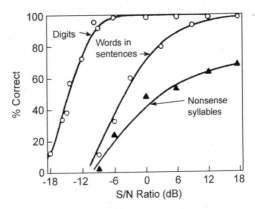

Figure 14.17 Psychometric functions showing the effects of test materials. *Source*: From Miller, Heise, and Lichten (1951), with permission of *J. Exp. Psychol.*

and 0.7 s for large rooms) and a SNR of +15 dB (ANSI S12.60, 2002; ASHA, 2004).

Nonacoustic Considerations

Speech perception depends on more than just the acoustical parameters of the speech signal. In their classical study, Miller, Heise, and Lichten (1951) asked subjects to discriminate (1) words in sentences, (2) digits from 0 to 9, and (3) nonsense (meaningless) syllables. A psychometric function was generated for each type of test material, showing percent correct performance as a function of SNR (Fig. 14.17). Note that the digits were audible at softer levels (lower SNRs) than were the words in sentences, which were in turn more accurately perceived than the nonsense syllables. We observe this result in several ways. First, at each SNR in the figure, percent-correct performance is best for the digits, less good for the words in sentences, and poorest for the syllables. Conversely, the subjects were able to repeat 50% of the digits at a level 17 dB softer than that needed to reach 50% correct for the monosyllables. Second, a small increase in SNR resulted in a substantial increase in digit discrimination but a much smaller improvement for the syllables, with improvement for word identification lying between these. Finally, notice that digit discrimination becomes asymptotic at 100% correct at low levels. On the other hand, words in sentences do not approach 100% intelligibility until the SNR reaches 18 dB, and monosyllable discrimination fails to attain even 70% at the highest SNR tested. Thus, we find that more redundant materials are more intelligible than the less redundant ones. In other words, we need only get a small part of the signal to tell one digit from another, whereas there is little other information for the subject to call upon if part of a nonsense syllable is unclear. For example, if one hears "-en" and knows in advance that the test item is a digit, the test is inordinately easier than when the initial sound might be *any* of the 25 or so consonants of English. Word redundancy falls between the exceptionally high redundancy of the digits and the rather minimal redundancy of the nonsense syllables. As expected, Miller and associates found that words were more intelligible in a sentence than when presented alone, which also reflects redundancy afforded by the context of the test item.

In a related experiment, Miller et al. (1951) obtained intelligibility measures for test vocabularies made up of 2, 4, 8, 16, 32, or 256 monosyllabic words, as well as for an "unrestricted" vocabulary of approximately 1000 monosyllables. The results were similar to those just described. The fewer the alternatives (i.e., the more redundant or predictable the message), the better the discrimination performance. As the number of alternatives increases, greater intensity (a higher SNR) was needed in order to obtain the same degree of intelligibility.

It should be clear from these classical examples that the perception of speech involves *top-down* processes as well as *bottom-up* processes.

SPEECH PERCEPTION THEORIES AND APPROACHES

Many theories and models explaining the nature of speech perception have been proposed over the years, and we will give an overview of some of the key features of several of these theories here. Students interested in pursuing these issues will find a number of contemporary reviews which approach the topic and its issues from a variety of perspectives (e.g., Jusczyk and Luce, 2002; Diehl et al., 2004; Remez, 2005; Galantucci et al., 2006; Pardo and Remez, 2006; Massaro and Chen, 2008). Notice while reading this material that most approaches to speech perception involve the interplay of both the incoming signal (*bottom-up processing*) as well as higher level cognitive influences (*top-down processing*).

Models Implicating the Production System
Motor Theory
Perhaps the most widely known speech perception theory is Liberman's **motor theory**, the details of which have evolved over the years (Liberman, 1996; Liberman et al., 1957, 1967; Liberman and Mattingly, 1985, 1989; Mattingly and Liberman, 1988; Liberman and Whalen, 2000). Recall that coarticulation causes a particular phonetic element to have different acoustical characteristics depending on its context (e.g., different formant transitions for /d/ in /di/ vs. /du/). Motor theory proposes that speech perception involves identifying the *intended speech gestures* (effectively the neuromotor instructions to the articulators) that resulted in the acoustical signal produced by the speaker and heard by the listener. In other words, we perceive the invariant intended phonetic gestures (e.g., release of the alveolar closure in /di/ and /du/) that are encoded in the variable acoustical signals. This perceptual process involves biologically evolved interactions between the speech *perception and production* systems, and is accomplished by a *specialized speech* or *phonetic module (mode)* in the central nervous system.

Direct Realist Theory
The **direct realist theory** developed by Fowler and colleagues (e.g., Fowler, 1986, 1991, 1996; Galantucci et al., 2006) is related to motor theory but certainly distinct from it. It is similar to motor theory in the sense that direct realist theory involves the perception of speech gestures and incorporates interactions with the motor system in speech perception. However, it differs from motor theory by making use of the sound signal reaching the listener to recover the *actual* articulatory gestures that produced them (as opposed to intended gestures), and does not involve a biologically specialized phonetic module.

Analysis-by-Synthesis
The speech production system is also involved in the **analysis-by-synthesis theory** (e.g., Stevens and Halle, 1967; Stevens, 1972), although the process is somewhat different from those of the motor and direct realist theories. Here, the perceptual decision about the speech signal is influenced by considering the articulatory manipulations that the listener might use to produce them, with the decision based on which of these gives the best match to the signal.

General Auditory Approaches
The **general auditory approaches** (Diehl et al., 2004) include a variety of descriptions and theories that address speech perception in terms of *auditory capabilities* and *perceptual learning* rather than the gesture perception and related mechanisms involved in the motor and direct realist theories. Having already addressed some of the findings supporting the notion that speech perception makes use of general auditory capabilities rather than a speech-specific phonetic module, let us turn our attention to the contribution of perceptual learning (for concise reviews see, e.g., Jusczyk and Luce, 2002; Diehl et al., 2004).

The effects of perceptual learning on speech perception is illustrated by comparing the speech sound discriminations of younger versus older infants. Recall that adults typically discriminate speech sound differences across the phoneme categories of their language, but not within these categories. Infants less than about six months of age can discriminate speech sounds within or across the phoneme categories of their language environment, but they become less responsive to differences falling within the phoneme categories of their language over the course of the next year or so (Werker, Gilbert, Humphrey, and Tees, 1981; Werker and Tees, 1984; Best, McRoberts, and Sithole, 1988; Pegg and Werker, 1997). As conceptualized by Kuhl and colleagues (e.g., Kuhl, 1991; Kuhl, Williams, Lacerda, et al., 1992), infants over about six months of age begin to employ phoneme category prototypes, which act as **perceptual magnets**. Here, speech patterns relatively close to the prototype are perceptually drawn to it and thus perceived as the same, whereas speech patterns sufficiently far from the prototype are perceived as different.

Fuzzy Logical Model of Perception

The **fuzzy logical model of perception** (**FLMP**; e.g., Ogden and Massaro, 1978; Massaro, 1987, 1998. Massaro and Chen, 2008) may be viewed as an example of a general auditory approach. Unlike the gesture perception approach of the motor and direct realist theories, the FLMP involves evaluating the auditory (and visual) features [2] of the stimulus and comparing them to prototypes of alternative speech categories in the listener's long term memory. Speech perception in this model involves three processes. (1) The evaluation process involves analyzing the features of the signal. The term "fuzzy" is used because the features are valued along a continuum from 0 to 1.0 instead being assessed on an all-or-none (present/absent) basis. (2) The integration process involves comparing the features with possible prototypes in the listener's long-term memory. (3) A decision is then made, which involves choosing the prototype with the best match to the features.

Word Recognition Models

Let us now briefly consider a number of speech perception models that concentrate on word recognition.

Prototype and Exemplar Models

Some word recognition approaches involve comparing the acoustical characteristics of the speech signal (as opposed abstract representations like phonetic features) to internalized perceptual references in the listener's long-term memory. In the **Lexical Access from Spectra (LAFS) model** (Klatt, 1989), the incoming speech spectra are compared to learned prototypes or templates. On the other hand, **exemplar models** involve comparing the incoming signal to all existing instances of the category in the listener's long-term memory (Johnson, 1997).

Logogen Model

The **Logogen model** (Morton, 1969) envisions the existence of recognition units called **logogens**.[3] The activation levels of the logogens increase as they accumulate acoustic, visual, and semantic information from the incoming signal, and a given logogen is triggered once its activation level reaches a certain threshold, at which point the corresponding word is recognized by the listener. Logogens associated with more commonly encountered words have lower thresholds so that higher frequencies words are more likely to be recognized than lower thresholds words.

Cohort Model

Word recognition in the **Cohort model** (Marslen-Wilson and Welsh, 1978; Marslen-Wilson and Tyler, 1980) involves progres-

sively reducing the viable alternatives in the listener's lexicon until a decision can be reached and is based on both a bottom-up analysis of the sound pattern and top-down considerations such as syntactic and semantic constraints on the possible alternatives. Consider the word *remarkable*. The /r/ activates a *cohort* of all words in the listener's lexicon beginning with that sound. Then, the cohort is progressively narrowed with each successive aspect of the word over time. For example, /ri/ limits the cohort to words beginning with /ri/ (*read*, *real*, *recent*, *relax*, *remarkable*, etc.); /rim/ narrows the cohort to words like *ream*, *remember*, *remark*, *remarkable*, etc.; /rimɑrk/ limits it to just *remark*, *remarks*, *remarked*, *remarking*, and *remarkable*; and /rimɑrkə/ finally reduces the cohort to *remarkable* (which is thus chosen). It is noteworthy that the various competing alternatives do not inhibit each other at each stage of the analysis. For example, activation of *remarkable* by /rim/ does not affect activation of *remember*, which falls out of the corpus when the stimulus analysis reaches /rimɑrk/. Bottom-down considerations are easily understood by considering how the cohort of possible alternatives is delimited by semantic and syntactic considerations when the word *remarkable* appears in different sentences (e.g., *That magic trick was remarkable.* vs. *The remarkable event that I will describe is....*).

Trace Model

The **Trace model** of word recognition (Elman and McClelland, 1986; McClelland and Elman, 1986; Elman, 1989) is a connectionist model, which means that it involves interconnected elements that influence each other. The elements of a connectionist model are called *units*, which can be activated to a greater or lesser degree, and the connections between the units are called *links*. Signals from *excitatory* links increase a unit's activation level, and signals from *inhibitory* links decrease the activation level. The recognition of a particular word in the Trace model involves three levels of units (features, phonemes, and word), with interactions both within and across these levels. Interactions within a particular level are inhibitory so that the representation of one unit (e.g., /t/ at the phoneme level, or *bite* at the word level) prevents activation of competing units (e.g., /g/ or /m/ at the phoneme level, or *sight* at the word level). On the other hand, interactions across levels are excitatory (e.g., the representation of voicelessness at the feature level enhances the representation of voicelessness at other levels as well).

Shortlist Model

The **Shortlist model** (Norris, 1994) is a bottom-up connectionist approach to word recognition. In this two-stage model, the incoming speech signal activates a "short list" of viable word choices on a bottom-up basis (that is analogous to Cohort but unlike Trace), which are then subjected to inhibitory competition (that is unlike Cohort but similar to Trace).

---

[2] Consideration of the auditory and visual features of the stimulus allows FLMP to account for the McGurk effect.

[3] The term *logogen* was coined by Hallowell Davis based on *logos* for *word* and *genus* for *birth* (Morton (1969).

CHAPTER 14

Neighborhood Activation Model

The **neighborhood activation model** (**NAM**; Luce, 1990; Kirk et al., 1995; Luce and Pisoni, 1998) attempts to account for how lexical neighborhoods and word frequency affect the identification of a word. The **lexical neighborhood** of a word is comprised of similar sounding alternatives. Words that have many similar sounding alternatives have *dense lexical neighborhoods*, and words with few similar sounding alternatives have *sparse lexical neighborhoods* (Luce, 1990; Kirk et al., 1995; Luce and Pisoni, 1998). Confusions are more likely to occur when there are many viable (similar sounding) alternatives, so that words with denser lexical neighborhoods are more difficult to recognize than other words with sparser lexical neighborhoods. **Word frequency** comes into play because we are significantly biased in favor of more frequently occurring words over those of lower frequency (e.g., Rosenzweig and Postman, 1957). According to the NAM, the sound patterns of a word are compared to acoustic–phonetic representations in the listener's memory. The probability of a representation being activated depends the degree to which it is similar to the stimulus. The next step is a lexical selection process among the words in memory that are potential matches to the stimulus, which is biased according to word frequency. A connectionist variation of NAM called **PARSYM** (Luce, Stephen, Auer, and Vitevitch, 2000; Auer and Luce, 2005) also accounts for probabilities of occurrence of different allophones in a various positions.

Speech Intelligibility and Acoustical Measurements

Speech intelligibility under given conditions can be estimated or predicted using a number of acoustical methods, such as the articulation index and the speech transmission index. The **articulation index** (**AI**) was introduced by French and Steinberg (1947). The AI estimates speech intelligibility by considering how much of the speech signal is audible above the listener's threshold as well as the signal-to-noise ratio. In its original formulation, the basic concept of the AI involves the use of 20 contiguous frequency bands, each of which contributes the same proportion (0.05 or 5%) to the overall intelligibility of the message. These bands are then combined into a single number from 0 to 1.0, which is the articulation index.

In general, a given band is given full credit if all of the speech signal it contains is above threshold and also has a high enough signal-to-noise ratio. Assuming that the speech level in a band is well above threshold, then it would receive given full credit (0.05) if its SNR is at least +18 dB, and would receive partial credit for poorer SNRs down to −12 dB, where that band's contribution is zero. The resulting part of the band's potential value of 0.05 is its contribution; the sum of the 20 values (one from each band) becomes the AI, which therefore has a range between 0 and 1.0. (The interested reader should consult the sources mentioned in this section for details of how to calculate the various versions of the AI.)

French and Steinberg's original AI, which employed 20 equally weighted bandwidths, has been modified in various ways

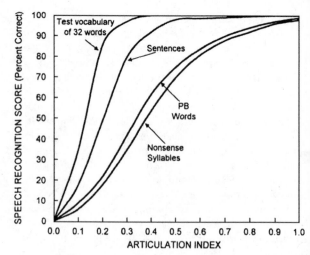

Figure 14.18 Relationship between the articulation index and speech recognition scores for selected speech materials. *Source*: Based on Kryter (1962b, 1985) and ANSI (1969, R1986).

since its original description (e.g., Beranek, 1947; Kryter, 1962a, 1962b, 1985; ANSI S3.5-1969, [R1986]; Pavlovic, Studebaker, and Sherbecoe, 1986; Pavlovic, 1987; ANSI S3.5-1997[R2007]; Rhebergen and Versfeld, 2005). The current version, known as the **speech intelligibility index** (**SII**) involves the use of standard third-octave and octave-bands, adjustments in importance weightings given to each band, as well as other modifications (ANSI S3.5 1997[R2007]).

The articulation index and the speech intelligibility are reasonably good predictors of actual speech recognition performance for a variety of speech materials (e.g., Kryter, 1962a, 1962b, 1985; Rhebergen and Versfeld, 2005). Figure 14.18 shows some examples of the way in which the AI is related to intelligibility scores for various kinds of speech materials. Notice that an AI of 0.5 corresponds to speech recognition scores of about 70% for nonsense syllables, 75% for phonetically balanced (PB) monosyllabic test words, 97% for sentences, and 100% when the test vocabulary is limited to only 32 words. The student should consider these differences in light of the discussion of the effects of test materials (and Fig. 14.17) earlier in this chapter. Beranek (1954/1986) proposed that the conditions for speech communication can be guesstimated as probably satisfactory when the AI is higher than 0.6 and most likely unsatisfactory when the AI is lower than 0.3. According to the material in Fig. 14.18 an AI of 0.6 is associated with speech recognition scores of approximately 98% for sentences and 85% for words, whereas speech intelligibility falls to about 80% for sentences and 45% for words when the AI is only 0.3.

The SII is based on the use a steady noise, but speech communication often occurs against a background of noise that fluctuates over time. To address this limitation, Rhebergen and Versfeld (2005) developed a modification of the SII for that can be used with fluctuating noises. Fundamentally, their

272

modification involves obtaining individual SII values within many successive time frames, which are then averaged to arrive at the overall SII value. They found that their approach produces more appropriate SII values for fluctuating noises and the same results as the standard SII for steady noises. With this method, Rhebergen and Versfeld showed that 50% correct sentence reception in noise occurs when the SII is 0.35, corresponding to SNRs of about −4.5 dB for steady noises and −12 dB for fluctuating noises.

The articulation index has been applied to the speech recognition of the hearing-impaired in a variety of ways. Although this topic is outside of the current scope, the interested student will find numerous papers dealing with this topic throughout the current literature (e.g., Pavlovic et al., 1986; Steeneken and Houtgast, 1980; Kamm et al., 1985; Humes et al., 1986; Pavlovic, 1988, 1991).

Beranek (1954/1986) introduced a simplified modification of the articulation index that estimates the amount of noise that will just allow speech communication to take place at various levels of vocal effort and distances between the talker and listener, is known as the **speech interference level (SIL)**. The SIL is simply the average of the noise levels that occur in three or four selected bands. The 500, 1000, 2000, and 4000 Hz octave bands are used in the current standard version of the SIL (ANSI, 1977, R1986). Several informative discussions of the SIL are available to the interested reader (e.g., Beranek, 1954/1986; Webster, 1978; ANSI-S3.14-1977 (R1997); Lazarus, 1987).

Another approach to estimate speech intelligibility from acoustical measurements is the **speech transmission index (STI)**, which is based upon the **modulation transfer function (MTF)**. This technique was originated by Steeneken and Houtgast (1980). In addition to their work, the interested reader should also refer to informative sources (e.g., Humes et al., 1986; Anderson and Kalb, 1987; Schmidt-Nielsen, 1987; Steeneken, 2006; van Wijngaarden and Drullman, 2008). An important advantage of the STI is that it accounts for the effects of all kinds of noises and distortions that affect the speech signal, including reverberation and other aberrations that occur over time.

Determining the STI begins by obtaining MTF results in the octave-bands from 125 to 8000 Hz. These results are used to produce a *transmission index* for each of the octave-bands, which are in turn adjusted by weighting factors that account for the importance of each band for speech communication. The weighted results are then combined to arrive at an STI, which can range in value from 0 to 1.0. Fig. 14.19 shows the STI and speech recognition performance for reprehensive kinds of test materials.

The **rapid speech transmission index (RASTI)** is an efficient and relatively simple method for making STI measurements using special instrumentation designed for this purpose (e.g., Bruel and Kjaer, 1985; IEC, 1987). A loudspeaker is placed in the room or other environment being tested at the location where a talker would be, and a microphone is placed at the

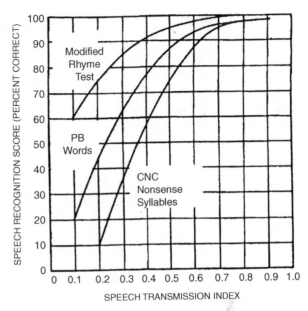

Figure 14.19 Relationship between the speech transmission index and speech recognition scores for selected speech materials. *Source*: Adapted from Anderson and Kalb (1987) with permission of *J. Acoust. Soc. Am.*

listener's location. The signal arriving at the microphone thus incorporates all of the ways in which the original signal has been modified by the noise, reverberation, and other acoustical features of the room. The RASTI equipment then provides the results as a value ranging from 0 to 1.0. Orfield (1987) proposed that relative speech intelligibility may be inferred from the outcome of RASTI testing as follows: RASTI values of 0.75 or higher may be considered *excellent*; 0.6–0.74 are *good*; 0.45–0.59 are *fair*; 0.3–0.44 are *poor*; and values of 0.29 or lower are considered *bad*.

CLEAR SPEECH

We know from common experience that we sometimes modify the way we talk when trying to maximize the clarity of our speech. This kind of speech is appropriately called **clear speech** (Picheny, Durlach, and Braida, 1985). Clear speech is used when we are trying to make our speech as intelligible as possible for the benefit of a hearing-impaired listener, or perhaps when speaking under adverse acoustical conditions.

The acoustical characteristics and perceptual impact of clear speech have been described in considerable detail (Picheny et al., 1985, 1986, 1989; Moon and Lindblom, 1994; Payton et al., 1994; Schum, 1996; Uchanski et al., 1996; Liu and Zeng, 2004, 2006; Krause and Braida, 2002, 2004; Liu, Del Rio, Bradlow, and Zeng, 2004; Kain, Amano-Kusumoto, and Hosom, 2008). Several of the acoustical distinctions between clear and conversational speech may be seen by comparing the two spectrograms

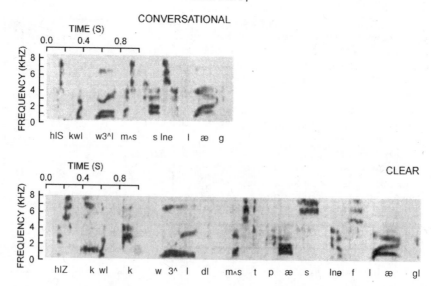

Figure 14.20 Spectrographic examples of conversational speech (above) and clear speech (below) produced by the same talker. *Source*: From Picheny, Durlach, and Braida (1986), with permission of the American Speech-Language-Hearing Association.

in Fig. 14.20. Clear speech involves a decrease in speaking rate so that it is slower or longer in duration than conversational speech. However, the durational difference is more than simply a matter of talking slowly. The increased duration of clear speech is due to *both* the insertion of more and longer pauses *and* increases in the durations of many of the individual speech sounds. In addition, instead of a uniform lengthening of all speech sounds, duration increases depend on the characteristics of the phonemes and their acoustical contexts. Moreover, there also tends to be greater variation in fundamental frequency and a greater degree of temporal modulation. Differences in the nature of the phonemes produced during clear and conversational speech are seen, as well. For example, all stop bursts and most final position consonants are released in clear speech, whereas this usually does not occur in conversational speech. Also, there are much less vowel modifications (e.g., vowel reduction) in clear speech than in conversational speech.

Another distinction is that clear speech involves greater amplitudes in the higher frequencies, with increased intensity for obstruent sounds, especially for the stops, which can be as much as 10 dB higher than in conversational speech. Related to this is the point that the relative power of consonants to vowels (consonant-to-vowel ratio) increases during clear speech. This contrasts with what occurs during loud conversational speech, where the consonant-to-vowel ratio decreases.

Does clear speech successfully accomplish its goal of providing improved intelligibility? The answer to this question is clearly yes. Improved speech intelligibility for clear speech compared to conversational speech has been a uniform finding under a variety of listening situations, including such adverse conditions as noise and/or reverberation, and these advantages are enjoyed by normal-hearing people as well as those with

hearing loss and learning disabilities (Picheny et al., 1985, 1989; Payton et al., 1994; Schum, 1996; Uchanski et al., 1996; Helfer, 1997; Bradlow and Bent, 2002; Ferguson and Kewley-Port, 2002; Gagne et al., 1995; Krause and Braida, 2002; Bradlow, Kraus, and Hayes, 2003; Liu et al., 2004).

REFERENCES

Abramson, AS, Lisker, L. 1970. *Discriminability along the voicing continuum: Cross-language tests.* Proceedings of the Sixth International Congress on Phonetic Science. Prague, Czech Republic: Academia, 569–573.

American National Standards Institute (ANSI). 1986. *S3.5-1969 (R1986): American national standard methods for the calculation of the articulation index.* New York, NY: ANSI.

American National Standards Institute (ANSI). 1997. *ANSI-S3.14-1977(R1997): American national standard for rating noise with respect to speech interference.* New York, NY: ANSI.

American National Standards Institute (ANSI). 2002. *S12.60-2002 Acoustical performance criteria, design requirements, and guidelines for schools.* New York, NY: ANSI.

American National Standards Institute (ANSI). 2007. *S3.5-1997(R2007) American national standard methods for calculation of the speech intelligibility index.* New York, NY: ANSI.

American Speech-Language-Hearing Association (ASHA). 2004. Acoustics in educational settings: Position statement. Available at http://www.asha.org/about/leadership projects/LC/spring04/ LCAHS12004PS.htm.

Anderson, BW, Kalb, JT. 1987. English verification of the STI method for estimating speech intelligibility of a communications channel. *J Acoust Soc Am* 81, 1982–1985.

Arkebauer, JH, Hixon, TJ, Hardy, JC. 1967. Peak intraoral air pressure during speech. *J Speech Hear Res* 10, 196–208.

Auer, ET Jr, Luce, PA. 2005. Probabilistic phonotactics in spoken word recognition. In: DB Pisoni, RE Remez (eds), *The Handbook of Speech Perception*. Oxford, MA: Blackwell, 610–630.

Beasley, DS, Maki, JE. 1976. Time- and frequency-altered speech. In: EC Carterette, MP Friedman (eds.), *Handbook of Perception. Vol. 7: Language and Speech*. New York, NY: Academic Press, 419–458.

Beasley, DS, Schwimmer, S, Rintelmann, WF. 1972. Intelligibility of time-compressed CNC monosyllables. *J Speech Hear Res* 15, 340–350.

Behrens, S, Blumstein, SE. 1988. On the role of the amplitude of the fricative noise in the perception of place of articulation in voiceless fricative consonants. *J Acoust Soc Am* 84, 861–867.

Benson, R, Whalen, DH, Richardson, M, Swainson, B, Clark, VP, Lai, S, Liberman, AM. 2001. Parametrically dissociating speech and nonspeech perception in the brain using fMRI. *Brain Lang* 78, 364–396.

Beranek, LL. 1947. The design of communication systems. *IRE Proc* 35, 880–890.

Beranek, LL. 1954/1986. *Acoustics*. New York, NY: Acoustical Society of America.

Berlin, CI, McNeil, MR. 1976. Dichotic listening. In: NJ Lass (ed.), *Contemporary Issues in Experimental Phonetics*. New York, NY: Academic Press, 327–387.

Berlin, CI, Lowe-Bell, SS, Cullen, JK, Thompson, CL, Loovis, CF. 1973. Dichotic speech perception: An interpretation of right-ear advantage and temporal-offset effects. *J Acoust Soc Am* 53, 699–709.

Bertoncini, J, Bijeljas-Babic, R, Jusczyk, P, Kennedy, L, Mehler, J. 1988. An investigation of young infants' perceptual representations of speech sounds. *J Exp Psychol: Gen* 117, 21–33.

Best, CT, McRoberts, GW, Sithole, NM. 1988. Examination of perceptual reorganization for nonnative speech contrasts: Zulu click discrimination by English-speaking adults and infants. *J Exp Psychol Hum Percept Perform* 14, 345–360.

Blumstein, SE, Stevens, KN. 1979. Acoustic invariance in speech production: Evidence from measurements of the spectral characteristics of stop consonants. *J Acoust Soc Am* 66, 1001–1017.

Blumstein, SE, Stevens, KN. 1980. Perceptual invariance and onset spectra for stop consonants indifferent vowel environments. *J Acoust Soc Am* 67, 648–662.

Blumstein, SE, Isaacs, E, Mertus, J. 1982. The role of gross spectral shape as a perceptual cue to place of articulation in initial stop consonants. *J Acoust Soc Am* 72, 43–50.

Bolt, RH, MacDonald, AD. 1949. Theory of speech masking by reverberation. *J Acoust Soc Am* 21, 577–580.

Bradlow, AR, Bent, T. 2002. The clear speech effect for nonnative listeners. *J Acoust Soc Am* 112, 272–284.

Bradlow, AR, Kraus, N, Hayes, E. 2003. Speaking clearly for children with learning disabilities: Sentence perception in noise. *J Speech Lang Hear Res* 46, 80–97.

Broadbent, DE. 1954. The role of auditory localization in attention and memory span. *J Exp Psychol* 47,191–196.

Broadbent, DE. 1956. Successive responses to simultaneous stimuli. *Q J Exp Psychol* 8, 145–152.

Bruel and Kjaer. 1985. *The modulation transfer function in room acoustics. RASTI: A tool for evaluating auditoria.* Technical Review No. 3-1985. Massachusetts: Bruel & Kjaer.

Byrne, D, Dillon, H, Tran, K, Arlinger, K, Cox, R, Hagerman, B, Hetu, R, Kei, J, Lui, C, Kiessling, J, Kotby, MN, Nasser, N, El Kholy, AH, Nakanishi, Y, Oyer, H, Powell, R, Stephens, D, Meredith, R, Sirimanna, T, Tavartkiladze, G, Frolenkov, GI, Westerman, S, Ludvigsen, C. 1994. An international comparison of long-term average speech spectra. *J Acoust Soc Am* 96, 2108–2120.

Calearo, C, Lazzaroni, A. 1957. Speech intelligibility in relation to the speed of the message. *Laryngoscope* 67, 410–419.

Campbell, GA. 1910. Telephonic intelligibility. *Philos Mag* 19, 152–159.

Colin, C, Radeau, M, Soquet, A, Demolin, D, Colin, F, Deltenre, P. 2002. Mismatch negativity evoked by the McGurk–MacDonald effect: A phonetic representation within short-term memory. *Clin Neurophysiol* 113, 495–506.

Colin, C, Radeau, M, Soquet, A, Deltenre, P. 2004. Generalization of the generation of an MMN by illusory McGurk percepts: Voiceless consonants. *Clin Neurophysiol* 115, 1989–2000.

Cooper, FS, Delattre, PC, Liberman, AM, Borst, JM, Gerstman, LJ. 1952. Some experiments on the perception of synthetic speech sounds. *J Acoust Soc Am* 24, 597–617.

Cooper, WE, Blumstein, SA. 1974. A "labial" feature analyzer in speech perception. *Percept Psychophys* 15, 591–600.

Cox, RM, Moore, JN. 1988. Composite speech spectrum for hearing aid gain prescriptions. *J Speech Hear Res* 31, 102–107.

Cullen, JK, Thompsen, CL, Hughes, LF, Berlin, CI, Samson, DS. 1974. The effects of various acoustic parameters on performance in dichotic speech perception tasks. *Brain Lang* 1, 307–322.

Cutting, JE, Rosner, BS. 1974. Categories and boundaries in speech and music. *Percept Psychophys* 16, 564–570.

Darwin, CJ. 1971. Dichotic backward masking of complex sounds. *Q J Exp Psychol* 23, 386–392.

Delattre, PC, Liberman, AM, Cooper, FS. 1955. Acoustic loci and transitional cues for consonants. *J Acoust Soc Am* 27, 769–773.

Delattre, PC, Liberman, AM, Cooper, FS, Gerstman, LJ. 1952. An experimental study of the acoustic determinants of vowel color; Observations on one- and two-formant vowels synthesized from spectrographic patterns. *Word* 8, 195–210.

Diehl, RL, Lotto, AJ, Holt, LL. 2004. Speech perception. *Ann Rev Psychol* 55, 149–179.

Dooling, RJ, Best, CT, Brown, SD. 1995. Discrimination of synthetic full-formant and sinewave /ra-la/ continua by budgerigars (*Melopsittacus undulatus*) and zebra finches (*Taeniopygia guttata*). *J Acoust Soc Am* 97, 1839–1846.

Egan, JP. 1948. Articulation testing methods, *Laryngoscope* 58, 955–981.

Egan, JP, Wiener, FM. 1946. On the intelligibility of bands of speech in noise. *J Acoust Soc Am* 18, 435–441.

Eimas, P. 1974. Auditory and linguistic processing of cues for place of articulation by infants. *Percept Psychophys* 16, 513–521.

Eimas, P, Corbit, JD. 1973. Selective adaptation of linguistic feature detectors. *Cogn Psychol* 4, 99–109.

Eimas, P, Siqueland, P, Jusczyk, P, Vigorito, J. 1971. Speech perception in infants. *Science* 171, 303–306.

Elangovan, S, Stuart, A. 2008. Natural boundaries in gap detection are related to categorical perception of stop consonants. *Ear Hear* 29, 761–774.

Elman, JL. 1989. Connectionist approaches to acoustic/phonetic processing. In: WD Marslen-Wilson (ed.), *Lexical Representation and Process*. Cambridge, MA: MIT Press, 227–260

Elman, JL, McClelland, JL. 1986. Exploiting lawful variability in the speech wave. In: JS Perkell, DH Klatt (eds.), *Invariance and Variability in Speech Processes*. Hillsdale, NJ: Erlbaum, 360–380.

Fairbanks, G. 1958. Test of phonemic differentiation: The rhyme test. *J Acoust Soc Am* 30, 596–600.

Fairbanks, G, Kodman, F. 1957. Word intelligibility as a function of time compression. *J Acoust Soc Am* 29, 636–641.

Fant, G. 1970. *Acoustic Theory of Speech Perception*. The Hague: Mouton.

Ferguson, SH, Kewley-Port, D. 2002. Vowel intelligibility in clear and conversational speech for normal-hearing and hearing-impaired listeners. *J Acoust Soc Am* 112, 259–271.

Ferrand, CT. 2007. *Speech Science*. 2nd ed. Boston, MA: Allyn and Bacon.

Fischer-Jorgensen, E. 1954. Acoustic analysis of stop consonants. *Misc Phonet* 2, 42–59.

Flanagan, JL. 1958. Some properties of the glottal sound source. *J Speech Hear Res* 1, 99–116.

Flanagan, JL. 1972. *Speech Analysis Synthesis and Perception*. New York, NY: Springer-Verlag.

Fletcher, H. 1953. *Speech and Hearing in Communication*. New York, NY: Van Nostrand.

Fletcher, H, Steinberg, JC. 1929. Articulation testing methods. *Bell Sys Tech J* 8, 848–852.

Formby, C, Barker, C, Abbey, H, Raney, JJ. 1993. Detection of silent temporal gaps between narrow-band noise markers having second-formant like properties of voiceless stop/vowel combinations. *J Acoust Soc Am* 93, 1023–1027.

Fowler, CA. 1986. An event approach to the study of speech perception from a direct realist perspective. *J Phon* 14, 3–28.

Fowler, CA. 1991. Auditory perception is not special: We see the world, we feel the world, we hear the world. *J Acoust Soc Am* 89, 2910–2915.

Fowler, CA. 1996. Listeners do hear sounds, not tongues. *J Acoust Soc Am* 99, 1730–1741.

Fowler, CA, Rosenblum, LD. 1991. Duplex perception: A comparison of monosyllables and slamming doors. *J Exp Psychol Hum Percept Perform* 16, 742–754.

French, NR, Steinberg, GC. 1947. Factors governing the intelligibility of speech. *J Acoust Soc Am* 19, 90–114.

Fry, D, Abramson, A, Eimas, P, Liberman, AM. 1962. The identification and discrimination of synthetic vowels. *Lang Speech* 5, 171–189

Fujimura, O. 1962. Analysis of nasal consonants. *J Acoust Soc Am* 34, 1865–1875.

Furui, S. 1986. On the role of spectral transition for speech perception. *J Acoust Soc Am* 80, 1016–1025.

Gagne, J, Querengesser, C, Folkeard, P, Munhall, K, Mastern, V. 1995. Auditory, visual and audiovisual speech intelligibility for sentence-length stimuli: An investigation of conversational and clear speech. *Volta Rev* 97, 33–51.

Galantucci, B, Fowler, CA, Turvey, MT. 2006. The motor theory of speech perception reviewed. *Psychon Bull Rev* 13, 361–377.

Gelfand, SA. 1998. Optimizing the reliability of speech recognition scores. *J Speech Lang Hear Res* 41, 1088–1102.

Gelfand, SA, Hochberg, I. 1976. Binaural and monaural speech discrimination under reverberation. *Audiology* 15, 72–84.

Gelfand, SA, Silman, S. 1979. Effects of small room reverberation upon the recognition of some consonant features. *J Acoust Soc Am* 66, 22–29.

Guerlekian, JA. 1981. Recognition of the Spanish fricatives /s/ and /f/. *J Acoust Soc Am* 79 1624–1627.

Haggard, MP, Ambler, S, Callow, M. 1970. Pitch as a voicing cue. *J Acoust Soc Am* 47, 613–617.

Halle, M, Hughes, GW, Radley, JPA 1957. Acoustic properties of stop consonants. *J Acoust Soc Am* 29, 107–116.

Harris, KS. 1958. Cues for the discrimination of American English fricatives in spoken syllables. *Lang Speech* 1, 1–7.

Harris, KS, Hoffman, HS, Liberman, AM, Delattre, PC, Cooper, FS. 1958. Effect of third formant transitions on the perception of the voiced stop consonants. *J Acoust Soc Am* 30, 122–126.

Harris, RW, Reitz, ML. 1985. Effects of room reverberation and noise on speech discrimination by the elderly. *Audiology* 24, 319–324.

Hawkins, JE, Stevens, SS. 1950. The masking of pure tones and of speech by white noise. *J Acoust Soc Am* 22, 6–13.

Heinz, JM, Stevens, N. 1961. On the properties of voiceless fricative consonants. *J Acoust Soc Am* 33, 589–596.

Helfer, KS. 1992. Aging and the binaural advantage in reverberation and noise. *J Speech Hear Res* 35, 1394–1401.

Helfer, KS. 1994. Binaural cues and consonant perception in reverberation and noise. *J Speech Hear Res* 37, 429–438.

Helfer, KS. 1997. Auditory and auditory-visual perception of clear and conversational speech. *J Speech Lang Hear Res* 40, 432–443.

Hillenbrand, J, Getty, LA, Clark, MJ, Wheeler, K. 1995. Acoustic characteristics of American English vowels. *J Acoust Soc Am* 97, 3099–3111.

Hirsh, IJ, Davis, H, Silverman, SR, Reynolds, ER, Eldert, E, Benson, RW. 1952. Development of materials for speech audiometry. *J Speech Hear Dis* 17, 321–337.

House, AS. 1957. Analog studies of nasal consonants. *J Acoust Soc Am* 22, 190–204.

House, AS, Fairbanks, G. 1953. The influence of consonant environment upon the secondary characteristics of vowels. *J Acoust Soc Am* 25, 105–113.

House, A, Williams, C, Hecker, H, Kryter, A. 1965. Articulation-testing methods: Consonantal differentiations with a close-response set. *J Acoust Soc Am* 37, 158–166.

Hughes, GW, Halle, M. 1956. Spectral properties of fricative consonants. *J Acoust Soc Am* 28, 303–310.

Humes, LE, Dirks, DD, Bell, TS, Ahlstrom, C, Kincaid, GE. 1986. Application of the Articulation index and the speech transmission index to the recognition of speech by normal hearing and hearing-impaired listeners. *J Speech Hear Res* 29, 447–462.

International Electrotechnical Commission (IEC). 1987. *Publ. 268: Sound system equipment part 16: Report on the RASTI method for objective rating of speech intelligibility in auditoria.*

Jassem, W. 1965. The formants of fricative consonants. *Lang Speech* 8, 1–16.

Johnson, K. 1997. Speech perception without speaker normalization: An exemplar model. In: K Johnson, JW Mullennix (eds.), Talker Variability in Speech Processing. San Diego, CA: Academic, 145–165.

Jongman, A. 1985. Duration of fricative noise as a perceptual cue to place and manner of articulation in English fricatives. *J Acoust Soc Am* 77(Suppl 1), S26.

Josse, G, Mazoyer, B, Crivello, F, Tzourio-Mazoyer, N. 2003. Left planum temporale: An anatomical marker of left hemispheric specialization for language comprehension. *Brain Res Cogn Brain Res* 18, 1–14.

Jusczyk, PW, Luce, PA. 2002. Speech perception and spoken word recognition: Past and present. *Ear Hear* 23, 2–40.

Kain, A, Amano-Kusumoto, A, Hosom, JP. 2008. Hybridizing conversational and clear speech to determine the degree of contribution of acoustic features to intelligibility. *J Acoust Soc Am* 124, 2308–2319.

Kamm, CA, Dirks, DD, Bell, TS. 1985. Speech recognition and the articulation index for normal and hearing impaired listeners. *J Acoust Soc Am* 77, 281–288.

Kent, RD, Read, C. 2002. *The Acoustic Analysis of Speech*, 2nd ed. New York, NY: Delmar.

Kewley-Port, D. 1983. Time-varying features as correlates of place of articulation in stop consonants. *J Acoust Soc Am* 73, 322–335.

Kewley-Port, D, Luce, PA. 1984. Time-varying features of stop consonants in auditory running spectra: A first report. *Percept Psychophys* 35, 353–360.

Kimura, D. 1961. Cerebral dominance and the perception of verbal stimuli. *Can J Psychol* 15, 166–171.

Kimura, D. 1964. Left-right differences in the perception of melodies. *Q J Exp Psychol* 16, 355–358.

Kimura, D. 1967. Functional asymmetry of the brain in dichotic listening. *Cortex* 3, 163–178.

Kirk, KI, Pisoni, DB, Osberger, MJ. 1995. Lexical effects on spoken word recognition by pediatric cochlear implant users. *Ear Hear* 16, 470–481.

Knudsen, VO. 1929. The hearing of speech in auditoriums. *J Acoust Soc Am* 1, 56–82.

Koenig, W, Dunn, HK, Lacy, LY. 1946. The sound spectrograph. *J Acoust Soc Am* 17, 19–49.

Krause, JC, Braida, LD. 2002. Investigating alternative forms of clear speech: The effects of speaking rate and speaking mode on intelligibility. *J Acoust Soc Am* 112, 2165–2172.

Krause, JC, Braida, LD. 2004. Acoustic properties of naturally produced clear speech at normal speaking rates. *J Acoust Soc Am* 115, 362–378.

Kryter, KD. 1962a. Methods for the calculation and use of the articulation index. *J Acoust Soc Am* 34, 1689–1697.

Kryter, KD. 1962b. Validation of the articulation index. *J Acoust Soc Am* 34, 1698–1702.

Kryter, KD. 1985. *The Effects of Noise on Man*, 2nd ed. New York, NY: Academic Press.

Kuhl, PK. 1991. Human adults and human infants show a 'perceptual magnet effect' for the prototypes of speech categories, monkeys do not. *Percept Psychophys* 50, 93–107.

Kuhl, PK, Miller, JD. 1975. Speech perception by the chinchilla: Voice–voiceless distinctions in alveolar plosive consonants. *Science* 190, 69–72.

Kuhl, PK, Miller, JD. 1978. Speech perception by the chinchilla: Identification functions for synthetic VOT stimuli. *J Acoust Soc Am* 63, 905–917.

Kuhl, PK, Padden, DM. 1982. Enhanced discriminability at the phonetic boundaries for the voicing feature in macaques. *Percept Psychophys* 32, 542–550.

Kuhl, PK, Padden, DM. 1983. Enhanced discriminability at the phonetic boundaries for the place feature in macaques. *J Acoust Soc Am* 73, 1003–1010.

Kuhl, PK, Williams, KA, Lacerda, F, Stevens, KN, Lindblom, B. 1992. Linguistic experience alters phonetic perception in infants by 6 months of age. *Science* 255, 606–608.

Kurowski, K, Blumstein, SE. 1987a. Acoustic properties for place of articulation in nasal consonants. *J Acoust Soc Am* 81, 1917–1927.

Kurowski, KM, Blumstein, SE. 1987b. In: MK Huffman, RA Krakow (eds.), *Nasals, Nasalization, and the Velum*. New York, NY: Academic, 197–222.

Kurowski, K, Blumstein, SE. 1993. Acoustic properties for the perception of nasal consonants. In: MK Huffman, R Krakow (eds.), *The Feature Nasal: Phonetic Bases and Phonological Implications*. Academic Press, 197–222.

Ladefoged, P, Broadbent, DE. 1957. Information conveyed by vowels. *J Acoust Soc Am* 29, 98–104.

Lazarus, H. 1987. Prediction of verbal communication in noise: A development of generalized SIL curves and the quality of communication, Part 2. *Appl Acoust* 20, 245–261.

Liberman, AM. 1996. *Speech: A Special Code.* Cambridge, MA: MIT Press.

Liberman, AM, Cooper, FS, Shankweiler, DB, Studdert-Kennedy, M. 1967. Perception of the speech code. *Psychol Rev* 74, 431–461.

Liberman, AM, Delattre, PC, Cooper, FS, Gerstman, LJ. 1954. The role of consonant–vowel transitions in the perception of the stop and nasal consonants. *Psychol Monogr* 68, 1–13.

Liberman, AM, Delattre, PC, Gerstman, LJ, Cooper, FS. 1956. Tempo of frequency as a cue for distinguishing classes of speech sounds. *J Exp Psychol* 52, 127–137.

Liberman, AM, Harris, KS, Hoffman, HS, Griffith, BC. 1957. The discrimination of speech sounds within and across phoneme boundaries. *J Exp Psychol* 54, 358–368.

Liberman, AM, Harris, KS, Kinney, KA, Lane, HL. 1961. The discrimination of relative onset of certain speech and non-speech patterns. *J Exp Psychol* 61, 379–388.

Liberman, AM, Mattingly, IG. 1985. The motor theory of speech perception revised. *Cognition* 21, 1–36.

Liberman, AM, Mattingly, IG. 1989. A specialization for speech perception. *Science* 243, 489–494.

Liberman, AM, Whalen, DH. 2000. On the relation of speech to language. *Trends Cogn Sci* 4, 187–196.

Licklider, JCR. 1946. Effects of amplitude distortion upon the intelligibility of speech. *J Acoust Soc Am* 18, 429–434.

Licklider, JCR, Bindra, D, Pollack, I. 1948. The intelligibility of rectangular speech waves. *Am J Psychol* 61, 1–20.

Licklider, JCR, Pollack, I. 1948. Effects of differentiation, integration, and infinite peak clipping upon the intelligibility of speech. *J Acoust Soc Am* 20, 42–51.

Lieberman, P. 1973. On the evaluation of language: A unified view. *Cognition* 2, 59–94.

Lindblom, B, Studdert-Kennedy, M. 1967. On the role of formant transitions in vowel recognition. *J Acoust Soc Am* 42, 830–843.

Lisker, L. 1957a. Closure duration and the intervocalic voiced-voiceless distinction in English. *Language* 33, 42–49.

Lisker, L. 1957b. Minimal cues for separating /w,r,l,y/ in intervocalic position. *Word* 13, 256–267.

Lisker, L, Abramson, AS. 1964. Cross-language study of voicing in initial stops: Acoustical measurements. *Word* 20, 384–422.

Lisker, L, Abramson, AS. 1967. Some effects of context on voice onset time in English stops. *Lang Speech* 10, 1–28.

Lisker, L, Abramson, AS. 1970. *The voicing dimension: Some experiments in comparative phonetics.* Proceedings of the Sixth International Congress on Phonetic Science. Prague, Czech Republic: Academia, 563–567.

Liu, S, Zeng, FG. 2006. Temporal properties in clear speech perception. *J Acoust Soc Am* 120, 424–432.

Liu, S, Rio, ED, Bradlow, AR, Zeng, F-G. 2004. Clear speech perception in acoustic and electric hearing. *J Acoust Soc Am* 116, 2374–2383.

Luce, PA. 1990. *Neighborhoods of Words in the Mental Lexicon.* Research on Speech Perception Tech. Report 6. Bloomington, IL: Indiana University.

Luce, PA, Pisoni, DB. 1998. Recognizing spoken words: The neighborhood activation model. *Ear Hear* 19, 1–36

Luce, PA, Stephen, DG, Auer, ET Jr, Vitevitch, MS. 2000. Phonetic priming, neighborhood activation, and PARSYN. *Percept Psychophys* 62, 615–625.

MacDonald, J, McGurk, H. 1978. Visual influences on speech perception processes. *Percept Psychophys* 24, 253–257.

Mäkelä, AM, Alku, P, May, PJ, Mäkinen, V, Tiitinen, H. 2005. Left-hemispheric brain activity reflects formant transitions in speech sounds. *Neuroreport* 16, 549–553.

Mäkelä, AM, Alku, P, Tiitinen, H. 2003. The auditory N1m reveals the left-hemispheric representation of vowel identity in humans. *Neurosci Lett* 353, 111–114.

Malecot, A. 1956. Acoustic cues for nasal consonants. *Language* 32, 274–284.

Marslen-Wilson, WD, Tyler, LK. 1980. The temporal structure of spoken language understanding. *Cognition* 8, 1–71.

Marslen-Wilson, WD, Welsh, A. 1978. Processing interactions during word-recognition in continuous speech. *Cogn Psychol* 10, 29–63.

Massaro, DW. 1987. *Speech Perception by Ear and Eye: A Paradigm for Psychological Inquiry.* Hillsdale, NJ: Erlbaum.

Massaro, DW. 1998. *Perceiving Talking Faces: From Speech Perception to a Behavioral Principle.* Cambridge, MA: MIT Press.

Massaro, DW, Chen, TH. 2008. The motor theory of speech perception revisited. *Psychon Bull Rev* 15, 453–457.

Mattingly, IG, Liberman, AM. 1988. Specialized perceiving systems for speech and other biologically significant sounds. In: GMG Edelman, WE Gall, WM Cowen (eds.), *Auditory Function: Neurological Bases of Hearing.* New York, NY: Wiley, 775–793.

McClelland, JL, Elman, JL. 1986. The TRACE model of speech perception. *Cogn Psychol* 18, 1–86.

McGurk, H, MacDonald, J. 1976. Hearing lips and seeing voices. *Nature* 264, 746–747.

Miller, GA. 1947. The masking of speech. *Psychol Bull* 44, 105–129.

Miller, GA. 1951. *Language and Communication.* New York, NY: McGraw-Hill.

Miller, JD. 1989. Auditory-perceptual interpretation of the vowel. *J Acoust Soc Am* 85, 2114–2134.

Miller, GA, Licklider, JCR. 1950. The intelligibility of interrupted speech. *J Acoust Soc Am* 22, 167–173.

Miller, GA, Heise, GA, Lichten, W. 1951. The intelligibility of speech as a function of the context of the test materials. *J Ex Psychol* 41, 329–335.

Miller, JL, Kent, RD, Atal, BS. (eds.) 1991. *Papers in Speech Communication: Speech Perception.* New York, NY: Acoustical Society of America.

Miller, GA, Nicely, PA. 1955. An analysis of perceptual confusions among some English consonants. *J Acoust Soc Am* 27, 338–352.

Miller, MI, Sachs, MB. 1983. Representation of stop consonants in the discharge patterns of auditory-nerve fibers. *J Acoust Soc Am* 74, 502–517.

Miller, JD, Wier, CC, Pastore, RE, Kelly, WJ, and Dooling, RJ. 1976. Discrimination and labeling of noise-buzz sequences with varying noise-lead times: An example of categorical perception. *J Acoust Soc Am* 60, 410–417.

Mirabile, PJ, Porter, RJ. 1975. *Dichotic and monotic interaction between speech and nonspeech sounds at different stimulus-onset-asynchronies.* Paper at 89th Meeting of the Acoustical Society of America, Austin, Texas.

Mitler, JD, Wier, CC, Pastore, R, Kelly, WJ, Dooling, RJ. 1976. Discrimination and labeling of noise-buzz sequences with varying noise-lead times: An example of categorical perception. *J Acoust Soc Am* 60, 410–417.

Moon, S, Lindblom, B. 1994. Interaction between duration, context, and speaking style in English stressed vowels. *J Acoust Soc Am* 96, 40–55.

Morton, J. 1969. Interaction of information in word recognition. *Psychol Rev* 76, 165–178.

Möttönen, R, Krause, CM, Tiippana, K, Sams, M. 2002. Processing of changes in visual speech in the human auditory cortex. *Brain Res Cogn Brain Res* 13, 417–425.

Näätänen, R. 2001. The perception of speech sounds by the human brain as reflected by the mismatch negativity (MMN) and its magnetic equivalent (MMNm). *Psychophysiology* 38, 1–21.

Nabelek, AK. 1976. Reverberation effects for normal and hearing-impaired listeners. In: SK Hirsh, DH Eldredge, IJ Hirsh, SR Silverman (eds.), *Hearing and Davis: Essays Honoring Hallowell Davis.* St. Louis, MO: Washington University Press, 333–341.

Nabelek, AK, Dagenais, PA. 1986. Vowel errors in noise and in reverberation by hearing impaired listeners. *J Acoust Soc Am* 80, 741–748.

Nabelek, AK, Letowski, TR. 1985. Vowel confusions of hearing-impaired listeners under reverberant and nonreverberant conditions. *J Speech Hear Dis* 50, 126–131.

Nabelek, AK, Letowski, TR, Tucker, FM. 1989. Reverberant overlap- and self-masking in consonant identification. *J Acoust Soc Am* 86, 1259–1265.

Nabelek, AK, Mason, D. 1981. Effect of noise and reverberation on binaural and monaural word identification by subjects with various audiograms. *J Speech Hear Res* 24, 375–383.

Nabelek, AK, Nabelek, IV. 1994. Room acoustics and speech perception. In: J Katz (ed.), *Handbook of Clinical Audiology*, 4th ed. Baltimore, MD: Williams & Wilkins, 624–637.

Nabelek, AK, Pickett, JM. 1974. Reception of consonants in a classroom as affected by monaural and binaural listening, noise, reverberation and hearing aids. *J Acoust Soc Am* 56, 628–639.

Nabelek, AK, Robinette, LN. 1978. Reverberation as a parameter in clinical testing. *Audiology* 17, 239–259.

Nearey, TM. 1989. Static, dynamic, and relational properties in vowel perception. *J Acoust Soc Am* 2088–2113.

Nelson, DA, Marler, P. 1989. Categorical perception of a natural stimulus continuum: Birdsong. *Science* 244, 976–978.

Nelson, PB, Nittrouer, S, Norton, SJ. 1995. "Say-stay" identification and psychoacoustic performance of hearing-impaired listeners. *J Acoust Soc Am* 97, 1830–1838.

Nittrouer, S,. 1992 Age-related difference in perceptual effects of formant transitions with syllables and across phoneme boundaries. *J Phonet* 20, 351–382.

Nittrouer, S, Studdert-Kennedy, M. 1987. The role of coarticulatory effects in the perception of fricatives by children and adults. *J Acoust Soc Am* 86, 1266–1276.

Norris, DG. 1994. SHORTLIST: A connectionist model of continuous speech recognition. *Cognition* 52, 189–234.

O'Connor, JD, Gerstman, LJ, Liberman, AM, Delattre, PC, and Cooper, FS. 1957. Acoustic cues for the perception of initial /w,j,r,l/ in English. *Word* 13, 24–43.

Ogden, GC, Massaro, DW. 1978. Integration of featural information in speech perception. *Psychol Rev* 85, 172–191.

Ohde, RN, Haley, KL, Barnes, CW. 2006. Perception of the [m]-[n] distinction in consonant–vowel (CV) and vowel–consonant (VC) syllables produced by child and adult talkers. *J Acoust Soc Am* 119, 1697–1711.

Ohde, RN, Haley, KL, Vorperian, HK, McMahon, C. 1995. A developmental study of the perception of onset spectra for stop consonants in different vowel environments. *J Acoust Soc Am* 97, 3800–3812.

Orfield, SJ 1987. The RASTI method of testing relative intelligibility. *Sound Vibr* 21(12), 20–22.

Pardo, JS, Remez. 2006. The perception of speech. In: M Traxler, MA Gernsbacher (eds.), *The Handbook of Psycholinguistics*, 2nd ed. New York, NY: Academic, 201–248.

Pavlovic, CV. 1987. Derivation of primary parameters and procedures for use in speech intelligibility predictions. *J Acoust Soc Am* 82, 413–422.

Pavlovic, CV. 1988. Articulation index predictions of speech intelligibility in hearing aid selection. *ASHA* 30(6/7), 63–65.

Pavlovic, CV. 1991. Speech recognition and five articulation indexes. *Hear Inst* 42(9), 20–23.

Pavlovic, CV, Studebaker, GA, Sherbecoe, RL. 1986. An articulation index based procedure for predicting the speech recognition performance of hearing-impaired individuals. *J Acoust Soc Am* 80, 50–57.

Payton, KL, Uchanski, RM, Braida, LD. 1994. Intelligibility of conversational and clear speech in noise and reverberation for listeners with normal and impaired hearing. *J Acoust Soc Am* 95(3), 1581–1592.

Pearsons, KS, Bennett, RL, Fidell, S. 1977. *Speech levels in various noise environments*. EPA Report 600/1-77-025. Washington, D.C.: Environmental Protection Agency.

Pegg, JE, Werker, JF. 1997. Adult and infant perception of two English phones. *J Acoust Soc Am* 102, 3742–3753.

Peterson, GE. 1952. The information-bearing elements of speech. *J Acoust Soc Am* 24, 629–637.

Peterson, GE, Barney, HL. 1952. Control methods used in a study of the vowels. *J Acoust Soc Am* 24, 175–184.

Peterson, GE, Lehiste, I. 1962. Revised CNC lists for auditory tests. *J Speech Hear Dis* 27, 62–70.

Phillips, DP. 1999. Auditory gap detection, perceptual channels, and temporal resolution in speech perception. *J Am Acad Audiol* 10, 343–354.

Phillips, DP, Taylor, T, Hass, SE, Carr, MM, Mossop, JE. 1997. Detection of silent intervals between noises activating different perceptual channels: Some properties of "central" gap detection. *J Acoust Soc Am* 101, 3694–3705.

Picheny, MA, Durlach, NI, Braida, LD. 1985. Speaking clearly for the hard of hearing I: Intelligibility differences between clear and conversational speech. *J Speech Hear Res* 28, 96–103.

Picheny, MA, Durlach, NI, Braida, LD. 1986. Speaking clearly for the hard of hearing II: Acoustic characteristics of clear and conversational speech. *J Speech Hear Res* 29, 434–446.

Picheny, MA, Durlach, NI, Braida, LD. 1989. Speaking clearly for the hard of hearing III: An attempt to determine the contribution of speaking rate to differences in intelligibility of clear and conversational speech. *J Speech Hear Res* 32, 600–603.

Pickett, JM. 1999. *The Acoustics of Speech Communication*. Boston, MA: Allyn and Bacon.

Pisoni, DB. 1977. Identification and discrimination of the relative onset time of two component tones: Implications for voicing perception in stops. *J Acoust Soc Am* 61, 1352–1361.

Pisoni, DB, McNabb, SD. 1974. Dichotic interactions and phonetic feature processing. *Brain Lang* 1, 351–362.

Porter, RJ. 1975. Effect of delayed channel on the perception of dichotically presented speech and nonspeech sounds. *J Acoust Soc Am* 58, 884–892.

Potter, RK, Kopp, GA, Green, HC. 1947. *Visible Speech*. New York, NY: Van Nostrand.

Powers, GL, Speaks, C. 1973. Intelligibility of temporally interrupted speech. *J Acoust Soc Am* 54, 661–667.

Price, C, Thierry, G, Griffiths, T. 2005. Speech-specific auditory processing: Where is it? *Trends Cogn Sci* 9, 271–276.

Raphael, LJ. 1972. Preceding vowel duration as a cue to the perception of the voicing characteristics of word-final consonants in American English. *J Acoust Soc Am* 51, 1296–1303.

Raphael, LJ, Borden, GJ, Harris, KS. 2007. *Speech Science Primer*, 5th ed. Baltimore, MD: Lippincott Williams & Wilkins.

Remez, RE. 2005. Perceptual organization of speech. In: DB Pisoni, RE Remez (eds.), *The Handbook of Speech Perception*. Oxford, MA: Blackwell, 28–50.

Remez, RE, Rubin, PE, Berns, SM, Pardo, JS, Lang, JM. 1994. On the perceptual organization of speech. *Psychol Rev* 101, 129–156.

Remez, RE, Rubin, PE, Pisoni, DB, Carrell, TD. 1981. Speech perception without traditional speech cues. *Science* 212, 947–950.

Repp, BR. 1984. Categorical perception: Issues, methods, findings. In: N Lass (ed.), *Speech and Language: Advances in Basic Research and Practice*, Vol. 10. New York, NY: Academic Press, 243–335.

Repp, BR, Lin, HB. 1989. Acoustic properties and perception of stop consonant release transients. *J Acoust Soc Am* 85, 379–396.

Rhebergen, KS, Versfeld, NJ. 2005. A Speech Intelligibility Index-based approach to predict the speech reception threshold for sentences in fluctuating noise for normal-hearing listeners. *J Acoust Soc Am* 117, 2181–2192.

Rosenzweig, MR, Postman, L. 1957. Intelligibility as a function of frequency of usage. *J Exp Psychol* 54, 412–422.

Ryalls, J. 1996. *A Basic Introduction to Speech Perception*. San Diego, CA: Singular.

Sacia, CE, Beck, CJ. 1926. The power of fundamental speech sounds. *Bell Sys Tech J* 5, 393–403.

Saint-Amour, D, DeSanctis, P, Molholm, S, Ritter, W, Foxe, JJ. 2007. Seeing voices: High-density electrical mapping and source-analysis of the multisensory mismatch negativity evoked during the McGurk illusion. *Neuropsychologica* 45, 587–597.

Sams, M, Aulanko, R, Hämäläinen, M, Hari, R, Lounasmaa, OV, Lu, ST, Simola, J. 1991. Seeing speech: Visual information from lip movements modifies activity in the human auditory cortex. *Neurosci Lett* 127, 141–145.

Sawusch, JR, Jusczyk, PW. 1981. Adaptation and contrast in the perception of voicing. *J Exp Psychol Hum Percept Perform* 7, 408–421.

Sawusch, JR, Pisoni, D. 1974. On the identification of place and voicing features in synthetic stop consonants. *J Phonet* 2, 181–194.

Schmidt-Nielsen, A. 1987. Comments on the use of physical measures to assess speech intelligibility. *J Acoust Soc Am* 81, 1985–1987.

Schouten, MEH, vanHessen, AJ. 1992. Modeling phoneme perception. I: Categorical perception. *J Acoust Soc Am* 92, 1841–1855.

Schum, DJ. 1996. Intelligibility of clear and conversational speech of young and elderly talkers. *J Am Acad Audiol* 7, 212–218.

Searle, CL, Jacobson, JZ, Rayment, SG. 1979. Stop consonant discrimination based on human audition. *J Acoust Soc Am* 79, 799–809.

Shankweiler, D, Studdert-Kennedy, M. 1967. Identification of consonants and vowels presented to the left and right ears. *Q J Exp Psychol* 19, 59–63.

Sharf, DJ. 1962. Duration of post-stress intervocalic stops preceding vowels. *Lang Speech* 5, 26–30.

Shtyrov, Y, Pihko, E, Pulvermüller, F. 2005. Determinants of dominance: Is language laterality explained by physical or linguistic features of speech? *Neuroimage* 27, 37–47.

Slis, IH. 1970. Articulatory measurements on voiced, voiceless and nasal consonants. *Phonetica* 24, 193–210.

Steeneken, HJM. 2006. *Speech Transmission Index (STI): Objective Speech Intelligibility Assessment*. Available at http://www.steeneken.nl/sti.html (accessed April 29, 2008).

Steeneken, HJM, Houtgast, T. 1980. A physical method for measuring speech-transmission quality. *J Acoust Soc Am* 67, 318–326.

Stevens, KN. 1972. The quantal nature of speech: Evidence from articulatory-acoustic data. In: EE David, PB Denes (eds.), *Human Communication: A Unified View*. New York, NY: McGraw-Hill, 51–66.[check the surname]

Stevens, KN, Blumstein, SE. 1978. Invariant cues for place of articulation in stop consonants. *J Acoust Soc Am* 64, 1358–1368.

Stevens, KN, Halle, M. 1967. Remarks on analysis by synthesis and distinctive features. In: W Wathem-Dunn (ed.), *Models for the Perception of Speech and Visual Form*. Cambridge, MA: MIT Press, 88–102.

Stevens, KN, House, AS. 1955. Development of a quantitative description of vowel articulation. *J Acoust Soc Am* 27, 484–493.

Stevens, KN, House, AS. 1961. An acoustical theory of vowel productions and some of its implications. *J Speech Hear Res* 4, 302–320.

Stevens, KN, House, AS. 1963. Perturbation of vowel articulations by consonantal context: An acoustical study. *J Speech Hear Res* 6, 111–128.

Stevens, KN, Klatt, DH. 1974. The role of formant transitions in the voiced–voiceless distinctions for stops. *J Acoust Soc Am* 55, 653–659.

Stevens, SS, Miller, J, Truscott, I. 1946. The masking of speech by sine waves, square waves, and regular and modulated pulses. *J Acoust Soc Am* 18, 418–424.

Strange, W. 1989a. Dynamic specification of coarticulated vowels spoken in sentence context. *J Acoust Soc Am* 2135–2153.

Strange, W. 1989b. Evolving theories of vowel perception. *J Acoust Soc Am* 85, 2081–2087.

Strevens, P. 1960. Spectra of fricative noise in human speech. *Lang Speech* 3, 32–49.

Studdert-Kennedy, M, Shankweiler, D. 1970. Hemispheric specialization for speech perception. *J Acoust Soc Am* 48, 579–594.

Studdert-Kennedy, M, Shankweiler, D, Schulman, S. 1970. Opposed effects of a delayed channel on perception of dichotically and monotically presented CV syllables. *J Acoust Soc Am* 48, 599–602.

Takata, Y, Nabelek, AK. 1990. English consonant recognition in noise and in reverberation by Japanese and American listeners. *J Acoust Soc Am* 88, 663–666.

Tartter, VC, Eimas, PD. 1975. The role of auditory and phonetic feature detectors in the perception of speech. *Percept Psychophys* 18, 293–298.

Tervaniemi, M, Hugdahl, K. 2003. Lateralization of auditory-cortex functions. *Brain Res Brain Res Rev* 43, 231–246.

Tiffany, WR. 1953. Vowel recognition as a function of duration, frequency modulation and phonetic context. *J Speech Hear Disord* 18, 289–301.

Uchanski, RM, Choi, SS, Braida, LD, Reed, CM, Durlach, NI. 1996. Speaking clearly for the hard of hearing IV: Further studies of speaking rate. *J Speech Hear Res* 39, 494–509.

van Wijngaarden, SJ, Drullman, R. 2008. Binaural intelligibility prediction based on the speech transmission index. *J Acoust Soc Am* 123, 4514–4523.

Walley, AC, Carrell, TD. 1983. Onset spectra and formant transitions in the adult's and child's perception of place of articulation in stop consonants. *J Acoust Soc Am* 73, 1011–1022.

Webster, JC. 1978. Speech interference aspects of noise. In: DM Lipscomb (ed.), *Noise and Audiology*. Baltimore, MD: University of Park Press, 193–228.

Werker, JF, Gilbert, JHV, Humphrey, K, Tees, RC. 1981. Developmental aspects of cross language speech perception. *Child Dev* 52, 349–53.

Werker, JF, Tees, RC. 1984. Cross-language speech perception: Evidence for perceptual reorganization during the first year of life. *Infant Behav Dev* 7, 49–63.

Whalen, DH, Liberman, AM. 1987. Speech perception takes precedence over nonspeech perception. *Science* 237, 169–171.

Whalen, DH, Benson, R, Richardson, M, Swainson, B, Clark, VP, Lai, S, Mencl, WE, Fulbright, RK, Constable, RT, Liberman, AM. 2006. Differentiation of speech and nonspeech processing within primary auditory cortex. *J Acoust Soc Am* 119, 575–581

Wood, CC. 1975. Auditory and phonetic levels of processing in speech perception: Neurophysiological and information-processing analyses. *J Exp Psychol* 104, 133.

Wood, CC, Goff, WR, Day, RS. 1971. Auditory evoked potentials during speech perception. *Science* 173, 1248–1251.

Author Index

Abbagnaro, LA, 237
Abbas, PJ, 111, 112
Abbey, H, 264
Abel, SM, 178
Abeles, M, 129
Abelson, RP, 146
Abramson, A, 264
Abramson, AS, 259, 264
Adamonis, J, 133
Ades, HW, 134
Adrian, ED, 80
Ahad, PA, 234
Ahlstrom, C, 273
Ahroon, WA, 180
Ahveninen, J, 126
Aitkin, IM, 122, 125, 129
Aitkin, J, 44
Aitkin, LM, 125, 126
Alexander, GC, 157
Algazi, VR, 237
Alku, P, 263
Allen, JB, 157, 248
Allon, N, 123
Altschuler, R, 97
Altschuler, RA, 42, 129
Amano-Kusumoto, A, 273
Ambler, S, 260
Amitay, S, 155
Ananthanarayan, AK, 132
Andersen, RA, 125
Anderson, BW, 273
Anderson, DJ, 105, 106, 107, 108, 109, 111, 113, 115, 117, 125, 129, 226
Anderson, RA, 45
Anson, BJ, 31
Aoyagi, M, 133
Arbogast, TL, 179, 201, 234
Arieh, Y, 212
Arkebauer, JH, 259
Arlinger, K, 265, 266
Armand, F, 222
Arne, BC, 197
Arruda, M, 241
Aschoff, A, 42, 122
Ashe, JH, 42
Ashmore, JE, 97
Atal, BS, 257
Atteave, F, 223
Auer, ET, Jr, 272
Aulanko, R, 265
Avan, P, 42

Avendano, C, 237
Avinash, G, 93
Axelsson, A, 34, 35

Babkoff, H, 199
Bachem, A, 222, 223
Backus, AS, 122
Backus, ASN, 57
Bacon, SP, 173, 176, 177, 197, 198, 199
Bacon, SR, 173
Bader, CR, 96, 97
Baer, T, 209
Bagasan, B, 132
Ballenger, WL, 243
Baran, JA, 41, 44, 122
Barany, E, 55, 56, 59
Barker, C, 264
Barlam, D, 34
Barnes, CW, 262
Barney, HL, 258, 259
Barone, P, 125, 126
Barren, M, 131
Barret, N, 34
Barrett, DJK, 126
Bartolome, V, 42
Batra, R, 125
Bauer, BB, 237
Beagley, HC, 117
Beasley, DS, 268
Beauchamp, JW, 227
Bechara Kachar, B, 78
Beck, CJ, 265
Beck, J, 218
Beedle, RK, 66
Begault, DR, 243
Behrens, S, 261, 262
Bekesy, G, 28, 31, 51, 53, 54, 55, 56, 58, 59, 72, 74, 75, 76, 77, 80, 84, 87, 88, 105, 151, 167, 218, 225, 243
Bell, TS, 273
Belliveau, JW, 126
Belmore, SM, 44
Benbasset, CA, 179
Benes, SC, 155
Benevento, LA, 125
Bennett, KB, 179
Bennett, M, 53
Bennett, RL, 266
Benson, DA, 125, 126
Benson, R, 265
Benson, RR, 130
Benson, RW, 266

Bent, T, 274
Beranek, K, 42
Beranek, LL, 1, 272, 273
Berbel, P, 129
Berg, K, 199
Berger, H, 166
Berger, KW, 227
Berglund, G, 211
Berglund, V, 211
Berkley, DA, 246, 248
Berlin, CI, 93, 262, 263
Berns, SM, 264
Bernstein, LR, 175, 241
Bertoncini, J, 264
Bertrand, D, 96, 97
Besing, J, 177, 178
Best, CT, 264, 270
Best, L, 131
Best, V, 241
Beurg, M, 37
Bharucha, JJ, 130, 222
Biddulph, R, 174, 231, 232
Bieser, A, 123
Bijeljas-Babic, R, 264
Bilger, RC, 180, 181, 189, 191, 192
Billone, MC, 78, 82, 91
Bilsen, FA, 224, 226
Bindra, D, 267
Birdsall, TG, 161
Birk, JL, 130, 222
Blauert, J, 51, 235, 237, 243, 244
Block, MG, 66
Blodgett, HC, 247
Blom, S, 62
Blumstein, SA, 264
Blumstein, SE, 260, 261, 262
Bode, DL, 151, 155
Bohne, BA, 30
Bolt, RH, 245, 269
Bonding, P, 210, 211
Bonmassar, G, 126
Borden, GJ, 257
Borg, E, 44, 62, 63, 67, 68
Boring, EG, 220
Borst, JM, 259, 262
Bos, CE, 190
Botros, A, 221
Botte, MC, 213
Boucher, BL, 133
Boudreau, JC, 124, 127, 128
Boudreau, JD, 126
Bouman, MA, 171
Bowers, JN, 243
Boyle, AJ, 87, 88

Boyle, JE, 88
Bradlow, AR, 273, 274
Braida, LD, 172, 173, 273, 274
Brandt, JF, 170, 211, 212
Brantley, MA, 175
Bray, CW, 83
Bredberg, G, 34
Breebaart, J, 250
Bregman, AS, 234
Bretscher, A, 37
Broadbent, DE, 232, 259, 262
Bronkhorst, AW, 237, 239, 241, 243
Browman, CP, 209
Brown, CF, 133
Brown, DK, 133
Brown, MC, 45, 78, 112, 135
Brown, ME, 179
Brown, RB, 124, 127, 128
Brown, SD, 264
Brownell, WE, 37, 38, 96, 97
Bruel, 273
Brugge, JE, 105, 106, 107, 108, 109, 129
Brugge, JF, 105, 111, 113, 115, 125, 129, 226
Brughera, A, 234
Brungart, DS, 243
Brunso-Bechtold, 42, JK
Brunso-Bechtold, JK, 42
Buchanan, JL, 243
Buchsbaum, G, 220, 221
Buchwald, JS, 131
Buell, TN, 241, 247
Buining, E, 200
Burck, W, 170
Burger, JF, 245
Burgio, PA, 117
Burkard, R, 133
Burkhard, RF, 131
Burns, EM, 93, 96, 135, 222, 224
Buss, E, 197, 201
Butler, R, 237, 238
Butler, RA, 80, 134, 238, 243
Buunen, TJF, 226
Buus, S, 155, 173, 177, 207, 209, 210, 211, 212
Byrne, AJ, 173, 232
Byrne, D, 265, 266

Caird, D, 124, 125
Calabro, A, 34
Calearo, C, 268
Callaghan, BP, 201, 202
Callow, M, 260
Campbell, GA, 266
Campbell, M, 226
Campbell, RA, 153, 154, 173, 178, 225

Campbell, RS, 170
Canevet, G, 209, 213
Cant, NB, 41, 124, 126
Cárdenas, J, 133
Cardozo, B, 226
Carhart, R, 60, 151, 155, 198, 199, 249
Carlile, S, 241
Carlson, L, 42
Carlyon, RP, 197, 224
Carlyon, RR, 173
Carney, LH, 114, 122
Carr, M, 177, 178
Carr, MM, 264
Carrell, TD, 261, 264
Carricondo, F, 42
Carrier, SC, 240
Caspary, DM, 42, 124
Cassady, M, 126
Casseday, JH, 122, 124, 134
Causse, R, 231
Chadwick, RS, 78
Chain, F, 134
Chamberlain, SC, 34, 122
Champagne, SC, 133
Champlin, CA, 197
Chan, JC, 124
Chan, JCK, 124
Chandler, DW, 243
Chatterjee, M, 199
Chavasse, P, 231
Cheatham, MA, 9, 81, 82, 85, 86, 88,
    91, 97
Cheathan, MS, 83, 85
Chen, J, 234
Chen, TH, 257, 270, 271
Chendru, F, 134
Cherry, C, 232
Cherry, EC, 232, 233
Cheung, HC, 35
Chistovich, LA, 194
Chmiel, R, 133
Chocolle, R, 200, 220
Choi, SS, 273, 274
Chow, K, 41
Chow, KL, 44
Chum, RA, 111
Churcher, BG, 207, 231
Clarey, JC, 125, 126
Clark, G, 133
Clark, M, 227
Clark, MJ, 258
Clark, VP, 265
Clark, WW, 180
Clarke, S, 43, 44

Clifton, RK, 244, 245, 247
Cochran, P, 243
Cody, AR, 181
Cohen, A, 224
Cohen, L, 133
Cohen, MF, 167
Cokely, CG, 199
Coker, N, 133
Colburn, HS, 201, 235, 244, 247
Coleman, PD, 125, 243, 244
Colin, C, 265
Colin, F, 265
Collet, L, 135
Collins, LM, 155
Comegys, TH, 34
Comis, SD, 35, 78
Cone-Wesson, B, 133
Constable, RT, 265
Cook, ND, 224
Coomb, CH, 146
Coopens, AB, 1
Cooper, FS, 258, 259, 260, 262, 264, 270
Cooper, NP, 93, 111
Cooper, WA, 213
Corbit, JD, 264
Corey, DP, 35, 37, 76, 78, 79
Counter, SA, 67, 68, 154, 170
Covell, WP, 57
Covey, E, 122
Cowan, JA, 155
Cox, PG, 170, 211, 212
Cox, PH, 243
Cox, R, 265, 266
Cox, RM, 157, 265, 266
Cranford, J, 134
Crawford, AC, 35, 88, 97
Creelman, CD, 152, 154, 155, 211
Creten, WL, 56, 57
Creutzfeldt, O, 123
Crivello, F, 263
Crouch, EC, 34
Crow, G, 132
Cudahy, E, 173
Cullen, JK, 262, 263
Culling, JF, 234, 250
Cunningham, D, 62
Curtis, TH, 248
Cutting, JE, 264
Cynader, MS, 123, 129

Dadson, RS, 166, 167, 168, 207
Dagenais, PA, 245, 269
Dale, AM, 130
Dallos, D, 97

Dallos, P, 9, 30, 37, 56, 57, 58, 62, 63, 66, 78, 80, 81, 82, 83, 84, 85, 86, 88, 91, 97, 104, 117, 118, 119, 199, 249
Dallos, PJ, 80, 88
DalSasso, A, 32
Damianopoulus, EN, 200
Daniloff, TG, 224
Darwin, CJ, 114, 241, 263
Dasheiff, R, 132
David, EE, Jr, 1
Davies, H, 231
Davis, A, 34
Davis, H, 32, 74, 77, 78, 80, 81, 82, 83, 84, 85, 103, 105, 111, 117, 131, 168, 189, 266
Day, RS, 263
de Ribaupierre, F, 122, 123
de Ribaupierre, Y, 122
Dear, SP, 180, 181
Dear, SR, 35
Deatherage, B, 82, 85
Deatherage, BH, 82, 85, 189, 199
Deatheredge, BH, 247
deBoer, E, 190, 226
Decraemer, WF, 55
Degutte, B, 136
Dekker, TN, 93, 94
Delattre, PC, 258, 259, 260, 262
Delgutte, B, 114, 247
Deliwala, PS, 201
Deltenre, P, 265
DeMaio, J, 240
Demany, L, 222, 223
Demolin, D, 265
Deng, L, 114
Derbyshire, A, 80
DeRibaupierre, E, 125
DeRibaupierre, Y, 125
deRibaupierre, Y, 96, 97
DeRosier, DJ, 35
DeSanctis, P, 265
Desmedt, JE, 129
Dethlefs, DL, 201, 202
DeVenecia, RK, 45, 135
DeVidi S, 133
Devore, S, 126
Dhar, S, 167
Diamond, IT, 44, 45, 130, 134
Dickson, EDD, 168
Diehl, RL, 257, 264, 270
Dillon, H, 265, 266
Dimitriadis, EK, 78
Dimitrijevic, A, 133
Dirks, D, 62, 63, 64, 65
Dirks, DD, 67, 155, 167, 168, 200, 213, 273
Dixon, RM, 244

Dixon, WJ, 152
Djupesland, G, 61, 62, 63
Dobie, R, 133
Dodds, LW, 38, 90, 91
Dolan, DF, 93, 97, 135, 136, 137
Dolan, TR, 247, 248
Don, M, 131
Donaldson, JA, 29, 31
Dooley, GJ, 178, 179
Dooling, RJ, 264
Dorman, MF, 179
Dosanjh, DS, 180
Doucet, J, 199
Doughty, JM, 170
Downs, MR, 167
Druga, R, 134
Drullman, R, 273
Dubno, JR, 155
Dubrovsky, NA, 125
Ducarne, B, 134
Duclaux, R, 135
Duda, RO, 237, 243
Duifhuis, H, 88, 196, 199
Dunlop, CW, 122, 125, 129
Dunn, HK, 258
Dunn, J, 42
Duquesnoy, AJ, 155
Durieux-Smith, 133, A
Durlach, NI, 172, 173, 235, 245, 247, 248, 249, 250, 273, 274
Durrant, JD, 78, 82, 91, 132
Dye, RH, 241
Dye, RH, Jr, 239, 240

Eady, HR, 235, 239, 240
Ebata, M, 244
Egan, JP, 160, 164, 189, 213, 266
Eggermont, JJ, 83, 117
Ehmer, RH, 187, 188, 189
Ehret, G, 41, 43, 44
Eimas, P, 264
Eimas, PD, 264
Ekman, E, 211
El Kholy, AH, 265, 266
Elangovan, S, 177, 178, 264
Elberling, C, 94
Eldert, E, 266
Eldredge, DH, 80, 82, 85, 189
Eldridge, DH, 82, 117
Elliot, E, 167
Elliot, PB, 161
Elliott, DN, 180, 181, 213
Elliott, LL, 197, 198, 199
Elman, J, 271, L
Emmerson, PL, 155

Engstrom, H, 34, 38, 40
Escourolle, R, 134
Evans, EE, 111, 123
Evans, EF, 87, 88, 117
Evans, J, 134–135
Evans, MG, 97
Evans, TR, 199
Everest, FA, 1
Eybalin, M, 74

Faingold, CL, 42
Fairbanks, G, 261, 266, 268
Fakler, B, 97
Fant, G, 257, 262
Farley, GR, 111, 226
Fastl, H, 197, 199, 209, 218, 219, 224
Faure, PA, 122
Fausti, SA, 166
Fay, RF, 41
Fay, RR, 30, 78, 122, 126
Feddersen, WE, 236, 237
Feinmesser, M, 131
Feldman, A, 61, 62, 63
Feldman, RS, 239
Feldtkeller, J, 211
Ferguson, SH, 198, 199, 274
Fernandes, MA, 196
Fernandez, C, 80, 82, 84, 85, 105
Ferrand, CT, 257
Ferraro, J, 83, 85
Ferraro, JA, 43
Festen, JM, 226
Feth, LL, 199
Fettiplace, R, 35, 37, 78, 79, 88, 97
Fex, J, 42, 97, 135
Fidell, S, 192, 266
Fields, JM, 215
Filion, PR, 173, 174
Finck, A, 187
Findlay, JM, 155
Fingerhood, BJ, 55, 60
Finlayson, PG, 124
Fischer-Jorgensen, E, 259
Fisher, HG, 239
Fisher, JF, 134
Fishken, D, 231
Fitzgibbons, PJ, 177
Fitzpatrick, DC, 125
Flanagan, JL, 257, 258
Flanigin, H, 131
Fletcher, H, 66, 189, 190, 191, 192, 207, 210, 231, 257, 265, 266, 267
Fletcher, J, 167
Flock, A, 35, 37, 76, 80, 88, 97

Flock, B, 35, 37, 97
Florentine, M, 155, 173, 177, 207, 209, 210, 211, 212
Flottrop, G, 61, 62, 63, 191, 211
Folkeard, P, 274
Folsom, R, 133
Forbes, SM, 152, 155
Forest, TG, 176, 177
Formby, C, 157, 198, 199, 264
Formby, C, 168, 175, 176, 177
Forrest, TG, 175
Fowler, CA, 257, 264, 270
Foxe, JJ, 265
Franssen, NV, 246
Fraser, W, 180, 181
Fraser, WD, 213
Freda, JS, 199
Freedman, RA, 1
Freedman, SJ, 239
Fremouw, T, 122
French, NR, 272
Frey, AR, 1
Frey, RH, 166
Freyman, RL, 174, 244, 245, 247
Frishkopf, L, 131
Frisina, RD, 122
Frolenkov, GI, 265, 266
Frost, J, 133
Fry, D, 264
Fuchs, PA, 35
Fujimura, O, 262
Fujisawa, TX, 224
Fulbright, RK, 265
Funnell, WRL, 55
Furness, DN, 35, 38
Furst, M, 220, 221
Furui, S, 260
Fuse, T, 133

Gacek, RR, 40
Gagne, J, 274
Gago, G, 125
Galaburda, A, 43
Galambos, R, 103, 111, 122, 126, 128, 135, 224
Galantucci, B, 257, 270
Galbraith, G, 132
Gales, RS, 190
Gallum, FJ, 201, 234, 241
Gamble, T, 114
Gannon, WJ, 83
Gao, J, 97
Gardi, J, 132
Gardner, MB, 51, 168, 237, 243, 244
Gardner, RS, 51
Gardner, WR, 208

Garner, CA, 96
Garner, WR, 170, 224
Gehlbach, G, 42
Geisler, C, 131
Geisler, CD, 78, 79, 87, 93, 96, 111, 114, 125, 129, 135
Gelfand, SA, 17, 21, 27, 61, 62, 66, 67,.88, 155, 180, 192, 245, 266, 269
Gengel, RW, 170, 171, 180
Gerson, A, 226
Gerstman, LJ, 258, 259, 260, 262
Getty, LA, 258
Gifford, M, 135, L
Gifford, ML, 135, 136
Gil-Loyzaga, P, 42
Gilbert, JHV, 270
Gilkey, RH, 155
Gilman, S, 62, 63, 64, 65
Giovanetti, H, 197, 198
Glantz, J, 200
Glasberg, BJ, 192, 193
Glasberg, BR, 192, 197, 209, 210, 224
Glasberg, R, 194, 195, 196
Glaser, EM, 132
Glassberg, BR, 177
Glattke, TJ, 93, 94
Glendenning, KK, 42, 124, 125, 129
Glorig, A, 167, 180, 181
Glueckert, R, 30
Gockel, HE, 224
Godfrey, D, 42
Godfrey, DA, 122, 126
Goff, WR, 263
Goldberg, A, 132
Goldberg, JM, 124, 126, 127, 128, 129, 134
Goldberg, JP, 172, 173
Goldstein, DP, 249
Goldstein, JL, 218, 220, 221, 222, 225, 226
Goldstein, L, 198, 199
Goldstein, MH, 116, 117, 129, 130
Goldstein, MH, Jr, 123
Goldstein, R, 117
Golob, EJ, 131
González, A, 133
Goode, RL, 60
Goodman, DA, 156
Goodyear, RJ, 37
Gordon, JW, 227
Gordon-Salant, S, 177
Gorga, MP, 95, 96
Gorga, MR, 111
Goude, G, 227
Grantham, DW, 198, 239, 240, 243, 244, 245, 247
Grasse, KL, 125
Gray, GA, 157

Greated, C, 222
Green, DM, 155, 172, 173, 174, 175, 176, 177, 190, 192, 197, 201, 231, 232, 233, 237, 239, 240, 247, 249
Green, HC, 258
Green, KW, 61
Greenbaum, H, 208
Greenbaum, HB, 111
Greenberg, GZ, 164
Greenberg, S, 122
Greene, DM, 160
Greenwood, DD, 126, 129, 189, 190, 191, 218
Grey, JM, 227
Griffith, BC, 270
Griffiths, T, 263
Grigsby, SS, 155
Groen, JJ, 233
Groff, JA, 135
Grose, JH, 197, 201
Gross, EE, 1
Gross, NB, 125
Grundfest, H, 74
Gu, X, 233
Guerlekian, JA, 261
Gueta, R, 34
Guinan, J, 55
Guinan, JJ, 45, 91, 103, 126, 135, 136
Guinan, JJ, Jr, 45, 97, 126, 127, 135, 136
Guinan, SS, 126, 127
Guirao, M, 208, 209
Guo, MH, 97, 135
Guttman, N, 248
Guzman, SJ, 244, 247

Haas, H, 244
Hackett, TA, 43
Hackney, CM, 35, 37, 38, 78, 79, 97
Hafter, ER, 240, 241, 247
Hagerman, B, 265
Haggard, MP, 196, 260
Hake, HW, 189
Haley, KL, 260, 262
Hall, DA, 126
Hall, JL, 130, 155, 157, 220, 221
Hall, JW, 131, 133, 196, 197, 201, 211, 212, 225, 226
Hall, S, 177, 178
Hall, SE, 123
Halle, M, 259, 260, 261, 270
Hallett, M, 44, 130
Hämäläinen, M, 126, 265
Hamernick, R, 62, 63, 111, 112
Hamernick, RP, 109
Hamernik, RP, 180
Hamilton, PM, 190
Hammershoi, D, 241

Hardy, JC, 259
Harford, ER, 66
Hari, R, 265
Harris, D, 91
Harris, DM, 199
Harris, GG, 240
Harris, JD, 173, 174, 231, 243
Harris, KS, 257, 260, 261, 263, 264, 270
Harris, LB, 198, 199
Harris, RW, 269
Harrison, JM, 45
Harrison, WA, 135
Hartmann, WM, 234, 235, 246, 247
Harvey, AR, 42
Hascall, VC, 34
Hass, SE, 264
Hatch, DR, 197
Hato, N, 60
Hatoh, T, 223
Hawkey, DJC, 155
Hawkins, DB, 157
Hawkins, JE, 189, 190, 191, 268
Hawley, ML, 234
Hayashi, T, 224
Hayes, E, 274
Hazelton, DW, 125
He, DZZ, 97
Healy, EW, 197
Hebrank, J, 237
Hecker, H, 266
Hecox, KE, 132
Hedlun, JM, 233
Heffner, HE, 134
Heffner, RS, 134
Heinz, JM, 261
Heinz, MG, 175
Heise, GA, 269, 270
Helfer, KS, 269, 274
Helfert, RH, 42, 122, 129
Heller, LM, 241
Hellman, R, 61, 66, 213
Hellman, RP, 156, 157, 208, 209, 210, 231
Hellweg, FC, 123
Helmholtz, H, 27, 53, 54, 55
Henderson, D, 62, 63, 111, 112, 180
Henderson, JL, 177
Hendrick, MS, 198
Henning, GB, 174, 241, 245, 249
Henning, GR, 247
Hensen, V, 60
Henson, MM, 32
Henson, OW, Jr, 32, 45
Heppelmann, G, 135
Herdman, AT, 133

Hesse, A, 155
Hetu, R, 265, 266
Hewitt, PG, 1
Hicks, ML, 197
Hildreth, KM, 83
Hill, NI, 241
Hill, TJW, 222
Hillenbrand, J, 258
Hinchcliffe, R, 135
Hind, JE, 105, 106, 107, 108, 109, 111, 113, 115, 123, 125, 126, 129, 226, 237
Hinton, K, 155
Hirokawa, N, 35
Hirsh, IJ, 172, 177, 178, 180, 181, 189, 231, 247, 248, 249, 266
Hixon, TJ, 259
Hochberg, I, 269
Hoffman, HS, 260, 270
Holley, MC, 37, 96, 97
Holt, LL, 257, 264, 270
Honrubia, V, 83, 84, 85
Hood, JD, 168, 212, 213
Horn, AG, 244
Horonjeff, R, 192
Horst, JW, 226
Hosom, JP, 273
House, A, 266
House, AS, 258, 259, 261, 262
Houtgast, T, 192, 196, 243, 273
Houtsma, AJM, 172, 173, 225, 226, 227
Howard, J, 76, 78
Howard, JH, 179
Howe, ME, 45
Hsieh, CY, 42
Hsueh, KD, 180
Huang, CM, 131
Hubbard, AE, 135
Hudspeth, AJ, 76, 78
Huerta, MF, 43, 45
Huffman, RF, 45
Hugdahl, K, 263
Hughes, GB, 26
Hughes, GW, 259, 260, 261
Hughes, JR, 122, 126, 128
Hughes, JW, 170
Hughes, LF, 262, 263
Huis in't Veld, F, 132
Huizing, EH, 60
Humes, LE, 199, 273
Humes, LR, 221
Humphrey, K, 270
Hung, I, 62, 63
Hunter, C, 42
Hutson, KA, 124, 129
Hyvarinen, J, 126

Imaizumi, K, 130
Imig, TJ, 44, 125, 126, 129
Ingham, JG, 200
Irons, WA, 125, 126
Irvine, DRF, 122, 125, 126
Irwin, A, 155
Isaacs, E, 260
Iurato, S, 32
Ivarsson, C, 125
Iverson, P, 227

Jääskeläinen, IP, 126
Jacobs, J, 88
Jacobs, R, 76, 78
Jacobson, JZ, 260
Janata, P, 130, 222
Janisch, R, 34
Jannetta, PJ, 131
Janssen, T, 135
Jasper, H, 135
Jassem, W, 261
Javel, E, 226
Javell, E, 111
Jefferies, DJR, 35
Jeffress, LA, 124, 173, 236, 237, 240, 247, 248, 250
Jeng, PS, 157
Jenison, RL, 241
Jenkins, DB, 32
Jensen, CB, 241
Jepsen, O, 61, 66, 67
Jerger, J, 61, 62, 63, 64, 133, 134, 173
Jerger, S, 134
Jesteadt, W, 95, 155, 172, 173, 174, 179, 196, 199, 207, 231, 232, 233
Jewett, DL, 131
Jia, S, 97
Job, RFS, 215
John, JE, 131
John, M, 133
John, MS, 133
Johnsen, NJ, 94
Johnson, GW, 88
Johnson, K, 249, 271
Johnson, PW, 43, 44
Johnson, TA, 96
Johnstone, BM, 87, 88, 90, 91, 92, 109, 181
Johnstone, JR, 85, 87, 88
Jones, EG, 43, 45, 130
Jones, K, 96
Jones, KO, 213
Jongman, A, 261
Joris, PX, 122, 124
Josse, G, 263

Jusczyk, P, 264
Jusczyk, PW, 257, 264, 270

Kaas, JH, 43
Kachar, B, 96, 97
Kaernbach, C, 155
Kain, A, 273
Kalb, JT, 273
Kalinec, F, 96
Kameoka, A, 223
Kamm, C, 67
Kamm, CA, 273
Kane, EC, 126
Kanno, Y, 123, 126
Kapadia, S, 135
Kaplan, H, 62, 63, 64, 65
Karaseva, TA, 134
Karlovich, R, 61
Karlovich, TS, 63
Karol, EA, 44
Kato, T, 60, 63
Katsuki, Y, 109, 122, 123, 126
Kawase, T, 136
Kazmierczak, P, 78
Kearny, JK, 173
Kei, J, 265, 266
Keithley, EM, 104, 126, 127
Kelly, JB, 134
Kelly, JP, 90
Kelly, K, 212
Kelly, WJ, 179, 264
Kemp, DT, 93, 111, 135
Kenedy, DT, 87
Kennedy, HJ, 97
Kennedy, L, 264
Kent, RD, 257, 259
Kettner, RE, 125
Kewley-Port, D, 260, 274
Keys, J, 231
Khanna, SM, 54, 55, 56, 60, 88, 89, 90
Kiang, NY, 103, S
Kiang, NYS, 39, 87, 91, 103, 105, 109, 110, 111, 112, 114, 116, 117, 122, 126, 135, 137
Kidd, G, 199, 201, 202, 234
Kidd, G, Jr, 175, 179
Kidd, GK, 234
Kiessling, J, 265, 266
Killan, EC, 135
Killion, MC, 166, 167
Kim, DO, 112, 135
Kim, Y, 133
Kimura, D, 262
Kimura, R, 82, 85
Kimura, RS, 32

Kincaid, GE, 273
King, AJ, 207, 231, 241
King, JH, 166, 167, 168
King, LE, 243
King, WM, 199
King-Smith, PE, 155
Kingsbury, BA, 207
Kinney, KA, 263, 264
Kinsler, LE, 1
Kiren, T, 133
Kirk, KI, 272
Kistler, DJ, 237, 238, 239, 241, 248
Kitzes, LM, 125, 126
Kjaer, 273
Klöcker, N, 97
Klatt, DH, 264, 271
Klink, R, 74
Klinke, R, 124, 125
Klockhoff, I, 61
Klumpp, RG, 235, 239, 240
Knight, PL, 129
Knudsen, VO, 172, 174, 269
Kobrack, H, 60
Kobrak, H, 126
Kochhar, RK, 237
Kodman, F, 268
Koehnke, J, 177, 178
Koenig, AH, 248
Koenig, W, 258
Kohlrausch, A, 197, 250
Koike, Y, 133
Kollmeier, B, 155
Konishi, T, 80, 109, 135
Kontsevich, LL, 155
Kopp, GA, 258
Korezak, P, 131
Kotby, MN, 265, 266
Kotowski, P, 170
Kowalchuk, D, 177
Kramer, M, 196
Krantz, DH, 164
Krantz, FW, 168
Kraus, N, 274
Krause, CM, 265
Krause, JC, 273, 274
Krishnan, A, 132
Kroesen, M, 215
Kros, CJ, 37, 79, 80
Krumhansl, C, 227
Krumhansl, CL, 227
Kryter, A, 266
Kryter, KD, 134, 180, 214, 215, 272
Kuhl, PK, 264, 270
Kuhn, GF, 237

Kulkarni, A, 235
Kuriyagawa, M, 223
Kurowski, K, 262
Kurtovic, H, 245
Kuwada, S, 125
Kwan, KY, 35, 37, 78, 79

Lacerda, F, 270
Lacy, LY, 258
Ladefoged, P, 259
Lai, S, 265
Lamb, M, 177
Lane, CE, 187, 188
Lane, HL, 263, 264
Lang, JM, 264
Langford, TL, 248
Lasky, EZ, 173
Lawrence, CL, 248, 249
Lawrence, M, 23, 28, 35, 53, 54, 74, 78, 81, 82, 83, 220
Lawton, DW, 51
Lazarus, H, 273
Lazzaroni, A, 268
Leak-Jones, PA, 41
Leakey, DM, 232
Ledden, PJ, 130
LeDouz, JE, 42
Lee, CC, 130
Lee, J, 197
Leek, MR, 155, 179
Legouix, JP, 83, 111, 116, 117, 220
Lehiste, I, 266
Lehman, JR, 199
Lehnhardt, E, 233
Leman, M, 130, 222
Leonard, CM, 199
Leonard, DGB, 88, 89, 90
LePage, EL, 92
Leshowitz, B, 173
Letowski, TR, 269
Levänen, S, 126
Levelt, WJM, 223
Levi, E, 133
Levine, RA, 135, 137
Levitt, H, 151, 152, 154, 155, 249
Levy, ET, 243
Lewis, N, 62, 63, 64
Lewy, EH, 126
Lhermitte F, 134
Li, L, 234
Li, W, 234
Li, XF, 42
Liang, L, 123
Liberman, AM, 257, 258, 259, 260, 262, 263, 264, 265, 270

Liberman, MC, 38, 39, 40, 41, 45, 86, 90, 91, 97, 103, 104, 111, 112, 113, 114, 126, 135, 136
Liberman, NC, 91
Lichte, H, 170
Lichten, W, 269, 270
Licklider, JCR, 225, 233, 247, 249, 267, 268
Liden, G, 61
Lieberman, P, 259
Lilly, DJ, 63
Lim, DJ, 32, 33, 35
Lim, LS, 173
Lin, FH, 126
Lin, HB, 261
Lindblom, B, 259, 270, 273
Lindsay, JR, 60
Lins, O, 133
Lins, OG, 133
Lisker, L, 259, 260, 262, 264
Lister, J, 177, 178
Litovsky, RY, 234, 244, 245, 247
Little, AD, 243
Liu, S, 273, 274
Lochner, JPA, 244, 245
Loeb, M, 67
Loeffler, JD, 129
Logue, AW, 209
Lombardino, LJ, 199
Lomber, SG, 126
Long, GR, 167
Long, K, 97
Lonsbury-Martin, BL, 93, 94
Loovis, CF, 262, 263
Lorente de Nó, R, 63
Lotto, AJ, 257, 264, 270
Lounasmaa, OV, 265
Lowe-Bell, SS, 262, 263
Lowry, OH, 29
Lowy, K, 58
Lu, ST, 265
Lu, T, 123
Luce, PA, 257, 260, 270, 272
Ludvigsen, C, 265, 266
Ludwig, J, 97
Lufti, RA, 196
Lui, C, 265, 266
Luk, GD, 45
Lurie, M, 80
Lüscher, E, 173
Lynn, G, 198
Lyons, MJ, 44

MacDonald, AD, 245, 269
MacDonald, J, 265
Machiki, K, 34

Mackenzie, E, 155
Macmillan, NA, 245
Macpherson, EA, 239, 241
Madigan, R, 155
Madison, LD, 97
Mäkelä, AM, 263
Maki, JE, 268
Mäkinen, V, 263
Makous, JC, 238
Malecot, A, 262
Malhotra, S, 126
Malmquist, C, 200
Mangabeira-Albarnaz, PL, 200
Manganari, E, 199
Manley, GA, 88
Manoussaki, D, 78
Mapes-Riordan, D, 212
Marcotti, W, 37
Marcus, DC, 30
Margolis, R, 61, 66
Margolis, RH, 56, 57, 61
Marks, LE, 209, 210, 212, 231, 232, 249
Marks, LM, 157
Marlborough, K, 243, 245
Marler, P, 264
Marshall, L, 155
Marslen-Wilson, WD, 271
Martens, WL, 243
Martin, BA, 131
Martin, GK, 93, 94
Martin, V, 133
Maruyama, N, 122
Marvit, P, 155
Mas-terton, RB, 42
Mason, CR, 173, 175, 179, 201, 234
Mason, D, 269
Massaro, DW, 257, 265, 270, 271
Masta, RI, 78, 135
Mastern, V, 274
Masterson, RB, 125
Masterton, RB, 42, 124, 134
Matsuoka, H, 44
Mattingly, IG, 265, 270
Mauldin, L, 62, 63, 64
May, PJ, 263
Mayer, AM, 187
Mazelová, J, 134
Mazoyer, B, 263
McAdams, S, 227
McAuliffe, DR, 84, 105
McBride, LM, 61, 62
McCall, D, 245, 247
McCandless, G, 131
McClelland, JL, 271

McCollough, JK, 63
McDonald, LP, 114
McFadden, D, 93, 94, 197, 211, 212, 240, 241, 247
McGee, J, 111
McGee, T, 196
McGill, WJ, 172, 173
McGregor, P, 244
McGurk, H, 265
McKay, J, 126
McKenna, NM, 45
McMahon, C, 260
McMurtry, PL, 243
McNabb, SD, 263
McNeil, MR, 262
McRoberts, GW, 270
Mehler, J, 264
Mehrgardt, S, 51, 52
Meiselman, C, 213
Meiselman, CH, 156, 157, 209
Meissner, WA, 213
Melcher, JR, 130
Mellers, BA, 156
Mellert, V, 51, 52
Melnick, W, 180, 181
Mencl, WE, 265
Mendelson, ES, 60
Mendelson, JR, 123, 125
Meneguzzi, S, 227
Merchán, MA, 129
Meredith, R, 265, 266
Merrill, P, 243, 245
Mershon, DH, 243
Mertus, J, 260
Merzenich, M, 132
Merzenich, MM, 45, 125, 129, 199
Mesulam, MM, 44
Metherate, R, 42
Metz, O, 50, 61, 62, 66
Metz, PJ, 248
Meyer, DR, 134
Meyer, LB, 224
Meyer, ME, 187
Meyer, MF, 220
Michelse, K, 129
Middlebrooks, JC, 51, 237, 238, 239, 241
Miedema, HME, 215
Miller, CE, 32
Miller, GA, 211, 212, 257, 267, 268, 269, 270
Miller, JD, 57, 180, 181, 259, 264, 268
Miller, JL, 257
Miller, JM, 29
Miller, MI, 114, 260
Miller, S, 155
Milligan, RA, 78

Mills, AW, 235, 239, 240, 241, 242
Mills, JH, 180
Milroy, R, 192
Mimpen, AM, 155
Minckler, J, 42, 43
Minifie, FD, 213
Mirabile, PJ, 263
Miskiewicz, A, 213
Misrahy, GS, 83
Mitler, JD, 264
Molholm, S, 265
Molin, EJE, 215
Møller, A, 61, 62
Møller, AR, 41, 44, 56, 61, 62, 66, 67, 122, 131
Møller, H, 241
Molnar, CE, 111, 112
Montgomery, A, 157
Montgomery, HC, 168
Mood, AM, 152
Moody, DB, 91
Moon, S, 273
Moore, BCJ, 172, 173, 174, 177, 178, 179, 188, 192, 193, 194, 195, 196, 197, 198, 199, 209, 210, 224, 225, 227
Moore, DR,, 155
Moore, JK, 42, 131
Moore, JN, 265, 266
Moore, RF, 1
Moran, LM, 133
Morera, C, 32
Morest, DK, 43, 45, 126
Morgan, CT, 224
Morgan, DE, 67, 155, 213
Morgan, DW, 167, 168
Morgon, A, 135
Morton, J, 271
Mossop, JE, 177, 178, 264
Mott, JB, 114
Mott, JT, 135
Möttönen, R, 265
Moulin, A, 135
Mountain, DC, 75, 135
Moushegian, G, 132, 240
Moushegian, GM, 122
Moxon, EC, 103, 111, 135, 137
Mrsic-Flogel, TD, 241
Muesch, H, 209
Muir, K, 176, 177
Muir, PJ, 133
Mukherjee, S, 44
Mukherjee, SK, 130
Müller, J, 135
Muller, U, 78
Müller-Preuss, P, 123
Mulligan, BE, 248

Mulligan, MJ, 248
Mulroy, MJ, 35
Munhall, K, 274
Munson, W, 231
Munson, WA, 66, 167, 207, 210
Murray, E, 35
Murugasu, E, 97, 135, 136
Musicant, A, 237, 238, 243
Musiek, FE, 41, 42, 44, 122

Näätänen, R, 131, 265
Nabelek, AK, 245, 269
Nabelek, IV, 269
Nachmias, J, 173
Nadol, JB, Jr, 38, 39, 41
Naidu, RC, 75
Nakanishi, Y, 265, 266
Nam, J-H, 37
Narayan, SS, 88, 91, 92, 93
Nasser, N, 265, 266
Naunton, R, 60
Nearey, TM, 259
Nedzelnitsky, V, 56, 57
Nedzelski, J, 133
Neeley, ST, 95
Neely, ST, 96, 135
Neff, DL, 179, 201, 202
Neff, WD, 44, 134, 135, 243
Neilsen, DW, 135
Nelson, DA, 174, 264
Nelson, PB, 264
Neutzel, JM, 241
Newman, EB, 156, 218, 231, 237, 239, 244
Nicely, PA, 267, 268
Nieder, B, 212
Nieder, I, 136
Nieder, P, 136
Nielsen, DW, 109
Nielsen, SH, 243, 244
Nielsen, SS, 60
Niimi, K, 44
Nimmo-Smith, I, 192
Nimura, T, 244
Noble, W, 239
Nodar, RH, 42
Nomoto, M, 109
Norat, MA, 91
Nordlund, B, 237
Nordmark, JO, 174
Norris, BE, 45, 122, 126, 127
Norris, DG, 271
Norris, JC, 200
Northern, JL, 167

Northrop, CC, 39, 103, 112
Norton, SJ, 95, 135, 196, 264
Nudo, RJ, 124
Nuttall, AL, 66, 78, 93, 97, 135, 136, 137

O'Connor, JD, 262
O'Loughlin, BJ, 194
O'Toole, AJ, 179
Odenthal, DW, 83
Ogden, GC, 271
Ohde, RN, 260, 262
Ohgushi, K, 223
Ohyama, K, 30
Old?eld, SR, 51
Oldfield, SR, 238
Oliver, D, 97
Oliver, DL, 43, 45
Oliver, ME, 112
Olson, RK, 223
Onsan, ZA, 175
Orfield, SJ, 273
Osberger, MJ, 272
Osborne, M, 35
Osborne, MP, 78
Osborne, MR, 35
Osterhammel, P, 132
Ostroff, J, 133
Owren, MJ, 178, 179
Oxenham, AJ, 199
Oyer, H, 265, 266
Ozdamar, O, 117, 118, 119

Padden, DM, 264
Palmer, A, 114, 122
Palmer, AA, 111
Palmer, AR, 43, 44, 114
Palmer, SE, 234
Pandya, DN, 44, 130
Pang, XD, 235
Parasuraman, R, 179
Pardo, JS, 264, 270
Park, TJ, 124
Parker, J, 133
Parker, PA, 51, 238
Parli, J, 42
Pasanen, EG, 241
Pastore, R, 264
Pastore, RE, 198, 199, 264
Paterson, DN, 197
Patterson, J, 175
Patterson, RD, 188, 192, 193, 196, 224, 225, 226
Patuzzi, R, 79, 88, 90, 91, 92, 96, 109, 111, 181
Pavlovic, CV, 272, 273
Payton, KL, 273, 274

Peake, WT, 55, 80, 103, 117, 135
Pearce, JR, 1
Pearsons, KS, 214, 266
Pegg, JE, 270
Pelli, DG, 155
Penfield, W, 134–135, 135
Penner, MJ, 173, 177, 199
Pentland, A, 155
Pérez Abalo, M, 133
Perez-Abalo, MC, 133
Perlman, HB, 60
Perrett, S, 239
Perrott, DR, 242, 243, 245
Peters, RW, 177, 224, 225, 226
Petersen, J, 243
Petersen, MR, 178, 179
Peterson, APG, 1
Peterson, GE, 258, 259, 266
Peterson, JL, 61
Petralia, R, 42
Petty, JW, 213
Pfaller, K, 30
Pfeiffer, RR, 57, 111, 122
Phillips, DP, 123, 125, 134, 177, 178, 264
Phillips, R, 42
Picardi, MC, 155, 175
Picheny, MA, 273, 274
Pichora-Fuller, MK, 177
Pickett, JM, 257, 269
Pickler, AG, 231
Pickles, JO, 35, 76, 78, 88
Pike, CL, 35
Pillon, B, 134
Piskorski, P, 167
Pisoni, DB, 178, 263, 264, 272
Plack, CJ, 224
Planert, N, 238
Plenge, G, 51, 237
Plomp, R, 155, 171, 177, 220, 223, 224, 225, 226, 227, 237
Plourde, G, 133
Poirier, P, 125
Pollack, I, 199, 207, 231, 239, 267
Pollack, J, 60
Poole, JD, 168
Popel, AS, 37, 38, 96
Popelka, G, 61, 66
Popelka, S, 61, 62, 66, 67
Popper, AN, 30, 41, 78
Popper, N, 122, 126

Porter, RJ, 263
Postman, L, 272
Potter, AB, 60
Potter, RK, 258
Poulsen, T, 207, 212
Powell, R, 265, 266
Powell, TPS, 45, 130
Powers, GL, 268
Pratt, H, 131, 132
Preuss, AP, 123
Preuss, TM, 43
Price, C, 263
Probst, R, 93, 94
Proctor, B, 26, 30
Prosek, RA, 157
Pugh, JE, Jr, 117
Puil, E, 42
Puleo, JS, 199
Pulvermüller, F, 263
Puranik, CS, 199
Purcell, D, 133
Purcell, DW, 133

Qu, H, 234
Querengesser, C, 274

Raab, DH, 134, 172, 173
Rabiner, LR, 154, 155, 248, 249
Rabinowitz, WM, 67, 173, 243
Raczkowski, D, 44, 45
Radeau, M, 265
Radley, JPA, 259, 260
Raij, T, 126
Rainey, D, 197
Rajan, R, 126
Rakerd, B, 246, 247
Rance, G, 133
Raney, JJ, 264
Raphael, LJ, 257, 260
Rappaport, BZ, 166
Rask-Andersen, H, 30
Rasmussen, GL, 5, 40, 45
Rasmussen, T, 135
Ravizza, R, 134
Ravizza, RJ, 44
Rayment, SG, 260
Raynor, S, 78, 82, 91
Read, C, 257, 259
Reale, RA, 44, 125, 129
Recio, A, 88, 91, 92, 93
Reed, CM, 273, 274
Reeves, A, 197, 198
Reger, SN, 66
Reitz, ML, 269

Relkin, EM, 199
Remez, RE, 264, 270
Remond, MC, 111, 117
Remus, JJ, 155
Repp, BR, 261, 264
Révész, G, 222
Reynolds, ER, 266
Reynolds, GS, 231
Rhebergen, KS, 272
Rho, JM, 39, 103, 112
Rhode, WS, 87, 88, 91, 92, 93, 111, 122, 123, 125
Rhys Evans, RH, 35
Ricci, AJ, 37
Rich NC, 41
Rich, NC, 88, 91, 92, 93, 109, 111
Richard, G, 173
Richards, AM, 211, 212
Richards, F, 133
Richards, V, 247
Richards, VM, 201, 202
Richardson, GP, 37
Richardson, M, 265
Rickards, F, 133
Rickards, FW, 133
Riesz, RR, 172, 173
Rigopulos, A, 235
Rintelmann, WF, 268
Rio, ED, 273, 274
Riopelle, AJ, 67
Ritsma, R, 225, 226
Ritsma, RJ, 94, 224
Ritter, W, 265
Rivier, F, 43, 44
Roberts, B, 194, 195, 196
Roberts, WM, 76, 78
Robertson, CE, 199
Robertson, D, 42, 45, 92
Robinette, LN, 245, 269
Robinette, MS, 93, 94
Robinson, DE, 147, 247, 248
Robinson, DW, 166, 167, 207, 208, 209
Robles, L, 78, 88, 91, 92, 93, 97, 111
Rockel, AJ, 43, 45
Romand, R, 41, 42, 43, 44
Romano, MN, 131
Ronald, A, 78
Ronken, DA, 175–176
Rooney, BJ, 134
Rose, JE, 44, 105, 106, 107, 108, 109, 111, 113, 115, 122, 125, 126, 128, 129, 226
Rose, M, 239
Rosen, BR, 130
Rosen, S, 199
Rosenblith, W, 131

Rosenblith, WA, 51, 174
Rosenblum, LD, 264
Rosenblut, B, 82, 85
Rosenzweig, MR, 134, 244, 272
Rosler, G, 67, 68
Rosner, BS, 264
Rosowski, JJ, 56
Ross, C, 42
Ross, DA, 51, 52
Ross, L, 155
Ross, S, 66
Rossing, TD, 1, 222
Roth, GL, 125
Roth, RL, 237
Rouiller, E, 122
Rouiller, EM, 122, 124
Rousso, I, 34
Rowan, D, 155
Rowland, RC, 231
Rowley, RR, 208
Rubin, PE, 264
Rudell, AP, 131
Rudmose, W, 167
Ruggero, MA, 41, 78, 88, 91, 92, 93, 97, 109, 111
Ruhm, H, 131
Runge, PS, 239
Rupert, AL, 122, 132
Ruppersberg, JP, 97
Russell, IJ, 78, 80, 81, 85, 86, 88, 89, 97, 111, 135, 136
Rutherford, 73, W
Ryalls, J, 257
Ryan, AF, 34, 35
Ryan, S, 135
Rybalko, N, 134
Ryugo, DK, 38, 39, 41, 103, 112

Saberi, K, 199, 201, 202, 243, 245
Sachs, MB, 103, 109, 110, 111, 112, 114, 115, 116, 122, 136, 260
Sacia, CE, 265
Sahley, SL, 42
Saint-Amour, D, 265
Sakaguchi, H, 78
Salt, AN, 30
Salvi, R, 111, 112
Sams, M, 126, 265
Samson, DS, 262, 263
Samson, FK, 125
Samson, FR, 126
Sandel, TT, 236, 237
Sanders, JB, 1
Sando, I, 126, 127
Sanides, F, 43
Santi, PA, 41
Santos-Sacchi, J, 80, 88, 96, 97

Saul, L, 80

Saunders, JC, 35, 180, 181

Savel, S, 197

Savio, G, 133

Sawusch, JR, 264

Sayers, BMcA, 232, 233

Scarrow, I, 155

Schacht, J, 29, 30, 34, 74, 79, 80, 81, 97

Schacknow, RN, 173

Schaefer, TH, 190

Schalk, TB, 111

Scharf, B, 22, 61, 66, 187, 191, 192, 197, 198, 209, 210, 212, 213, 218, 231

Scharlock, DP, 134

Schechter, MA, 166

Schellenberg, EG, 223

Scherg, M, 131, 133

Schlauch, RS, 207

Schloth, E, 167

Schmidt, PN, 83

Schmidt-Nielsen, 273, A

Schmiedt, RA, 109, 180, 181

Schmitt, U, 97

Schneider, BA, 177, 234

Schneider, ME, 35, 180, 181

Schnupp JWH, 241

Schooneveldt, GP, 197

Schorn, K, 194

Schouten, JF, 224, 225, 226

Schouten, MEH, 264

Schreiber, RC, 104, 126, 127

Schreiner, C, 123

Schreiner, CE, 123, 129, 130

Schrott-Fisher, A, 30

Schubert, ED, 249

Schulman, AI, 164

Schulman, S, 262, 263

Schulte, U, 97

Schultz, MC, 249

Schum, DJ, 273

Schwartz, DW, 42

Schwartz, IR, 42

Schwartzkopff, J, 122

Schwimmer, S, 268

Scott, KR, 243

Searle, CL, 260

Sears, RE, 88

Seebeck, A, 224

Seewann, M, 226

Sellick, PM, 78, 80, 81, 85, 86, 88, 89, 90, 91, 92, 109

Sellick, RM, 111

Semal, C, 223

Semple, MN, 125

Sereno, MI, 130

Sergeant, RL, 243

Sewell, WE, 103

Sewell, WF, 74, 91

Shah, P, 175

Shailer, MJ, 177, 192, 224

Shamma, S, 114, 122

Shanks, JE, 63

Shankweiler, D, 262, 263

Shankweiler, DB, 264, 270

Sharbrough, F, 134

Sharf, DJ, 259

Shaw, EAG, 51, 52, 167, 237, 238

Shaw, WA, 218, 231

Sheft, S, 234

Shelton, BR, 155

Shen, W, 97

Shepard, RN, 222

Sherbecoe, RL, 272, 273

Sherlock, LP, 198, 199

Sherlock, P, 157, 168

Sherrick, CE, Jr, 177, 178, 200

Shewaker, CA, 190

Shinabarger, EW, 83

Shinn-Cunningham, BG, 241, 244, 245

shinn-Cunningham, BG, 126

Shneck, RZ, 34

Shoeny, ZG, 82, 85, 91

Shower, EG, 174, 231, 232

Shtyrov, Y, 263

Sieben, UK, 155

Siegel, JH, 135

Silberberg, Y, 34

Silkes, SM, 114

Silman, S, 61, 62, 66, 67, 245, 269

Silverman, CA, 62

Silverman, SR, 266

Simmons, DD, 40, 41, 103

Simmons, FB, 57, 66, 67

Simola, J, 265

Simpson, WA, 155

Simpson, WE, 243

Sinex, DG, 114

Sinnott, JM, 178, 179

Siqueland, P, 264

Sirimanna, T, 265, 266

Sirinathsinghji, DJ, 42

Sithole, NM, 270

Sivian, LJ, 166, 167, 231

Sjostrand, F, 40

Sklar, DL, 180, 181

Slepecky, N, 97

Slepecky, NB, 29, 32, 34, 35, 37

Slepian, JZ, 135

Slis, IH, 260

Small, A, 224, 225
Small, AM, 170, 178, 187, 194, 198, 211, 212, 213, 224, 225, 226
Smiarowski, RA, 199
Smith, CA, 29, 40, 82, 85
Smith, DW, 91
Smith, HD, 66, 67
Smith, JC, 177, 178
Smith, MA, 197
Smith, PH, 122, 124
Smith, RL, 105, 122, 199
Smoorenburg, G, 226
Smoorenburg, GF, 221
Smurzynski, J, 227
Snead, CR, 129
Snyder, RL, 45
Sohmer, HS, 80, 131, 132
Sokolich, WG, 109
Sondhi, MM, 248
Sone, T, 244
Soquet, A, 265
Sorensen, MF, 241
Sovijarvi, ARA, 126
Spatz, W, 45
Speaks, C, 268
Speaks, CE, 1
Spencer, H, 34
Spieth, W, 189
Spiropoulos, CS, 80
Spitzer, MW, 125
Spoendlin, H, 38, 39, 40, 41
Spoor, A, 83
Squires, KC, 132
Stanford, TR, 125
Stanton, ME, 174
Stapells, DR, 131, 133
Starr, A, 66, 131, 233
Stebbins, W, 91, C
Steel, KR, 33, 35, 78
Steeneken, HJM, 223, 273
Steinberg, GC, 272
Steinberg, JC, 168, 266, 267
Stellmack, MA, 173, 232, 241
Stenfelt, S, 60
Stephen, DG, 272
Stephens, D, 265, 266
Stephens, SDG, 212
Stepp, CE, 53
Stern, RM, 124
Stevens, JC, 157, 208, 209, 211, 212
Stevens, KN, 174, 258, 259, 260, 264, 270
Stevens, N, 261
Stevens, SS, 66, 146, 156, 157, 189, 190, 191, 207, 208, 209, 211, 218, 224, 231, 237, 239, 268
Stillman, RD, 132

Stinton, MR, 51
Stokinger, TE, 213
Stoll, G, 226
Stonecypher, JF, 248
Strange, W, 259
Stream, RW, 167
Strelioff, D, 35
Strevens, P, 261
Strickland, EA, 93, 96, 197
Strominger, NL, 134
Strong, W, 227
Strutz, J, 45
Strybel, TZ, 243, 245
Stuart, A, 177, 178, 264
Studdert-Kennedy, M, 259, 261, 262, 263, 264, 270
Studebaker, GA, 208, 213, 272, 273
Suga, N, 109, 123, 126
Sulahian, J, 132
Summerfield, Q, 250
Summers, IR, 222
Sundby, A, 62, 63
Supowit, A, 155
Suter, CM, 132
Sutton, S, 131, 199
Suzuki Y, 133
Swainson, B, 265
Swets, JA, 160, 161, 164, 190
Swiderski, N, 133
Syka, J, 134
Synder, RL, 41
Szalda, K, 133

Takahashi, GA, 197
Takahashi, T, 32
Takata, Y, 269
Tal, E, 34
Talavage, TM, 130
Talmadge, CL, 167
Tang, Z, 201, 202
Tanner, WP, Jr, 161, 190
Tartter, VC, 264
Tasaki, I, 80, 83, 116, 117
Tavartkiladze, G, 265, 266
Taylor, IM, 157
Taylor, KJ, 87, 88
Taylor, MM, 152, 154, 155
Taylor, T, 177, 178, 264
Teas, DC, 117, 125, 126, 135, 236, 237
Tees, RC, 270
Teffeteller, S, 192
Tennigkeit, F, 42
Terhardt, E, 191, 192, 224, 226
Terkildsen, K, 60, 132

Tervaniemi, M, 263
Thallinger, G, 34
Thalmann, I, 34
Thalmann, R, 30, 34
Theodore, LH, 161
Thierry, G, 263
Thomas, M, 130
Thompson, CL, 262, 263
Thompson, GC, 42
Thompson, PO, 190
Throop, J, 243
Thurlow, WR, 224, 225, 226, 239
Thwing, EJ, 213
Tietze, G, 63
Tiffany, WR, 259
Tiippana, K, 265
Tiitinen, H, 263
Tillman, T, 249
Tillmann, B, 130, 222
Tilney, LG, 35
Tilney, MS, 35
Tobias, JV, 231, 233
Todd, MA, 244
Tokita, J, 78
Tollin, DJ, 245
Tomlin, D, 133
Tonndorf, J, 54, 55, 56, 58, 59, 60, 74, 77, 88
Torick, EL, 237
Toros-Morel, A, 122
Tos, M, 27
Townsend, TH, 249
Trahiotis, C, 124, 241
Tran, K, 265, 266
Trehub, SE, 177, 223
Tremblay, KL, 131
Truscott, I, 268
Tsuchitani, C, 124, 127, 128
Tsuchitani, CC, 126
Tubis, A, 93, 96, 167
Tucker, FM, 269
Tucker, J, 243
Tukey, JW, 146
Tunturi, AR, 129
Turner, CW, 173, 174, 199
Turner, RG, 35
Turvey, MT, 257, 270
Tyler, CW, 155
Tyler, LK, 271
Tzourio-Mazoyer, N, 263

Uchanski, RM, 175, 273, 274
Ulehlova, J, 34
Ulehlova, L, 34
Ulfendahl, M, 37, 97

Urbas, JV, 123
Utter, G, 35

Vaillancourt, MM, 52, 237
Valdés, J, 133
van Bergeijk, WA, 1
van de Par, S, 250
Van Den Brink, G, 167, 226
Van Der Werff, KR, 133
van Horn, JD, 130, 222
van Noorden, 227, L
Van Roon, P, 133
van Wee, B, 215
VanCamp, J, 56, 57
vanHessen, AJ, 264
vanWijngaarden, SJ, 273
Versfeld, NJ, 272
Veuillet, E, 135
Vicente-Torres, A, 42
Viemeister, NF, 172, 173, 176, 177, 198, 199, 224, 232
Vigorito, J, 264
Villchur, E, 167
Vingrys, AJ, 155
Vitevitch, MS, 272
Voldrich, L, 34
Volkmann, J, 156, 218
Vollrath, MA, 35, 37, 78, 79
von Bismark, G, 227, 248
von Klitzing, R, 197
vonCramon, D, 131
vonHelmholtz, H, 72
Vorperian, HK, 260
Vos, H, 215
Voss, SE, 53

Wagenaars, WM, 243
Wagner, E, 212
Wagner, W, 135
Waldegger, S, 97
Walden, BE, 157
Walker, E, 131
Wallace, MN, 43, 44
Wallach, H, 239, 244
Walley, AC, 261
Walsh, EJ, 111
Walsh, JL, 209
Walton, J, 199
Walzl, EM, 129
Wang, C, 234
Wang, C-Y, 78, 82, 91
Wang, X, 123
Wang, XQ, 122
Wangemann, P, 29, 30, 74, 79, 80, 81
Ward, PH, 83, 84, 85
Ward, WD, 180, 181, 222, 223, 224

Warr, WB, 45, 122, 124, 135
Warren, ML, 135
Watanabe, T, 122
Watson, AB, 155
Watson, CS, 57, 147, 170, 171, 179, 180
Weber, DL, 192, 196, 199
Weber, K, 37
Webster, DB, 122
Webster, DL, 192
Webster, FA, 248
Webster, JC, 233, 250, 273
Webster, WB, 41
Webster, WR, 122, 125, 129
Wedin, L, 227
Wegel, RL, 167, 187, 188
Weikers, NJ, 134
Weinrich, S, 237
Weiss, TE, 35, 80
Wenthold, R, 42
Wenthold, RJ, 42
Wenzel, EM, 235, 241
Werker, JF, 270
Wernick, JS, 233
Wersall, J, 34, 38
Westerman, LA, 105
Westerman, S, 265, 266
Wetherill, GB, 151, 152, 154
Wever, EG, 23, 28, 53, 54, 73, 74, 80, 81, 82, 83
Wezel, DL, 227
Whalen, DH, 264, 265, 270
Wheeler, K, 258
Wheeler, LJ, 168
Wheeler, PA, 1
Whitcomb, MA, 122
White, LJ, 197
White, SD, 166, 167, 231
Whitehead, ML, 93, 94
Whitfield, IC, 113, 115, 123, 129, 134
Whitworth, RH, 240, 247
Wickesberg, RE, 125
Widin, GP, 199
Wiederhold, ML, 135
Wiener, FM, 51, 52, 167, 266
Wiener, FN, 57
Wier, CC, 172, 173, 174, 207, 231, 232, 233, 264
Wightman, EL, 93, 94
Wightman, FL, 66, 196, 224, 226, 237, 238, 239, 240, 241, 248
Wild, T, 60
Wiley, T, 61
Wiley, TL, 63
Williams, C, 266
Williams, D, 155
Williams, KA, 270
Williston, JS, 131

Wilson, JP, 85, 87, 88
Wilson, JR, 167
Wilson, RH, 56, 57, 61, 62, 63, 168, 198, 199
Wilson-Kubalek, EM, 78
Winer, JA, 41, 43, 44, 45, 130
Winslow, RL, 136
Winter, IM, 92, 114
Winther, F, 61, 62
Wit, HP, 94
Wittenberg, A, 235
Witzel, T, 126
Wojtczak, M, 172, 173
Wolberg, Z, 123
Wood, CC, 263
Woodford, C, 62, 63
Woods, WS, 201, 235
Woodworth, RS, 235
Woolsey, CN, 44, 129, 130, 134
Wrege, KS, 126
Wright, A, 34, 35
Wright, BA, 199, 201, 202, 233
Wright, D, 237
Wright, HN, 170, 199, 213
Wroton, HW, 179
Wu, M-L, 29
Wu, X, 97, 234
Wu, Y, 234
Wynne, B, 42

Yang, X, 244
Yantis, PJ, 220
Yates, GK, 88, 92, 181
Yela, M, 134
Yeni-Komshian, GH, 123
Yeshurun, Y, 123
Yin, TCT, 122, 124, 125
Yoshie, N, 117
Yost, WA, 199, 212, 234, 239, 240, 244, 247, 249
Young, ED, 114, 115, 116
Young, HD, 1
Zahorik, P, 243, 244
Zajic, G, 97
Zakrisson, JE, 62
Zeng, FG, 273, 274
Zenner, HP, 97, 135
Zheng, J, 97
Zimmerman, U, 97
Zubin, J, 131
Zuo, J, 97
Zurek, PM, 93, 94, 245
Zwicker, E, 167, 191, 192, 194, 197, 199, 209, 211, 218, 219, 220, 221, 224
Zwislocki, JJ, 34, 53, 57, 60, 61, 62, 88, 109, 156, 157, 170, 173, 174, 200, 208, 209, 210, 211, 231, 239

Subject Index

A-weighting network (see Weighting networks)
Absolute (perfect) pitch, 223
Absolute magnitude estimation, 156
Absolute magnitude production, 156
Absolute refractory period (see Refractory period)
Absolute sensitivity, 147, 149, 166–168, 170 (see also Threshold)
Acceleration, 2, 18
Accessory structures, 74
Accommodation theory, 67
Acoustic emissions (see Otoacoustic emissions)
Acoustic reflex, 28, 44, 60–61, 62, 66, 67, 68
Acoustic reflex arc, 44–45
Acoustic stria, 42
Acoustic theory of speech production, 257, 258
Acoustics, 1
Across-fiber tuning curves, 118, 119
Action potential (AP), 74, 83, 103
Active processes in cochlea, 90, 95, 96, 135 (see also Cochlear micromechanics)
Adaptation, 63, 64, 65, 105, 213, 214 (see also Loudness adaptation)
Adaptive procedures, 151–155
Aditus ad antrum, 20, 26
Afferent neurons and system (see Auditory neuron, Auditory pathways)
Affricates, 259, 262
Air conduction, 58, 60
All-or-none response, 73
Allophones, 257, 272 (see also Phonemes)
Alveolars, 259, 260, 262
Amplitude, 11, 12, 15, 117, 132, 133, 220, 246, 262
Amplitude modulation (AM), 172, 173, 176
Amplitude-latency function of action potential, 117
Ampullae, 30
Anechoic, 237, 243, 246
Analysis-by-synthesis, 270
Ankle connectors, 37
Annulus, 23, 54
Anterior auditory field (see Auditory cortex)
Anteroventral cochlear nucleus (see Cochlear nucleus)
Anticipation, 148
Antihelix, 23
Antinodes, 16
Antitragus, 23
Antrum, 20
Aperiodic waves, 11, 13 (see also Complex waves, Noise, Waves)
Area (see Auditory cortex)
Area AI (see Auditory cortex)
Area AII (see Auditory cortex)

Area AIII (see Auditory cortex)
Area ratio, 53–54
Articulation index (AI), 272, 273
Articulation score (see Speech recognition)
Artificial mastoid, 169
Ascending series (or run), 147
Aspiration, 257, 259
ASSR (see Auditory steady-state response)
Asymptotic threshold shift (ATS), 180
Attic (see Epitympanic recess)
Audiogram, 169, 170
Audiology, 130, 169
Audiometer and Audiometry, 168, 170 (see also Audiology, Hearing level, Hearing loss)
Audiometric standards (see Hearing level)
Auditory area (see Auditory cortex)
Auditory brainstem response (see Short latency response)
Auditory cortex, 43, 44, 123, 125–126, 130, 133, 134, 135
Auditory evoked potentials, 130–133
Auditory filter, 190, 192, 193, 225
Auditory frequency analysis (see Auditory filter, Critical band, Frequency selectivity, Pitch, Tuning)
Auditory nerve, 20, 30, 38, 44, 74, 103–119
Auditory neuron (see Auditory nerve)
Auditory pathways, 122–137
Auditory radiations, 43
Auditory scene analysis, 233–234
Auditory steady-state response (ASSR), 132–133
Auditory streaming (see Auditory scene analysis)
Auditory theories of speech perception (see General auditory speech perception approaches)
Aural beats (see Beats)
Aural harmonics, 220 (see also Beats, Combination tones, Distortion)
Auricle (see Pinna)
AVCN (see Cochlear nucleus)
AVE SP (see Summating potential)
Average acceleration, 2
Average velocity, 1, 2
Averaged localized synchronized rate (ALSR), 115, 116
Averaging, 116, 131, 157
Azimuth, 51, 52, 126, 156, 235, 239, 244
Azimuth effect, 52

B-weighting network (see Weighting networks)
Backward masking, 198, 199 (see also Forward masking, Temporal masking)
Balance system (see Vestibular system)
Band-pass filter, 15, 16
Band-reject filter, 15, 16
Bandwidth, 15, 61, 87, 189, 190, 266

Bark scale, 191

Basic quantities, 1

Basilar membrane (and Cochlear partition), 30, 31, 32, 72, 74, 75, 76, 78, 86, 90, 93, 113

Bass, 207

Beats, 172, 188, 192, 219–221, 232 (see also Binaural beats, Best beats, Binaural fusion, Combination tones, Distortion)

Best beats, 219, 220

Best beats method, 220

Best frequency (see Characteristic frequency)

Beta (β), 162

Bias, 147, 152, 156, 157

Bilabials, 259, 260

BILD (see Masking level differences)

Binaural beats, 233

Binaural coding, 123–126

Binaural fusion, 232–233

Binaural hearing, 51, 231

Binaural intelligibility level differences (BILD) (see MLD for speech)

Binaural interference, 241

Binaural masking level differences (BMLD (see Masking level differences)

Binaural summation, 231, 232

Binaural unmasking (see Masking level differences)

Blood supply to cochlea, 34, 35, 81

Bone conduction, 58–60

Bony labyrinth, 28

Bottom-up processing, 270

Bounce effect (in TTS), 181

Brachium of inferior colliculus, 43

Bracketing method, 149

Brainstem auditory evoked response (see Short latency response)

BUDTIF, 153–154

BUDYEN, 154

Build-up units, 246

Bushy cells, 122

C-weighting network (see Weighting networks)

Cancellation, 12, 58, 250

Cancellation method, 220

Capacitance probe, 54, 88

Carhart's notch, 60

Catch trials, 150, 160, 161, 164

Categorical perception, 263–264

Category scales, 156

Center clipping, 267

Center frequency (of filter), 15, 192, 193

Central auditory nervous system (CANS) (see Auditory pathways)

Central auditory system (see Auditory pathways)

Central masking, 199–200

Central nervous system (CNS) (see Auditory pathways)

Cents, 222

Cerebellum, 20, 45

Cerebral dominance (see Hemispheric lateralization)

Ceruminous glands, 23–24

cgs system/units (see also MKS system/units)

Characteristic delay, 124, 125

Characteristic frequency (CF) (see also Tuning)

Chemical mediators, 74, 80

Chopper units, 122

Chorda tympani nerve, 27 (see also Facial nerve)

Chords, 223, 224

Chroma, 222, 223

Cilia, 34, 78, 81 (see also Hair cells)

Cilia cross-links (see Cross-links)

Claudius cells, 33

Clear speech, 273–274

Click pitch, 170 (see also Pitch, Tonality)

Clifton effect, 245, 246–247 (see also Precedence effect)

Clinical method of limits, 149

Closed set, 266

CMR (see Comodulation masking release)

CNV (see Contingent negative variation)

Cochlea, 20, 28, 30–34, 38, 45, 53, 58, 72, 77, 83, 87, 90, 93, 97, 104, 105, 116, 126, 225

Cochlear amplifier, 96–97, 135

Cochlear aqueduct, 30

Cochlear duct (see Scala media)

Cochlear echo (see Otoacoustic emissions)

Cochlear electrical potentials, 79–86

Cochlear fluids, 52, 53, 58, 80 (see also Endolymph, Perilymph)

Cochlear frequency map, 86, 104

Cochlear micromechanics, 96 (see also Active processes, Cochlear frequency selectivity, Tuning)

Cochlear microphonic (CM), 58, 66, 78, 80, 81, 82, 83, 84, 86, 111, 116, 135 (see also Receptor potentials)

Cochlear models, 76

Cochlear nerve (see Auditory nerve)

Cochlear nucleus (CN), 42, 117, 122, 126

Cochlear partition (see Basilar membrane)

Cochlear tuning (see Cochlear frequency selectivity, Cochlear micromechanics, Tuning)

Cochleariform process, 26, 28

Cocktail party effect, 233

Coefficient of friction, 3

Cognates, 259

Cohort model, 271

Combination tones, 72, 188, 192, 219–221

Commissural fibers of Probst, 43

Commissure of inferior colliculus, 42, 43

Common fate (see Auditory scene analysis)

Comodulated bands, 196

Comodulation masking release (CMR), 196–197

Complex waves, 13–15

Compound action potential (CAP), 115, 131, 136 (see also Whole-nerve action potential)
Compression, 7, 9, 58
Concha, 23
Concurrent minimum audible angle (CMAA), 242 (see also Minimal audible angle)
Conductive mechanism, 51–68
Cone of confusion, 242
Confidence rating methods, 164
Confusion scales (see Discriminability scales)
Consonance, 223
Consonants, 114, 223, 259–262, 265
Consonant-to-vowel ratio, 274
Context, 28, 64, 88, 90, 175, 200, 219, 222, 270
Contingent negative variation (CNV), 131
Continuous pedestal, 172, 173
Contractile proteins, 37
Conversational speech, 273–274 (see also Clear speech)
Corpus callosum, 44
Correct rejection, 160, 163
Correction for guessing, 160
Cortical ablation effects (see Cortical sound discrimination)
Cortical evoked potentials (see Long latency response)
Cortical sound discrimination, 134–135
Corticofugal pathways, 45
Cost, 163
Coupler-referred MAP (MAPC), 166, 167
Cristae, 29
Criterion, 161, 162, 163, 164
Critical band, 61, 191, 192, 202, 210, 223 (see also Auditory filter, Critical ratio)
Critical band rate scale (see Bark scale)
Critical duration, 212
Critical ratio, 191 (see also Critical band, Masking)
Cross-hearing, 199
Cross-links, 35
Cross-modality matching, 157
Crossed olivocochlear bundle (COCB) (see Olivocochlear bundle)
CTCF (Continuous tone at its characteristic frequency), 110, 111
Cubic difference tone, 95, 220–221
Curved-membrane mechanism, 54–55
Curved membrane principle (see Curved-membrane mechanism)
Cut-off frequency (of filter), 15, 190
Cuticular plate, 34, 35, 37
Cycle, 11, 13, 73, 76, 113
Cycles per second (cps), 11, 188 (see also Hertz)
Cytoarchitecture of auditory cortex, 125–126
d' (d prime), 161, 163
Damping, 7, 19, 72
dB (see Decibels)
dB-A (see Weighting networks)

dB-B (see Weighting networks)
dB-C (see Weighting networks)
dc fall (see Summating potential)

DCN (see Cochlear nucleus)
Deafness (see Hearing loss)
Decibels (dB), 4, 5, 15, 171, 177
Decision axis, 160, 162, 164
Deiters' cells, 32, 33, 34, 38
Descending series (or run), 147, 148, 149
Desensitization-interference-injury protection theory (of acoustic reflex), 168
Dichotic listening, 262–263
DIF SP (see Summating potential)
Difference limen (DL), 149, 171, 218, 231 (see also Just noticeable difference)
Difference tones, 95, 220, 221, 225
Differential sensitivity, 147, 149, 164, 171–179, 231–232
Diphthongs, 257
Direct scaling, 155–157
Directional hearing, 234–244
Direct Realist Theory, 270
Discharge patterns (see Firing patterns)
Discriminability scales, 156
Discrimination score (see Speech recognition)
Discrimination suppression (see Precedence effect)
Displacement, 1, 2, 3, 10, 11, 16, 17, 18, 78, 136
Dissonance, 223–224
Distortion, 55, 60, 225, 245, 273
Distortion product otoacoustic emissions (see Otoacoustic emissions)
Distortional bone conduction, 59
Dorsal cochlear nucleus (see Cochlear nucleus)
Doubling rule, 153
Down rule, 154
Ductus reuniens, 30
Duplex perception, 264
Duplex theory, 235
Duration effects, 170–171 (see also Temporal discrimination, Temporal summation)
Dyne, 3

Ear canal, 20, 23–24
Eardrum, 24–25 (see also Tympanic membrane)
Earlobe, 23
Earphones, 166, 210, 235, 239, 244, 247
Echo suppression, 244, 247
Echo suppression (see Precedence effect)
Echo threshold (see Precedence effect)
Echoes, 237
Echolocation (in bats), 126
Ectosylvian area (Ep) (see Auditory cortex)
Ectosylvian sulcus (see Auditory cortex)
Effective area of eardrum, 54

Effective quiet, 180
Efferent neurons and system, 40 (see also Olivocochlear bundle)
Eighth (cranial) nerve (see Auditory nerve)
Elastic modulus, 3
Elasticity, 3, 7
Electrodes, 80, 83, 132
Electroencephalographic response (EEG), 130
Electromyographic response (EMG), 62
Elevation, 51, 235, 237
Endocochlear potential (EP), 80, 135
Endolymph, 29, 31, 79, 80
Endolymphatic duct, 30
Endolymphatic fluid (see Endolymph)
Endolymphatic sac, 30
Energetic masking, 200, 201, 202
Energy, 4, 161, 171
Epitympanic recess, 20, 27
Equal loudness contours, 66, 207, 211 (see also Phons)
Equal loudness levels (see Phons)
Equal noisiness contours, 207
Equal pitch distances, 218
Equal temperament, 221, 222
Equalization-cancellation model of MLDs, 250
Equilibrium, 3
Equivalent rectangular filter, 192
Erg, 4
Eustachian tube, 25, 26, 28
Event-related potentials, 131
Evoked auditory potentials, 130–133
Evoked otoacoustic emissions (see Otoacoustic emissions)
Evoked potentials (see Evoked auditory potentials)
Evoked responses (see Evoked auditory potentials)
Excitation (see Excitatory responses)
Excitation pattern, 113, 188 (see also Traveling wave)
Excitatory responses, 122, 124
Exemplar models, 271
Expectation, 66, 265
External auditory meatus (see Ear canal)

Facial nerve, 28, 44
False alarm, 153, 160, 161, 162, 163
Fatigue (see Post-stimulatory fatigue)
Features, 271
Feedback, 66, 96, 175
Feeling, threshold of, 168
FFR (see Frequency-following response)
Fifth (cranial) nerve (see Trigeminal nerve)
Figure-ground (see Auditory scene analysis)
Filter, 15–16, 190 (see also Auditory filter)
Filtered speech, 263
Firing patterns, 103, 104–109, 122
Firing rate, 103, 111, 115, 124, 135
First wavefront principle (see Precedence effect)

Flanking bands (see Off-frequency bands)
Fletcher-Munson curves (see Equal loudness contours, Phons)
Force, 1, 2, 3, 54
Formant transitions, 260
Formants, 114, 257, 258
Forward masking, 196, 198, 199 (see also Backward masking, Temporal masking)
Fossa incudis, 26, 28
Fourier analysis, 14, 72, 226
Fourier's theorem, 14
Fractionalization, 156 (see also Ratio production)
Franssen effect, 246 (see also Precedence effect)
Frequency, 9, 11, 13, 14, 17, 18, 166, 176, 181, 258
Frequency coding, 74, 103–111 (see also Tuning)
Frequency discrimination, 72, 87, 134, 174–175
Frequency-following response (FFR), 132
Frequency modulation, 132, 174
Frequency selectivity, 86–91, 190–194
Frequency theory (see Temporal theory)
Frication, 262, 267
Fricatives, 259, 261–262
Friction, 3, 7, 18
Fundamental frequency, 13, 72, 109, 224, 225, 226, 257, 274
Fusiform cells, 122, 123
Fuzzy logical model of perception (FLMP), 271

Gap detection, 177, 264
Gap detection threshold, 134, 177
Gated pedestal, 173
Gaussian noise (see White noise)
General auditory speech perception approaches, 264, 270
Generator potential, 74
Gestalt grouping factors (see Auditory scene analysis)
Glides, 262 (see also Semivowels)
Glottis, 262
Good continuation (see Auditory scene analysis)

Haas effect (see Precedence effect)
Habenula perforata, 32, 38
Habituation, 148, 149
Hair bundle motor, 97 (see also Somatic motor)
Hair cell activation, 76–78
Hair cell motility (see Cochlear micromechanics)
Hair cells, 34–38
Half-power point, 15, 87
Halving rule, 153
Harmonic distortion (see Distortion)
Harmonic motion, 6–11 (see also Simple harmonic motion)
Harmonicity (see Auditory scene analysis)
Harmonics, 13, 219–221
Head movement, 239, 242
Head-related transfer function (HRTF), 51, 52, 237
Head shadow, 51, 235, 236
Hearing level, 169–170

Hearing loss, 60, 135, 168, 170
Helicotrema, 31, 75
Helix, 21, 23, 222
Hemispheric lateralization, 262
Hensen's body, 33, 35
Hensen's cells, 33
Hensen's stripe (see also Tectorial membrane)
Hertz (Hz), 11
Heschl's gyrus (see Auditory cortex)
Heterophonic loudness balance (see Loudness balance)
High-pass filter, 15, 16, 60, 267
Hit, 160
Hooke's law, 3
Horseradish peroxidase (HRP), 39, 86, 103
HRP (see Horseradish peroxidase)
HRTF (see Head-related transfer function)
Hybrid adaptive procedures, 155

IC (see Inferior colliculus)
Ideal observer, 162, 163
IHC (see Hair cells)
IIDs (see Interaural intensity differences)
ILDs (see Interaural level differences)
Impedance, 17–18, 52
Impedance matching transformer (see Middle ear transformer mechanism)
Incus, 27, 28, 53, 55
Induced Loudness Reduction (ILR), 212 (see also Loudness recalibration)
Inertia, 2, 7, 53, 59
Inertial bone conduction, 59 (see also Bone conduction)
Inferior colliculus (IC), 42, 122, 125, 129
Informational masking, 179, 200–202 (see also Stimulus uncertainty)
Inhibition (see Inhibitory responses)
Inhibitory areas, 110, 111
Inhibitory responses, 124, 135
Inner ear, 20, 28–38, 45, 59, 72 (see also Cochlea)
Inner hair cells (see Hair cells)
Innervation of the cochlea, 40 (see also Auditory nerve)
Input-output (I-O) function, 81, 82, 112, 197
Insert receivers, 168, 186
Instantaneous acceleration, 2
Instantaneous amplitude, 11, 12
Instantaneous velocity, 2
Insular area (INS) (see Auditory cortex)
Intensity, 4, 5
Intensity coding, 111–114, 115
Intensity discrimination, 172–174
Intensity image, 240
Intensity level (IL), 5, 6, 103, 207
Interaural intensity differences (see Interaural level differences)
Interaural intensity discrimination (see Interaural intensity differences, Interaural level differences)

Interaural level differences (ILD), 123, 124, 235, 249
Interaural phase differences (see Interaural time differences)
Interaural phase discrimination (see Interaural time differences)
Interaural time differences (ITD), 123, 124, 235, 236, 237, 240, 241 (see also Interaural intensity differences)
Internal auditory meatus (canal), 20, 40
Internal spiral sulcus, 32
Interruption rate, 225, 268
Intertragal incisure, 23
Interval of uncertainty, 149
Interval scale, 146
Intracellular potential (IP), 80, 88
Intracellular receptor potentials (see Receptor potentials)
Intrastrial fluid, 29
Invariance in speech perception, 270 (see also Variance in speech perception)
Inverse square law, 4, 6, 243
Iso-amplitude curves (see Tuning curves)
Isofrequency bands, 129
Iso-velocity curves (see Tuning curves)
ITD (see Interaural time differences)

Jewett bumps (see Short latency response)
Joule, 3
Just (diatonic) scale, 222
Just noticeable difference (jnd), 147, 149, 171, 208 (see also Difference limen)

Kemp echo (see Otoacoustic emissions)
Kinetic energy, 4
Kinocilium, 34 (see also Cilia, Stereocilia)

Lag effect, 263
Larynx, 257
Laser inferometry, 88, 91
Late auditory evoked response, 130
Lateral inhibition, 88
Lateral lemniscus (LL), 42–43, 129
Lateral superior olive (LSO) (see Superior olivary complex)
Lateralization (see Lateralization and localization)
Lateralization and localization, 235, 239 (see also Directional hearing)
Lateralization model of MLDs, 250
Length, 1
Lexical Access from Spectra (LAFS) model, 271
Limbic system, 44, 131
Limbus, 32, 33
Lip position and rounding, 258, 262
Liquids, 262 (see also Semivowels)
LL (see Lateral lemniscus)
Lobe (see Earlobe)
Lobule (see Earlobe)
Localization (see Lateralization and localization)

Localization dominance (see Precedence effect)

Locus of second formant transition, 260, 261

Logogens, 271

Logogen model, 271

Long latency response, 131, 132

Longitudinal shear (see Shear)

Longitudinal waves, 9

Long-term average speech spectrum (LTASS), 265–266 (see also Speech spectrum)

Loudness, 65, 66, 146, 207–215

Loudness adaptation, 212–214

Loudness balance, 155, 211, 213, 231

Loudness discomfort level (LDL) (see Uncomfortable loudness levels)

Loudness Level, 207–208, 209 (see also Phons)

Loudness of complex sounds, 66, 146, 157, 207

Loudness recalibration, 212 (see also Induced Loudness Reduction)

Loudness recruitment, 65, 66

Loudness scaling, 156, 208 (see also Sones)

Loudness summation, 210, 211, 231, 249

Low pitch, 218, 224

Lower limen, 149

Low-pass filter, 15, 16, 91, 267, 268–269

LSO (see Superior olivary complex)

MAA (see Minimal audible angle)

Mach bands, 88

MAF (see Minimal audible field)

Magnitude estimation, 156–157, 208

Magnitude production, 156–157, 208

Magnitude scaling, 211 (see also Ratio scaling)

Malleus, 25, 26, 27, 53, 55

MAMA (see Minimum audible movement angle

Mandible, 20

Manner of articulation, 259

Manubrium (see Malleus)

MAP (see Minimal audible pressure)

MAPC (see Coupler-referred MAP)

Marginal net (see Tectorial membrane)

Masking, 187–202, 269

Masking audiograms (see Masking patterns)

Masking level differences (MLDs), 199, 247–250

Masking patterns, 187, 188, 194

Mass, 1, 7, 18

Mass reactance, 18

Mastoid air cells, 53

Mastoid antrum (see Antrum)

Mastoid portion (of temporal bone), 20

Mastoid process, 20 (see also Mastoid portion)

Maximum likelihood methods, 155

McGurk effect (illusion), 264, 265, 271

McGurk-MacDonald effect (see McGurk effect [illusion])

Measurement methods, 146–147

Measurement scales, 146

Mechanoelectrical transduction, 37, 78–79

Mechanoelectrical transduction (MET) channels, 79

Medial efferent acoustic reflex, 135

Medial geniculate body (MGB), 43, 44, 122, 125, 129

Medial plane, 51, 235

Medial superior olive (MSO) (see Superior olivary complex)

Mels, 218 (see also Pitch scales)

Membranous labyrinth, 28, 29, 30, 31

Metathetic continua, 156

MET channels (see Mechanoelectrical transduction [MET] channels)

Method of adjustment, 149

Method of constants (constant stimuli), 149–151, 164

Method of limits, 147–149

MGB (see Medial geniculate body)

Middle auditory evoked response (see Middle latency response)

Middle ear, 20, 23–28 (see also Tympanic cavity)

Middle ear transformer mechanism, 53, 56, 72

Middle ear response, 56–58

Middle ear transformer (see Middle ear transformer mechanism)

Middle latency response, 131

Midline lateralization, 239

Minimal audible angle (MAA), 239, 241, 242

Minimal audible field (MAF), 231

Minimum audible pressure (MAP), 166, 167

Minimum audible levels, 166–167 (see also Absolute sensitivity, Threshold)

Minimum audible movement angle (MAMA), 243

Minimum integration time (see Temporal resolution)

Mismatch negativity, 131

Miss, 160

Missing 6 dB, 167

Missing fundamental, 72, 224, 225, 226

MKS system/units, 1 (see also cgs system/units)

MLD (see Masking level differences)

Mode of vibration, 17

Modiolus, 30, 77

Modulation depth, 176, 177

Modulation frequency (see Modulation rate)

Modulation rate, 132, 133, 176

Modulation transfer function (MTF), 273

Modulus, 156

Momentum, 2

Monaural spectral cues (see Spectral cues)

Monopolar cells, 122

Mössbauer technique, 88

Motor theory, 270

MSO (see Superior olivary complex)

Müller's doctrine of specific nerve energies, 72

Multiple generators, 131, 132

Multiple-interval forced choice methods, 151, 164
Music, 207, 223, 235

N-interval forced-choice, 164
Nasal cavity, 257
Nasal murmur, 262
Nasality, 267, 269
Nasals, 259, 262, 265
Natural frequency, 72, 75 (see also Resonant frequency)
Near miss to Weber's law, 173, 174 (see also Weber's law)
Negative baseline shift (see Summating potential)
Negative reactance (see Stiffness reactance)
Neighborhood activation model, 272
Net force, 3
Net reactance, 18
Neural coding, 66, 105, 113, 233, 247
Newton, 2
Nodes, 16
Noise, 160, 192, 215, 237, 243, 247
Noisiness, 214–215
Nominal scale, 146
Nonauditory factors, 160, 166
Nonclassical auditory pathways, 44
Nonlinear response of cochlea, 53, 72, 92, 96
Nonlinearities (see Distortion)
Nonsimultaneous masking (see Temporal masking)
Normal hearing (see Hearing level)
Normalized firing rate, 115, 116
Notched noise, 194
Noy(s), 214

Occlusion effect, 60
Octave equivalence, 222
Octopus cells, 122
Off-frequency bands, 196
Off-frequency listening, 193, 194
Off-set time disparities (see Precedence effect)
OHC (see Hair cells)
Ohms, 17
Ohm's auditory law, 72
Olivocochlear bundle (OCB), 38, 40, 45 (see also Efferent neurons and system)
On (onset) units, 122
On-signal band, 196
Onset spectra, 260
Onset time disparities (see Precedence effect)
Open set, 266
Ordered metric scale, 146
Ordinal scale, 146
Organ of Corti, 20, 29, 32, 33, 37, 38, 40, 76, 80, 81
Osseotympanic bone conduction, 60
Osseous labyrinth (see Bony labyrinth)
Osseous spiral lamina, 30–31, 32, 78
Ossicles (see Ossicular chain)

Ossicular chain, 27–28, 55, 59, 60 (see also Incus, Malleus, Stapes)
Ossicular fixation theory, 67
Ossicular lag bone conduction (see Inertial bone conduction)
Ossicular lever mechanism, 56
Otoacoustic emissions, 93–96, 135
Otosclerosis, 59
Ototoxic drugs and effects, 78, 82
Outer ear, 20, 51–58, 60
Outer hair cells (see Hair cells)
Outer spiral bundle (see Innervation of the cochlea)
Oval window, 20, 26, 28, 53, 55, 60
Overlap masking, 269
Overshoot, 7, 197–198, 220
Overtones, 223

P3 response (see P300 response)
P300 response, 131
Pain threshold, 168
Palatals, 262
Pars flaccida, 25
Pars principalis (see Medial geniculate body)
PARSYM (see Neighborhood activation model)
Pars tensa, 25
Partial masking, 187
Partials, 223
Partially ordered scale, 146
Partition scales (see Category scales)
Pascal (Pa), 4
Pattern recognition, 226
Pausers units, 122
Payoff, 163
Peak amplitude, 11, 87 (see also Amplitude)
Peak clipping, 267 (see also Distortion)
Peak-to-peak amplitude, 11, 12, 76 (see also Amplitude)
Pendulum analogy, 75 (see also Traveling wave)
Perceived noise decibels (PNdB), 214
Perceived noisiness (see Noisiness)
Perceived temporal order, 178, 264
Perceptual magnet (effect), 270
Perceptual theory (of acoustic reflex), 67
Perfect pitch (see Absolute pitch)
Peri-stimulus time histogram (PSTH), 122, 123
Perilymph, 29, 31
Perilymphatic fluid (see Perilymph)
Period, 11, 13
Period histogram, 107, 109
Periodic waves, 11, 14, 15 (see also Complex waves, Waves)
Periodicity pitch, 224, 225
Periodicity theory (see Frequency theory)
Permanent threshold shift (PTS), 180, 181
Persistence, 149
Perstimulatory adaptation (see Loudness adaptation)

Parameter estimation by sequential testing (PEST), 152–153, 155

Petrous portion (of temporal bone), 20, 28, 30

Phalangeal cells, 34

Phantom sound, 237, 244

Phase, 10, 12, 247

Phase angle, 9, 10

Phase-locking, 103, 107, 113, 115, 247, 248 (see also Time-locking)

Phon curves (see Equal loudness contours)

Phoneme boundaries (see Categorical perception)

Phonemes, 257, 271, 274

Phonetic elements, 257, 270

Phonetic module (see Speech [or phonetic] module [mode])

Phons, 207, 209 (see also Equal loudness contours)

Physical quantities, 1–4

Physiological noise, 68, 167

Pillar cells (see Tunnel of Corti)

Pillars of Corti (see Tunnel of Corti)

Pilot experiments, 148

Pinna, 21, 23, 25, 51

Pinna cues (see Spectral cues)

Pitch, 146, 156, 218–227
  ambiguity, 226
  of complex sounds, 224–227

Pitch scales, 218 (see also Mels)

Pitch shift, 224, 226

Place of articulation, 259, 260, 262

Place principle, 53, 84, 219 (see also Place theory)

Place theory, 53 (see also Place principle)

Place-volley theory, 73–74

Plausibility hypothesis, 246

PNdB (see Perceived noise decibels)

Point of subjective equality (PSE), 149, 150

Positive reactance (see Mass reactance)

Posteroventral cochlear nucleus (see Cochlear nucleus)

Post-masking (see Forward masking)

Post-stimulatory fatigue (see Temporary threshold shift)

Post-stimulus time (PST) histogram, 105

Potential energy, 4

Power, 4

Power level, 5

Power law (see Stevens' power law)

Precedence effect, 244–247

Pregnance (see Auditory scene analysis)

Pre-masking (see Backward masking)

Pressure, 4, 6

Prestin, 97 (see also Somatic motor)

Prestin motor (see Somatic motor)

Primary auditory area, AI (see Auditory cortex)

Primary-like units, 122

Primitive processes (see Auditory scene analysis)

Profile analysis, 175, 176

Promontory, 26, 116

Protection theory, 67

Prothetic continua, 156

Prototype models, 271

Proximity (see Auditory scene analysis)

PST (see Post-stimulus time histogram)

PSTH (see Peri-stimulus time histogram)

Psychoacoustic tuning curves (PTCs), 91, 194–196 (see also Frequency selectivity, Tuning, Tuning curves)

Psychoacoustics, 146

Psychological magnitude balance (PMB), 157

Psychometric functions, 148, 150, 152, 154, 155, 269

Psychophysical tuning curves (see Psychoacoustic tuning curves)

Psychophysics, 146

Pulsed tones, 172, 174

Pure tone, 12, 62, 105, 172, 187, 201, 219 (see also Harmonic motion, Simple harmonic motion)

PVCN (see Cochlear nucleus)

Pyramidal eminence, 26, 28

Pythagorean scale, 222

Q, 15 (see also Q_{10dB}, Tuning)

Q_{10dB}, 87, 88 (see also Q, Tuning)

Radial fibers (see Innervation of the cochlea)

Radial shear (see Shear)

Random noise (see White noise)

Rapid speech transmission index (RASTI), 273

Rarefaction, 8, 9, 10

Rasmussen's bundle (see Olivocochlear bundle)

RASTI (see Rapid speech transmission index)

Rate-level function, 111, 113, 114, 135, 136

Ratio estimation, 156

Ratio production, 156, 218 (see also Fractionalization)

Ratio scale, 146, 156, 208

Ratio scaling, 208

REA (see Right ear advantage)

Reactance, 18, 19, 56

Receiver operating characteristic (ROC), 163

Receptor potentials, 74, 79, 80, 85, (see also Cochlear microphonic, Summating potential)

Recognition score (see Speech recognition)

Redundancy, 269–270

Reference equivalent threshold force level (RETFL), 169

Reference equivalent threshold sound pressure level (RETSPL), 168, 169

Reference values (for pressure, intensity), 1, 5, 168, 169, 170

Refractory period, 73

Reinforcement, 12

Reissner's membrane, 31, 32, 34

Relative refractory period (see Refractory period)

Remote masking, 189, 199

Repetition pitch, 224

Residue pitch, 224

Resistance, 3, 7, 18, 19, 81
Resonance theory, 72, 73 (see also Place theory)
Resonant frequency, 17, 51, 56, 60, 75, 260 (see also Natural frequency)
Resonators, 72 (see also Filters)
Response area (see Tuning curves)
Response perseveration, 149
Response proclivity, 147, 160
Rest, 1
Resting potentials, 79, 80
Restoring force, 3, 7, 8
RETFL (see Reference equivalent threshold force level)
Reticular lamina, 33, 78, 81
Reticular system, 131
RETSPL (see Reference equivalent threshold sound pressure level)
Reverberation, 243, 269, 273
Reverberation effects on speech, 269
Reverberation time, 269
Right ear advantage (REA), 262
ROC curve (see Receiver operating characteristic)
Rods of Corti (see Tunnel of Corti)
Root-mean-square (RMS) amplitude, 11, 12
Rosenthal's canal, 38, 126, 127
Roughness, 220, 223
Round window, 26, 30, 31, 53, 58, 83
Roving levels, 175
Run, 147, 148, 149, 152

Saccule, 20, 30
Scaphoid fossa, 23
Scala media (and Cochlear duct), 20, 31, 80, 81, 83, 85
Scala tympani, 29, 30, 31, 59, 80, 81, 85
Scala vestibuli, 31, 59, 79, 81, 85
Scalar quantities, 1
Scaling, 157
Schema-based processes (see Auditory scene analysis)
Sebaceous glands, 23
Second filter hypothesis, 88 (see also Tuning)
Second formant transitions (see Formant transitions)
Secondary auditory area AII (see Auditory cortex)
Secondary combination tones, 221
Selective adaptation, 264
Self-masking, 269
Semicircular canals, 20, 28, 30
Semitones, 222, 224
Semivowels (see also Glides, Liquids)
Sensation level, 259, 262, 265
Sensitivity, 103, 125, 160, 163 (see also Absolute sensitivity, Differential sensitivity)
Sensory capability, 147
Sensory receptor action, 74
Sensory transduction process (see Transduction process)
Series (see Run)

Seventh (cranial) nerve (see Facial nerve)
Shaft connectors, 36, 37
Sharpening (see Tuning)
Shear, 77 (see also Traveling wave)
Short latency response, 131
Shortlist model, 271
SI system/units (see MKS system/units)
Sibilants, 262
Side-branch resonator, 262
Signal averaging (see Averaging)
Signal-to-noise ratio, 68, 131, 249, 250, 263, 266, 272
SII (see Speech intelligibility index)
Similarity (see Auditory scene analysis)
Simple harmonic motion, 8 (see also Harmonic motion)
Simple up-down method, 152, 154
Sine wave, 9 (see also Harmonic motion, Simple harmonic motion)
Sine wave speech, 264
Sinusoid (see Sine wave)
Sinusoidal motion, 10, 75 (see also Simple harmonic motion, Sine wave)
Sinusoidal wave (see Sine Wave)
Slope of filter, 15
Smearing, 269 (see also Reverberation)
SOC (see Superior olivary complex)
Somatic motor, 97 (see also Hair bundle motor, Prestin)
Sones, 209, 210 (see also Loudness, Loudness scaling)
Sound field to eardrum transfer function, 51
Sound pressure level (SPL), 5, 6, 57, 58, 88, 167, 207, 209
Sound quality (see Timbre)
Sound source determination (see Auditory scene analysis)
Sound source identification, 243
Source-filter theory, 258
SP (see Summating potential)
Spatial orientation, 51, 134
Spatial release from masking, 234
Spatial unmasking (see Spatial release from masking)
Specificity of senses concept (see Mueller's doctrine)
Spectral cues, 123, 237, 241
Spectral pitch, 226
Spectrogram, 258, 260, 261, 265
Spectrum, 14, 15, 115, 132, 226, 243
Spectrum level, 189
Speech bandwidth (see Filtered speech)
Speech discrimination (see Speech recognition)
Speech intelligibility, 266–270, 272–273, 274 (see also Speech recognition)
Speech intelligibility index (SII), 272–273
Speech interference level (SIL), 273
Speech interruption, 267
Speech masking, 268
Speech mechanism, 257 (see also Vocal tract)
Speech (or phonetic) module (mode), 264, 270
Speech perception, 257, 264, 269, 270, 271

Speech power, 265

Speech recognition, 266, 272, 273 (see also Speech intelligibility)

Speech sound confusions and errors, 269

Speech sounds (see Phonemes, Phonetic elements)

Speech spectrum, 115, 249, 265 (see also Long term average speech spectrum, Spectrograms)

Speech transmission index (STI), 273

Speech, neural coding of, 114

Speech-time fraction, 267–268

Spike potential (see Action potential)

Spiral fibers (see Innervation of the cochlea)

Spiral ganglia, 38

Spiral ganglion frequency map, 104

Spiral ligament, 32, 34

Spontaneous discharge rate (see Spontaneous rate)

Spontaneous firing rate (see Spontaneous rate)

Spontaneous otoacoustic emissions (see Otoacoustic emissions)

Spontaneous rate (SR), 103, 105, 112

Squamous portion (of Temporal bone), 20

Square waves, 13

Staircase method (see Simple up-down method)

Standing waves, 16–17, 76, 169

Stapedius muscle and tendon, 28

Stapedius reflex (see Acoustic reflex)

Stapes, 27, 28, 53, 77

Statoacoustic nerve (see Auditory nerve)

Stellate cells, 122

Step size, 148, 149, 152, 153

Stereocilia, 34, 35, 37, 76, 77 (see also Cilia)

Stereophony, 235

Stevens' power law, 209

Stiffness, 66, 75

Stiffness gradient, 75 (see also Basilar membrane, Traveling wave)

Stiffness reactance, 18, 53, 56

Stimulated otoacoustic emissions (see Otoacoustic emissions)

Stimulus novelty, 123

Stimulus persistence, 149

Stimulus uncertainty, 179 (see also Informational masking)

Stimulus-response matrix, 160, 161

Stop burst spectrum, 260

Stops, 259, 260, 262, 263, 269

Strain, 3

Stream fusion (see Auditory scene analysis)

Stream integration (see Auditory scene analysis)

Stream segregation (see Auditory scene analysis)

Stress, 3

Stria vascularis, 29, 34, 80

Styloid process (of temporal bone), 20

Subarachnoid space, 30

Successiveness, 177

Summating potential (SP), 84–86, 135 (see also Receptor potentials)

Summation tone, 220

Summing localization (see Precedence effect)

Superior olivary complex (SOC), 42, 43, 123–125, 127–128

Suprasylvian gyrus (see Auditory cortex)

Suprasylvian sulcus (see Auditory cortex)

Sylvian fringe area SF (see Auditory cortex)

Synchronous discharges, 105, 115

Système International d'Unités (see MKS system/units)

Tectorial membrane, 32, 33, 34, 35, 78

Tegmen tympani, 20, 25

Telephone theory (see Temporal theory)

Temporal auditory acuity, 175, 177 (see also Temporal resolution)

Temporal bone, 20–21, 28, 58, 60

Temporal coding, 218

Temporal discrimination, 175, 177, 178–179

Temporal distortion, 267–268

Temporal integration (see Temporal summation)

Temporal lobe (see Auditory cortex)

Temporal masking, 198–199 (see also Backward masking, Forward masking)

Temporal modulation transfer function (TMTF), 176, 177

Temporal pattern discrimination, 134

Temporal resolution, 175–178

Temporal summation, 62–63, 64, 170, 171

Temporal theory, 73

Temporary threshold shift (TTS), 179–181, 213

Temporomandibular joint, 20

Tenseness, 258

Tension, 224

Tensor palatini muscle, 27

Tensor tympani muscle and tendon, 26, 28

Theories of hearing, 72–74

Theory of signal detection (TSD), 153, 160–164

Third formant transitions (see Formant transitions)

Third window, 59

3-dB down point

Threshold (see Absolute sensitivity, Sensitivity)

Threshold microstructure, 167

Threshold shift, 180, 187, 189, 198, 200

Tickle threshold, 168

Timbre, 227

Time image, 240

Time-averaged holography, 54

Time-compression (see Speeded speech)

Time-intensity trade, 62

Time-locking, 105 (see also Phase-locking)

Tip-links, 36, 37, 78, 79

Tolerance threshold, 168

Tonality, 166, 170 (see also Pitch)

Tone color (see Timbre)

Tone height, 222
Tongue position, 258
Tonotonicity (see Tonotopic organization)
Tonotopic organization, 126–130
Topographic brain map, 132
Top-down processing, 270
Torus tubarius, 26
Touch threshold, 168
Trace model, 271
Tracking method, 151, 194
Tragus, 23
Transduction links, 79 (see also Cross-Links)
Transduction pores (see Mechanoelectrical transduction [MET] channels)
Transduction process, 74, 78
Transfer function, 51, 56, 57, 58, 210
Transformed up-down methods, 154
Transients, 13, 170
Transverse waves, 9
Trapezoid body, 42, 45
Traveling wave, 58, 74–76, 77, 83, 85, 86, 96, 113
Treble, 207
Triangular fossa, 23
Trigeminal nerve, 28, 44
TSD (see Theory of signal detection)
TTS (see Temporary threshold shift)
Tubes, vibratory responses of, 96
Tuning, 19, 72, 87 (see also Frequency selectivity)
Tuning curves, 86, 87, 91, 103, 104, 126
Tuning fork, vibration of, 6, 7
Tunnel of Corti, 32, 38
Two-alternative forced-choice methods, 154, 164
Two-interval forced-choice (2IFC) methods, 153, 176, 201, 231
Two-tone inhibition (see Two-tone suppression)
Two-tone suppression, 92, 93, 109–111
Tympanic cavity, 25–27, 28 (see also Middle ear)
Tympanic membrane, 20, 24, 51, 57 (see also Eardrum)
Tympanic notch, 27
Tympanic portion (of temporal bone), 20
Tympanum (see Middle ear)
Type I auditory neurons (see Auditory nerve)
Type II auditory neurons (see Auditory nerve)

Umbo, 25, 55
Uncertainty, 199, 202
Uncomfortable loudness level (UCL) (see Uncomfortable loudness levels)
Uncomfortable loudness levels, 167, 168
Uncrossed olivocochlear bundle (UOCB) (see Olivocochlear bundle)
Up rule, 154
Upper limen, 149

Upward spread of masking, 187, 189, 192
Utricle, 20, 30

Value, 163
Variable resistance model, 82 (see also Cochlear microphonic)
Variance in speech perception, 257 (see also Invariance in speech perception)
VAS (see Virtual auditory space)
Vector model of MLDs (see Lateralization model of MLDs)
Vector quantities, 1
Vector theory (see Lateralization model of MLDs)
Velars, 259, 260
Velocity, 1, 2, 3
Velum, 259, 260, 262
Ventral cochlear nucleus (see Cochlear nucleus)
Vestibular nerve, 30
Vestibular system, 130
Vestibule, 28, 30, 59
Vestibulocochlear nerve (see Auditory nerve)
Vibration, 6, 7
Virtual auditory space (VAS), 241
Virtual pitch, 224, 225, 226, 227
Virtual sound (see Virtual auditory space)
Vocal cords (see Vocal folds)
Vocal folds, 257
Vocal tract, 257, 258, 259, 260, 261262 (see also Speech mechanism)
Voice onset time (VOT), 259
Voicing, 259, 262, 263, 269
Volley principle (see Place-volley theory)
VOT (see Voice onset time)
Vowels, 114, 115, 257–259, 265

Watt, 4
Waveform, 9, 10, 11, 13, 14
Wavelength, 9, 17
Waves, 11, 12, 13, 131
Weber fraction, 171, 172, 173, 175, 179, 191
Weber's law, 172, 173, 174, 175
Weighting networks, 207, 208
Wever-Brey effect (see Cochlear microphonic)
White noise, 13, 14, 15, 172, 189, 190, 192, 249
Whole-nerve action potential, 113, 115–119 (see also Compound action potential)
Woodworth model, 236
Work, 3, 4

Yes-no methods, 164
Young's modulus, 3
Zona arcuata, 32
Zona pectinata, 32
Zwislocki coupler, 93
Zygomatic process (of temporal bone), 20